Sleepiness

Causes, Consequences and Treatment

Edited by

Michael J. Thorpy
Michel Billiard

CAMBRIDGE UNIVERSITY PRESS

CAMBRIDGE UNIVERSITY PRESS
Cambridge, New York, Melbourne, Madrid, Cape Town,
Singapore, São Paulo, Delhi, Dubai, Tokyo, Mexico City

Cambridge University Press
The Edinburgh Building, Cambridge CB2 8RU, UK

Published in the United States of America by
Cambridge University Press, New York

www.cambridge.org
Information on this title: www.cambridge.org/9780521198868

© Cambridge University Press 2011

This publication is in copyright. Subject to statutory exception and to the provisions of relevant collective licensing agreements, no reproduction of any part may take place without the written permission of Cambridge University Press.

First published 2011

Printed in the United Kingdom
at the University Press, Cambridge

A catalog record for this publication is available from the British Library

Library of Congress Cataloging in Publication data
Sleepiness : causes, consequences, and treatment / edited by Michael J. Thorpy, Michel Billiard.
   p. ;   cm.
Includes bibliographical references and index.
ISBN 978-0-521-19886-8 (hardback)
1. Drowsiness.   I. Thorpy, Michael J.   II. Billiard, M. (Michel)
[DNLM: 1. Disorders of Excessive Somnolence. WL 108]
RC547.5.S55   2011
616.8′4982 – dc22   2010037672

ISBN 978-0-521-19886-8 Hardback

Cambridge University Press has no responsibility for the persistence or accuracy of URLs for external or third-party internet websites referred to in this publication, and does not guarantee that any content on such websites is, or will remain, accurate or appropriate.

Every effort has been made in preparing this book to provide accurate and up-to-date information which is in accord with accepted standards and practice at the time of publication. Although case histories are drawn from actual cases, every effort has been made to disguise the identities of the individuals involved. Nevertheless, the authors, editors and publishers can make no warranties that the information contained herein is totally free from error, not least because clinical standards are constantly changing through research and regulation. The authors, editors and publishers therefore disclaim all liability for direct or consequential damages resulting from the use of material contained in this book. Readers are strongly advised to pay careful attention to information provided by the manufacturer of any drugs or equipment that they plan to use.

Contents

List of contributors vii
Foreword xi
Preface xv
Abbreviations xvii

Section 1 – Introduction

1 **Epidemiology of excessive sleepiness** 3
  Maurice M. Ohayon

2 **Neurochemistry of excessive sleepiness** 14
  Seiji Nishino and Masashi Okuro

3 **Functional neuroimaging of disorders of sleepiness** 29
  Eric A. Nofzinger

4 **Clinical evaluation of the patient with excessive sleepiness** 36
  Imran M. Ahmed and Michael J. Thorpy

5 **Objective measures of sleepiness** 50
  Michael H. Bonnet and Donna L. Arand

6 **Subjective measures of sleepiness** 60
  Christopher L. Drake

7 **Cognitive effects of sleepiness** 72
  Melinda L. Jackson and Hans P. A. Van Dongen

8 **Motor vehicle driving and excessive sleepiness** 82
  Anna Anund and Göran Kecklund

9 **Medico-legal consequences of excessive sleepiness** 92
  Charles F. P. George

Section 2 – Sleep Disorders and Excessive Sleepiness

10 **Sleep deprivation: biomarkers for identifying and predicting individual differences in response to sleep loss** 101
   Namni Goel and David F. Dinges

11 **Narcolepsy** 111
   Astrid van der Heide and Gert Jan Lammers

12 **Idiopathic hypersomnia** 126
   Michel Billiard

13 **Kleine–Levin syndrome** 136
   Isabelle Arnulf

14 **Menstrual-related hypersomnia** 147
   Fiona C. Baker

15 **Sleepiness due to sleep-related breathing disorders** 154
   Jean-Louis Pepin, Sandrine H. Launois, Renaud Tamsier and Patrick Levy

16 **Daytime sleepiness in insomnia patients** 168
   Yinghui Low and Andrew D. Krystal

17 **Sleepiness in advanced and delayed sleep phase disorders** 176
   Scott S. Campbell and Patricia J. Murphy

18 **Shift work disorder and sleepiness** 186
   Torbjörn Åkerstedt

19 **Sleepiness in healthcare workers** 204
   Brian Abaluck and Christopher P. Landrigan

v

20 **Sleepiness in the military: operational implications and research imperatives** 215
Thomas J. Balkin

21 **Time-zone transitions and sleepiness** 225
Jim Waterhouse

22 **Restless legs syndrome and periodic limb movements and excessive sleepiness** 238
Anil N. Rama, Rajive Zachariah and Clete A. Kushida

23 **Long sleepers** 249
Catherine S. Fichten and Eva Libman

24 **Sleepiness in children** 262
Sanjeev V. Kothare and Joseph Kaleyias

Section 3 – Medical, Psychiatric and Neurological Causes of Sleepiness

25 **Depression and sleepiness: a chronobiological approach** 279
Sarah Laxhmi Chellappa and Christian Cajochen

26 **Aging, Alzheimer's disease and sleepiness** 292
Jennifer L. Martin and Sonia Ancoli-Israel

27 **Excessive daytime sleepiness in Parkinson's disease** 301
David B. Rye

28 **Myotonic dystrophy and sleepiness** 316
Luc Laberge and Yves Dauvilliers

29 **Post-traumatic sleepiness** 329
Christian R. Baumann

30 **Genetic disorders and sleepiness** 335
Sona Nevsimalova

31 **Brain tumors, infections, and other CNS causes of sleepiness** 351
Mari Viola-Saltzman and Nathaniel F. Watson

32 **Hypothyroidism and other endocrine causes of sleepiness** 364
Hideto Shinno

33 **Toxic and metabolic causes of sleepiness** 375
Fabio Cirignotta and Fabio Pizza

34 **Excessive sleepiness due to medications and drugs** 386
Paula K. Schweitzer

Section 4 – Therapy of Excessive Sleepiness

35 **Amphetamines, methylphenidate and excessive sleepiness** 401
Una D. McCann

36 **Modafinil/armodafinil in the treatment of excessive daytime sleepiness** 408
Renee Monderer and Michael J. Thorpy

37 **Sodium oxybate for the treatment of excessive sleepiness** 421
Neil T. Feldman

38 **Caffeine and other alerting agents** 430
William D. S. Killgore

39 **Histamine receptor (H$_3$R) antagonists, hypocretin agonists, and other novel alerting agents** 444
Meredith Broderick and Christian Guilleminault

40 **Behavioral and psychiatric treatments for sleepiness** 452
Shelby F. Harris and Michael J. Thorpy

Index 462

Color plates are to be found between pp. 334 and 335.

Contributors

Brian Abaluck
Harvard Work Hours, Health, and Safety Group, Division of Sleep Medicine, Department of Medicine, Brigham and Women's Hospital, Harvard Medical School, and Division of Sleep Medicine, Harvard Medical School, Boston, MA, USA

Imran M. Ahmed
Sleep–Wake Disorders Center, Montefiore Medical Center and Albert Einstein College of Medicine, Bronx, NY, USA

Torbjörn Åkerstedt
Stress Research Institute, Stockholm University, and Clinical Neuroscience, Karolinska institutet, Stockholm, Sweden

Sonia Ancoli-Israel
Professor of Psychiatry, University of California, San Diego, La Jolla, CA, USA

Anna Anund
Swedish National Road and Transport Research Institute, Linköping, Sweden

Donna L. Arand
Dayton Department of Veterans Affairs Medical Center, Wright State University, and Kettering Medical Center, Dayton, OH, USA

Isabelle Arnulf
National Reference Center for Narcolepsy, Idiopathic Hypersomnia and Kleine–Levin Syndrome, Sleep Disorders Unit and UMR 975, Pitié-Salpêtrière Hospital (APHP), Paris 6 University, Paris, France

Fiona C. Baker
Center for Health Sciences, SRI International, Menlo Park, CA, USA, and Honorary Senior Research Fellow, Brain Function Research Group, School of Physiology, University of the Witwatersrand, Johannesburg, South Africa

Thomas J. Balkin
Department of Behavioral Biology, Walter Reed Army Institute of Research Silver Spring, MD, USA

Christian R. Baumann
Department of Neurology, University Hospital Zurich, Switzerland

Michel Billiard
Department of Neurology, Gui de Chauliac Hospital, University Hospital, Montpellier, France

Michael H. Bonnet
Dayton Department of Veterans Affairs Medical Center, Wright State University, and Kettering Medical Center, Dayton, OH, USA

Meredith Broderick
Stanford University Sleep Medicine Program, Stanford, CA, USA

Christian Cajochen
Centre for Chronobiology, Psychiatric University Clinics, Basel, Switzerland

Scott S. Campbell
Laboratory of Human Chronobiology, Department of Psychiatry, Weill Cornell Medical College, White Plains, NY, USA

Sarah Laxhmi Chellappa
Centre for Chronobiology, Psychiatric University Clinics, Basel, Switzerland, and The CAPES Foundation/Ministry of Education of Brazil, Brazil

Fabio Cirignotta
Department of Neurological Sciences, University of Bologna, Italy

List of contributors

Yves Dauvilliers
Department of Neurology, Gui de Chauliac, Hospital University Hospital, CHU Montpellier, Montpellier, Inserm U888, Montpellier, France

David F. Dinges
Division of Sleep and Chronobiology, Department of Psychiatry, University of Pennsylvania School of Medicine, Philadelphia, PA, USA

Christopher L. Drake
Henry Ford Hospital Sleep Disorders and Research Center, and Department of Psychiatry and Behavioral Neurosciences, Wayne State College of Medicine, Detroit, MI, USA

Neil T. Feldman
St. Petersburg, St. Peters burg Sleep Disorders Center, Fl, USA

Catherine S. Fichten
Behavioral Psychotherapy and Research Unit, Jewish General Hospital, Montreal, Quebec, Canada

Charles F. P. George
University of Western Ontario, London Health Sciences Centre, South Street Hospital, London, ON, Canada

Namni Goel
Division of Sleep and Chronobiology, Department of Psychiatry, University of Pennsylvania School of Medicine, Philadelphia, PA, USA

Christian Guilleminault
Stanford University Sleep Medicine Program, Stanford, CA, USA

Shelby F. Harris
Sleep–Wake Disorders Center, Montefiore Medical Center and Albert Einstein College of Medicine, Bronx, NY, USA

Melinda L. Jackson
Sleep and Performance Research Center, Washington State University, Spokane, WA, USA

Joseph Kaleyias
Department of Pediatrics, Division of Pediatric Neurology, University Hospital of Patras, Medical School of Patras, Greece

Göran Kecklund
Stress Research Institute, Stockholm University, Stockholm, Sweden

William D. S. Killgore
Neuroimaging Center, McLean Hospital, Harvard Medical School, Belmont, MA, USA

Sanjeev V. Kothare
Department of Neurology, Division of Epilepsy and Clinical Neurophysiology, Center for Pediatric Sleep Disorders, Children's Hospital, Harvard Medical School, Boston, MA, USA

Andrew D. Krystal
Insomnia and Sleep Research Laboratory, Department of Psychiatry and Behavioral Sciences, Duke University School of Medicine, Durham, NC, USA

Clete A. Kushida
Stanford University Center of Excellence for Sleep Disorders, Stanford, CA, USA

Luc Laberge
Université du Québec à Chicoutimi, Saguenay, Québec, Canada

Gert Jan Lammers
Department of Neurology and Clinical Neurophysiology, Leiden University Medical Center, Leiden, The Netherlands

Christopher P. Landrigan
Harvard Work Hours, Health, and Safety Group, Division of Sleep Medicine, Department of Medicine, Brigham and Women's Hospital, Harvard Medical School, Division of Sleep Medicine, Harvard Medical School, and Division of General Pediatrics, Department of Medicine, Children's Hospital Boston, Harvard Medical School, Boston, MA, USA

Sandrine H. Launois
INSERM ERI17, HP2 Laboratory, Université Joseph Fourier, Faculté de Médecine, and CHU, Hôpital A. Michallon, Laboratoire du sommeil, Pôle Rééducation et Physiologie, Grenoble, France

Patrick Levy
INSERM ERI17, HP2 Laboratory, Université Joseph Fourier, Faculté de Médecine, and CHU, Hôpital A.

List of contributors

Michallon, Laboratoire du sommeil, Pôle Rééducation et Physiologie, Grenoble, France

Eva Libman
Behavioral Psychotherapy and Research Unit, Jewish General Hospital, Montreal, Quebec, Canada

Yinghui Low
Duke-NUS School of Medicine and Insomnia and Sleep Research Laboratory, Department of Psychiatry and Behavioral Sciences, Duke University School of Medicine, Durham, NC, USA

Jennifer L. Martin
Adjunct Assistant Professor, University of California, Los Angeles, Department of Medicine and Research Health Scientist, VA Greater Los Angeles Healthcare System, Geriatric Research, Education and Clinical Center, Los Angeles, CA, USA

Una D. McCann
Department of Psychiatry, The Johns Hopkins School of Medicine, Baltimore, MD, USA

Renee Monderer
Sleep–Wake Disorders Center, Montefiore Medical Center and Albert Einstein College of Medicine, Bronx, NY, USA

Patricia J. Murphy
Laboratory of Human Chronobiology, Department of Psychiatry, Weill Cornell Medical College, White Plains, NY, USA

Sona Nevsimalova
Department of Neurology, 1st Faculty of Medicine, Charles University, Prague, Czech Republic

Seiji Nishino
Sleep and Circadian Neurobiology Laboratory, Stanford University School of Medicine, Palo Alto, CA, USA

Eric A. Nofzinger
Sleep Neuroimaging Research Program, University of Pittsburgh School of Medicine, Pittsburgh, PA, USA

Maurice M. Ohayon
Stanford Sleep Epidemiology, School of Medicine, Stanford University, Stanford, CA, USA

Masashi Okuro
Sleep and Circadian Neurobiology Laboratory, Stanford University School of Medicine, Palo Alto, CA, USA

Jean-Louis Pepin
INSERM ERI17, HP2 Laboratory, Université Joseph Fourier, Faculté de Médecine, and CHU, Hôpital A. Michallon, Laboratoire du sommeil, Pôle Rééducation et Physiologie, Grenoble, France

Fabio Pizza
Department of Neurological Sciences, University of Bologna, Italy

Anil N. Rama
Stanford University Center of Excellence for Sleep Disorders, Stanford, CA, USA

David B. Rye
Professor of Neurology and Director, Emory Healthcare Program in Sleep Medicine Atlanta, GA, USA

Paula K. Schweitzer
Sleep Medicine and Research Center, St. Luke's Hospital, Chesterfield, MO, USA

Hideto Shinno
Associate Professor, Department of Neuropsychiatry, Kagawa University School of Medicine, Ikenobe, Miki, Kita, Kagawa, Japan

Renaud Tamsier
INSERM ERI17, HP2 Laboratory, Université Joseph Fourier, Faculté de Médecine, and CHU, Hôpital A. Michallon, Laboratoire du sommeil, Pôle Rééducation et Physiologie, Grenoble, France

Michael J. Thorpy
Sleep–Wake Disorders Center, Montefiore Medical Center and Albert Einstein College of Medicine, Bronx, NY, USA

Astrid van der Heide
Department of Neurology and Clinical Neurophysiology, Leiden University Medical Center, Leiden, The Netherlands

Hans P. A. Van Dongen
Sleep and Performance Research Center, Washington State University, Spokane, WA, USA

List of contributors

Mari Viola-Saltzman
Department of Neurology, Loyola University Medical Center, Maywood, IL, USA

Jim Waterhouse
Research Institute for Sport and Exercise Sciences, Liverpool John Moores University, Liverpool, UK

Nathaniel F. Watson
Department of Neurology, University of Washington, Seattle, WA, USA

Rajive Zachariah
Stanford University Center of Excellence for Sleep Disorders, Stanford, CA, USA

Foreword

Sleep research has made numerous discoveries that have enhanced the quality of human functioning across the 24-hour day. However, none compare to the potential impact of the insights that have been gained about Sleepiness as a biological drive state, and Excessive Sleepiness as an important symptom in public health and patient care. This volume assembles the research on normal and pathological sleepiness. Individual chapters address the measurement of sleepiness in the clinic, the "field" and the research laboratory. Other chapters address the various causes of sleepiness and the morbidity associated with excessive sleepiness. Finally, societal self-treatment for variants in normal sleepiness as well as medical treatment of excessive sleepiness in sleep disorder populations is addressed.

The term "sleepiness" is used to describe the normal biological drive for sleep. The ecological value of the sensation of sleepiness is to inform the individual that functioning is compromised and sleep is needed to correct this. Excessive sleepiness is used to describe a biological drive for sleep whose intensity is such that there is an inability to stay awake, and hence a high propensity to fall asleep even in situations that are inappropriate, interfer with activities of daily living, and can be harmful to the individual.

Sleepiness is mediated by homeostatic drive variables including time since the last sleep period, as well as the duration and continuity of previous sleep and especially the last sleep period. Importantly, circadian processes modulate the timing of sleepiness across the 24-hour day. These two determinants are the major causes of sleepiness in the general population. Most people are sleepy because they do not sleep enough on a nightly basis, are severely sleep-deprived for a single night, or because they are trying to work late into the night (i.e. at a down phase in their circadian rhythm). In contrast, excessive sleepiness is caused by inadequate sleep at night, circadian rhythm disorders, drugs, as well as sleep, medical, and psychiatric disorders. Inadequate sleep at night is probably the most common cause of sleepiness. Among the general population, insufficient duration of sleep at night is thought to be the cause of excessive sleepiness. In contrast, among patients, and the elderly population, it is the fragmentation of sleep which leads to excessive sleepiness. Importantly, in clinical populations, a variety of pathologies as well as their treatments also give rise to excessive sleepiness. In this volume, individual chapters will address each of these causes of sleepiness and define how parametric variations in these factors impact the degree of sleepiness.

The pervasiveness of sleepiness in our society is evidenced by two societal indicators. These are oversleeping on weekends and caffeine consumption. Caffeine is the most widely used central nervous system (CNS) active drug in the world. In North America, 80–90% of adults regularly use caffeine. Caffeine is the only CNS drug that can be legally purchased by children. In a study of children and adolescents, it was found that 98% ingest caffeine at least once a week. Not only is caffeine widely used, but the brands of coffees with the highest caffeine content are the most widely consumed brands. In addition, there are numerous "energy drinks" (a variety of different beverages with high caffeine content) routinely advertised in national media and commonly consumed by adolescents. Oversleeping on weekends is another indicator of pervasiveness of sleepiness. According to polls conducted by the National Sleep Foundation, the average adult sleeps approximately 7 h per night on weekdays, but 8 h per night on weekends. Importantly, in several laboratory studies it was found that requiring subjects to stay in bed for 8 h a night for several nights increases their level of alertness as determined by the Multiple Sleep Latency Test (MSLT).

Another important consideration in understanding sleepiness relates to the concepts of masking and misattribution. Masking refers to the fact that there are many variables which make individuals underestimate their level of sleepiness relative to their actual physiological state of sleepiness. Factors such as motivation, stress, and level of activity all mask our sleepiness. We have all had the experience of being engrossed in a task and it is not until we finish that we have a sense of overwhelming exhaustion or sleepiness. Similarly, when traveling on long journeys across multiple time zones you may not feel sleepy until you get into your room and see your bed. When these masking effects cease there is a sense of sleepiness often referred to as unmasking. What is interesting is that most individuals who deny sleepiness claim that a variety of situations make them sleepy. A group of sleep apnea patients who denied sleepiness reported that driving cars, watching television, going to church, and attending meetings all made them sleepy. We know that these factors do not cause sleepiness per se, but rather they unmask the sleepiness associated with their sleep apnea. In a National Sleep Foundation Poll, 90% of adult Americans reported that boredom makes them sleepy. Today we understand that there was a basal level of sleepiness in these individuals which was unmasked, not created, by the boring situation.

The existence of these masking phenomena raises an important clinical question. Namely, how does a clinician detect, evaluate severity of sleepiness and determine the effectiveness of treatment when patients are, at times, not aware of their own state of sleepiness? It is critical for the clinician, the employer and researcher to appreciate the importance of and the appropriate use of various measures of sleepiness. Historically, level of sleepiness has been assayed by introspection. The chapter on subjective sleepiness chronicles for the reader the evolution of subject-/patient-based scales. These have evolved from non-specific measures of mood to specific assays of subjective sleep propensity. In addition, laboratory studies have focused on the use of measuring various aspects of human performance as a measure of degree of sleepiness. These measures have been hypothesized to have the most direct application to industrial situations (e.g. transportation, shift work, health delivery systems). The seminal work of Carskadon and Dement in the development of the MSLT, often referred to as the gold standard measure of sleepiness, enabled research on sleepiness to dramatically expand. Since that initial description, variants of the MSLT and other physiological assays (e.g. evoked potentials) have advanced our ability to clinically identify and manage patients as well as to study sleepiness in the laboratory.

The importance of understanding sleepiness derives not only from its high prevalence, but also from the fact that it has significant associated morbidity. The early research on the effects of sleepiness focused on its effects on psychomotor performance in general and the frequency of lapses in performance specifically. There are seminal studies both in the USA and Europe that demonstrated that sleep-deprived subjects showed significant impairments. These effects were most clearly seen on long monotonous tasks (not different from driving) and the impairments seen were lapses. Lapses are short periods (less than a second) where people fail to respond to the environment. These lapses can have disastrous impact on behaviors such as highway driving, and other jobs that require sustained attention. Subsequent research has broadened the area of inquiry and demonstrated memory deficits, increased risk-taking behavior and impairments in executive function that are also associated with sleepiness. More recently, the focus has moved from the behavioral consequences of sleepiness to physiological consequences. Sleepiness has been shown to be associated with a variety of physiological functions including increased pain sensitivity and blunted arousal responses. These have significant implications. For example, in patients with sleep apnea, the degree of sleepiness correlates with the time to arousal and the resumption of breathing and hence with degree of hypoxemia.

As we look to the future, there are clear gaps in our knowledge which demand further research. An area of great need is in therapeutics. Historically, the pharmacological treatment of excessive sleepiness has consisted of medical treatment with dopaminergics and self-management with caffeine. In terms of medical management, modafinil was the first medication used for treating sleepiness which did not work primarily through dopamine. As we learn more about the neuropharmacology of sleep–wake systems, new therapeutic targets such as histamine and orexin need to be pursued. In terms of self-management, as higher-caffeine-containing substances become available and are used by larger segments of the population, we need to understand their abuse liability, severity and nature of withdrawal symptoms, effects on sleep, and the development of tolerance. Importantly in the area of patient management, there is a need to learn how to treat the underlying disorders, not simply excessive sleepiness as a symptom. Also, in terms of patient care, it is important to understand the causes of sleepiness.

Foreword

What are the causes of refractory sleepiness in successfully treated obstructive sleep apnea (OSA) patients? Are there subgroups of patients with affective disorders who are truly sleepy, not simply reporting sleepiness? If they are truly sleepy, what mediates their sleepiness? Among shift workers, why do some shift workers report and exhibit sleepiness while others do not? Generally, as we try to understand chronic sleepiness, two questions are critical. What are the genes that differentiate individuals who show significant impairment from the various causes of sleepiness from those who do not? Also, are there adaptive mechanisms to decrease the accumulation of sleepiness? If so, what are they and how do they minimize the consequences of sleepiness across time?

One of the greatest needs in the sleep field is a reliable, valid, rapidly derived measure of sleepiness. The ability to rapidly and accurately determine alcohol concentration levels from the breath has facilitated research on the effects of alcohol, and produced regulations about driving and fitness for duty associated with alcohol consumption. Clearly, a biological assay for sleepiness would have profound effects on patient care and public safety.

Research is said to be a social enterprise in that the value of a research finding, in part, depends on the degree of its dissemination to the medical or general community. The greatest need in the area of sleepiness is education. The void in knowledge about sleepiness exists at all levels of our society. In terms of medical education, it is the view of most people in the sleep field that if a patient were to present to a clinician with sleepiness-related symptoms (e.g. tired, fatigued, can't get started), the most likely diagnosis would be depression and the most likely treatment would be an antidepressant medication. Before the awareness of sleep apnea by the general medical community, most apnea patients were diagnosed as depressed. Similarly, profound sleepiness was thought to be narcolepsy. In fact, in the medical literature one can find drugs that make people sleepy referred to as narcoleptogenic drugs. Clearly, sleepiness is a very common symptom in medicine and physicians need to have education on identifying and diagnosing the cause of the sleepiness, and treatment of that cause as well as symptomatic management of sleepiness. I can think of no medical intervention which improves patients' overall quality of life as much as treating daytime sleepiness. OSA, narcolepsy and other excessive sleepiness patients describe their treatment as a rebirth saying, "I am alive again."

Finally, the greatest need is for public education. Estimates suggest that 20% of the adult US population experience sleepiness at a level that puts them at risk for a car accident. The expanding degree of caffeine consumption, the number of sleepiness-related car accidents, and the frequency of oversleeping on weekends all attest to the need to educate the general population about sleepiness, its causes, dangers and appropriate coping skills. Children from primary school through high school learn about exercise and nutrition because of their importance for long-term health outcomes. On the other hand, an adolescent who is chronically sleep-deprived because of school start times, extracurricular activities, part-time jobs and the availability of the Internet receives no education about sleep, sleep need, changes in sleep need across the lifespan, consequences of insufficient sleep, the interaction of sleep loss and alcohol, and effective countermeasures for drowsy driving; this despite the fact that adolescents are at an increased risk of a car accident in the short term. How is a teenaged driver supposed to know that when he feels sleepy while driving, opening the window or raising the volume on the radio will be of no use, while taking a nap will help?

This volume contains information about what we know about causes, consequences, and treatments for sleepiness. This information is not only important to physicians, but also to all individuals to develop sleep practices which optimize the quality and duration of their lives.

Thomas Roth PhD
Detroit, MI, 2010

Preface

Sleepiness is a widespread condition in modern society, in part because sleep deprivation is so pervasive among adolescents and young adults, and increasing rates of obesity have led to sleep-related breathing disorders. However, many disorders that cause sleepiness are now recognized ranging from behavioral to medical, neurological and psychiatric causes. *Sleepiness: Causes, Consequences and Treatment* details the important pathophysiological and clinical features of most disorders of excessive sleepiness.

The understanding of sleepiness in modern times is punctuated by a series of clinical, laboratory and therapeutic landmarks. Clinically, one of the first and most well-known descriptions was of Joe – the fat, sleepy boy who snored loudly; described in *The Posthumous Papers of the Pickwick Club*, by Charles Dickens in 1836 [1]. The condition of a 47-year-old male with "an irresistible and incessant propensity to sleep" was referred to as narcolepsy by Gelineau in 1880 [2]. Then Kleine, in 1925, described a 13-year-old boy who abruptly became drowsy after a febrile illness and displayed cognitive peculiarities for a period of 3 weeks with a similar episode 14 days later [3]; a condition referred to in 1942 by Critchley and Hoffman as the Kleine–Levin syndrome [4]. In 1923, von Economo described excessive sleepiness in patients with encephalitis lethargica that was associated with lesions in the tegmentum and posterior hypothalamus [5]. In the 1950s, Roth described sleepiness, different from narcolepsy, that subsequently was called idiopathic hypersomnia [6]. In 1978, Guilleminault and Dement edited a book entitled *Sleep Apnea Syndromes*, disorders causing sleepiness involving at least 5% of the population [7], and the same year, Lugaresi and colleagues edited a book entitled *Hypersomnia with Periodic Apneas* [8].

Electrophysiological laboratory testing of excessive sleepiness began in 1978 when Carskadon and Dement introduced the multiple sleep latency test to quantify sleepiness [9]. It was some years later in 1991 when a widely useful questionnaire to evaluate the degree of subjective sleepiness, the Epworth sleepiness scale, was developed by Johns [10]. In the late 1990s, discoveries led to the finding that hypocretin, a neuropeptide, is reduced or absent in patients with narcolepsy and cataplexy.

Finally, active pharmacological treatments of sleepiness have evolved from early amphetamines, such as benzedrine [11], to more recently developed and approved agents for narcolepsy, such as gamma-hydroxybutyrate [12] and modafinil [13].

Today, after years of disdain, clinicians recognize the importance of the complaint of sleepiness and the impact on cognitive functions and quality of life. Governmental authorities are increasingly concerned about the role of sleepiness in industrial, road, rail, sea or air accidents, yet no book has ever been published which solely focuses on the causes, consequences and treatment of sleepiness.

Sleepiness: Causes, Consequences and Treatment accumulates the most recently available information on sleepiness and is written by top specialists in the field, including sleep disorders physicians and sleep researchers, from the USA, Europe, Canada and Japan. The chapters are arranged in four major sections: an introductory section, a primary sleep disorders section, a medical, psychiatric and neurological section, and a therapeutic section.

The Introductory section comprises chapters on the epidemiology, neurochemical and neuroimaging of sleepiness, clinical evaluation of the patient, objective and subjective tests of sleepiness, consequences, including the cognitive effects, motor vehicle driving risks and the medico-legal implications. The second section presents the primary disorders of sleepiness such as sleep deprivation, narcolepsy, other central nervous system hypersomnias, pediatric causes of sleepiness, sleep-related breathing disorders, and circadian rhythm disorders, including shift work and sleepiness in the military. The third section details those medical, neurological, psychiatric, genetic, endocrine, toxic, and metabolic disorders that can cause sleepiness, as well as the effects of medications. The final and fourth section presents chapters on the medications used to treat sleepiness including the stimulants, modafinil, sodium oxybate, and newer alerting agents under investigation, as well as caffeine effects and behavioral treatments of sleepiness.

This volume is intended primarily for sleep disorders specialists and sleep researchers; however, it is suitable for neurologists, psychiatrists, and any researcher interested in the interdisciplinary field of sleep medicine. It will be of use for neurology and psychiatry residents and fellows, clinical psychologists, neuropsychologists, house officers, medical students and mental health and social workers who want to get an understanding of the importance and diagnostic features of excessive sleepiness. Also, this book is important for governmental agencies who are involved in public safety, particularly those in the transportation and occupational areas. In addition, military specialists concerned about fatigue will find this book of great interest along with the legal profession because of the medico-legal implications of excessive sleepiness.

We are greatly indebted to all the authors who have contributed to this book and we are appreciative of the help of the staff of Cambridge University Press in getting this publication in print so quickly so that the contents are up-to-date and current. As research into sleepiness is rapidly advancing, it is anticipated that future editions of this volume, *Sleepiness: Causes, Consequences and Treatment* will take these developments into account.

Michael Thorpy
Michel Billiard

References

1. **Dickens C**. *The Posthumous Papers of the Pickwick Club*. London: Chapman and Hall, 1836.
2. **Gelineau J**. De la narcolepsie. *Gazette des Hôpitaux*, 1880; **53**:626–28, 635–37.
3. **Kleine W**. Periodische Schlafsucht. *Monatsschrift fur Psychiatrie und Neurologie*, 1925; **57**:285–320.
4. **Critchley M**, **Hoffman H**. The syndrome of periodic hypersomnolence and morbid hunger (Kleine–Levin Syndrome). *BMJ*, 1942; **1**:137–39.
5. **von Economo C**. Encephalitis lethargica. *Wien Med Wochenschr*, 1923; **73**:777–82.
6. **Roth B**. *Narkolepsie a Hypersomnie s Hlediska Fysiologie Spanku*. Praha, Statni Zdravonicke Nakladtelstvi, 1957.
7. **Guilleminault C**, **Dement W**, eds. *Sleep Apnea Syndromes*. New York, NY: Alan Liss, Inc., 1978.
8. **Lugaresi E**, **Coccagna G**, **Mantovani M**, eds. *Hypersomnia with Periodic Apneas*. New York, NY: Spectrum Publications, 1978.
9. **Richardson G**, **Carskadon M**, **Flagg W**, et al. Excessive daytime sleepiness in man: multiple sleep latency measurements in narcoleptic and control subjects. *Electroencephalogr Clin Neurophysiol*, 1978; **45**:621–27.
10. **Johns MW**. A new method for measuring daytime sleepiness: the Epworth sleepiness scale. *Sleep*, 1991; **14**:540–45.
11. **Prinzmetal M**, **Bloomberg W**. The use of benzadrine for the treatment of narcolepsy. *JAMA*, 1935; **105**:2051–54.
12. **Broughton R**, **Mamelak M**. Gamma-hydroxybutyrate in the treatment of compound narcolepsy; a preliminary report. In: Guilleminualt C, Dement W, Passouant P, Eds. *Narcolepsy*. New York, NY: Spectrum, 1976: 659–67.
13. **Bastuji H**, **Jouvet M**. Treatment of hypersomnia with modafinil [in French]. *Presse Med*, 1986; **15**:1330–31.

Abbreviations

5-HIAA	5-hydroxyindoleacetic acid	EOG	electrooculogram
AAS	ascending arousal system	ES	excessive sleepiness
ACGME	Accreditation Council for Graduate Medical Educations	ESS	Epworth sleepiness scale
		FASPS	familial advanced sleep phase syndrome
ACh	acetylcholine	FSS	Fatigue Severity Scale
AD	adenosine	GHB	γ-hydroxybutyrate
ADEM	acute disseminated encephalomyelitis	GPCR	G-protein-coupled receptor
AHI	apnea–hypopnea index	HEEDNT	head, eyes, ears, nose, throat
ASL	arterial spin labeling	HH	hypnagogic hallucinations
ASPD	advanced sleep phase disorder	HLA	human leukocyte antigen
Bas	Brodmann areas	HMSN	hereditary motor and sensory polyneuropathies
BDI	Beck Depression Inventory		
BF	basal forebrain	HOMA	homeostasis model assessment
BiPAP	bilevel positive airway pressure	HOS	hours of service
CAP	cyclic alternating pattern	HPA	hypothalamic–pituitary–adrenal
CF	cystic fibrosis	HRQoL	health-related quality of life
CGI-C	Clinical Global Impression Scale of Change	HTP	hypothalamo-pituitary–thyroid
		HVA	homovanillic acid
CHD	coronary heart disease	ICC	intraclass correlation coefficients
CMT	Charcot–Marie–Tooth disease	ICSD	International Classification of Sleep Disorders
CNS	central nervous system		
COPD	chronic obstructive pulmonary disease	IGF BP	insulin-like growth factor binding protein
CPAP	continuous positive airway pressure		
CPT	continuous performance test	IH	idiopathic hypersomnia
CSA	central sleep apnea	IOM	Institute of Medicine
CSF	cerebrospinal fluid	IPF	idiopathic pulmonary fibrosis
CSR	chronic sleep restriction	ISWT	irregular sleep–wake type
DA	dopamine	IVIg	intravenous immunoglobulin
DIMS	difficulty initiating or maintaining sleep	KDS	Karolinska drowsiness score
		KLS	Kleine–Levin syndrome
DLMO	dim light melatonin onset	KSS	Karolinska sleepiness scale
DMD	Duchenne muscular dystrophy	LC	locus coeruleus
DOPAC	dihydroxyphenylacetic acid	LHA	lateral hypothalamic area
DS	Digit Span (test)	MCH	melanin-concentrating hormone
DSPD	delayed sleep phase disorder	MHAT	Mental Health Assessment Team
DSPS	delayed sleep phase syndrome	MHPG	3-methoxy-4-hydroxyphenylglycol
DSST	digit symbol substitution task	MIRS	muscular impairment rating scale
EDS	excessive daytime sleepiness	MMSE	mini mental status examination
EDSS	expanded disability status scale	MS	multiple sclerosis
EEG	electroencephalography	MSL	mean sleep latency
EMG	electromyogram		

List of abbreviations

MSLT	multiple sleep latency test	REM	rapid eye movement
mTBI	mild traumatic brain injury	RES	residual excessive sleepiness
MWT	maintenance of wakefulness test	RLS	restless legs syndrome
NAFLD	non-alcoholic fatty liver disease	SAFTE	sleep, activity, fatigue and task effectiveness
NARP	neuronal activity-regulated pentraxin	SBAR	situation background assessment recommendation
NCL	neuronal ceroid lipofuscinosis	SCA	spinocerebellar ataxias
NCV	nerve conduction velocity	SCN	suprachiasmatic nucleus
NE	norepinephrine	SD	sleep deprivation
NHP	Nottingham Health Profile	SDB	sleep-disordered breathing
NIAV	non-invasive assisted ventilation	SEM	slow eye movements
NORD	National Organization of Rare Disorders	SLSJ	Saguenay–Lac-Saint-Jean
NREM	non-REM	SMA	spinal muscular atrophies
OAD	obstructive airway disease	SMS	Safety Management System
OEF	Operation Enduring Freedom	SO	sodium oxybate
OIF	Operation Iraqi Freedom	SOL	sleep onset latency
OSA	obstructive sleep apnea	SOREMP	sleep onset REM period
OSAS	obstructive sleep apnea syndrome	SPECT	single-photon emission computed tomography
OSLeR	Oxford sleep resistance test	SPMS	sleep/performance management system
PAP	positive airway pressure	SSRI	selective serotonin reuptake inhibitor
PASAT	Paced Auditory Serial Addition Task	SSS	stanford sleepiness scale
PBC	primary biliary cirrhosis	SURT	surrogate reference task
PCS	post-concussion syndrome	SWA	slow-wave activity
PD	Parkinson's disease	SWD	Shift Work Disorder
PDSS	pediatric daytime sleepiness scale	SWE	slow-wave energy
PET	positron emission tomography	SWMT	Sternberg Working Memory Task
PFC	prefrontal cortex	SWP	sleep–wake predictor
PLMA	periodic leg movement arousal index	SWS	slow-wave sleep
PLMI	periodic leg movement index	SXB	sodium oxybate
PLMS	periodic limb movements in sleep	TBI	traumatic brain injury
PMDD	premenstrual dysphoric disorder	TIB	time in bed
POMS	profile of mood states	TMN	tuberomamillary nucleus
PPN	pedunculopontine tegmental	TMS	transcranial magnetic stimulation
PPT/LDT	pedunculopontine and laterodorsal tegmental nuclei	TPM	the three process model of alertness
PRC	phase-response curve	TSD	total sleep deprivation
PSD	partial sleep deprivation	TSH	thyroid-stimulating hormone
PSG	polysomnography	TST	total sleep time
PSQI	Pittsburg sleep quality index	UARS	upper airway resistance syndrome
PSQ-SS	pediatric sleep questionnaire, sleepiness scale	VAS	visual analogue scale
PST	pupillographic sleepiness test	VLPO	ventrolateral preoptic nucleus
PTT	pulse transit time	VNS	vagus nerve stimulator
PUI	pupillary unrest index	VNTR	variable number tandem repeat
PVT	psychomotor vigilance test	vPAG	ventral periaqueductal gray matter
RAS	reticular activating system	WASO	wake time after sleep onset
RBD	REM sleep behavior disorder	WRAIR	Walter Reed Army Institute of Research
rCBF	regional cerebral blood flow		
RDI	respiratory disturbance index		

Section 1: Introduction

Section 1 Chapter 1

Introduction

Epidemiology of excessive sleepiness

Maurice M. Ohayon

The epidemiology of excessive sleepiness has received less attention than insomnia. Several factors have contributed to this situation: (1) there is no clear definition of what is excessive sleepiness; and (2) excessive sleepiness is not a diagnosis. There is a growing trend in the popular media to label excessive sleepiness as a distinct disorder, but to date, in the classifications, it remains a symptom or a consequence of a sleep disorder, of a physical illness, or of a mental disorder. Therefore, studying prevalence, incidence and risk factors for excessive daytime sleepiness bears little impact on the development of new treatments for this symptom.

However, as we will see, excessive sleepiness is very common in the general population. It is a disabling symptom that adversely affects the quality of life of individuals in various areas of functioning, and it is a good indicator of the presence of health problems.

In the latest edition of the International Classification of Sleep Disorders (ICSD-II), excessive sleepiness is an essential symptom to the diagnosis of 3 types of sleep disorders: hypersomnia, narcolepsy, and behaviorally induced insufficient sleep syndrome, totaling 12 different diagnoses. However, with the exception of narcolepsy, these sleep disorders have rarely been studied in the general population.

Definitions of excessive sleepiness

Table 1.1 presents a summary of excessive sleepiness definitions used in epidemiological studies. There are 14 definitions used for a total of about 40 epidemiological studies assessing excessive sleepiness. There are several important limitations when attempting to compare the different studies. (1) Some studies have assessed the excessive sleep quantity, but the majority of studies have focused on the sleep propensity during wakefulness, i.e. excessive sleepiness. The earliest studies were mostly focused on excessive sleep quantity. In the studies of the past decade, daytime sleepiness has referred to sleep propensity in situations of diminished attention. (2) The terms hypersomnia and excessive sleepiness are often used interchangeably. Hypersom-

Table 1.1 Definitions of excessive sleepiness used in epidemiological studies

	Description	# of studies using that definition
1	Hypersomnia	1
2	Sleeping too much	6
3	Falling asleep during the day	1
4	Frequent feeling of sleepiness during the day or evening that requires taking a nap	1
5	Usually sleepy in the daytime	2
6	Tendency to sleep all day	1
7	Strong need to sleep during the day	1
8	Presence of sleepiness during the previous month, ≥3d/wk	8
9	Sleepiness independent of meal times	1
10	Moderate/severe daytime sleepiness	9
11	Daytime sleepiness often or very often	2
12	Consider themselves more clearly tired than others Daily experience of desire to sleep during normal activities Feel tired every day	1
13	Tendency to fall easily asleep during the day ≥3 d/wk Periods of sudden and irresistible sleep ≥3 d/wk	5
14	Epworth Sleepiness Scale	1

Sleepiness: Causes, Consequences and Treatment, ed. Michael J. Thorpy and Michel Billiard. Published by Cambridge University Press. © Cambridge University Press 2011.

1. Introduction

nia is a broader terminology that encompasses excessive sleep quantity or sleep propensity during wakefulness.

(3) Another aspect that makes comparisons difficult is that the time frame (for example, past week, past month, past year), frequency, severity and duration are inconsistently assessed. (4) The evaluation of the symptom is mostly limited to a single question, which differs from one study to the other. Consequently, the variance in results across studies does not make it possible to reach any definite conclusions in the matter.

Prevalence of excessive sleep quantity

A total of six studies have assessed excessive amount of sleep [1–6]. It should be noted that these studies have assessed the perception of sleeping too much or getting too much sleep. None of these studies has compared the reported sleep duration with the perception of sleeping too much. The prevalence of sleeping too much ranged between 2.8 and 9.5% in the general population with one exception: a study with young adults reported a prevalence of 16.3% [3].

Prevalence of excessive sleepiness

Eight studies have assessed excessive sleepiness, asking simply about its presence or absence using one question. An Italian study asked about the presence of "sleepiness independent of meal times" in a sample of 5713 individuals aged 3 years and older living in the Republic of San Marino. They found a prevalence of 8.7% [7]. An American study conducted with 2187 subjects aged 18 years and older in Tucson (Arizona, USA) got a prevalence of 12.3% of men and 11.7% of women falling asleep during the day [8]. Three elderly studies assessed the presence of excessive daytime sleepiness by asking the participants if they were "usually sleepy in the daytime." A first study using 5201 subjects 65 years and older from the Cardiovascular Health Study (baseline evaluation 1989–1990) reported a prevalence of 17% of men and 15% of women being "usually sleepy in the daytime" [9]. The 1993–94 evaluation included 4578 adults aged 65 and older; being "usually sleepy in the daytime" was reported by 20% of the sample in this second evaluation [10]. Using the same question, Foley et al. [11] obtained a prevalence of 7.7% in a sample of 2346 Japanese-American men. A Canadian study using a national sample of 1659 elderly who underwent a clinical examination obtained a prevalence of 3.9% of subjects who had a tendency to sleep all day [12]. However, sleep disturbance questions were part of the physician's assessment of depression, which may have contributed to the low prevalence of excessive sleepiness in that particular sample. A Mexican study of 1000 adult participants ($\geq$18 years of age) reported a prevalence of 21.5% of participants who experienced a "strong need to sleep during the day" [4]. In Japan, 28 714 participants ($\geq$20 years of age) of the Active Survey of Health and Welfare were assessed for excessive sleepiness with the following question: "Do you fall asleep when you must not sleep (for example, when you are driving a car)?" A total of 2.5% of the sample answered positively to that question [13] (Table 1.2).

Frequency of excessive sleepiness was assessed with two different approaches. Some studies have used a subjective graduated scale ranging from never to very often or always, while others have used the number of days per week with excessive sleepiness. A Swedish study involving 3557 adults aged between 30 and 65 years reported a prevalence of 5.2% of men and 5.5% of women being often or very often sleepy during the daytime [14]. A Polish study asked its 1186 participants aged between 38 and 67 how often they felt sleepy and wanted to fall asleep in the daytime: 26.1% answered "often" but only 2.5% of the sample reported interference with their activities [15]. Another Japanese study reported that 15% of its nationally representative sample of 3030 participants ($\geq$20 years of age) reported feeling "often" or "always" excessively sleepy during the daytime [16]. Martikainen et al. [17] found that 9.8% of their 1190 Finnish respondents, aged between 36 and 50 years, reported being "clearly more tired than others," experiencing a "daily desire to sleep in the course of normal activities" or feeling "very tired daily."

When using a frequency per week in a sample of European adults aged between 20 and 45 years, Janson et al. [18] obtained a prevalence of 20.6% of daytime sleepiness occurring at least 3 days per week and 5% of daily daytime sleepiness. Hublin et al. [19] found a 9% prevalence of daytime sleepiness occurring daily or almost daily in the Finnish twin cohort of 11 354 twins aged between 33 and 60 years. Ohayon et al. [20] used two definitions of sleepiness in a 5-country sample of 18 980 individuals aged 15 years and over. When asked if they had a tendency to fall asleep easily during the daytime and almost anywhere, 4% of the participants answered it occurred at least 3 days per

1. Epidemiology of excessive sleepiness

Table 1.2 Prevalence of excessive sleepiness in the general population

Authors	N	Age	Definition	Prevalence (%) (M/F)
Karacan et al. [53] Alachua county, Florida, USA, 1976	1645	≥18	Hypersomnia	0.3
Bixler et al. [1] Los Angeles, USA, 1979	1006	≥18	Sleep too much	4.2
Klink and Quan [8] Tucson, USA, 1987	2187	≥18	Falling asleep during the day	12.3/11.7
Ford and Kamerow [2] Baltimore, Durham, Los Angeles, USA, 1989	7954	≥18	Sleep too much lasting 2 weeks or more, and professional consultation, sleep-enhancing medication intake, or interferes a lot with daily life	2.8/3.5
Hays et al. [54] North Carolina, USA, 1996	3962	≥65	Frequent feeling of sleepiness during the day or evening that requires taking a nap	25.2
Enright et al. [9] Forsyth, Sacramento, Washington, Pittsburgh counties, USA, 1996	5201	≥65	Usually sleepy in the daytime	17.0/15.0
Foley et al. [11] Island of Oahu, Hawai, USA, 2001	2346 men	71–93	Usually sleepy in the daytime	7.7
Rockwood et al., [12] Canada, 2001	1659	65–99	Tendency to sleep all day	3.9
Téllez-Lòpez et al. [4] Monterrey, Mexico, 1995	1000	≥18	— Getting too much sleep — Strong need to sleep during the day	9.5 21.5
Hara et al. [21] Bambui, Brazil, 2004	1066	≥18	Presence of sleepiness during the previous month, ≥3d/wk	16.8
Lugaresi et al. [7] San Marino, Italy, 1983	5713	≥3	Sleepiness independent of meal times	8.7
Gislason et al. [22] Uppsala, Sweden, 1987	3201 men	30–69	Moderate daytime sleepiness Severe daytime sleepiness	16.7 5.7
Liljenberg et al. [14] Gävleborg and Kopparberg counties, Sweden, 1988	3557	30–65	Daytime sleepiness often or very often	5.2/5.5
Martikainen et al. [17] Tampere, Finland, 1992	1190	36–50	— Consider themselves more clearly tired than others, or — Daily experience of desire to sleep during normal activities, or — Feel tired every day	9.8
Janson et al. [18] Reykjavik, Iceland Uppsala and Göteborg, Sweden, Antwerp, Belgium, 1995	2202	20–45	Daytime sleepiness ≥3 days/week	11–21
Hublin et al. [19] Finland, 1996	11/354	33–60	Daytime sleepiness every or almost every day	6.7/11.0
Asplund [55] Västerbotten and Norrbotten, Sweden, 1996	6143	≥65	— Often sleepy during the day — Often naps in daytime	32.0/23.2 29.4/14.4
Ohayon et al. (5) United Kingdom, 1997	4972	≥15	Feel sleepy during the day: A lot or greatly, ≥1 month Moderately, ≥1 month	4.4/6.6 21.5/17.9

(cont.)

1. Introduction

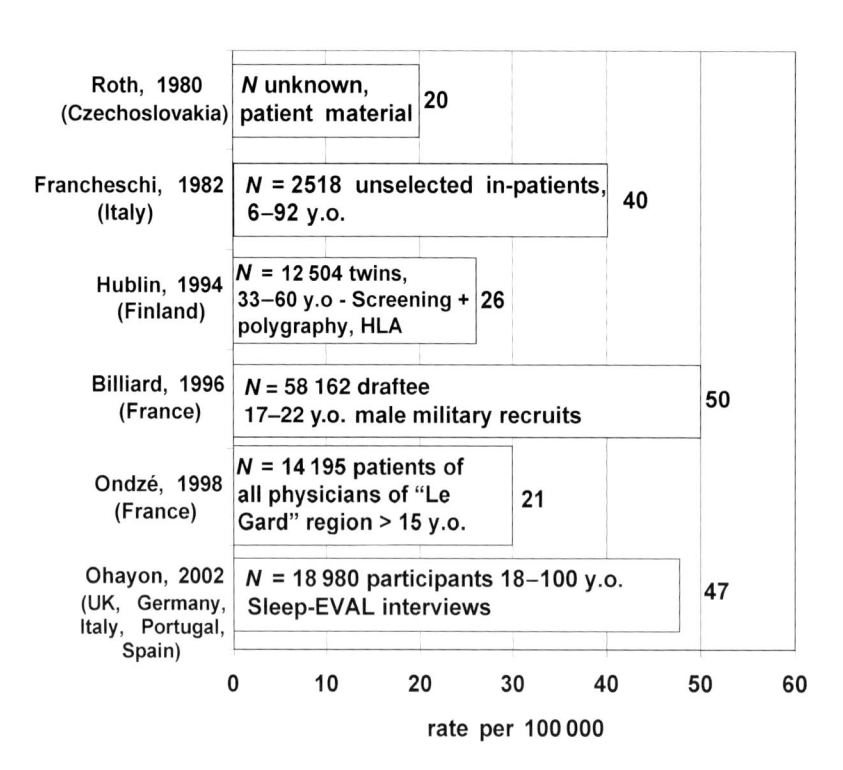

Figure 1.1 Prevalence of narcolepsy in Europe.

insufficient sleep syndrome was likely to be lower than 4% in that sample. Another study, conducted in Japan [16], evaluated insufficient sleep by asking subjects if they got as much sleep as they needed. A total of 23.1% answered negatively to that question, of which 31.3% had daytime sleepiness. Consequently, the combination of insufficient sleep and daytime sleepiness was present in about 7.2% of their adult sample. Again, no differential diagnosis was applied. One study conducted in the UK [5] applied strict differential diagnosis and found a prevalence of insufficient sleep syndrome at 1.1% in their sample.

Narcolepsy, although very rare, has received greater attention. However, reliable estimates of narcolepsy in the general population are difficult to achieve. It requires scanning a large number of individuals to obtain sufficient precision in the prevalence. Consequently, most of the studies have extrapolated the prevalence of narcolepsy to the general population using clinical samples, specific community groups or advertisements. Only three studies calculated the prevalence of narcolepsy in samples representative of the general population. According to these studies, the prevalence varies from 20 to 67 per 100 000 inhabitants in Europe (Figure 1.1) [29, 31–35] and North America (Figure 1.2) [36–39].

In Asian countries (Figure 1.3), a study performed in Japan set this rate at 590 per 100 000 inhabitants [40], and another Japanese study set this rate at 160 per 100 000 inhabitants [41]. In Hong Kong, this prevalence was estimated to be between 1 and 40 narcoleptics per 100 000 inhabitants [42]. Another study performed with Jews in Israel, a population known for its low rate of human leukocyte antigen (HLA-DR2), a predisposing marker for narcolepsy, set the prevalence at 0.23 per 100 000 inhabitants [43].

Among the studies based on representative general community samples, the oldest study was performed in Saudi Arabia [44]. Nearly all inhabitants, aged 1 year or older, of the Thugbah community were interviewed. A total of 23 227 individuals participated in face-to-face interviews. A neurologist subsequently evaluated all participants with abnormal responses in the questionnaire. Narcolepsy was found in 40 per 100 000, 0.04% of the sample (95% confidence interval, 0.014–0.066%).

A study [20] was conducted with representative samples of five European countries (the UK, Germany, Italy, Portugal and Spain). A total of 18 980 individuals, aged 15 years and over, were interviewed by telephone. Using the minimal criteria proposed

Figure 1.2 Prevalence of narcolepsy in North America.

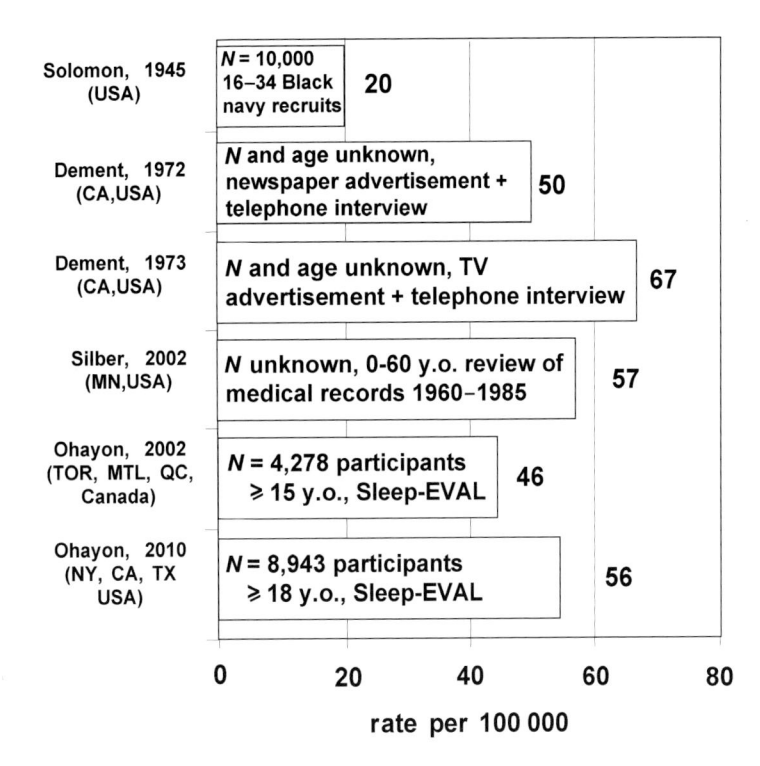

Study	Details	Rate per 100,000
Solomon, 1945 (USA)	N = 10,000; 16–34 Black navy recruits	20
Dement, 1972 (CA, USA)	N and age unknown, newspaper advertisement + telephone interview	50
Dement, 1973 (CA, USA)	N and age unknown, TV advertisement + telephone interview	67
Silber, 2002 (MN, USA)	N unknown, 0–60 y.o. review of medical records 1960–1985	57
Ohayon, 2002 (TOR, MTL, QC, Canada)	N = 4,278 participants ≥ 15 y.o., Sleep-EVAL	46
Ohayon, 2010 (NY, CA, TX USA)	N = 8,943 participants ≥ 18 y.o., Sleep-EVAL	56

Figure 1.3 Prevalence of narcolepsy in Asia.

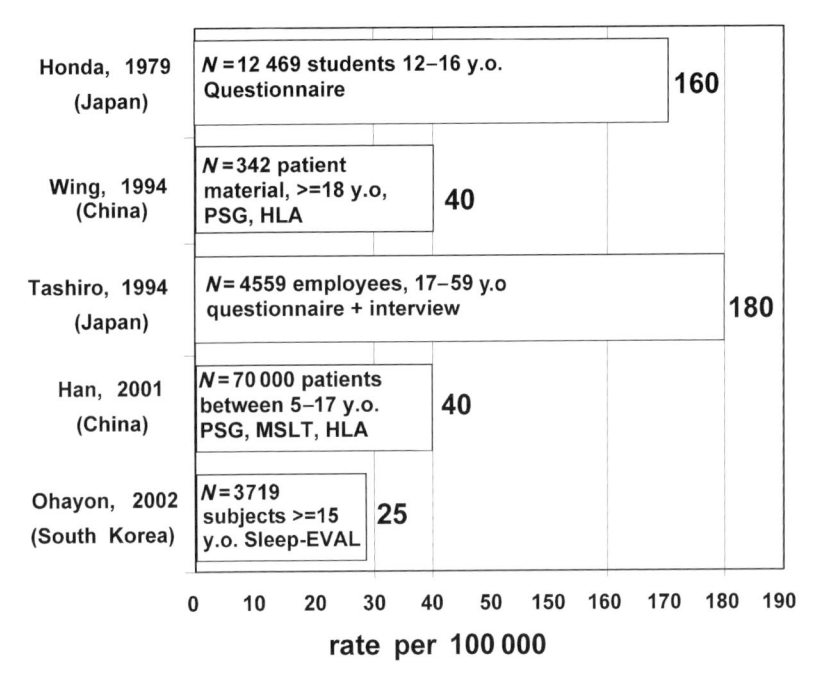

Study	Details	Rate per 100,000
Honda, 1979 (Japan)	N = 12 469 students 12–16 y.o. Questionnaire	160
Wing, 1994 (China)	N = 342 patient material, >=18 y.o, PSG, HLA	40
Tashiro, 1994 (Japan)	N = 4559 employees, 17–59 y.o questionnaire + interview	180
Han, 2001 (China)	N = 70 000 patients between 5–17 y.o. PSG, MSLT, HLA	40
Ohayon, 2002 (South Korea)	N = 3719 subjects >=15 y.o. Sleep-EVAL	25

by the International Classification of Sleep Disorders (ICSD), a prevalence of narcolepsy of 47 per 100 000, 0.047% (95% confidence interval, 0.016–0.078%) was observed.

Wing et al. [45] conducted a telephone study using a general population sample of 9851 adults aged between 18 and 65 years. Participants answered a validated Chinese version of the Ullanalina

Narcolepsy Scale. Subjects with positive scores on the Ullanalina Narcolepsy Scale ($n = 28$) were invited to a clinical interview and further testing (polysomnography, MSLT and human leukocyte antigen (HLA) typing). Three subjects refused supplemental evaluation. Three subjects were identified as narcoleptics. This sets the prevalence of narcolepsy at 34 per 100 000, 0.034% (95% CI: 0.021–0.154%) in Hong Kong.

Limitations from existing classifications pose serious difficulties in studying narcolepsy in the general population. The use of too large criteria inflates the prevalence. For example, the narcolepsy symptoms (automatic behavior, sleep paralysis and hypnagogic hallucinations) are too poorly defined to be useful in epidemiology. Recurrent intrusions of elements of REM sleep into the transition between sleep and wakefulness are highly prevalent in the general population: 6.2% for sleep paralysis and 24.1% for hypnagogic hallucinations [20]. This indicates that these symptoms are not specific to narcolepsy.

Relationship with cognitive deficits and mortality

Two epidemiological studies have linked excessive sleepiness to cognitive deficits. In a study involving 2346 Japanese-American men aged between 71 and 93 years, Foley et al. [11] found that men who reported excessive sleepiness at baseline were twice as likely to be diagnosed with dementia three years later than those without daytime sleepiness. In another study involving 1026 subjects aged 60 years or older, Ohayon and Vechierrini [24] found that after controlling for age, gender, physical activity, occupation, organic diseases, use of sleep or anxiety medication, sleep duration and psychological well-being, subjects with excessive sleepiness were twice as likely to have attention–concentration deficits, difficulties in orientation and memory problems than did the others.

Some general population studies have investigated the mortality risks associated with excessive sleepiness. The study of Hays et al. [46] assessed mortality risks in a sample of 3962 elderly individuals (65 years and older). In that study, excessive sleepiness was defined by the presence of naps during the daytime. They found that individuals who reported napping most of the time had a mortality risk of 1.73.

Another study [12] found a small increased mortality risk (1.89) from daytime sleepiness in their elderly sample. However, this risk was non-significant when they adjusted the model for age, depression, cognitive deficits, and illness.

Factors associated with excessive sleepiness

Unlike insomnia symptoms, excessive sleepiness is generally not gender-related. Whether its prevalence increases or decreases with age is not clear, as both trends have been observed [4, 20, 22, 23].

Excessive sleepiness can be caused by various factors such as poor sleep hygiene [5, 19], work conditions [5], and psychotropic medication use [5, 19, 23].

Excessive sleepiness has been found to be associated also with sleep-disordered breathing [5, 18, 19, 23], psychiatric disorders, especially depression [2, 3, 5, 19, 23], and physical illnesses [5, 18, 23].

Conclusions

From these epidemiological studies, it is clear that a uniform operational definition of excessive sleepiness is still missing. None of these epidemiological studies used a standardized questionnaire to assess daytime sleepiness. Worst, excessive sleepiness was mostly evaluated on the basis of a single question, which was formulated differently from one study to the other. In such circumstances, it is difficult to reach any definite conclusions.

Excessive sleep quantity is an associated symptom in depressive disorders in the DSM-IV classification. However, no epidemiological study has investigated such a relationship, even though mental disorders are present in about 10% of sleepy individuals who consult in sleep disorders clinics; between 10 and 75% of depressed patients complain of sleeping too much. Few polysomnographic studies have been performed with patients having a mood disorder in relationship to excessive sleep quantity or excessive sleepiness. The Multiple Sleep Latency Test (MSLT) did not reveal abnormalities in the daytime sleep latency [47]. Several clinical studies have also pointed out the high occurrence of subjective excessive sleepiness in association with mental disorders, organic disorders, or both. This high comorbidity may hide a more complex problem based on the definition of excessive sleepiness.

For now, only the Multiple Sleep Latency Test (MSLT) objectively measures excessive sleepiness and is considered the gold standard. The MSLT, however, must be administered in a sleep laboratory, therefore limiting its uses in epidemiological studies unless a subsample is invited to perform this examination in a sleep laboratory. Consequently, it is very highly desirable that a self-administered questionnaire be developed in order to assess excessive sleepiness. If it is done, however, it should be kept in mind that we would pass from an objective measure to a subjective measure of excessive sleepiness. One of the most commonly used self-administered sleepiness scales is the Epworth scale [48]. Unfortunately, studies that measured the agreement between this scale and MSLT revealed a poor agreement between them [49].

Few of the epidemiological studies have reported results by ethnic group, or indicated the ethnic makeup of their sample. In fact, there have been almost no data published on ethnocultural differences in excessive sleepiness in the USA or elsewhere [20, 50]. Some investigators have interpreted data from the Human Relations Area Files as indicating that certain aspects of sleep, such as daytime napping may occur more in some cultural groups [51], but epidemiologic data on such cross-cultural differences are actually quite rare. A recent study of college students in Mexico City found no support for the "siesta culture" concept, characterized by a strong tendency for daytime naps and daytime sleepiness [52]. More similarities than differences were noted between the sample from Mexico and samples from other countries on sleep patterns.

In summary, there are yet several areas that need to be clarified regarding excessive sleepiness in the general population. First, an operational definition needs to be developed so that it can be used in general population studies. Once the agreement is made on the definition of excessive sleepiness and the criteria necessary to confirm its presence, several questions would still remain: how can we differentiate daytime sleepiness from fatigue? To what extent do these two concepts overlap? Is daytime sleepiness always a cause of fatigue, or can daytime sleepiness occur without fatigue? To what extent can subjective daytime sleepiness assessment be compared with objective daytime sleepiness assessment? How can we distinguish between the different causes of excessive sleepiness?

Acknowledgments

MMO was supported by a NIH grant (#5R01NS044199) and an educational grant from Cephalon Inc.

References

1. **Bixler E O**, **Kales A**, **Soldatos C R**, et al. Prevalence of sleep disorders in the Los Angeles metropolitan area. *Am J Psychiatry*, 1979; **136**:1257–62.

2. **Ford D E**, **Kamerow D B**. Epidemiologic study of sleep disturbances and psychiatric disorders. An opportunity for prevention? *JAMA*, 1989; **262**:1479–84.

3. **Breslau N**, **Roth T**, **Rosenthal L**, et al. Sleep disturbance and psychiatric disorders: a longitudinal epidemiological study of young adults. *Biol Psychiatry* 1996; **39**:411–18.

4. **Téllez-Lòpez A**, **Sánchez E G**, **Torres F G**, et al. Hábitos y trastornos del dormir en residentes del área metropolitana de Monterrey. *Salud Mental* 1995; **18**:14–22.

5. **Ohayon M M**, **Caulet M**, **Philip P**, et al. How sleep and mental disorders are related to complaints of daytime sleepiness. *Arch Intern Med* 1997; **157**:2645–52.

6. **Roberts R E**, **Shema S J**, **Kaplan G A**. Prospective data on sleep complaints and associated risk factors in an older cohort. *Psychosom Med* 1999;**61**:188–96.

7. **Lugaresi E**, **Cirignotta F**, **Zucconi M**, et al. Good and poor sleepers: an epidemiological survey of the San Marino population. In: Guilleminault C, Lugaresi E, Eds. *Sleep/Wake Disorders: Natural History, Epidemiology, and Long-Term Evolution*. New York, NY: Raven Press, 1983: 1–12.

8. **Klink M**, **Quan S F**. Prevalence of reported sleep disturbances in a general adult population and their relationship to obstructive airways diseases. *Chest*, 1987; **91**:540–46.

9. **Enright P L**, **Newman A B**, **Wahl P W**, et al. Prevalence and correlates of snoring and observed apneas in 5,201 older adults. *Sleep* 1996; **19**:531–38.

10. **Whitney C W**, **Enright P L**, **Newman A B**, et al. Correlates of daytime sleepiness in 4578 elderly persons: the Cardiovascular Health Study. *Sleep* 1998; **21**:27–36.

11. **Foley D**, **Monjan A**, **Masaki K**, et al. Daytime sleepiness is associated with 3-year incident dementia and cognitive decline in older Japanese-American men. *J Am Geriatr Soc* 2001; **49**:1628–32.

12. **Rockwood K**, **Davis H S**, **Merry H R**, et al. Sleep disturbances and mortality: results from the Canadian Study of Health and Aging. *J Am Geriatr Soc* 2001; **49**:639–41.

13. **Kaneita Y**, **Ohida T**, **Uchiyama M**, et al. Excessive daytime sleepiness among the Japanese general population. *J Epidemiol* 2005; **15**:1–8.

14. **Liljenberg B**, **Almqvist M**, **Hetta J**, et al. The prevalence of insomnia: the importance of

operationally defined criteria. *Ann Clin Res* 1988; **20**:393–98.

15. **Zielinski J**, **Zgierska A**, **Polakowska M**, *et al.* Snoring and excessive daytime somnolence among Polish middle-aged adults. *Eur Respir J* 1999; **14**: 946–50.

16. **Liu X**, **Uchiyama M**, **Kim K**, *et al.* Sleep loss and daytime sleepiness in the general adult population of Japan. *Psychiatry Res.* 2000; **93**: 1–11.

17. **Martikainen K**, **Hasan J**, **Urponen H**, *et al.* Daytime sleepiness: a risk factor in community life. *Acta Neurol Scand* 1992; **86**:337–41.

18. **Janson C**, **Gislason T**, **De Backer W**, *et al.* Daytime sleepiness, snoring and gastro-oesophageal reflux amongst young adults in three European countries. *J Intern Med* 1995; **237**:277–85.

19. **Hublin C**, **Kaprio J**, **Partinen M**, *et al.* Daytime sleepiness in an adult Finnish population. *J Intern Med* 1996; **239**:417–23.

20. **Ohayon M M**, **Priest R G**, **Zulley J**, *et al.* Prevalence of narcolepsy symptomatology and diagnosis in the European general population. *Neurology* 2002; **58**:1826–33.

21. **Hara C**, **Lopes Rocha F**, **Lima-Costa M F**. Prevalence of excessive daytime sleepiness and associated factors in a Brazilian community: the Bambuí study. *Sleep Med* 2004; **5**:31–36.

22. **Gislason T**, **Almqvist M**, **Erikson G**, *et al.* Prevalence of sleep apnea syndrome among Swedish men – an epidemiological study. *J Clin Epidemiol* 1988; **41**:571–76.

23. **Nugent A M**, **Gleadhill I**, **McCrum E**, *et al.* Sleep complaints and risk factors for excessive daytime sleepiness in adult males in Northern Ireland. *J Sleep Res* 2001; **10**:69–74.

24. **Ohayon M M**, **Vecchierini M F**. Daytime sleepiness and cognitive impairment in the elderly population. *Arch Intern Med* 2002; **162**:201–08.

25. **Bixler E O**, **Vgontzas A N**, **Lin H M**, *et al.* Excessive daytime sleepiness in a general population sample: the role of sleep apnea, age, obesity, diabetes, and depression. *J Clin Endocrinol Metab* 2005; **90**: 4510–15.

26. **Souza J C**, **Magna L A**, **Reimao R**. Excessive daytime sleepiness in Campo Grande general population, Brazil. *Arq Neuropsiquiatr* 2002; **60**:558–62.

27. **Takegami M**, **Sokejima S**, **Yamazaki S**, *et al.* An estimation of the prevalence of excessive daytime sleepiness based on age and sex distribution of Epworth sleepiness scale scores: a population based survey [in Japanese]. *Nippon Koshu Eisei Zasshi* 2005; **52**:137–45.

28. **Baldwin C M**, **Kapur V K**, **Holberg C J**, *et al.* Sleep Heart Health Study Group. Associations between gender and measures of daytime somnolence in the Sleep Heart Health Study. *Sleep* 2004; **27**:305–11.

29. **Ohayon M M**, **Ferini-Strambi L**, **Plazzi G**, *et al.* Frequency of narcolepsy symptoms and other sleep disorders in narcoleptic patients and their first-degree relatives. *J Sleep Res* 2005; **14**:437–45.

30. **Hublin C**, **Kaprio J**, **Partinen M**, *et al.* Insufficient sleep – a population-based study in adults. *Sleep* 2001; **24**:392–400.

31. **Hublin C**, **Kaprio J**, **Partinen M**, *et al.* The prevalence of narcolepsy: an epidemiological study of the Finnish Twin Cohort. *Ann Neurol* 1994; **35**:709–16.

32. **Roth B**, (Eng. Trans.), **Broughton R**. *Narcolepsy and Hypersomnia*. Chapter 10. Basel: Karger, 1980.

33. **Franceschi M**, **Zamproni P**, **Crippa D**, *et al.* Excessive daytime sleepiness: a 1-year study in an unselected inpatient population. *Sleep* 1982; **5**:239–47.

34. **Billiard M**, **Alperovich A**, **Perot C**, *et al.* Excessive daytime sleepiness in young men: prevalence and contributing factors. *Sleep* 1987; **10**:297–305.

35. **Ondzé B**, **Lubin S**, **Lavendier B**, *et al.* Frequency of narcolepsy in the population of a French "département". *J Sleep Res* 1998; 7:193.

36. **Solomon P**. Narcolepsy in negroes. *Dis Nerv Syst* 1945; **6**:176–83.

37. **Dement W**, **Zarcone W**, **Varner V**, *et al.* The prevalence of narcolepsy. *Sleep Res* 1972; **1**:148.

38. **Dement W C**, **Carskadon M**, **Ley R**. The prevalence of narcolepsy II. *Sleep Res* 1973; **2**:147.

39. **Silber M H**, **Krahn L E**, **Olson E J**, *et al.* The epidemiology of narcolepsy in Olmsted County, Minnesota: a population-based study. *Sleep* 2002; **25**:197–202.

40. **Honda Y**. Census of narcolepsy, cataplexy and sleep life among teenagers in Fujisawa city. *Sleep Res* 1979; **8**:191.

41. **Tashiro T**, **Kanbayashi T**, **Iijima S**, *et al.* An epidemiological study on prevalence of narcolepsy in Japanese. *J Sleep Res* 1992; **1**(Suppl):228.

42. **Wing Y K**, **Chiu H F**, **Ho C K**, *et al.* Narcolepsy in Hong Kong Chinese – a preliminary experience. *Aust N Z J Med* 1994; **24**:304–06.

43. **Lavie P**, **Peled, R**. Letter to the Editor: Narcolepsy is a rare disease in Israel. *Sleep* 1987; **10**:608–09.

44. **al Rajeh S**, **Bademosi O**, **Ismail H**, *et al.* A community survey of neurological disorders in Saudi Arabia: the Thugbah study. *Neuroepidemiology* 1993; **12**:164–78.

45. **Wing Y K**, **Li R H**, **Lam C W**, *et al.* The prevalence of narcolepsy among Chinese in Hong Kong. *Ann Neurol* 2002; **51**:578–84.

46. **Hays J C, Blazer D G, Foley D J**. Risk of napping: excessive daytime sleepiness and mortality in an older community population. *J Am Geriatr Soc* 1996; **44**:693–98.

47. **Nofzinger E A, Thase M E, Reynolds C F** 3rd, *et al.* Hypersomnia in bipolar depression: a comparison with narcolepsy using the multiple sleep latency test. *Am J Psychiatry* 1991; **148**:1177–81.

48. **Johns M W**. A new method for measuring daytime sleepiness: the Epworth sleepiness scale. *Sleep* 1991; **14**:540–45.

49. **Olson L G, Cole M F, Ambrogetti A**. Correlations among Epworth sleepiness scale scores, multiple sleep latency tests and psychological symptoms. *J Sleep Res* 1998; **7**:248–53.

50. **Morin C M, Edinger J D**. Sleep disorders: evaluation and diagnosis. In: Turner SM, Hersen M, Eds. *Adult Psychopathology and Diagnosis* (3rd Ed.). New York: John Wiley & Sons, 1997: 483–507.

51. **Webb W B, Dinges D F**. Cultural perspectives on napping and the siesta. In: Dinges D F, Broughton R J, Eds. *Sleep and Alertness: Chronobiological, Behavioral and Medical Aspects of Napping*. New York, NY: Raven Press, 1989: 247–65

52. **Valencia-Flores M, Castano V A, Campos R M**, *et al.* The siesta culture concept is not supported by the sleep habits of urban Mexican students. *J Sleep Res* 1998; **7**:21–29.

53. **Karacan I, Thornby J I, Anch M**, *et al.* Prevalence of sleep disturbance in a primarily urban Florida county. *Soc Sci Med* 1976; **10**:239–44.

54. **Hays J C, Blazer D G, Foley D J**. Risk of napping: excessive daytime sleepiness and mortality in an older community population. *J Am Geriatr Soc* 1996; **44**:693–98.

55. **Asplund R**. Daytime sleepiness and napping amongst the elderly in relation to somatic health and medical treatment. *J Intern Med* 1996; **239**:261–67.

Section 1 Chapter 2

Introduction

Neurochemistry of excessive sleepiness

Seiji Nishino and Masashi Okuro

Introduction

In this review, our current understanding of the neurochemistry of excessive daytime sleepiness (EDS) is discussed. Human subjects with EDS have been reported across the millennia. For example, in an old Japanese picture book from the Heian period (794–1184 AC), *Illustrations of Some Peculiar Diseases*, Yamaino Soushi depicts a man with EDS (Figure 2.1) among his representations of 18 diseases. Interestingly, the note, pertaining to the man with hypersomnia explains that there are many different causes for EDS and that the cause of the depicted man's EDS is unknown. This same explanation may still be valid in the twenty-first century, as we have only recently begun to develop an understanding of the mechanisms/neurochemistry underlying some EDS disorders.

Our recent progress in understanding the pathophysiology of EDS is particularly indebted to the 1999 discovery of narcolepsy genes (i.e. hypocretin receptor and peptide genes) in animals and subsequent discovery (in 2000) of hypocretin ligand deficiency in idiopathic cases of human narcolepsy–cataplexy. The discovery in human narcolepsy led to (A) the establishment of a new diagnostic test (i.e. low cerebrospinal fluid (CSF) hypocretin-1 levels) and (B) the development of hypocretin replacements to be used in the treatment of hypocretin-deficient narcolepsy. Further refinement of this therapeutic option is the focus of current, ongoing research (see [1]).

The prevalence of primary hypersomnia, such as narcolepsy and idiopathic hypersomnia, is not high (0.05 and 0.005%, respectively), but the prevalence of symptomatic (secondary) hypersomnia may be much higher. For example, several million subjects in the USA suffer from chronic brain injury. Of these patients, 75% have sleep problems and about a half claim sleepiness [2]. By comparison, the prevalence of symptomatic narcolepsy is likely to be much smaller, and only about 120 of such cases have been reported in the literature in the past 30 years. Nevertheless, meta-analysis of these cases indicates that hypocretin deficiency may also partially explain the neurochemical mechanisms of both EDS and EDS associated with symptomatic cases of narcolepsy [3].

The recent discovery of hypocretin peptidergic systems in 1998, followed by the discovery of narcolepsy genes only a year later, immediately prompted and illuminated related studies, seeking specific understanding of the roles of hypocretin peptidergic systems in sleep regulation under both normal and pathological conditions.

Anatomical and functional studies demonstrate that the hypocretin systems integrate and coordinate the multiple wake-promoting systems (such as monoamine and acetylcholine systems) to keep subjects fully alert [4]. Histamine is one of these wake-active monoamines, and, notably, low CSF histamine levels are also found in narcolepsy with hypocretin deficiency [5, 6]. Since hypocretin neurons project and excite histamine neurons in the posterior hypothalamus, it is conceivable that impaired histamine neurotransmission may mediate sleep abnormalities in hypocretin-deficient narcolepsy. However, low CSF histamine levels were also observed in narcolepsy with normal hypocretin levels and in idiopathic hypersomnia, a primary hypersomnia not associated with hypocretin deficiency (and with REM sleep abnormalities). Thus, decreased histamine neurotransmission may be involved in the broader category of EDS than in hypocretin-deficient narcolepsy [6]. Since CSF histamine levels are normalized in EDS patients treated with wake-promoting compounds, low CSF histamine levels may be a new state marker for primary

---

Sleepiness: Causes, Consequences and Treatment, ed. Michael J. Thorpy and Michel Billiard. Published by Cambridge University Press. © Cambridge University Press 2011.

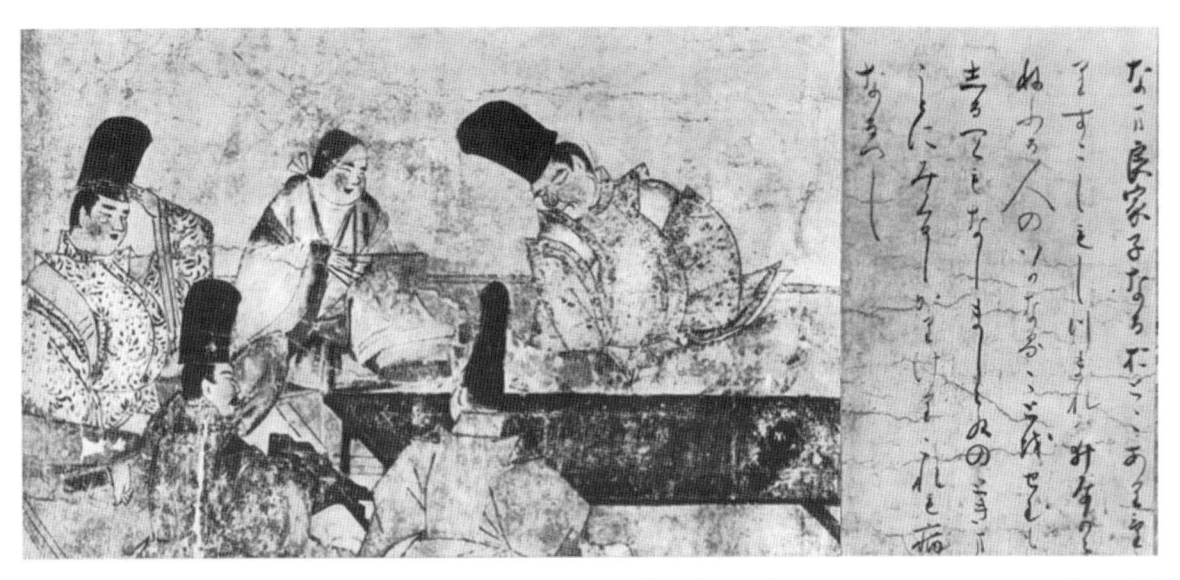

Figure 2.1 A man of hypersomnia (from Yamaino Soushi, Illustrations of Some Peculiar Diseases, published in Heian period (794–1184 AC) in Japan).

hypersomnia. The functional significance of this finding requires further study [6].

Since a large majority of patients with EDS are currently treated with pharmacological agents, further knowledge of the neurochemistry of EDS will likely lead to the development of new treatments and management strategies for patients with hypersomnia with various etiologies.

Basic sleep physiology and symptoms of narcolepsy

A brief discussion of basic sleep physiology and narcolepsy symptoms facilitates an understanding of the specific neurochemistry of hypersomnia. As narcolepsy is a prototypical EDS disorder and since the major pathophysiology of narcolepsy (i.e. deficiency in hypocretin neurotransmission) has recently been revealed, a discussion of the neurochemical aspects of narcolepsy will help establish a general understanding of neurochemistry in EDS.

Narcolepsy patients manifest symptoms specifically related to dysregulation of REM sleep [7]. In the structured, cyclic process of normal sleep, two distinct states – rapid eye movement (REM) and 4 stages (S1, S2, S3, S4) of non-REM (NREM) sleep – alternate sequentially every 90 min in a cycle repeating 4–5 times per night [8]. As electroencephalography (EEG) signals in humans indicate, NREM sleep, characterized by slow oscillation of thalamocortical neurons (detected as cortical slow waves) and muscle tonus reduction, precedes REM sleep, when complete muscle atonia occurs. Slow-wave NREM predominates during the early phase of normal sleep, followed by a predominance of REM during the later phase [8].

Notably, sleep and wake are highly fragmented in narcolepsy, and affected subjects cannot maintain long bouts of either state. Normal sleep physiology is currently understood as dependent upon coordination of the interactions of facilitating sleep centers and inhibiting arousal centers in the brain, such that stable sleep and wake states are maintained for specific durations [8]. An ascending arousal pathway, running from the rostral pons and through the midbrain reticular formation, promotes wakefulness [8, 9]. This arousal pathway may be composed of neurotransmitters (acetylcholine (ACh), norepinephrine (NE), dopamine (DA), excitatory amino acids), produced by brainstem and hypothalamic neurons (hypocretin/orexin and histamine) and also linked to muscle tonus control during sleep [8, 9]. Whereas full alertness and cortical activation require coordination of these arousal networks, effective sleep requires suppression of arousal by the hypothalamus [9]. Narcolepsy patients may experience major neurological malfunction of this control system.

Narcoleptics exhibit a phenomenon, termed short REM sleep latency or sleep onset REM period

(SOREMP), in which REM sleep is entered more immediately upon falling asleep than is normal [7]. In some cases, NREM sleep is completely bypassed and the transition to REM sleep occurs instantly [7].

Moreover, intrusion of REM sleep into wakefulness may explain the cataplexy, sleep paralysis and hypnogogic hallucinations, which are cardinal features symptomatic of narcolepsy. Significantly, however, whereas paralysis and hallucinations manifest in other sleep disorders (sleep apnea syndromes and disturbed sleep patterns in normal population) [10], cataplexy is pathognomic for narcolepsy [7]. As such, identifying cataplexy's unique pathophysiological mechanism emerged as potentially pivotal to describing the pathology underlying narcolepsy overall.

Discovery of hypocretin deficiency and postnatal cell death of hypocretin neurons

The significant roles, first, of hypocretin deficiency and, subsequently, of postnatal cell death of hypocretin neurons as the major pathophysiological process underlying narcolepsy with cataplexy emerged from a decade of investigation, employing both animal and human models. In 1998, the simultaneous discovery by two independent research groups of a novel hypothalamic peptide neurotransmitter (variously named hypocretin and orexin) proved pivotal [11, 12] (Figure 2.2A). These neurotransmitters are produced exclusively by thousands of neurons, which are localized in the lateral hypothalamus and project broadly to specific cerebral regions and more densely to others [13] (Figure 2.2B).

Within a year, Stanford researchers, using positional cloning of a naturally occurring familial canine narcolepsy model, identified an autosomal recessive mutation of hypocretin receptor 2 (Hcrtr2) responsible for canine narcolepsy, characterized by cataplexy, reduced sleep latency, and SOREMPs [14]. This finding coincided with the simultaneous observation of the narcolepsy phenotype, characterized by cataplexic behavior and sleep fragmentation, in hypocretin ligand-deficient mice (prepro-orexin gene knockout mice) [15]. Together, these findings confirmed hypcretins as principal sleep-modulating neurotransmitters and prompted investigation of hypocretin system involvement in human narcolepsy.

Although screening of patients with cataplexy failed to implicate hypocretin-related gene mutation as a major cause of human narcolepsy, narcoleptic patients did exhibit low CSF levels of hypocretin-1 [16] (Figure 2.3A). Postmortem brain tissue of narcoleptic patients, assessed through immunochemistry, radioimmunological peptide assays, and in-situ hybridization, revealed loss of hypocretin peptides and undetectable levels of hypocretin peptides or pre-hypocretin RNA (Figure 2.3B). Further, melanin-concentrating hormone neurons, normal to the same brain region [17], were observed intact, thus indicating that damage to hypocretin neurons and production is selective in narcolepsy, rather than due to generalized neuronal degeneration.

As a result of these findings, a diagnostic test for narcolepsy, based on clinical measurement of CSF hypocretin-1 and detected hypocretin ligand deficiency, is now available [18]. Whereas CSF hypocretin-1 concentrations above 200 pg/ml almost always occur in controls and patients with other sleep and neurological disorders, concentrations below 110 pg/ml are 94% predictive of narcolepsy with cataplexy [19]. As this represents a more specific assessment than the multiple sleep latency test (MSLT), CFS hypocretin-1 levels below 110 pg/ml are indicated in the ICSD-2 as diagnostic of narcolepsy with cataplexy [18].

Moreover, separate coding of "narcolepsy with cataplexy" and "narcolepsy without cataplexy" in the ICSD-2 underscores how discovery of specific diagnostic criteria now informs our understanding of narcolepsy's nosology; narcolepsy with cataplexy, as indicated by low CSF hypocretin-1, appears etiologically homogeneous and distinct from narcolepsy without cataplexy, exhibiting normal hypocretin-1 levels [19]. Further, the potential of hypocretin receptor agonists (or cell transplantation) in narcolepsy treatment is currently being explored, and CFS hypocretin-1 measures may be useful in identifying appropriate patients for a novel therapeutic option, namely hypocretin replacement therapy.

Soon after the discovery of human hypocretin deficiency, researchers identified specific substances and genes, such as dynorphin and neuronal activity-regulated pentraxin (NARP) [20] and, most recently, insulin-like growth factor binding protein 3 (IGF BP3) [21], which colocalize in neurons containing hypocretin (Figure 2.3C). These findings underscored selective hypocretin cell death as the cause of hypocretin deficiency (as opposed to transcription/biosynthesis

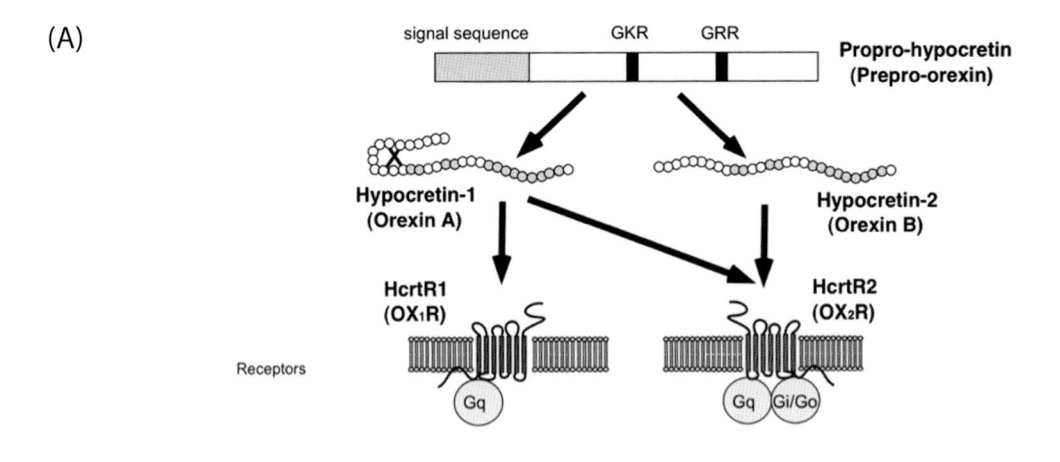

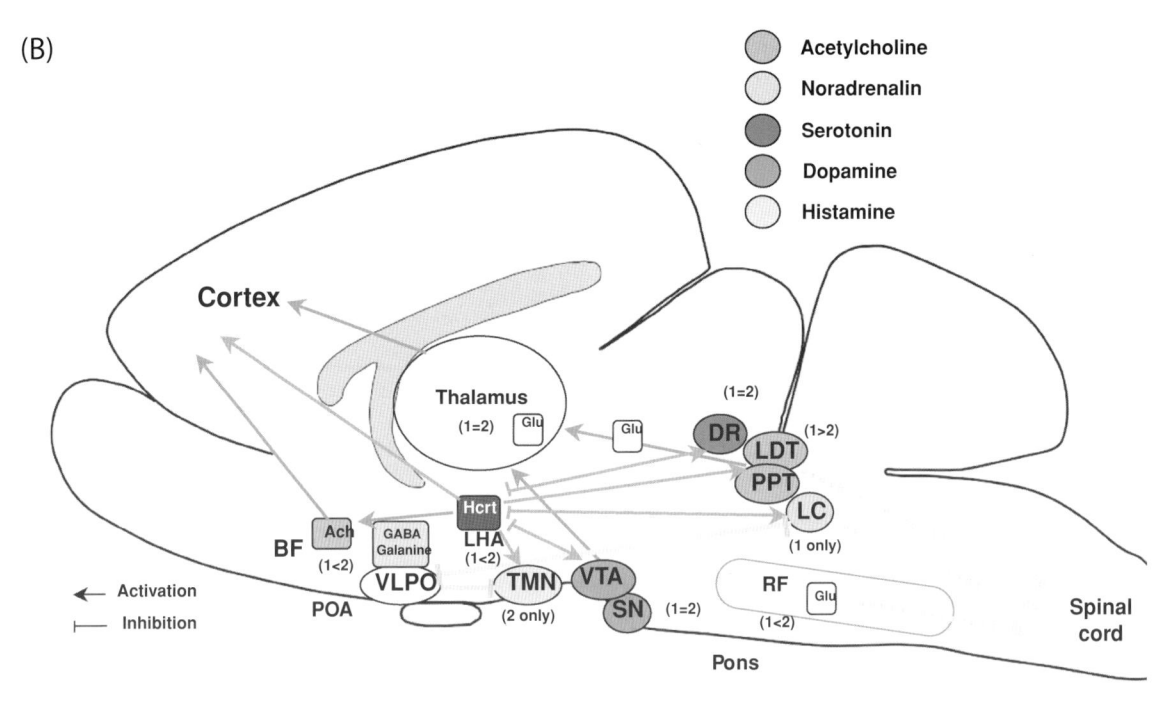

Figure 2.2 (a) Structures of mature hypocretin-1 (orexin-A) and hypocretin-2 (orexin-B) peptides. (b) Schematic representation of the hypocretin (orexin) system. (c) Projections of hypocretin neurons in the rat brain and relative abundances of hypocretin receptor 1 and 2. (a) The topology of the two intrachain disulfide bonds in orexin-A is indicated in the above sequence. Amino acid identities are indicated by shaded areas. (b) The actions of hypocretins are mediated via two G-protein-coupled receptors named hypocretin receptor-1 (Hcrtr1) and hypocretin receptor-2 (Hcrtr2), also known as orexin-1 (OX_1R) and orexin-2 (OX_2R) receptors, respectively. Hcrtr1 is selective for hypocretin-1, whereas Hcrtr2 is non-selective for both hypocretin-1 and hypocretin-2. Hcrtr1 is coupled exclusively to the G_q subclass of heterotrimeric G proteins, whereas in-vitro experiments suggest that Hcrtr2 couples with G_i/G_o, and/or G_q (adapted from [25]). (c) Hypocretin-containing neurons project to these previously identified monoaminergic and cholinergic and cholinoceptive regions where hypocretin receptors are enriched. The relative abundance of Hcrtr1 vs. Hcrtr2 in each brain structure was indicated in parenthesis (data from [4]). Impairments of hypocretin input may thus result in cholinergic and monoaminergic imbalance and generation of narcoleptic symptoms. Most drugs currently used for the treatment of narcolepsy enhance monoaminergic neurotransmission and adjust these symptoms.

VTA, ventral tegmental area; SN; substantia nigra; LC, locus coeruleus; LDT, laterodorsal tegmental nucleus; PPT, pedunculopontine tegmental nucleus; RF, reticular formation; BF, basal forebrain; VLPO, ventrolateral preoptic nucleus; LHA, lateral hypothalamic area; TMN; tuberomamillary nucleus; DR, dorsal raphe; Ach, acetylcholine; Glu, glutamate; GABA, gamma-aminobutyric acid; HI, histamine; DA, dopamine; NA, noradrenalin, 5-HT, serotonin. (See color plate section).

1. Introduction

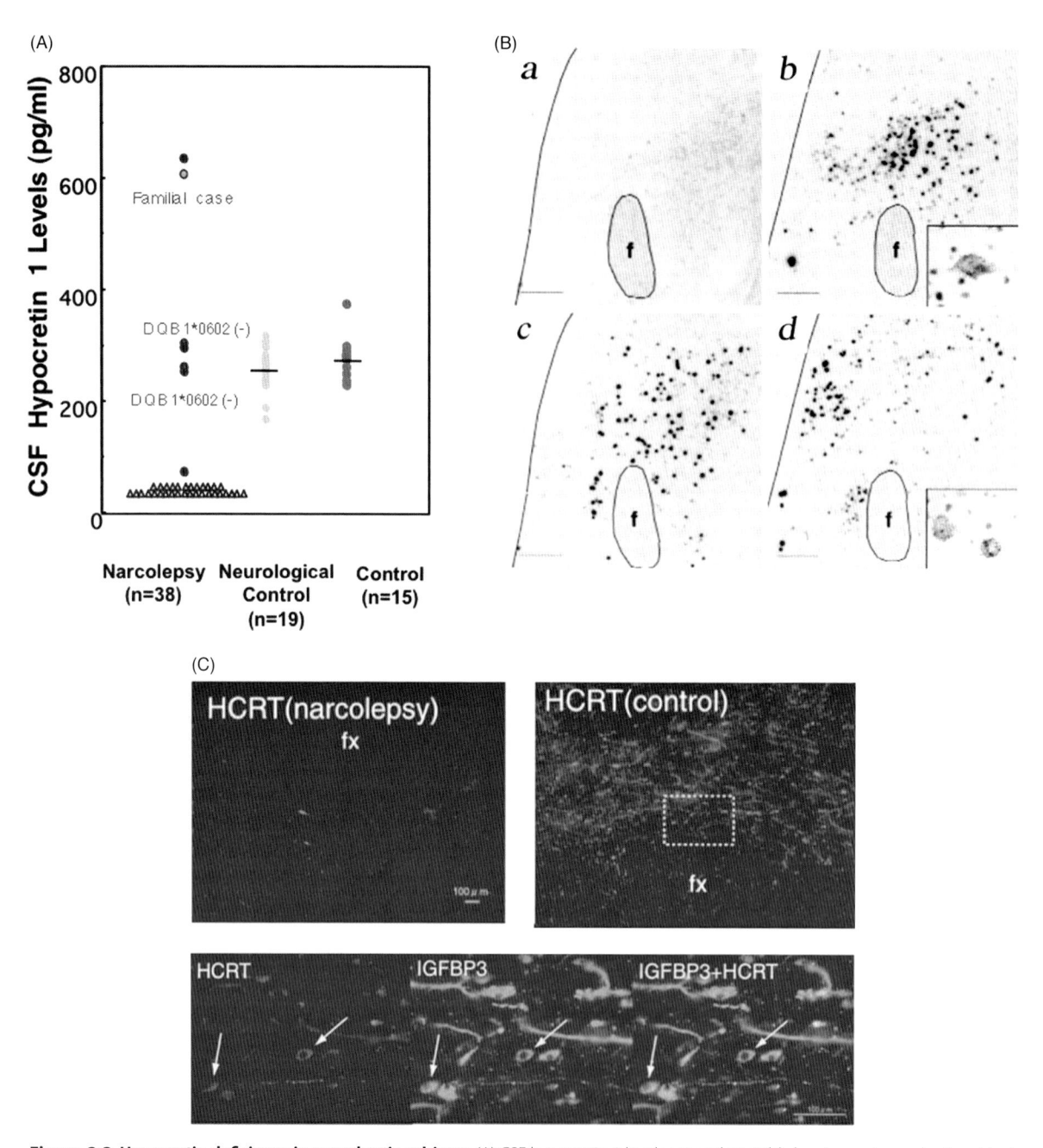

Figure 2.3 Hypocretin deficiency in narcoleptic subjects. (A) CSF hypocretin-1 levels are undetectably low in most narcoleptic subjects (84.2%). Note that two HLA DqB1*0602-negative and one familial case have normal or high CSF hypocretin levels. (B) Preprohypocretin transcripts are detected in the hypothalamus of control (b) but not in narcoleptic subjects (a). Melanin-concentrating hormone (MCH) transcripts are detected in the same region in both control (d) and narcoleptic (c) sections. (C) Colocalization of IGF BP3 in HCRT cells in control and narcolepsy human brain. Upper panel: Distribution of hypocretin cells and fibers in the perifornical area of human hypothalamus. (e) In control brains, HCRT cells and fibers were densely stained by an anti-HCRT monoclonal antibody (red fluorescence: VectorRed), while in narcolepsy brains, staining was markedly reduced. (f) Lower panel: HCRT immunoreactivity (g: red fluorescence) and IGF BP3 immunoreactivity (h: green fluorescence; Q-dot525) and a composite picture (i) arrows indicate HCRT cells colocalized with IGF BP3). Note non-neuronal autofluorescent elements. f and fx, fornix. Scale bar represents 10 mm (a–d), 500 mm in e and f, 100 mm in g–i (adapted from [17] and [21]). (See color plate section).

or hypocretin peptide processing problems), because these substances are also deficient in the postmortem brain lateral hypothalamic area (LHA) of hypocretin-deficient narcoleptic patients [20, 21]. Further, these findings, in view of the generally late onsets of sporadic narcolepsy compared with those of familial cases, suggest that postnatal cell death of hypocretin neurons constitutes the major pathophysiological process in human narcolepsy with cataplexy.

Idiopathic hypersomnia, hypocretin non-deficient primary hypersomnia

With the clear definition of narcolepsy (cataplexy and dissociated manifestations of REM sleep), it became apparent that some patients with hypersomnia suffer from a different disorder. In the late 1950s and early 1960s, Bedrich Roth was the first to describe a syndrome characterized by EDS: prolonged sleep and sleep drunkenness with the absence of "sleep attacks," cataplexy, sleep paralysis, and hallucinations. Although the terms "independent sleep drunkenness" and "hypersomnia with sleep drunkenness" were initially suggested [22], this syndrome is now categorized as idiopathic hypersomnia with and without long sleep time [18]. Idiopathic hypersomnia should not be considered synonymous with hypersomnia of unknown origin.

In the absence of systematic studies, the prevalence of idiopathic hypersomnia is unknown. Nosologic uncertainty causes difficulty in determining the epidemiology of the disorder. Recent reports from large sleep centers reported a 1:10 ratio of idiopathic hypersomnia to narcolepsy [23]. The age of onset of symptoms varies, but is frequently between 10 and 30 years. The condition usually develops progressively over several weeks or months. Once established, symptoms are generally stable and long-lasting, but spontaneous improvement in EDS may be observed in up to one-quarter of patients [23].

The pathogenesis of idiopathic hypersomnia is unknown. Hypersomnia usually starts insidiously. Occasionally, EDS is first experienced after transient insomnia, abrupt changes in sleep–wake habits, overexertion, general anesthesia, viral illness, or mild head trauma [23]. Despite reports of an increase in HLA DQ1, 11 DR5, Cw2, and DQ3, and of a decrease in Cw3, no consistent findings have emerged [23].

The most recent attempts to understand the pathophysiology of idiopathic hypersomnia relate to the potential role of the hypocretins. However, most studies suggest normal CSF levels of hypocretin-1 in idiopathic hypersomnia [19, 24]. Thus, it is now confirmed that the pathophysiology of idiopathic hypersomnia is distinct from that of narcolepsy.

How does hypocretin ligand deficiency cause narcolepsy phenotype?

Because hypocretin deficiency is a major pathophysiological mechanism in narcolepsy–cataplexy, some discussion of how hypocretin ligand deficiency may cause narcolepsy phenotype is warranted.

(A) hypocretin/orexin system and sleep regulation

Hypocretins/orexins were discovered by two independent research groups in 1998. One group called the peptides "hypocretin" because of their primary hypothalamic localization and similarities with the hormone "secretin" [12]. The other group called the molecules "orexin" after observing that central administration of these peptides increased appetite in rats [11].

Hypocretins/orexins (hypocretin-1 and hypocretin-2/Orexin A and Orexin B) are cleaved from a precursor preprohypocretin (prepro-orexin) peptide [11, 12, 25]). Hypocretin-1 with 33 residues contains 4 cysteine residues forming two disulfide bonds. Hypocretin-2 consists of 28 amino acids and shares similar sequence homology, especially at the C-terminal side, but has no disulfide bonds (a linear peptide) [11]. There are two G-protein-coupled hypocretin receptors – Hcrtr1 and Hcrtr2, also called orexin receptor 1 and 2 (OX_1R and OX_2R). The distinct distribution of these receptors in the brain is known: Hcrtr1 is abundant in the locus coeruleus (LC) and Hcrtr2 is found in the tuberomamillary nucleus (TMN) and basal forebrain. Both receptor types are found in the midbrain raphe nuclei and mesopontine reticular formation [4].

Hypocretins-1 and -2 are produced exclusively by a well-defined group of neurons localized in the lateral hypothalamus. The neurons project to the olfactory bulb, cerebral cortex, thalamus, hypothalamus and brainstem, particularly the LC, raphe nucleus, as well as to the cholinergic nuclei (the laterodorsal tegmental and pedunculopontine tegmental nuclei) and cholinoceptive sites (such as pontine reticular formation), which are thought to be important for sleep regulation [13, 25].

A series of recent studies have now shown that the hypocretin system is a major excitatory system, which affects the activity of monoaminergic [dopamine DA, NE, serotonin (5-HT) and histamine] and cholinergic systems, significantly affecting vigilance states [25, 26]. Thus, it is likely that a deficiency in hypocretin neurotransmission induces an imbalance between these classic neurotransmitter systems, with primary effects on sleep-state organization and vigilance.

Many measurable activities (brain and body) and compounds manifest rhythmic fluctuations over a 24-h period. Whether or not hypocretin tone changes with zeitgeber time was assessed by measuring extracellular hypocretin-1 levels in the rat brain across 24-h periods, using in-vivo microdialysis [27]. Hypocretin levels increase during the active periods and are highest at the end of the active period, with the levels declining at sleep onset (see also figure 2.5a). Furthermore, sleep deprivation increases hypocretin levels [27].

Recent electrophysiological studies have shown that hypocretin neurons are active during wakefulness and reduce their activity during slow wave sleep [28]. The neuronal activity during REM sleep is the lowest, but intermittent increases in the activity, associated with body movements or phasic REM activity, are observed [28]. In addition to this short-term change, the results of microdialysis experiments also suggest that basic hypocretin neurotransmission involves in slower changes; it fluctuates across the 24-h period and slowly builds up toward the end of the active period. Adrenergic LC neurons are typical wake-active neurons, involved in vigilance control, and it has recently been demonstrated that basic firing activity of wake-active LC neurons also significantly fluctuates across various circadian times [29].

Several acute manipulations, such as exercise, low glucose utilization in the brain, fasting, and forced wakefulness, increase hypocretin levels [26, 27, 30]. Therefore, it is hypothesized that a build-up/acute increase of hypocretin levels may counteract homeostatic sleep propensity, which typically increases during the daytime and during forced wakefulness [27, 30].

(B) hypocretin/orexin deficiency and narcoleptic phenotype

Human studies have demonstrated that the occurrence of cataplexy is closely associated with hypocretin deficiency [19]. Furthermore, the hypocretin deficiency was already observed at the very early stages of the disease (just after the onset of EDS), even before the occurrences of clear cataplexy. Occurrences of cataplexy are rare in acute symptomatic cases of EDS, associated with a significant hypocretin deficiency (see [3]); therefore, it appears that a chronic and selective deficit of hypocretin neurotransmission may be required for the occurrence of cataplexy. The possibility of the involvement of a secondary neurochemical change, related to the occurrence of cataplexy, cannot be ruled out. If some of these changes are irreversible, hypocretin supplement therapy may only have limited effects on cataplexy.

Sleepiness in narcolepsy is most likely due to the patients' difficulty in maintaining wakefulness as normal subjects do. The sleep pattern of narcoleptic subjects is also fragmented; they exhibit insomnia (frequent wakening) at night. This fragmentation occurs across 24 h, and, thus, the loss of hypocretin signaling likely plays a role in this vigilance stage stability (see [31]), but other mechanisms may also be involved in EDS in narcoleptic subjects. One of the most important characteristics of EDS in narcolepsy is that sleepiness is reduced, and patients feel refreshed after a short nap; however, this does not last long and patients become sleepy within a short period of time. The lack of hypocretin build up/increase, caused by circadian time and by various alerting stimulations (that normally enhance hypocretin tonus), may also play a role in EDS associated with hypocretin-deficient narcolepsy.

Mechanisms for cataplexy and REM sleep abnormalities, associated with impaired hypocretin neurotransmission, have been studied. Hypocretin significantly inhibits REM sleep in vivo, but could activate all brainstem REM-off raphe neurons, and REM-on cholinergic neurons as well as local GABAnergic neurons in vitro preparations. It is proposed that disinhibition (rather than disfacilitation) of REM-off monoaminergic neurons and stimulation of REM active cholinergic neurons, mediated through disfacilitation of inhibitory GABAnergic inert neurons (associated with impaired hypocretin neurotransmission), are proposed as abnormal manifestations of REM sleep.

Considerations for the pathophysiology of narcolepsy with normal hypocretin levels

The pathophysiology of narcolepsy with normal hypocretin-1 levels is currently debated. Over 90% of patients with narcolepsy without cataplexy exhibit normal CSF hypocretin-1 levels, yet they also present REM sleep abnormalities (i.e. SOREMS). Moreover, even when strict criteria for narcolepsy–cataplexy is applied, up to 10% of patients with narcolepsy–cataplexy show normal CSF hypocretin-1 levels. Considering the fact that occurrence of cataplexy is tightly associated with hypocretin deficiency, impaired hypocretin neurotransmission is still likely involved in narcolepsy with normal CSF hypocretin-1 levels. Conceptually, there are two potential explanations for these mechanisms: (1) specific impairment of hypocretin receptor and their downstream pathway, and (2) partial/localized loss of hypocretin ligand (yet exhibition of normal CSF levels). A good example for the first explanation is provided by Hcrtr2-mutated narcoleptic dogs, which exhibit normal CSF hypocretin-1 levels [32], while having full-blown narcolepsy. Thannickal et al. recently reported one narcolepsy without cataplexy patient, who had an overall loss of 33% of hypocretin cells (compared to normal) with maximal cell loss in the posterior hypothalamus [33]. This result is more supportive of the second hypothesis, but further case studies are needed.

Neurochemistry in symptomatic narcolepsy and EDS: hypocretin involvements

Narcolepsy symptoms can also occur during the course of other neurological conditions (i.e. symptomatic narcolepsy), and discovery of hypocretin ligand deficiency in idiopathic narcolepsy has led to new insights into the pathophysiology of symptomatic (or secondary) narcolepsy and EDS. In a recent meta-analysis, 116 symptomatic narcolepsy cases reported in the literature were analyzed [3]. As several authors have previously reported, inherited disorder ($n = 38$), tumors ($n = 33$), and head trauma ($n = 19$) are the three most frequent causes for symptomatic narcolepsy. Of the 116 cases, 10 are associated with multiple sclerosis (MS), one with acute disseminated encephalomyelitis, and relatively few with vascular disorders ($n = 6$), encephalitis ($n = 4$), degeneration ($n = 1$), and heterodegenerative disorder (autosomal dominant cerebrospinal ataxia with deafness, 3 cases in 1 family). Although it is difficult to rule out the comorbidity of idiopathic narcolepsy in some cases, literature review reveals numerous unquestionable cases of symptomatic narcolepsy [3]. These include cases with HLA-negative and/or late onset and cases where occurrence of narcoleptic symptoms parallels the rise and fall of the causative disease. Notably, one review of these cases (particularly those with brain tumors) clearly illustrates that the hypothalamus is most often involved [3].

Also, quite a few EDS cases without cataplexy or REM sleep abnormalities (defined as symptomatic cases) are associated with these neurological conditions [3]. While the same review lists about 70 symptomatic EDS cases, prevalence of symptomatic EDS is likely much higher. For example, several million US subjects suffered chronic brain injury, and 75% experienced sleep problems and about 50% reported sleepiness [2]. Thus, symptomatic EDS may have significant clinical relevance.

CSF hypocretin-1 measurement was also conducted in these symptomatic narcolepsy and EDS cases, and reduced CSF hypocretin-1 levels were noted in most with various etiologies [3]. EDS in these cases is sometimes reversible with an improvement of the causative neurological disorder or hypocretin status, thus suggesting a functional link between hypocretin deficiency and sleep symptoms in these patients.

Changes in other neurotransmitter systems in narcolepsy and idiopathic hypersomnia

(A) Narcolepsy in dogs and humans

Studies in humans with narcolepsy have shown a decrease in DA concentration in the CSF [34]. Studies on Hcrtr2-mutated narcoleptic dogs, performed before and after probenecid administration, demonstrated an altered DA turnover with significantly less

1. Introduction

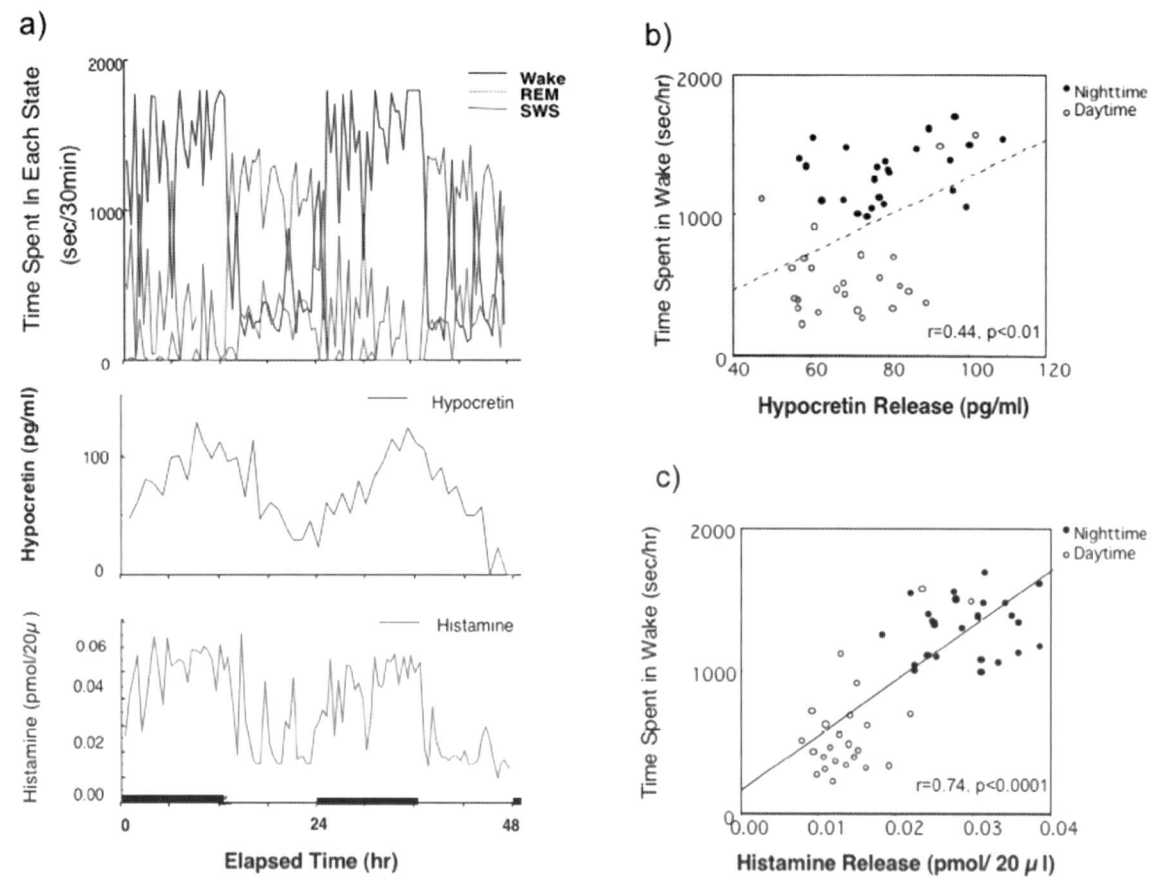

Figure 2.5 Fluctuation of extracellular hypocretin and histamine levels with changes in amount of wakefulness. Extracellular hypocretin and histamine levels simultaneously monitored in rats with sleep recordings under freely moving conditions using special floor-rotating rat chambers [30]. Changes in amount of wakefulness, hypocretin, and histamine levels were analyzed in 1-h time bins (the hypocretin levels were measured in 1-h time bins, while the mean of two consecutive 30-min bins were used for the histamine levels, see the Method). The dark periods are indicated by filled bars. (a) Typical data from one animal. Amount of wakefulness is displayed as s/h, while hypocretin and histamine concentrations are shown as pg/ml and pmol/20μl, respectively. (b, c) Correlations between time spent in wake and hypocretin/histamine releases in 4 rats. Filled symbols indicate data collected during dark periods. Extracellular histamine levels (c) are significantly (and positively) correlated with time spent in wakefulness across 24 h, while hypocretin levels (b) were clustered in light and dark periods, and the overall correlation between hypocretin levels and time spent in wakefulness is less significant. (See color plate section).

patterns of fluctuation in histamine levels are very similar to those of extracellular hypocretin levels in the lateral hypothalamus and thalamus, in rats [30].

In order to study physiological correlations of the hypocretin and histamine systems in relation to the control of vigilance, we have measured extracellular hypocretin and histamine levels simultaneously in rats with sleep recordings under freely moving conditions [50]. Two microdialysis probes were implanted in the brain (lateral hypothalamus for hypocretin measures and anterior preoptic area for histamine measures) of each rat. Microdialysis perfusates were collected in 30-min bins, and histamine and hypocretin assays were done on 1-h pooled bin samples. We found that both hypocretin-1 and histamine fluctuate significantly over 24-h periods and are high during active periods and low during resting periods (Figure 2.5). Histamine and hypocretin-1 levels seemed to fluctuate in correlation with amount of wakefulness, but histamine changed more rapidly than hypocretin-1. Correlations between amounts of wake, histamine levels, and hypocretin levels are presented in Figure 2.5b–c. As demonstrated previously [30], although hypocretin levels are positively correlated with the amount of wakefulness, the levels are rather clustered in two groups: the wakefulness amounts in respective time periods are very different during day and night even though the hypocretin levels are in a similar range. In contrast, histamine levels showed a better correlation with the amount of wakefulness over 24 h.

In addition to the changes in the extracellular histamine levels, we also observed that the CSF histamine levels exhibit clear diurnal fluctuations in rats: mean of the CSF histamine levels during the dark period was significantly higher than that during the light period [51]. After 6 h sleep deprivation from ZT0, CSF histamine levels increased significantly in comparison with controls whose sleep were not deprived. We also found that thioperamide (a H3 antagonist, 5 mg/kg, i.p.) significantly increased CSF histamine levels with little effects on locomotor activation. Since H3 autoreceptor antagonists are known to enhance terminal histamine releases from histaminergic neurons, the activity of neuronal histamine is likely to be reflected in the CSF histamine levels.

(B) Human narcolepsy and other idiopathic hypersomnia are also associated with decreased histaminergic neurotransmission

Since the results of our animal experiment suggest that CSF histamine levels at least partially reflect the central histamine neurotransmission and vigilance state changes, we evaluated the histaminergic neurotransmission in human narcolepsy using CSF. We conducted two clinical studies for evaluating the CSF histamine in narcolepsy. The first study included narcolepsy with low CSF hypocretin-1 ($\leq$110 pg/ml, $n = 34$, 100% with cataplexy), narcolepsy without low CSF hypocretin-1 ($n = 24$, 75% with cataplexy), and normal controls ($n = 23$) [5]. Narcoleptic subjects with and without hypocretin deficiency were included in order to determine if histamine neurotransmission is dependent on the hypocretin status of each subject. A significant reduction of CSF histamine levels was found in the cases with low CSF hypocretin-1, and levels were intermediate in other narcolepsy cases: mean CSF histamine levels were: 133.2 ± 20.1 pg/ml in narcoleptic subjects with low CSF hypocretin-1, 233.3 ± 46.5 pg/ml in patients with normal CSF hypocretin-1, and 300.5 ± 49.7 pg/ml in controls. Our results suggest the impaired histaminergic neurotrans-

mission in human narcolepsy, but this is not entirely dependent on the hypocretin-deficient status.

We also examined CSF histamine levels in narcolepsy and other sleep disorders in a Japanese population. This second clinical study included 67 narcolepsy subjects, 26 idiopathic hypersomnia (IH) subjects, 16 obstructive sleep apnea syndrome (OSAS) subjects, and 73 neurological controls [6].

We found significant reductions in CSF histamine levels in hypocretin-deficient narcolepsy with cataplexy (mean $\pm$ SEM; 176.0 ± 25.8pg/ml), hypocretin non-deficient narcolepsy with cataplexy (97.8 ± 38.4pg/ml), hypocretin non-deficient narcolepsy without cataplexy (113.6 ± 16.4pg/ml), and IH (161.0 ± 29.3pg/ml), while the levels in OSAS (259.3 ± 46.6pg/ml) did not differ statistically from those in the controls (333.8 ± 22.0pg/ml) (Figure 2.6). Low CSF histamine levels were mostly observed in non-medicated patients, and significant reductions in histamine levels were evident in non-medicated patients with hypocretin-deficient narcolepsy with cataplexy (112.1 ± 16.3pg/ml) and IH (143.3 ± 28.8pg/ml), while the levels in the medicated patients were in the normal range. Similar degrees of reduction, as seen in hypocretin-deficient narcolepsy with cataplexy, were also observed in hypocretin non-deficient narcolepsy and in IH, while those in OSAS (non-CNS hypersomnia) were not altered. These results confirmed the result of the first study, but further suggest that an impaired histaminergic system may be involved in mediating sleepiness in a much broader category of patients with EDS than hypocretin-deficient narcolepsy cases. The decrease in histamine in these subjects was more specifically observed in non-medicated subjects, suggesting that CSF histamine is a new biomarker, reflecting the degree of hypersomnia of central origin. It is not known if decreased histamine could either passively reflect or partially mediate daytime sleepiness in these pathologies. Further studies are essential, since central histamimetic compounds, such as H3 antagonists, may be developed as a new class of wake-promoting compounds for EDS with various etiologies.

Conclusion

This chapter described the current understanding of the neurochemistry for EDS with various etiologies. Although prevalence of primary hypersomnia, such as

1. Introduction

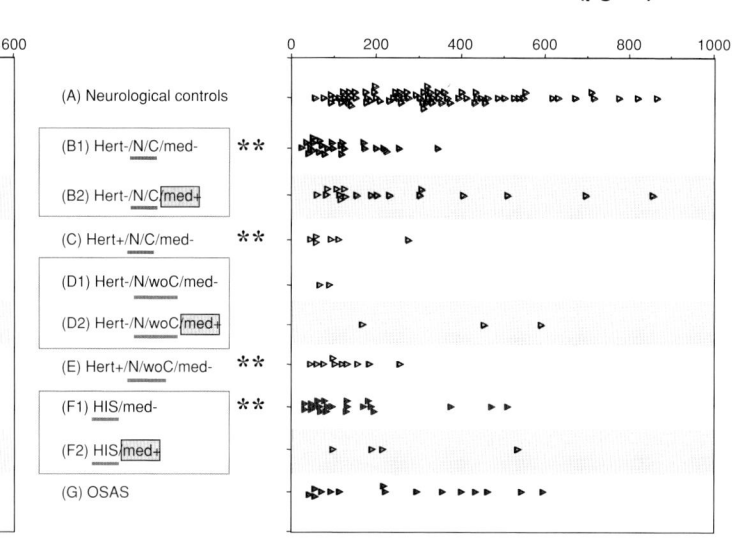

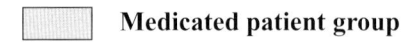

Figure 2.6 CSF Hcrt1 and histamine values for each individual with sleep disorders. CSF Hcrt1 (i: left panel) and histamine (ii: right panel) values for each individual are plotted. The patient groups are indicated as Group A to Group G from above. The results of the subjects with CNS stimulants (shadowed) and without CNS stimulants medication are presented separately in the figure. The vertical lines show mean values. The cut-off value of CSF hypocretin-1 level (less than or equal to 110 pg/ml) clearly segregated hypocretin deficiency from non-deficiency. None of the patients with idiopathic hypersomnia and OSAS showed hypocretin deficiency. We found significant reductions in CSF histamine levels in hypocretin-deficient (B: 176 ± 25.8 pg/ml) and non-deficient narcolepsy with cataplexy (C: 97.8 ± 38.4 pg/ml), hypocretin non-deficient narcolepsy without cataplexy (E: 113.6 ± 16.4 pg/ml) and IHS (F: 161.0 ± 29.3 pg/ml), while those in hypocretin-deficient narcolepsy without cataplexy (D: 273.6 ± 105 pg/ml) and OSAS (G: 259.3 ± 46.6 pg/ml) were not statistically different from those in the control range (A: 333.8 ± 22.0 pg/ml). The low CSF histamine levels were mostly observed in non-medicated patients, and significant reductions in histamine levels were observed only in non-medicated patients with hypocretin-deficient narcolepsy with cataplexy (B1: 112.1 ± 16.3 pg/ml) and IHS (F1: 143.3 ± 28.8 pg/ml). The levels in the medicated subjects are in the normal range (B2: 256.6 ± 51.7 pg/ml and F2: 259.5 ± 94.9 pg/ml). Non-medicated subjects had a tendency for low CSF histamine levels in hypocretin-deficient narcolepsy without cataplexy (D1: 77.5 ± 11.5 pg/ml) (adapted from [6]). (See color plate section).

narcolepsy and idiopathic hypersomnia, is not high, prevalence of symptomatic EDS is considerably high, and the pathophysiology of symptomatic EDS likely overlaps with that of primary hypersomnia.

Although much progress has been made regarding the pathophysiology and neurochemistry of EDS, this new knowledge is not yet incorporated in the development of new treatments, rendering further research absolutely critical.

References

1. **Nishino S, Okuro M, Kotorii N**, et al. Hypocretin/orexin and narcolepsy: new basic and clinical insights. *Acta Physiol (Oxf)* 2009; **198**:209–22.

2. **Verma A, Anand V, Verma N P**. Sleep disorders in chronic traumatic brain injury. *J Clin Sleep Med* 2007; **3**:357–62.

3. **Nishino S, Kanbayashi T**. Symptomatic narcolepsy, cataplexy and hypersomnia, and their implications in the hypothalamic hypocretin/orexin system. *Sleep Med Rev* 2005; **9**:269–310.

4. **Marcus J N, Aschkenasi C J, Lee C E**, et al. Differential expression of orexin receptors 1 and 2 in the rat brain. *J Comp Neurol* 2001; **435**:6–25.

5. **Nishino S, Sakurai E, Nevsimalova S**, et al. Decreased CSF histamine in narcolepsy with and without low CSF hypocretin-1 in comparison to healthy controls. *Sleep* 2009; **32**:175–80.

6. **Kanbayashi T, Kodama T, Kondo H**, et al. CSF histamine contents in narcolepsy, idiopathic hypersomnia and obstructive sleep apnea syndrome. *Sleep* 2009; **32**:181–87.

7. **Nishino S, Mignot E**. Pharmacological aspects of human and canine narcolepsy. *Prog Neurobiol* 1997; **52**:27–78.

8. **Nishino S, Taheri S, Black J**, et al. The neurobiology of sleep in relation to mental illness. In: Charney D S, Ed. *Neurobiology of Mental Illness*. New York, NY: Oxford University Press, 2004: 1160–79.

9. **Saper C B, Scammell T E, Lu J**. Hypothalamic regulation of sleep and circadian rhythms. *Nature* 2005; **437**:1257–63.

10. **Aldrich M S, Chervin R D, Malow B A**. Value of the multiple sleep latency test (MSLT) for the diagnosis of narcolepsy. *Sleep* 1997; **20**:620–29.

11. **Sakurai T, Amemiya A, Ishii M**, et al. Orexins and orexin receptors: a family of hypothalamic neuropeptides and G protein-coupled receptors that regulate feeding behavior. *Cell* 1998; **92**:573–85.

12. **De Lecea L, Kilduff T S, Peyron C**, et al. The hypocretins: hypothalamus-specific peptides with neuroexcitatory activity. *Proc Natl Acad Sci USA* 1998; **95**:322–27.

13. **Peyron C, Tighe D K, Van Den Pol A N**, et al. Neurons containing hypocretin (orexin) project to multiple neuronal systems. *J Neurosci* 1998; **18**:9996–10 015.

14. **Lin L, Faraco J, Li R**, et al. The sleep disorder canine narcolepsy is caused by a mutation in the hypocretin (orexin) receptor 2 gene. *Cell* 1999; **98**:365–76.

15. **Chemelli R M, Willie J T, Sinton C M**, et al. Narcolepsy in orexin knockout mice: molecular genetics of sleep regulation. *Cell* 1999; **98**:437–51.

16. **Nishino S, Ripley B, Overeem S**, et al. Hypocretin (orexin) deficiency in human narcolepsy. *Lancet* 2000; **355**:39–40.

17. **Peyron C, Faraco J, Rogers W**, et al. A mutation in a case of early onset narcolepsy and a generalized absence of hypocretin peptides in human narcoleptic brains. *Nat Med* 2000; **6**:991–97.

18. **ICSD-2**, editor. *ICSD-2-International Classification of Sleep Disorders, 2nd ed.: Diagnostic and Coding Manual*. Westchester, IL: American Academy of Sleep Medicine, 2005.

19. **Mignot E, Lammers G J, Ripley B**, et al. The role of cerebrospinal fluid hypocretin measurement in the diagnosis of narcolepsy and other hypersomnias. *Arch Neurol* 2002; **59**:1553–62.

20. **Crocker A, Espana R A, Papadopoulou M**, et al. Concomitant loss of dynorphin, NARP, and orexin in narcolepsy. *Neurology* 2005; **65**:1184–88.

21. **Honda M, Eriksson K S, Zhang S**, et al. IGFBP3 colocalizes with and regulates hypocretin (orexin). *PLoS ONE* 2009; **4**:e4254.

22. **Roth B**. *Narkolepsie und hypersomnie vom standpunkt der physiologie des schlafes*. Berlin: VEB Verlag Volk und Gesundheit, 1962.

23. **Bassetti C, Aldrich M S**. Idiopathic hypersomnia. A series of 42 patients. *Brain* 1997; **120**:1423–35.

24. **Bassetti C, Gugger M, Bischof M**, et al. The narcoleptic borderland: a multimodal diagnostic approach including cerebrospinal fluid levels of hypocretin-1 (orexin A). *Sleep Med* 2003; **4**:7–12.

25. **Sakurai T**. Roles of orexins in regulation of feeding and wakefulness. *NeuroReport* 2002; **13**:987–95.

26. **Willie J T, Chemelli R M, Sinton C M**, et al. To eat or to sleep? Orexin in the regulation of feeding and wakefulness. *Annu Rev Neurosci* 2001; **24**:429–58.

30. **Yoshida Y, Fujiki N, Nakajima T**, et al. Fluctuation of extracellular hypocretin-1 (orexin A) levels in the rat in relation to the light–dark cycle and sleep–wake activities. *Eur J Neurosci* 2001; **14**:1075–81.

28. **Lee M G, Hassani O K, Jones B E**. Discharge of identified orexin/hypocretin neurons across the sleep–waking cycle. *J Neurosci* 2005; **25**:6716–20.

29. **Aston-Jones G, Chen S, Zhu Y**, et al. A neural circuit for circadian regulation of arousal. *Nat Neurosci* 2001; **4**:732–38.

27. **Fujiki N, Yoshida Y, Ripley B**, et al. Changes in CSF hypocretin-1 (orexin A) levels in rats across 24 hours and in response to food deprivation. *NeuroReport* 2001; **12**:993–97.

31. **Saper C B, Chou T C, Scammell T E**. The sleep switch: hypothalamic control of sleep and wakefulness. *Trends Neurosci* 2001; **24**:726–31.

32. **Ripley B, Fujiki N, Okura M**, et al. Hypocretin levels in sporadic and familial cases of canine narcolepsy. *Neurobiol Dis* 2001; **8**:525–34.

33. **Thannickal T C, Nienhuis R, Siegel J M**. Localized loss of hypocretin (orexin) cells in narcolepsy without cataplexy. *Sleep* 2009; **32**:993–98.

34. **Montplaisir J, de Champlain J, Young S N**, et al. Narcolepsy and idiopathic hypersomnia: biogenic amines and related compounds in CSF. *Neurology* 1982; **32**:1299–302.

35. **Faull K F, Zeller-DeAmicis L C, Radde L**, et al. Biogenic amine concentrations in the brains of normal and narcoleptic canines: current status. *Sleep* 1986; **9**:107–10.

36. **Aldrich M S, Hollingsworth Z, Penney J B**. Dopamine-receptor autoradiography of human narcoleptic brain. *Neurology* 1992; **42**:410–15.

37. **Hublin C, Launes J, Nikkinen P**, et al. Dopamine D2-receptors in human narcolepsy: a SPECT study with 123I-IBZM. *Acta Neurol Scand* 1994; **90**: 186–89.

38. **Rinne J, Hublin C, Partinen M**, et al. PET study of human narcolepsy: no increase in striatal dopamine D2-receptors. *Neurology* 1995; **45**:1735–38.

39. **Mefford I N**, **Baker T L**, **Boehme R**, et al. Narcolepsy: biogenic amine deficits in an animal model. *Science* 1983; **220**:629–32.

40. **Nishino S**, **Fujiki N**, **Ripley B**, et al. Decreased brain histamine contents in hypocretin/orexin receptor-2 mutated narcoleptic dogs. *Neurosci Lett* 2001; **313**:125–28.

41. **Nishino S**, **Riehl J**, **Hong J**, et al. Is narcolepsy REM sleep disorder? Analysis of sleep abnormalities in narcoleptic Dobermans. *Neurosci Res* 2000; **38**:437–46.

42. **Eriksson K S**, **Sergeeva O**, **Brown R E**, et al. Orexin/hypocretin excites the histaminergic neurons of the tuberomammillary nucleus. *J Neurosci* 2001; **21**:9273–79.

43. **Yamanaka A**, **Tsujino N**, **Funahashi H**, et al. Orexins activate histaminergic neurons via the orexin 2 receptor. *Biochem Biophys Res Commun* 2002; **290**:1237–45.

44. **Faull K F**, **Guilleminault C**, **Berger P S**, et al. Cerebrospinal fluid monoamine metabolites in narcolepsy and hypersomnia. *Ann Neurol* 1983; **13**:258–63.

45. **Lin J S**. Brain structures and mechanisms involved in the control of cortical activation and wakefulness, with emphasis on the posterior hypothalamus and histaminergic neurons. *Sleep Med Rev* 2000; **4**:471–503.

46. **Haas H**, **Panula P**. The role of histamine and the tuberomamillary nucleus in the nervous system. *Nat Rev Neurosci* 2003; **4**:121–30.

47. **Huang Z L**, **Qu W M**, **Li W D**, et al. Arousal effect of orexin A depends on activation of the histaminergic system. *Proc Natl Acad Sci USA* 2001; **98**:9965–70.

48. **Mochizuki T**, **Yamatodani A**, **Okakura K**, et al. Circadian rhythm of histamine release from the hypothalamus of freely moving rats. *Physiol Behav* 1992; **51**:391–94.

49. **Strecker R E**, **Nalwalk J**, **Dauphin L J**, et al. Extracellular histamine levels in the feline preoptic/anterior hypothalamic area during natural sleep–wakefulness and prolonged wakefulness: an in vivo microdialysis study. *Neuroscience* 2002; **113**:663–70.

50. **Yoshida Y**, **Nishino S**, **Ishizuka T**, et al. Vigilance change, hypocretin and histamine release in rats before and after a histamine synthesis blocker (alpha-FMH) administration. *Sleep* 2005; **28**(Abstract Supplement):A18.

51. **Soya S**, **Song Y H**, **Kodama T**, et al. CSF histamine levels in rats reflect the central histamine neurotransmission. *Neurosci Lett* 2008; **430**:224–29.

Section 1 Chapter 3

Introduction

Functional neuroimaging of disorders of sleepiness

Eric A. Nofzinger

Introduction

In the past few decades, neuroimaging methods have emerged as a new way to assess brain function in health and pathology. These methods allow for the quantification of a variety of aspects of brain function including brain structure, metabolism, blood flow and receptor binding. Given that sleep is regulated by the brain and may ultimately serve brain function, these tools may provide important information regarding brain function during sleep and various levels of sleepiness. This chapter will review the use of neuroimaging studies that relate to the brain mechanisms of sleepiness.

Functional neuroimaging studies of healthy human sleep

Functional neuroimaging studies have revealed reliable broad changes in cerebral activity across the sleep–wake cycle. Globally, brain activity decreases from waking to NREM sleep, then increases to waking levels again during REM sleep [1–17]. Preclinical studies support a deafferentation of the cortex at the level of the thalamus and the occurrence of intrinsic thalamocortical electrical oscillations in NREM sleep. Studies across several laboratories and using various imaging methods have demonstrated that from waking to NREM sleep there are relative regional reductions in activity in heteromodal association cortex in the frontal, parietal and temporal lobes as well as in the thalamus. These studies support a role for NREM sleep in restoration/rejuvenation and/or growth in these networks. Preclinical work shows that REM sleep is associated with an electrophysiologically active cortex, with selective activation of cholinergic networks that originate in the brainstem and basal forebrain and that densely innervate limbic and paralimbic cortex. Consistent with this, in relation to waking and NREM sleep, REM sleep is associated with increased relative activity in the pontine reticular formation, as well as limbic (e.g. amygdala and hypothalamus) and paralimbic cortex (e.g. ventral striatum, anterior cingulate and medial prefrontal cortex). This suggests that REM sleep may play an important role in emotional behavior, given the important involvement of these structures in the regulation of affect and in motivated behavior.

The subjective experience of sleepiness may have diverse etiologies. Sleepiness is common following experimentally induced sleep deprivation. While this form of sleepiness may have some differentiating features from pathological sleepiness found in a variety of disorders, such as narcolepsy or sleepiness secondary to psychiatric disorders, it seems reasonable that there may be some overlaps in terms of the brain mechanisms of healthy sleepiness induced by sleep deprivation and the sleepiness of pathological disorders. Therefore, a brief review of the known brain mechanisms of sleep deprivation may provide some insights into the brain mechanisms of sleepiness in general.

Wu et al. [18] assessed regional cerebral metabolism using the [^{18}F]FDG method in healthy subjects before and after 32 h of sleep deprivation. They noted prominent decreases in metabolism in the thalamus, basal ganglia, temporal lobes, and cerebellum with increases in visual cortex. Whole-brain absolute metabolic rate was not different. Thomas et al. [19, 20] described the effects of 24, 48 and 72 h of sleep deprivation on waking regional cerebral metabolism assessed via [^{18}F]FDG positron emission tomography (PET), as well as alertness and cognitive performance. Sleep deprivation was associated with global declines in absolute cerebral metabolism. Regionally, these declines were most notable in frontoparietal cortex and in the thalamus.

Sleepiness: Causes, Consequences and Treatment, ed. Michael J. Thorpy and Michel Billiard. Published by Cambridge University Press. © Cambridge University Press 2011.

1. Introduction

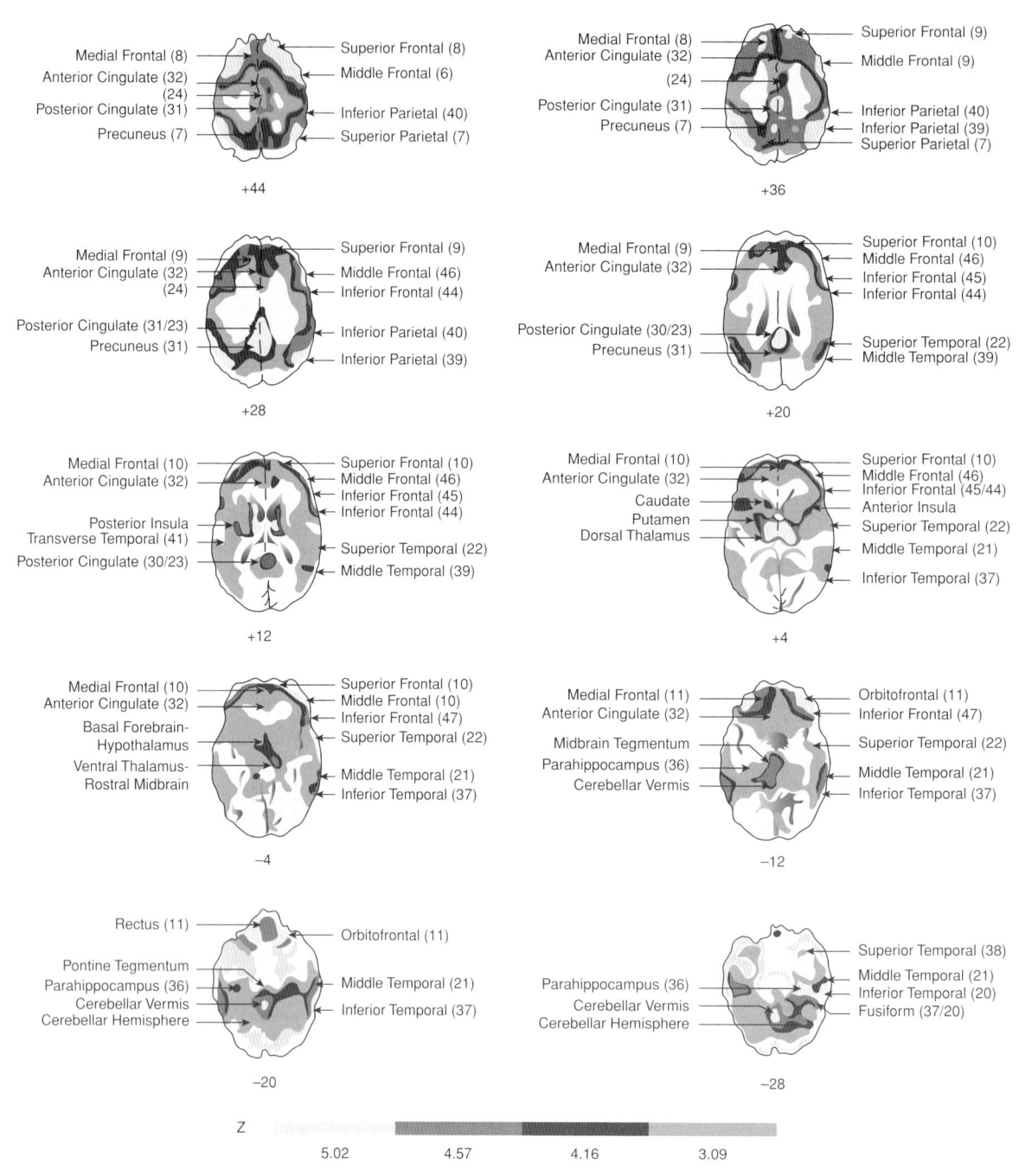

Figure 3.1 Significant decreases from baseline in absolute regional CMRglu during wakefulness and cognitive task performance after 24 h of sleep deprivation across 17 subjects. Deactivations are superimposed on a single subject's magnetic resonance imaging (MRI) template. Axial images are oriented in millimeters relative to the anterior commissure–posteriors (AC–PC) plane. The left/right hemispheres appear as the left/right sides of each image. Significant regions are color-coded to reflect thresholds for statistical probability levels: $5.02 = 0.001$ corrected, $4.57 = 0.01$ corrected, $4.16 = 0.05$ corrected, $3.09 = 0.001$ uncorrected. Thresholds for statistical significance are $Z \geq 3.09$ for regions predicted to decrease a priori (thalamus and prefrontal cortex) and/or previously published for short-term sleep deprivation effects on regional CMRglu (temporal cortex, thalamus, and cerebellum [18]), and $Z \geq 4.16$ for non-hypothesized regions. Statistically significant regions are neuroanatomically labeled and approximate Brodmann areas (BAs) are noted in parenthesis ( ). (See color plate section).

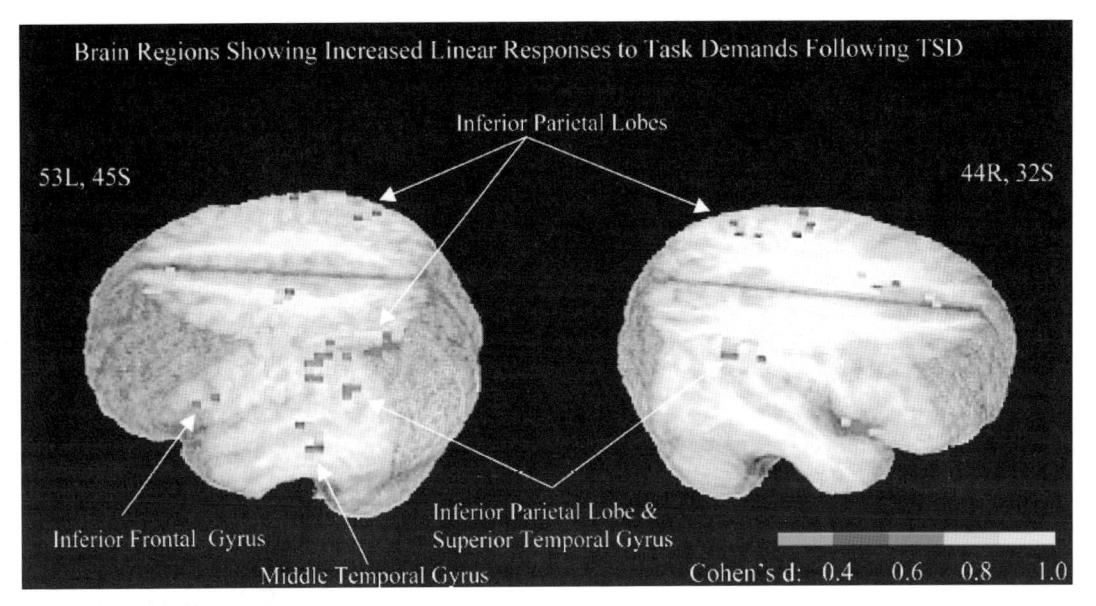

Figure 3.2 Brain regions showing increased linear responses to task demands following total sleep deprivation. Picture depicts the anatomic image averaged across all subjects as an underlay and the results of the main effect of total sleep deprivation (TSD) on the linear response to increasing task demands as the overlay. Functional data are color-coded per voxel by the effect size, Cohen's d, associated with the increased linear response following TSD compared to normal sleep. Only those voxels surviving our cluster threshold α protection method are shown. Each three-dimensional brain image has two slices removed. Left image: 53 mm left and 45 mm superior of the anterior commissure–posterior commissure line (AC–PC). Right image: 44 mm right and 32 mm superior of the AC–PC line. (See color plate section).

This is consistent with studies showing that the effects of sleep deprivation on slow-wave sleep are greatest in frontal EEG leads. Alertness and cognitive performance on a sleep deprivation-sensitive serial addition/subtraction test declined in association with the sleep deprivation-associated regional deactivations. These findings support the role for sleep in restoration of brain function in thalamocortical networks associated with higher-order cognition.

More recent reports focus on defining how the brain behaves in a sleep-deprived state. For example, Mu et al. [21] investigated the cerebral hemodynamic response to verbal working memory following sleep deprivation. Neuroimaging data revealed that, in the screening and rested states, the brain regions activated by the Sternberg working memory task were found in the left dorsolateral prefrontal cortex, Broca's area, supplementary motor area, right ventrolateral prefrontal cortex, and the bilateral posterior parietal cortexes. After 30 h of sleep deprivation, the activations in these brain regions significantly decreased, especially in the bilateral posterior parietal cortices.

Neuroimaging studies have been used to determine the neurobiological basis of individual differences in vulnerability to sleep deprivation. For example, Mu et al. [22] divided their sleep deprivation subjects into resilient and vulnerable subgroups based on subsequent performance following sleep deprivation. While both groups showed significant decreases in global brain activation compared to their rested group baseline, the sleep deprivation-resilient group had significantly more brain activation than did the sleep deprivation-vulnerable group at both the rested baseline and in the sleep-deprived states.

Investigators have also assessed the degree to which the brain is able to overcome the effects of sleep deprivation in order to perform more demanding tasks. These studies could have relevance for the clinical management of patients with narcolepsy. Drummond et al., for example [23], had subjects perform a modified version of Baddeley's logical reasoning task while undergoing functional magnetic resonance imaging before and after 35 h of total sleep deprivation (TSD). The task was modified to parametrically manipulate task difficulty. Subjects performed the same before and after TSD. Neuroimaging data revealed a linear increase in cerebral response with a linear increase in task demands in several brain regions after normal sleep. Even stronger linear responses were found after TSD in several brain regions, including bilateral

1. Introduction

inferior parietal lobes, bilateral temporal cortex, and left inferior and dorsolateral prefrontal cortex.

Also, Chee and Choo [24] assessed the neurobehavioral effects of 24 h of TSD on working memory in young healthy adults using functional magnetic resonance imaging (fMRI). Two tasks, one testing maintenance and the other manipulation and maintenance, were used. After sleep deprivation (SD), response times for both tasks were significantly slower. Performance was better preserved in the more complex task. Both tasks activated a bilateral, left hemisphere-dominant frontal–parietal network of brain regions reflecting the engagement of verbal working memory. In both states, manipulation elicited more extensive and bilateral (L > R) frontal, parietal, and thalamic activation. After SD, there was disproportionately greater activation of the left dorsolateral prefrontal cortex and bilateral thalamus when manipulation was required.

Narcolepsy

Narcolepsy is a sleep disorder characterized by recurrent daytime sleep attacks and often cataplexy, sleep onset paralysis and hypnagogic hallucinations. As there may be significant overlaps between the neurobiology of "sleepiness" in general and the disorder narcolepsy, it seems useful to review brain imaging studies of narcolepsy in order to further understand the neurobiology of sleepiness, per se. Recent advances have linked narcolepsy with altered function in the hypocretin system, a peptide produced in the posterior lateral hypothalamus that has activating properties and is functionally related to all known arousal systems in the central nervous system (CNS) [25–27]. The role of functional neuroimaging studies in human narcoleptic patients is in further clarifying the mechanisms of the extrahypothalamic manifestations of the illness, such as cataplexy, sleep attacks, and hypnogogic hallucinations. Few studies have been conducted to date. Hublin et al. [28] performed ^{123}I-iodobenzamide SPECT studies in narcoleptic patients and Parkinsonian controls. They found no differences in striatal/frontal D2 occupancy ratios between these two groups. Asenbaum et al. [29] assessed blood flow during waking and sleep onset REM periods in six narcoleptic patients using the HMPAO SPECT method. They found evidence for right hemispheric increased flow and thalamic decreased flow in REM sleep. Given the small sample sizes, they suggested that a replication of the findings was needed. Sudo et al. [30] assessed muscarinic cholinergic receptors in narcoleptic subjects using [^{11}C]N-methyl-4-piperidylbenzilate ([^{11}C]NMPB) both before and after pharmacotherapy. No differences were observed between patients and healthy subjects at baseline and minimal treatment effects were observed. Joo et al. [31] assessed cerebral glucose metabolism in 24 narcoleptic patients and 24 normal controls. They found cerebral glucose hypometabolism in hypothalamus–thalamus–orbitofrontal pathways in narcoleptic patients. Joo et al. [32] assessed cerebral perfusion in 25 narcoleptic patients and 25 normal controls using 99m Tc-ethylcysteinate dimmer single photon emission computed tomography (SPECT). They found reduced cerebral perfusion in bilateral anterior hypothalami, caudate nuclei, pulvinar nuclei of the thalamus, parts of the dorsolateral/ventromedial prefrontal cortices, parahippocampal gyri and cingulated gyri in narcoleptic patients. These findings were interpreted to be consistent with deficits in neural networks related to the hypocretin arousal pathway. As these arousal networks presumably also play a significant role in "sleepiness", these studies provide useful insights into the neurobiology of sleepiness.

Brenneis et al. [33] assessed regional brain volumes between narcoleptic patients and healthy controls. They found significant gray matter loss in the right prefrontal and frontomesial cortex of patients with narcolepsy. The comparison of cerebrospinal fluid partition detected an enlargement of subarachnoidal space of controls close to the prefrontal cortex. The volume reduction of gray matter in narcoleptic patients could indicate a disease-related atrophy pattern, although they suggested that these findings require replication in an independent drug-naive sample of patients. Eisensehr et al. [34] assessed the striatal presynaptic dopamine transporter and postsynaptic D2-receptors in seven patients with narcolepsy and seven control subjects using [^{123}I](N)-(3-iodopropene-2-yl)-2beta-carbomethoxy-3beta-(4-chlorophenyl) tropane and [^{123}I](S)-2-hydroxy-3-iodo-6-methoxy-([1-ethyl-2-pyrrolidinyl]methyl) benzamide SPECT. D2-receptor binding was elevated in narcolepsy ($p = 0.017$) and correlated with the frequency of cataplectic and sleep attacks ($R >$ or $= 0.844$, $p >$ or $= 0.017$). They propose that the human striatal dopaminergic system is altered in vivo in narcolepsy/cataplexy. Hong et al. [35] assessed cerebral perfusion using SPECT in

3. Functional neuroimaging

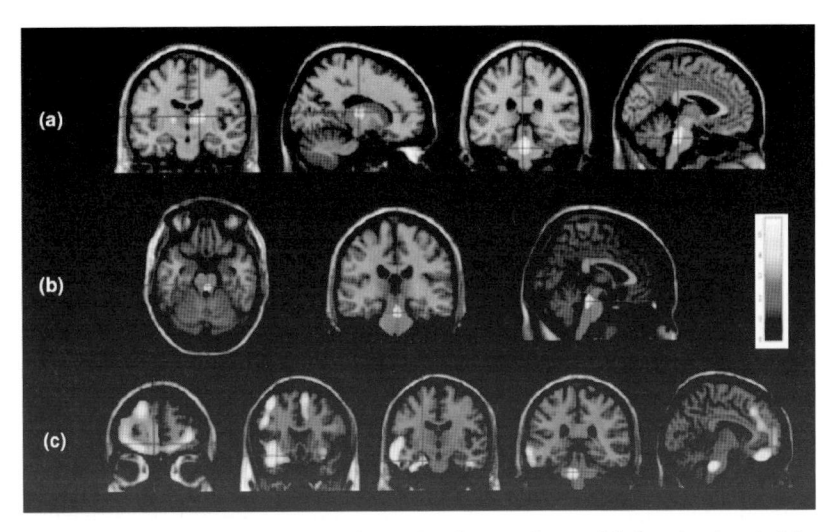

Figure 3.3 Brain regions showing significant rCBF changes after modafinil or placebo administration in healthy volunteers. (a) *On modafinil vs. Off modafinil*: Modafinil increased rCBF in bilateral thalami and in mid- and dorsal pons of the brainstem on T1 template overlaid MR coronal and sagittal images. (b) *On placebo vs. Off placebo*: Placebo increased rCBF in smaller regions in the mid- and dorsal pons of the brainstem on axial, coronal and sagittal images. (c) *On modafinil vs. On placebo:* Modafinil increased rCBF in bilateral orbitofrontal cortices, left dorsolateral prefrontal cortex (first imaging session from left side), left superior/middle frontal gyri, bilateral anterior insular gyri (second imaging session), left lateral and basal temporal areas (third imaging session), and in left anterior cingulate cortex, left mid- and dorsal pons of the brainstem (fourth and fifth imaging sessions in right side). Left to right panel order represents coronal images of the brain taken in the anterior to posterior direction. Left sides of images represent brain left sides. (a)–(c) were all significant at the uncorrected $P < 0.001$. (c) was also significant at FDR corrected $P < 0.05$. (See color plate section).

narcoleptic patients during baseline wake states, REM sleep and periods of cataplexy. They found activation of an amygdalo-cortico-basal ganglia brainstem circuit in cataplexy.

Narcolepsy pharmacotherapy and neuroimaging

Neuroimaging studies related to pharmacotherapy of narcolepsy may reveal insights into the neurobiology of "sleepiness".

A variety of compounds have been discovered with mechanisms of action that may affect sleep/wake regulation and that may play some role in the pathophysiology or treatment of narcolepsy and sleepiness. Testing in preclinical models suggest that these compounds may have novel mechanisms of action; however, the degree to which these mechanisms will translate into a clinical application are often unknown. Functional neuroimaging studies may identify the degree to which these compounds have beneficial mechanisms of action on brain structures that are known to regulate sleepiness in humans. One way of achieving this goal is to administer the compound to human subjects, then assess a functional neuroanatomic response to the compound and levels of sleepiness in humans, such as a blood flow or metabolic response. Further, these studies may help to determine the optimum dose of the compound in humans that maximizes beneficial effects of the compound, yet does not lead to adverse effects. The use of receptor ligands may clarify whether one compound has a unique mechanism of action on a specific receptor subtype that may not be shared by other compounds in its class and may therefore hold a therapeutic advantage over other agents. Finally, once a compound has been identified and shown to have effects in the CNS in humans, functional neuroimaging studies can then be used to determine the degree to which the compound reverses distinct alterations in neural function in a clinical population. The review below reveals some of the early studies in these areas of relevance to narcolepsy and sleepiness.

Receptor ligand studies

Cholinergic receptor density and distributions have been studied in narcolepsy and sleep-related movement disorders. Sudo *et al*. [30] assessed muscarinic cholinergic receptors in narcoleptic subjects using [^{11}C]NMPB both before and after pharmacotherapy. No differences were observed between patients and healthy subjects at baseline and minimal treatment effects were observed. Modafinil has been shown clinically to improve daytime sleepiness in patients with narcolepsy. Neuroimaging studies could be useful in clarifying the brain mechanisms of this agent in reversing the biology of sleepiness and possibly in the sleep attacks associated with narcolepsy. Joo et al. [36] assessed cerebral blood flow in healthy volunteers using SPECT before and after modafinil administration, a wake-promoting agent. They found increases in blood flow in bilateral thalami, dorsal pons, bilateral frontopolar, orbitofrontal, superior frontal, middle frontal gyri, short insular gyri, left cingulated gyrus, left middle/inferior temporal gyri, left parahippocampal gyrus and left pons consistent with the effects of this medication on arousal, emotion and executive function networks in the brain. Joo et al. [37] assessed the effects of modafinil on regional cerebral blood flow (rCBF) using SPECT in 43 narcoleptic patients. They found increased rCBF in the right dorsolateral and bilateral medial prefrontal cortices. Conversely, after modafinil administration, rCBF was decreased in bilateral precentral gyri, left hippocampus, left fusiform gyrus, bilateral lingual gyri, and cerebellum. There was no significant rCBF change after placebo administration.

They concluded that by a chronic administration of modafinil in narcoleptic patients, rCBF increased in the bilateral prefrontal cortices, whereas it decreased in left mesio/basal, temporal, bilateral occipital areas, and cerebellum. By extension, "sleepiness" could be inferred to result from alterations in these arousal networks that are affected by modafinil therapy.

Summary

Functional neuroimaging studies support a role for sleep in restoration/rejuvenation/growth in broad thalamocortical neural networks that play important roles in waking executive function, attention, concentration, working memory, and emotion regulation. Sleep deprivation studies show that there are reductions in metabolic activity in these regions during waking periods following sleep deprivation and these reductions are associated with the cognitive deficits and subjective experience of "sleepiness" experienced by these subjects. Pharmaceutical agents that produce alertness have been shown to increase activity in arousal networks that maintain generalized thalamocortical activity, reversing sleepiness associated with pathological conditions. "Sleepiness" therefore appears intimately related to a loss of function in diffuse thalamocortical networks.

Acknowledgments

Support for this work was provided by AG-020677; MH66227, MH61566, MH24652; and RR00056.

References

1. **Maquet P, Dive D, Salmon E**, et al. Cerebral glucose utilization during sleep–wake cycle in man determined by positron emission tomography and [^{18}F]2-fluoro-2-deoxy-d-glucose method. *Brain Res* 1990; **513**:136–43.

2. **Madsen P L, Holm S, Vorstrup S**, et al. Human regional cerebral blood flow during rapid-eye-movement sleep. *J Cereb Blood Flow Metab* 1991; **11**:502–07.

3. **Maquet P, Peters J, Aerts J**, et al. Functional neuroanatomy of human rapid-eye-movement sleep and dreaming. *Nature* 1996; **383**:163–66.

4. **Meyer J S, Hayman L A, Amano T**, et al. Mapping local blood flow of human brain by CT scanning during stable xenon inhalation. *Stroke* 1981; **12**:426–36.

5. **Heiss W D, Pawlik G, Herholz K**, et al. Regional cerebral glucose metabolism in man during wakefulness, sleep, and dreaming. *Brain Res* 1985; **327**:362–66.

6. **Buchsbaum M S, Gillin J C, Wu J**, et al. Regional cerebral glucose metabolic rate in human sleep assessed by positron emission tomography. *Life Sci* 1989; **45**:1349–56.

7. **Maquet P, Dive D, Salmon E**, et al. Cerebral glucose utilization during stage 2 sleep in man. *Brain Res* 1992; **571**:149–53.

8. **Hofle N, Paus T, Reutens D**, et al. Regional cerebral blood flow changes as a function of delta and spindle activity during slow wave sleep in humans. *J Neurosci* 1997; **17**:4800–08.

9. **Braun A R, Balkin T J, Wesenten N J**, et al. Regional cerebral blood flow throughout the sleep–wake cycle. An H$_2$(^{15})O PET study. *Brain* 1997; **120**:1173–97.

10. **Maquet P**. Positron emission tomography studies of sleep and sleep disorders. *J Neurol* 1997; **244**(Suppl 1):S23–28.

11. **Maquet P, Phillips C**. Functional brain imaging of human sleep. *J Sleep Res* 1998; **7**(Suppl 1):42–47.

12. **Maquet P**. Brain mechanisms of sleep: contribution of neuroimaging techniques. *J Psychopharmacol* 1999; **13**(Suppl 1):S25–28.

13. **Maquet P**. Functional neuroimaging of normal human sleep by positron emission tomography. *J Sleep Res* 2000; **9**:207–31.

14. **Nofzinger E A, Mintun M A, Wiseman M B**, et al. Forebrain activation in REM sleep: An FDG PET study. *Brain Res* 1997; **770**: 192–201.

15. **Nofzinger E A, Mintun M A, Price J**, et al. A method for the assessment of the functional neuroanatomy of human sleep using FDG PET. *Brain Res Prot* 1998; **2**:191–98.

16. **Nofzinger E A, Buysse D J, Miewald J M**, et al. Human regional cerebral glucose metabolism during non-rapid eye movement sleep in relation to waking. *Brain* 2002; **125**:1105–15.

17. **Kjaer T W, Law I, Wiltschiotz G**, et al. Regional cerebral blood flow during light sleep – a $H_2^{15}O$-PET study. *Sleep Res* 2002; **11**:201–07.

18. **Wu J C, Gillin J C, Buchsbaum M S**, et al. The effect of sleep deprivation on cerebral glucose metabolic rate in normal humans assessed with positron emission tomography. *Sleep* 1991; **14**:155–62.

19. **Thomas M, Sing H, Belenky G**, et al. Neural basis of alertness and cognitive performance impairments during sleepiness. I. Effects of 24 h of sleep deprivation on waking human regional brain activity. *J Sleep Res* 2000; **9**:335–52.

20. **Thomas M L, Sing H C, Belenky G**, et al. Neural basis of alertness and cognitive performance impairments during sleepiness II. Effects of 48 and 72 h of sleep deprivation on waking human regional brain activity. *Thalamus Rel Syst* 2003; **2**:199–229.

21. **Mu Q, Nahas Z, Johnson K A**, et al. Decreased cortical response to verbal working memory following sleep deprivation. *Sleep* 2005; **28**:55–67.

22. **Mu Q, Mishory A, Johnson K A**, et al. Decreased brain activation during a working memory task at rested baseline is associated with vulnerability to sleep deprivation. *Sleep* 2005; **28**:433–46.

23. **Drummond S P, Brown G G, Salamat J S**, et al. Increasing task difficulty facilitates the cerebral compensatory response to total sleep deprivation. *Sleep* 2004; **27**:445–51.

24. **Chee M W, Choo W C**. Functional imaging of working memory after 24 hr of total sleep deprivation. *J Neurosci* 2004; **24**:4560–67.

25. **Lin L, Faraco J, Li R**, et al. The sleep disorder canine narcolepsy is caused by a mutation in the hypocretin (orexin) receptor 2 gene. *Cell* 1999; **98**:365–76.

26. **Chemelli R M, Willie J T, Sinton C M**, et al. Narcolepsy in orexin knockout mice: molecular genetics of sleep regulation. *Cell* 1999; **98**:437–51.

27. **Nishino S, Ripley B, Overeem S**, et al. Hypocretin (orexin) deficiency in human narcolepsy. *Lancet* 2000; **355**:39–40.

28. **Hublin C, Launes J, Nikkinen P**, et al. Dopamine D2-receptors in human narcolepsy: a SPECT study with ^{123}I-IBZM. *Acta Neurol Scand* 1994; **90**:186–89.

29. **Asenbaum S, Zeithofer J, Saletu B**, et al. Technetium-99m-HMPAO SPECT imaging of cerebral blood flow during REM sleep in narcoleptics. *J Nucl Med* 1995; **36**:1150–55.

30. **Sudo Y, Suhara T, Honda Y**, et al. Muscarinic cholinergic receptors in human narcolepsy: a PET study. *Neurology* 1998; **51**:1297–302.

31. **Joo E Y, Tae W S, Kim J H**, et al. Glucose hypometabolism of hypothalamus and thalamus in narcolepsy. *Ann Neurol* 2004; **56**:437–40.

32. **Joo J H, Solano F X, Mulsant B H**, et al. Predictors of adequacy of depression management in the primary care setting. *Psychiatr Serv* 2005; **56**:1524–28.

33. **Brenneis C, Brandauer E, Frauscher B**, et al. Voxel-based morphometry in narcolepsy. *Sleep Med* 2005; **6**:531–36.

34. **Eisensehr I, Linke R, Tatsch K**, et al. Alteration of the striatal dopaminergic system in human narcolepsy. *Neurology* 2003; **60**:1817–19.

35. **Hong S B, Tae W S, Joo E Y**. Cerebral perfusion changes during cataplexy in narcolepsy patients. *Neurology* 2006; **66**:1747–49.

36. **Joo E Y, Tae W S, Jung K Y**, et al. Cerebral blood flow changes in man by wake-promoting drug, modafinil: a randomized double blind study. *J Sleep Res* 2008; **17**:82–88.

37. **Joo E Y, Seo D W, Tae W S**, et al. Effect of modafinil on cerebral blood flow in narcolepsy patients. *Sleep* 2008; **31**:868–73.

Section 1 Chapter 4

Introduction

Clinical evaluation of the patient with excessive sleepiness

Imran M. Ahmed and Michael J. Thorpy

Introduction

Sleepiness is defined as a physiologic drive toward sleep. It is a normal process that can occur briefly upon awaking after the major sleep period, after prolonged sustained wakefulness, or when awoken from the middle of one's natural sleep period. The term is often used interchangeably with the words "somnolence" or "drowsiness". Frequently, patients who complain of sleepiness do not use the word "sleepiness" to describe their symptoms, but use vague terms such as tired, fatigue, no energy, or other similar terminology. As it may affect diagnosis and treatment, the physician should differentiate between fatigue and true sleepiness. Fatigue is a feeling of tiredness that may be both physical and psychological, and it typically occurs in conditions such as depression or multiple sclerosis. Pure fatigue is not associated with significant daytime sleepiness, as there is no physiological drive for sleep, so on lying down sleep does not occur, but instead wakefulness and rest ensues [1–3]. People may describe themselves being "tired", "fatigued" or perhaps as "not having enough energy" after a period of physical activity; but sleep does not occur, i.e. the individual would not be sleepy. In a study of 190 obstructive sleep apnea (OSA) patients, only about 47% used the term "sleepiness" to describe their symptoms, while about 62% described themselves as having a "lack of energy", 61% reported feelings of "tiredness", and 57% used the term "fatigue". When these patients were asked to select the most prominent symptom, only about 22% chose "sleepiness" and most (about 40%) chose "lack of energy" [4].

Sleepiness is considered "excessive" when there is an increased quantity of sleep or an increased propensity towards sleep during waking hours making a person unable to remain awake or alert in situations where it is required. It often results in impairment of academic or occupational performance, and can cause social disturbances of mood and/or social adjustment [5]. Patients who have excessive sleepiness tend to have involuntary sleep episodes that occur during activities such as when relaxing in front of the television, when sitting quietly reading, while in a lecture, or at social events when the lights are dimmed. The sleep episodes when severe enough may also occur while the individual is eating, having a conversation, or driving. Driving while sleepy is an especially important topic and is discussed in another chapter of this book.

The term "hypersomnia" is often used synonymously with "excessive sleepiness"; however, it should be reserved to identify disorders that are associated with excessive sleepiness, such as idiopathic hypersomnia (IHS). There are many sleep disorders or sleep variants listed in the International Classification of Sleep Disorders, 2nd edition (ICSD-2) that clinically manifest as excessive sleepiness (Table 4.1). These disorders, which can be identified in each of the eight ICSD-2 classification groups, have a common feature in that they either shorten or fragment the major sleep period, or are a manifestation of central nervous system (CNS) dysfunction. In a relatively small study by Stepanski *et al.*, 4 groups of subjects, 15 with OSA, 15 with periodic limb movement disorder, 15 with insomnia, and 10 healthy volunteers with no sleep complaints were evaluated with polysomnograms and multiple sleep latency tests (MSLT). It was demonstrated that the total number of arousals correlated significantly with the severity of sleepiness [6]. In 2007, a rodent model duplicating the frequent arousals seen in severe sleep apnea patients also confirmed that sleep fragmentation seen in many sleep disorders are at least partially responsible for the symptom of excessive daytime sleepiness [7]. A large clinical study by Oksenberg

---

Sleepiness: Causes, Consequences and Treatment, ed. Michael J. Thorpy and Michel Billiard. Published by Cambridge University Press. © Cambridge University Press 2011.

4. Clinical evaluation

Table 4.1 Common differential diagnosis of excessive daytime somnolence

1. Behaviorally induced insufficient sleep syndrome (sleep deprivation)
2. Sleep-related breathing disorders, e.g. obstructive sleep apnea
3. Circadian rhythm disorders, e.g. delayed sleep phase type or advanced sleep phase type
4. Hypersomnia due to medical or psychiatric disorder or drug or substance
5. Narcolepsy with/without cataplexy
6. Idiopathic hypersomnia
7. Recurrent hypersomnia
8. Long sleeper
9. Environmental sleep disorder
10. Periodic limb movement disorder

Table 4.2 Medical and psychiatric disorders that can cause a complaint of excessive sleepiness

Congestive heart failure
Bronchial asthma
Kyphoscoliosis (neuromuscular disease, spondylitis, Marfan syndrome)
Endocrine abnormalities (e.g. excessive GH, hypothyroidism, diabetes mellitus)
Chronic renal insufficiency
Brain tumors
Strokes
Head trauma
Seizures, including subclinical seizures
Hereditary hemorrhagic telangiectasis
Infectious diseases (e.g. HIV, CNS lyme disease, trypanosomiasis)
Encephalopathies
Fibromyalgia
Chronic fatigue syndrome
Schizophrenia
Mood (depressive) disorders
Seasonal affective disorder
Conversion disorder
Factitious disorder
Somatoform disorder
Malingering

et al. comparing sleepy OSA patients with non-sleepy OSA patients also found a direct correlation with sleep fragmentation and excessive sleepiness [8]. Some disorders such as narcolepsy (with or without cataplexy), IHS, recurrent hypersomnia or long sleeper are associated with excessive sleepiness as a result of a suspected CNS abnormality [9–12]. Other disorders result in excessive sleepiness because the total sleep time is shortened, e.g. behaviorally induced insufficient sleep syndrome causes excessive sleepiness in individuals who get less than their biologically determined sleep requirement. Circadian rhythm sleep disorders, e.g. advanced sleep phase type and delayed sleep phase type, may manifest as sleepiness during the evening hours or morning hours, respectively. If a patient with a circadian rhythm disorder is awake when the body physiologically is trying to go to sleep, then the sleep drive will interfere with social or occupational functioning, and under these circumstances the resulting sleepiness can also be considered excessive. Drugs, alcohol, substances of abuse, certain medical, neurologic, and psychiatric disorders can cause excessive sleepiness either by fragmenting the major sleep period or by interfering with CNS sleep–wake mechanisms (Table 4.2).

The numerous causes of excessive sleepiness can become overwhelming to the general medical practitioner; accordingly, a systematic approach, which should include a careful sleep history taken from the patient and the patient's bed partner or caregiver, is necessary. Information about any comorbid illnesses, past medical history, psychosocial history, family history, physical examination and appropriate laboratory studies are valuable when forming a differential diagnosis. This chapter details the important elements in the clinical evaluation of patients with excessive sleepiness.

Epidemiology

About 65% of people have some type of sleep disturbance a few nights every month; 14% of the population surveyed have excessive daytime sleepiness at least a few days a week (2008 Sleep in America Poll, National Sleep Foundation, 1000 people surveyed). The demographics of the specific causes of excessive sleepiness will be discussed in detail in another chapter of this book (see Chapter 1). Briefly, although the exact statistics are not known, it is likely that behaviorally induced insufficient sleep syndrome is the most common cause of the daytime sleepiness occurring in up to 44% of the people surveyed (2008 Sleep in America Poll, National Sleep Foundation, 1000 people surveyed).

Table 4.3 Assessment of the patient with excessive sleepiness

Clinical interview
    Direct observation
    Frequency, nature, and impact of the sleepiness
    Perspective of spouse, family member, bed partner
    Thorough medical, psychiatric, family and psychosocial history

Questionnaires
    Epworth Sleepiness Scale (ESS)
    Karolinska Sleepiness Scale (KSS)
    Visual Analogue Scale of Sleepiness

Physical exam

Sleep studies
    Polysomnography (PSG)
    Multiple Sleep Latency Test (MSLT)
    Maintenance of Wakefulness Test (MWT)

Additional studies
    Blood tests (chemistry, endocrine, immune, etc.)
    Fiber-optic endoscopy
    Cephalometric X-rays
    Neuroimaging
    Electromyograms (EMG) and nerve conduction velocity (NCV) studies
    Electroencephalograms (EEG)

Table 4.4 Key inquiries in the evaluation of excessive sleepiness

Does the sleepiness occur only when the patient is in a quiet or monotonous situation or also when the patient is active?

Does the sleepiness occur during situations that would compromise the patient's or others' safety?

What is the patient's sleep–wake schedule?
    What time do they go to bed and get up on weekdays and weekends?

Inquire about other associated sleep features and other questions that may identify the cause of sleepiness
    Does the patient have discomfort in or jerking of the legs at night?
    Does the patient snore, gasp, choke, or stop breathing during sleep?
    Does the patient have cataplexy?

Determine if the patient is truly sleepy or just fatigued

What is happening during the night (e.g. causes of sleep fragmentation, such as periodic limb movements, etc.) and the following morning (e.g. awaking with a morning headache)?

Does the patient feel rested after a night's sleep?

Does the patient take naps?

What medications is the patient taking?

OSA is also a common cause of excessive sleepiness, occurring in 4% of men and 2% of women [13, 14]. Narcolepsy with cataplexy has a prevalence of 0.18–0.2% [9, 12, 15]. IHS is believed to be less common than narcolepsy, and recurrent hypersomnia may even be rarer, with only about 200 cases reported in the literature [9, 15].

Evaluation of the patient

The clinical evaluation of the patient with sleepiness involves clearly determining the patient's primary complaint, a careful sleep history followed by a medical, psychiatric, psychosocial and family history, physical examination, completion of appropriate sleep questionnaires, formulation of a differential diagnosis, and consideration of sleep studies and other medical tests (Table 4.3).

History

Chief complaint

Assessment begins with a careful and detailed evaluation of the presenting sleep complaint associated with excessive sleepiness (Table 4.4). As mentioned earlier, excessive sleepiness may manifest as symptoms other than sleepiness, and patients may report feeling tired, fatigued, and irritable or have other mood changes. In addition, patients may find that they are unable to carry out their usual daily activities involving housework or their occupation without a great increase in effort. In a questionnaire survey of 180 patients with narcolepsy and 180 matched controls, excessive sleepiness was at least partially to blame for statistically significant deleterious effects upon occupational performance, promotion, earning capacity, fear of or actual job loss, and increased disability insurance. Work or home accidents attributed to sleepiness or sleep (49%) were much more common in patients. There were also deleterious effects on education, recreation and personality related to disease [16]. Sleepiness can also manifest as difficulty with memory, concentration and attention, and can cause headaches or an abnormal feeling of fuzziness or grogginess that can occur throughout the day. There may be a depressive quality about these features, although the patient may or may not be significantly depressed [15].

Sometimes patients with significant sleepiness are not aware that they are sleepy; this typically occurs in disorders such as Parkinson's Disease (PD) [17]. The PD patient either may deny sleepiness, because of a lack of awareness of full alertness, or because they are unaware of episodes of falling asleep, and therefore a history from a bed partner or caretaker can be very helpful for collaborating or refuting the patient's statements on sleepiness.

Characterizing the excessive sleepiness

With the complaint in mind, a thorough history should be taken, including information on characterizing the sleepiness, assessing the patient's functional and psychological status, and differentiating between the various sleep disorders.

Does the sleepiness occur only when the patient is sedentary or when active? In order to determine the severity of sleepiness, the physician should determine whether the patient will tend to fall asleep easily, not only when in a sedentary activity such as watching television, using a computer or when reading, but also when they are active, such as while at work, during parties/other social gatherings or during sexual activity. A patient may deny sleepiness because it does not occur when active, yet the patient can fall asleep easily when sedentary. The American Academy of Sleep Medicine differentiated the severity of sleepiness into three categories: mild, moderate, and severe. Mild sleepiness included unwanted episodes of sleep that occurred during activities that required little attention, e.g. watching television. Moderate sleepiness was defined as having sleep episodes that involuntarily occurred during activities that required some attention, e.g. while sitting at a meeting. Severe sleepiness involves involuntary sleep episodes that occur during situations that require active attention, e.g. driving [18].

Does the sleepiness occur during situations that would compromise the patient's or others' safety, e.g. when driving? Of great importance is sleepiness while driving. The patient may report a tendency to doze off when waiting at red traffic lights or when in stop-and-go traffic, and as a consequence accidents occur. The accident may simply be the sleepy patient's car nudging the vehicle in front when the foot slips off the brake, usually not producing any significant motor vehicle damage, but the patient will arouse and become aware that it was caused by sleepiness. The accidents can, of course, be more severe and cause deaths as a result of falling asleep while traveling at higher speeds. The occurrence of sleepiness while driving is a medical emergency and all patients need to be thoroughly evaluated to determine the cause, and appropriate treatment should be instituted.

What is happening during the night and the following morning? Information on nocturnal sleep behavior is essential, such as whether the patient is restless, how frequently they have to get up to go to the bathroom at night, whether there is excessive sweating, whether there is abnormal movement activity or vocalization during sleep, or if they snore or have other abnormal breathing events. The sleep position may be helpful, as sleeping on the back can be associated with more severe apnea, and varied sleep positions are common in patients who have sleep apnea or insomnia. Whether the patient is rested, tired, fatigued or groggy upon awakening, and whether headaches occur on awakening may be indicative of poor sleep quality.

What is the sleep–wake schedule? The patient's bedtime, time to fall asleep, duration in bed and time of awakening help to determine circadian rhythm sleep disorders and determine sleep need. A person with delayed sleep phase type may complain of sleepiness when awoken in the morning (when awakening prior to completion of his habitual sleep period). A person with advanced sleep phase type, on the other hand, may complain of sleepiness towards the evening hours. A two-week assessment of the patient's bedtime and wake up time is useful to help identify these disorders. Furthermore, if a person is getting less sleep than the biologically determined sleep requirement, sleepiness will occur. The average adult needs about 7.5–8 h of sleep per 24-h period, regardless of environmental or cultural differences. In a large questionnaire study of 17 465 university students (90% of which responded to the survey), 63% reported sleeping an average of 7–8 h, 6% indicated sleeping less than 6 h, 15% reported an average of 6–7 h of sleep and 10% slept between 8 and 10 h, and 6% indicated sleeping for over 10 h a day [19].

Inquiries about other associated sleep features. Narcolepsy features, such as cataplexy, sleep paralysis and hypnagogic hallucinations will help determine whether narcolepsy is present [20]. The presence of snoring, gasping, choking or difficulty breathing at night may indicate OSA. Pain and discomfort or jerking of the legs in bed may suggest restless legs syndrome or periodic limb movement disorder.

Determine if the patient is truly sleepy. The distinction between fatigue and sleepiness is important, because if sleepiness is present the focus will be on sleep at night and specific sleep disorders, whereas if the primary complaint is one of fatigue without sleepiness the focus will be on an underlying medical or psychological problem.

However, some patients will have both fatigue and sleepiness as is often seen in patients with multiple sclerosis or depression who present with fatigue but also can suffer from sleep disorders such as OSA [14]. Patients with PD are often very sleepy during the daytime, but even when the sleepiness is relieved there can be fatigue that is not responsive to usual management of the sleep disorder [21].

Primary sleep disorders

When a patient presents with excessive daytime sleepiness, the differential diagnoses of the primary sleep disorders need to be considered. Daytime sleepiness could result if: (1) there were insufficient time allowed for sleep, (2) sleep occurs at a biologically appropriate time but not a socially appropriate time, (3) the nocturnal sleep is disrupted, (4) there is an organic or neurochemical dysfunction of the brain, (5) a medical or psychiatric disorder is present, or (6) as a result of a drug or other substance. In most cases, the likely diagnosis can be identified by the patient's history.

Sleep disorders such as insufficient sleep syndrome, narcolepsy, IHS, recurrent hypersomnia, and sleep-related breathing disorders need to be considered.

A history of excessive sleepiness with episodes of muscle weakness that occur in association with emotional stress (cataplexy) suggests narcolepsy with cataplexy until proven otherwise (see Chapter 11). Other features supportive of this diagnosis include sleep paralysis, hypnagogic hallucinations, and automatic behaviors. A diagnosis of narcolepsy without cataplexy is suggested when the aforementioned REM sleep phenomena (i.e. hypnagogic hallucinations and sleep paralysis) and REM sleep features on polysomnography occur in the absence of cataplexy. Secondary narcolepsy would be considered in patients with narcolepsy features and the presence of a neurological disorder that affects CNS function.

A history of excessive sleepiness (without REM features) that is present almost daily for at least 3 months suggests a diagnosis of IHS, if other causes of hypersomnia are ruled out by polysomnography (see Chapter 12). Although the history identifies the likely cause of excessive daytime sleepiness in most cases of narcolepsy or IHS, objective studies including a polysomnogram with or without an MSLT may be necessary to confirm the diagnosis or assess its severity [15].

A history of recurrent episodes of sleepiness lasting from 2 days to 4 weeks, occurring at least once a year, and normal alertness and cognition in between attacks is suggestive of a recurrent hypersomnia including Kleine–Levin syndrome and its variants or menstrual-related sleep disorder (see Chapters 13 and 14).

Symptoms of a sleep-related breathing disorder, e.g. OSA, should be identifiable on history by the presence of snoring, episodes of choking or gasping for air, witnessed apneic events, or if the person is a mouth breather (see Chapter 15). Understanding how the snoring affects the patient's bed partner is also important, as often patients who have very loud snoring will have moved out of the bedroom so as to prevent the snoring from disturbing the bed partner. Occasionally, it is the bed partner who moves out of the bedroom. The variation and the quality of the snoring are often essential in determining whether sleep apnea is present, as quiet episodes alternating with loud episodes of snoring will often indicate apnea [22]. Romero et al. reported that the symptom of snoring can identify sleep apnea in patients with a sensitivity, specificity, positive predictive value and negative predictive value of 82.6, 43.0, 84.7, and 39.6%, respectively [23]. The patient may not report episodes of apnea or gasping or choking; however, the bed partner may observe these events; thus, interviewing the bed partner about the patient's sleep behaviors is often helpful.

As a patient's weight greatly influences sleep apnea, historical information should be taken on the height and the weight of the patient, and the weight change over the previous 5 years, as well as any attempts of weight reduction [24].

Although not a common cause of excessive sleepiness, restless legs syndrome and periodic limb movement disorder should be included in the differential diagnosis (see Chapter 22).

Medical history

A detailed medical history should follow the sleep history, and should include the identification of cardiovascular and nasopharyngeal problems. A cardiac history should include determination of whether there is any evidence of heart failure, ischemic heart disease, hypertension, and leg edema. Cerebrovascular disease is also notable, as there is an increased prevalence of sleep apnea in patients with stroke [25, 26]. Metabolic disorders, such as thyroid disease or diabetes, can manifest as excessive sleepiness or disrupt nocturnal sleep [27–31]. Nocturnal pain syndromes including arthritis and peripheral neuropathy can disrupt nocturnal sleep and subsequently result in daytime fatigue and/or sleepiness [32, 33].

Patients who have chronic upper airway obstruction tend to be mouth breathers and inquiry as to whether they are an obligatory mouth breather may be helpful. It is also prudent to identify any history of rhinitis, nasal congestion, postnasal drip, sinus problems, prior tonsillar or adenoidal surgery or previous visits to see an otolaryngologist as this can suggest a etiology for a disrupted night's sleep.

Most prescription medications can either adversely affect sleep at night and/or cause impaired alertness during the daytime [34].

Psychiatric assessment

Sleepiness can occur as part of many psychiatric disorders; it can be due to the psychiatric disorder itself, due to a comorbid sleep disorder, or a consequence of psychopharmacotherapy (see Chapter 25). Accordingly, in any disorder of excessive sleepiness it is prudent to inquire about comorbid or prior history of psychiatric disorders, such as mood disorders, anxiety disorders, and psychotic disorders.

Mood disorders, such as major depressive disorder, dysthymic disorder, and bipolar disorder, can clinically manifest with excessive daytime sleepiness. Sleep disturbances in atypical depression (representing about 15–20% of cases) and some bipolar depression patients include excessive daytime sleepiness and/or prolonged nocturnal sleep [15, 35–37]. It is suggested that the excessive sleepiness noted in some of these depressed patients is related to other symptoms of anergic depression (e.g. lack of interest, withdrawal, decreased energy, or psychomotor retardation), rather than an increase in true sleep propensity [38]. Others speculate that the sleepiness may be a non-specific homeostatic coping response to the depressive disorder [39]. In anxiety disorders, on the other hand, excessive sleepiness is often secondary to disrupted nocturnal sleep [40], e.g. excessive sleepiness can occur in a patient having frequent nocturnal panic attacks. In psychotic disorders, such as schizophrenia, excessive daytime sleepiness is often reported clinically; however, it is usually not systematically assessed [41]. Excessive sleepiness in psychiatric disorders can also be due to a comorbid sleep disorder; some studies suggest that sleep disorders are more prevalent in psychiatric disorders, e.g. Hattori *et al.* documents a OSA prevalence of 59.4% in mood disorder patients [42].

Conversion disorders can also manifest as excessive sleepiness. A case of pseudo-narcolepsy was described by Hicks and Shapiro, where clinical and polysomnographic features of narcolepsy disappeared after disclosure of severe psychological stress [43]. In addition, as with any medical disorder, the clinician must remain vigilant for the possibility of factitious disorders or malingering [44, 45]; therefore, careful questioning about the patient's psychosocial circumstances is important. A request for stimulant medication in a patient who reports excessive sleepiness may be a manifestation of drug-seeking behavior.

As mentioned earlier, certain medications can result in excessive sleepiness, which is especially true for many medications used to manage psychiatric disorders. Certain serotonin reuptake inhibitors, tricyclic antidepressants, anti-anxiety and antipsychotics medications can result in excessive sleepiness [34].

Family/social history

The social history should be elicited, particularly relationships with other family members, and including determination of any financial, personal or social stresses that may contribute to sleep disturbance. A history that focuses on use of drugs and alcohol and the level of physical activity should be determined. Some sleep disorders including sleep apnea syndrome, narcolepsy, recurrent hypersomnia as well as restless legs syndrome, have a familial tendency [15].

Sleep questionnaires and sleep logs

Sleep questionnaires can be very helpful to rapidly collect extensive information regarding sleepiness severity and sleep–wake habits (see Chapter 6). The Epworth Sleepiness Scale is a valuable questionnaire for assessing the presence and severity of daytime sleepiness over a two-week period [46](Table 4.5). The patient scores the chance of dozing in eight typical everyday situations on a rating scale of 0 to 3 leading to a maximum score of 24. Patients with a score of 10 or higher should be considered to have abnormal daytime sleepiness, and those over 15 have severe daytime sleepiness. A visual analogue scale rating sleepiness on a line from 0 to 10 can be a simple but effective way of determining severity of sleepiness from "Fully Alert" to "Severely Sleepy" (Figure 4.1). Both scales can be useful for assessing sleepiness over time and to determine response to treatment.

Other sleep questionnaires such as the Pittsburgh Sleep Quality Index, the Stanford Sleepiness Scale, the Ullanalina Narcolepsy Scale, or the Karolinska Sleepiness Scale may be useful in some patients (Table 4.6).

Table 4.5 Epworth Sleepiness Scale

Indicate your chance of falling asleep under the following situations:

0 = no chance of dozing	1 = slight chance of dozing
2 = moderate chance of dozing	3 = high chance of dozing
Situation	Chance of dozing
1. Sitting and reading	_____
2. Watching television	_____
3. Sitting inactive in a public place (e.g. a theater or meeting)	_____
4. As a passenger in a car for an hour without a break	_____
5. Lying down to rest in the afternoon when circumstances permit	_____
6. Sitting and talking to someone	_____
7. Sitting quietly after a lunch without alcohol	_____
8. In a car, while stopped for a few minutes in traffic	_____

Abnormal >10, Severe Sleepiness >15

Table 4.7 Clinical evaluation of the patient with sleep disorders

Examination of head, eyes, ears, nose, throat (HEENT)

Features consistent with sleep-related breathing disorders:
  Crowded oropharynx: assess tonsils, soft palate, uvula, tongue
  Retrognathic or micrognathic, small maxilla, small oral space
  Chronic nasal congestion, enlarged turbinates, deviated nasal septum
  Enlarged thyroid
  Enlarged neck circumference (>17 inches in men and >16 inches in women >43 centimeters in men and >40 > centimeters in women)

Cardiovascular
  Hypertension
  Heart failure
  Ankle edema
  Distal pulses

Pulmonary
  Breathing pattern
  Auscultation of lungs

Neurologic
  Assess for CNS disease (e.g. Parkinson's disease, focal abnormalities due to CNS pathologies such as stroke or brain tumors)
  Assess for peripheral nerve disease (e.g. peripheral neuropathy, radiculopathy)

Table 4.6 Karolinska Sleepiness Scale

On a scale of 1 through 9, indicate how sleepy you are feeling:

1 = very alert
2
3 = Alert, normal level
4
5 = Neither alert nor sleepy
6
7 = Sleepy, but no effort to keep awake
8
9 = Very sleepy, great effort to keep awake, fighting sleep

A sleep log or diary that documents, over a period of approximately 2 weeks, the time of sleep onset, wake time and awakenings during the night as well as daytime naps, can help determine the circadian sleep pattern and the severity of the sleep difficulty. The sleep log can also help to quantify behavioral or other events that disrupt the major sleep period and that could contribute to the daytime sleepiness.

Physical exam

The physical examination ideally should be comprehensive and focus on respiratory, cardiovascular, gastrointestinal, endocrine and neurological evaluation (Table 4.7). However, the examination can be a focused examination if time does not allow a comprehensive physical, or if a full physical exam has recently been completed. The examination should always include determination of the patient's blood pressure and vital signs. Height and weight, Body Mass Index (BMI), and neck circumference should be obtained as well as a determination of the distribution of body fat (e.g. abdominal, neck, etc.) Thyroid size may prove relevant as thyroid enlargement can contribute to airway obstruction [47–51]. The upper airway evaluation should include determination of airway size, the presence and size of tonsillar tissue, tongue size, and the size and shape of the soft palate and uvula. If OSA is suspected, the patient should be referred to an otolaryngologist for endoscopic evaluation of the upper airway to determine the location and/or extent of obstruction present, particularly that in the posterior nasopharynx or oropharynx.

For the patient with restless legs syndrome (RLS), a neurological and vascular evaluation of the

Figure 4.1 Visual Analogue Scale of Sleepiness.

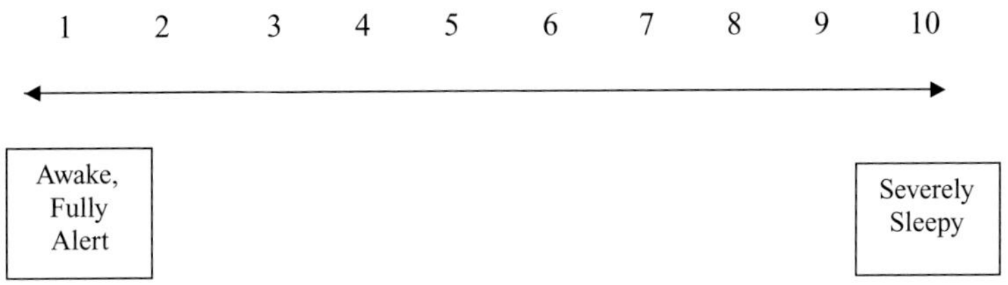

```
        1   2   3   4   5   6   7   8   9   10
            <----------------------------------->
            Awake,                    Severely
            Fully                      Sleepy
            Alert
```

circulation, motor and sensory function of the extremities may indicate a vascular problem, neuropathy, or a radiculopathy. Palpation of the distal pulses and an assessment of the presence of leg edema may suggest a vascular etiology for leg symptoms (e.g. vascular claudication) that is occasionally confused with RLS. Appropriate EMG and nerve conduction studies may be needed for further assessment of possible nerve lesions, while a lower-extremity ultrasound or other studies may be required to assess vascular disorders. A neurological examination is also important when evaluating narcolepsy, IHS, and REM sleep behavior disorder as focal abnormalities on exam may suggest an underlying neurologic disorder.

Laboratory investigations

Polysomnography

Objective evaluation of sleep involves polysomnographic monitoring, which is indicated in the evaluation of excessive sleepiness for most patients, unless insufficient sleep syndrome or a circadian rhythm sleep disorder is the suspected diagnosis. Patients with insomnia generally do not complain of excessive sleepiness (although fatigue is commonly reported) and, hence, a sleep study is not usually indicated [52] (see Chapter 16). The cause of the insomnia can often be determined from the history, and treatment can be initiated without the need for a sleep study evaluation. However, in some patients, particularly older patients, OSA or other disruptive nocturnal events may underlie the insomnia and therefore polysomnography may be necessary. These older patients may not initially complain of sleepiness, but a detailed history would usually elicit the presence of severe sleepiness. The severity of sleepiness, regardless of cause, can be assessed objectively with a multiple sleep latency test. It is clinically indicated in the evaluation of sleepiness especially when narcolepsy is suspected (discussed later in this chapter). It is performed immediately following overnight polysomnography with at least 6 h of sleep, but is not usually necessary when OSA is evident and considered the sole cause of the sleepiness.

In overnight polysomnography the patient typically is studied at the time and for the duration of the usual major sleep episode with measures of sleep, cardiac, respiratory parameters, and movement activity. Electrodes are applied to the head to record electroencephalogram (EEG), to the lower limbs and chin to record electromyogram (EMG), and near the eyes to record electrooculogram (EOG) activity. Additional leads and sensors measure ventilation via respiratory effort belts that respond to movements of the chest and abdomen, airflow and air pressure via sensors placed at the nose and mouth, oxygen saturation by means of an infrared oximeter, and a single lead of electrocardiography. Leg activity is also assessed by means of the EMG electrodes placed on the anterior tibialis muscle of each leg and the patient is videotaped throughout the recording for abnormal sleep behavior. Other measures such as end-tidal carbon dioxide concentration, or gastroesophageal pH, body position, or sounds of snoring can also be determined.

The polysomnographic information is typically stored in a digital form on a computer attached to a polysomnograph. The data can then be displayed on a computer screen for analysis. Typically, the recordings are performed and analyzed at a recording speed of 15 mm/s; however, this can be changed to 30 mm/s if abnormal epileptic activity is suspected [53].

The amount and percentage of each sleep stage is recorded as well as the degree of sleep fragmentation and the association with any abnormal sleep-related breathing events (i.e. apneas or hypopneas). Other causes of sleep fragmentation are also identified if possible, e.g. the presence of periodic limb movements or other abnormal disruptive movements/behaviors. The majority of all-night polysomnograms are utilized for the detection of OSA; therefore, an apnea/hypopnea index, which is the number of respiratory events per hour of sleep, is typically determined to assess severity of the sleep apnea. If OSA is detected, the patient may be required to return for a second night of polysomnography with nasal positive airway pressure

(PAP) to determine if it is an effective treatment modality.

Polysomnography is very useful for determining abnormal events that occur during specific sleep stages, such as sleep terrors that might arise out of slow-wave sleep, or periodic leg movements that typically occur during NREM sleep. Video monitoring along with EEG activity helps determine the clinical features of an abnormal event that occurs during sleep and help differentiate a parasomnia from an epileptic disorder [54].

Polysomnography also aids in the diagnosis of narcolepsy by documenting the absence of other causes of excessive sleepiness, such as sleep apnea, and is then followed by an MSLT, which if it demonstrates two or more sleep onset REM periods with a mean sleep latency of 8 min or less supports the diagnosis of narcolepsy. If other causes of sleepiness are identified on the polysomnogram, they need to be appropriately treated before a diagnosis of narcolepsy is confirmed.

Multiple Sleep Latency Test (MSLT)

An MSLT is performed during the main period of wakefulness to determine a patient's tendency to fall asleep and to confirm a diagnosis of narcolepsy [55] (also see Chapter 5). The MSLT consists of four or five brief nap opportunities at two-hourly intervals throughout the day, with the first nap occurring approximately 2 h after awakening in the morning and subsequent naps at two-hourly intervals. The patient is in a darkened room in sleepwear and asked to lie back, relax and to fall asleep if they would like to. Twenty minutes are allowed to achieve sleep and the average time to fall asleep across the four or five nap opportunities (mean sleep latency or MSL) and the stage of sleep that occurs are determined. Unfortunately, there is no large systematically gathered collection of normative MSLT data [56]; however, multiple studies have provided good approximations of normal values in certain populations. Levine et al. [57] and later Johns [58] collected and tabulated MSLT data from 176 normal sleepers and determined the MSL to be between 11.1 min (in subjects aged 18–29) and 12.5 min (in subjects aged 30–60) with an overall MSL of 11.5 ± 5.1 min. Other smaller studies calculated the MSL to be close to this value [59, 60]. Patients with severe sleepiness, on the other hand, fall asleep within a mean of 5 min (i.e. have an MSL of ≤5min) over the four or five nap opportunities and do not usually go into REM sleep [61]. Not uncommonly, one nap episode with REM sleep does occur in patients, but it is considered within the normal range; however, two or more naps with REM sleep is indicative of pathology [62–65]. If the patient has a normal amount and percentage of REM sleep at night and two or more sleep onset REM periods occur during the day, then this is highly suggestive of narcolepsy [65].

The MSLT is most useful in documenting sleepiness in a patient who might otherwise deny sleepiness, which is particularly useful in an older individual who may insist on driving a motor vehicle despite pleas to the contrary by family members who may have noticed severe daytime sleepiness. The objective measure of sleepiness may be helpful to illustrate to the patient that significant sleepiness is present or support family members requests that the patient not drive.

Maintenance of Wakefulness Test (MWT)

There is a variation of the MSLT called the Maintenance of Wakefulness Test (MWT) [66], which is performed in much the same way as the MSLT except that the patient is placed in a semi-reclining position in street clothes and asked to try to remain awake during four 40-min nap opportunities. The time from lights out to the onset of sleep (defined as three consecutive epochs of stage N1 sleep or any one epoch of stage N2, N3 or REM sleep) for each nap is recorded. There is even more limited data for MWT normative values than for the MSLT [67]. A total of 97.5% of the 64 normal subjects studied had a mean sleep latency of >8.0 min and 59% of normal subjects remained awake for the entire 40 min across each of four nap opportunities. Accordingly, a mean sleep latency < 8.0 min on the 40-min MWT is considered abnormal; values greater than this but less than 40 min are of uncertain significance [56, 68]. A patient's ability to remain awake is strongly supported by their ability to remain awake for the duration of each of the four nap opportunities (i.e. a MSL of 40 min) [56, 68].

The MWT is useful in determining the effects of treatment to relieve daytime sleepiness, or for determining the ability to be alert during employment [68]. For example, a patient who has been placed on alerting medications during the daytime, or a patient who has been treated by means of nasal CPAP, may undergo an MWT to demonstrate the ability to remain awake when desired. The test is also required annually by the Federal Aviation Administration (FAA) to determine fitness for work in pilots (www.faa.gov). Some employers require episodic MWT testing of OSA patients who are on CPAP to ensure daytime alertness.

Performance testing

The patient who is sleepy may be asked to complete various tests of performance, such as a psychomotor vigilance test (PVT), or other tests of cognitive ability. Although not typically used in clinical practice, research studies of sleepiness often employ these performance tests to assess the behavioral consequences of excessive sleepiness. The PVT measures patients' abilities to sustain attention by using the reaction time to successive stimuli to measure deficits in attention and performance [69]. In a study comparing two versions of the PVT on 21 patients, both versions demonstrated an increase in reaction time with increasing hours of wakefulness [70]. Cognitive assessment tests, e.g. mini mental status examination (MMSE) and the frontal assessment battery [71], are additional, quick and easy to administer tests that appraise patients' memory as well as executive functioning.

Oxford Sleepiness Resistance (OSLeR) Test

An alternative to the MWT is the Oxford Sleepiness Resistance (OSLeR) test that combines features of an MWT with the PVT [72]. The patient is seated in a dimly lit, quiet room for four 40-min sessions throughout the day. During the sessions, the patient is given a task for which reaction time is measured. More specifically, the subject is asked to press a switch in response to a light emitting diode (LED), which was lit for one second every three seconds. Both the switch and the light are connected to a computer that stores both the number of times the light was illuminated and whether a correct response was made. A failure to respond to three consecutive illuminations is suggestive of microsleep episodes (i.e. EEG sleep features of 3 s or less duration) and impaired attention, while a failure to respond to seven consecutive illuminations is indicative of sleep onset. The OSLER test was able to discriminate between normal subjects (average MSL of 39.8 min among 10 subjects) from patient with sleepiness due to OSA (average MSL 10.5 min among 10 patients) [73]; it is a reliable tool for the evaluation of a patient's ability to remain awake as well as vigilant, and is more convenient than the MWT as it does not require a polysomnograph.

Additional studies

Additional investigations may be required to assess any underlying disorders in patients with excessive sleepiness.

Blood and urine tests

The referring physician usually performs blood tests, particularly screening blood tests, prior to referral to the sleep specialist for evaluation of excessive sleepiness. Thyroid function tests in a patient with clinical features of hypothyroidism may confirm hypothyroidism as a cause of sleepiness. However, most patients with daytime sleepiness do not require routine thyroid testing, as the likelihood of a positive return is low [74]. Nevertheless, many clinicians obtain serum thyroid function studies in patients that are in a high-risk group for the development of hypothyroidism, e.g. women over the age of 60 [75].

Patients with features suggestive of RLS require biochemical screening to ensure that there is no evidence of renal impairment or other chemical abnormality. In addition, a serum ferritin level and iron studies should be determined [76]. A serum ferritin level of less than 50 μg/l or an iron saturation of less than 16% indicates a need for iron replacement therapy in a patient with RLS [76]. The serum ferritin level is more widely utilized as a measure of cerebral iron stores than the percent iron saturation.

Serum or urine screening for drugs is most helpful in people with unexplained daytime sleepiness, when drug abuse is the suspected cause. Illicit recreational drugs, such as cocaine, methylenedioxymethamphetamine (MDMA, "ecstasy"), marijuana, or opiates have a pronounced effect on sleep, either directly or indirectly. The sedating properties of opiates are well known and widely published. They inhibit the hypocretin system (responsible for arousal and maintenance of a wake state) by direct action on the cell bodies, reducing its spike frequency, causing hyperpolarization, and altering potassium and calcium ion currents [77]. MDMA is a popular recreational drug of abuse and a selective brain serotonin neurotoxin that can cause sleep disruption/sleepiness during withdrawal. MDMA may also indirectly cause sleepiness by possibly predisposing a patient to sleep apnea. McCann and others studied 71 medically healthy recreational MDMA users and 62 control subjects via polysomnography. Recreational MDMA users who had been drug-free for at least 2 weeks had significantly increased rates of obstructive sleep apnea and hypopnea compared with controls. The odds ratio (95% confidence interval) for sleep apnea in MDMA users during non-REM sleep was 8.5 (2.4–30.4). Severity of OSA was significantly related to lifetime MDMA exposure [78]. Cocaine is a serotonin–norepinephrine–dopamine reuptake inhibitor that increases wakefulness and suppresses REM sleep; acute cocaine withdrawal, similar to MDMA, is often associated with sleep disturbances such as fragmented nocturnal sleep and/or excessive sleepiness and unpleasant dreams [79]. Acute cannabis use appears to facilitate falling asleep and to increase Stage 4 sleep [79]; Jean-Louis *et al*. also demonstrated an association between marijuana use and students falling asleep in class [80]. Accordingly, drugs of abuse can cause sleepiness and testing should be undertaken if there is clinical suspicion of their use.

Electroencephalogram (EEG)

If sleep-related seizures or subclinical seizures are suspected, a routine EEG with sleep, hyperventilation and photic stimulation is required. If negative (i.e. no interictal epileptiform activity or electrographic seizures), then an EEG with sleep deprivation is necessary. Often the EEG can turn out normal even in patients known to have seizures. This is especially common with patients with mesial frontal lobe seizures [81]. Accordingly, after about three EEGs that are unrevealing, a prolonged daytime EEG or long-term video-EEG monitoring for 24 h or longer may be needed if seizures are clinically suspected. In some severe cases, invasive intracranial recording may be necessary.

Neuroimaging

Neuroimaging can help determine if a neurologic illness is associated with the excessive sleepiness [82] (see Chapter 3). MRI of the brain, especially with visualization of the brainstem, is valuable when looking for strategically located structural lesions that may cause, for instance, REM sleep behavior disorder. It may identify a third ventricle tumor (e.g. colloid cyst) that can cause intermittent episodes of lethargy (which is easily confused with sleepiness) [83]. In addition, an MRI of the brain with thin cuts through the temporal lobe is required for patients with seizures.

Other studies

Fiber-optic endoscopy of the upper airway can determine if there is obstruction in the nasopharynx, enlarged turbinates, small nasal choanae, enlarged adenoids or tonsils, or a prolapsing epiglottis. Cephalometric X-rays of a patient who has micrognathia or retrognathia can provide information that is helpful if upper airway surgery is contemplated.

EMG and nerve conduction velocity (NCV) studies may be required, as mentioned earlier, for better evaluation of a neuropathy or a radiculopathy that is mimicking RLS symptoms.

Pulmonary function tests can help identify and determine the severity of pulmonary disorders that may be responsible for the sleepiness; while a 12-lead EKG or 24-h holter monitoring can help identify ischemic heart disease or cardiac arrhythmias.

Management

A detailed discussion regarding management of individual disorders, including pharmaceutical therapy and other more specific behavioral therapies, is beyond the scope of this chapter and will be addressed in later chapters (see Chapters 35–40).

Primary treatment of the underlying disorder is essential, but in addition all patients should be educated about good sleep hygiene and be instructed to allow adequate time for sleep and to maintain a regular sleep–wake schedule. If fatigued, tired or sleepy during the daytime, the tendency is to go to bed early to try to get more sleep; as a result, the sleep–wake pattern often becomes disrupted and spread out over a larger portion of the day. Furthermore, sleep hygiene consists of not only controlling the sleep–wake timing, but also avoiding things that may be counter-productive to good sleep. The patient should avoid caffeinated beverages, such as sodas or coffee or tea, in the evening. Alcohol may be initially helpful to fall asleep at night, but then in the second half of the night usually causes sleep to become disrupted and is best avoided [84].

Medications that contribute to the excessive sleepiness should be changed if possible and/or their timing should be altered to coincide with the patient's natural sleep–wake cycle, e.g. taking sedating medications at bedtime. Most importantly, the underlying disorder(s) causing the sleepiness need(s) to be identified and treated appropriately. Often, pharmaceutical assistance is necessary to alleviate the symptom of excessive sleepiness. Medications can be prescribed to optimize nocturnal sleep when sleep is disrupted with subsequent improvement in daytime sleepiness (e.g. zolpidem, anxiolytics, sedating antidepressants, sodium oxybate, etc.) or to maintain wakefulness during the waking hours (e.g. modafinil, armodafinil, amphetamines, etc.).

Summary

The evaluation of the patient with excessive sleepiness requires that a detailed sleep history is taken with medical, psychiatric, and psychosocial factors considered, and a differential diagnosis developed. Once a clinical history has been taken and appropriate investigations, which often include polysomnography and an MSLT, have been performed, the physician is in a good position to understand the nature and treatment direction for most disorders that result in excessive sleepiness. It may be necessary to refer the patient to a consultant specialist, such as a psychiatrist or cardiologist, if an underlying medical or psychiatric illness is suspected.

References

1. **Lerdal A**. Energy, fatigue, and perceived illness in individuals with multiple sclerosis: a multimethod approach. Doctoral Dissertation, Department of Behavioral Science in Medicine, University of Oslo, Unipub AS, 2005.
2. **Lee K A, Lentz M J, Taylor D L**, et al. Fatigue as a response to environmental demands in women's lives. *Image J Nurs Sch* 1994; **26**:149–54.
3. **Lerdal A, Bakken L N, Kouwenhoven S E**, et al. Poststroke fatigue – a review. *J Pain Symptom Mgmt* 2009; **38**:928–49.
4. **Chervin R D**. Sleepiness, fatigue, tiredness, and lack of energy in obstructive sleep apnea. *Chest* 2000; **118**:372–79.
5. **Ohayon M M**. From wakefulness to excessive sleepiness: what we know and still need to know. *Sleep Med Rev* 2008; **12**:129–41.
6. **Stepanski E, Lamphere J, Badia P**, et al. Sleep fragmentation and daytime sleepiness. *Sleep* 1984; **7**:18–26.
7. **McKenna J T, Tartar J L, Ward C P**, et al. Sleep fragmentation elevates behavioral, electrographic and neurochemical measures of sleepiness. *Neuroscience* 2007; **146**:1462–73.
8. **Oksenberg A, Arons E, Nasser K**, et al. Severe obstructive sleep apnea: sleepy versus nonsleepy patients. *Laryngoscope* 2010; **120**:643–48.
9. **Frenette E, Kushida C A**. Primary hypersomnias of central origin. *Semin Neurol* 2009; **29**:354–67.
10. **Bove A, Culebras A, Moore J T**, et al. Relationship between sleep spindles and hypersomnia. *Sleep* 1994; **17**:449–55.
11. **Sforza E, Gaudreau H, Petit D**, et al. Homeostatic sleep regulation in patients with idiopathic hypersomnia. *Clin Neurophysiol* 2000; **111**: 277–82.
12. **Nishino S, Kanbayashi T**. Symptomatic narcolepsy, cataplexy and hypersomnia, and their implications in the hypothalamic hypocretin/orexin system. *Sleep Med Rev* 2005; **9**:269–310.
13. **Young T, Palta M, Dempsey J**, et al. The occurrence of sleep-disordered breathing among middle-aged adults. *N Engl J Med* 1993; **328**:1230–35.
14. **Stradling J R, Davies R J**. Sleep. 1: Obstructive sleep apnoea/hypopnoea syndrome: definitions, epidemiology, and natural history. *Thorax* 2004; **59**:73–78.
15. **American Academy of Sleep Medicine**. *International Classification of Sleep Disorders – 2*. Chicago, IL: American Academy of Sleep Medicine, 2005.
16. **Broughton R, Ghanem Q, Hishikawa Y**, et al. Life effects of narcolepsy in 180 patients from North America, Asia and Europe compared to matched controls. *Can J Neurol Sci* 1981; **8**:299–304.
17. **Merino-Andreu M, Arnulf I, Konofal E**, et al. Unawareness of naps in Parkinson's disease and in disorders with excessive daytime sleepiness. *Neurology* 2003; **60**:1553–54.
18. **The Report of an American Academy of Sleep Medicine Task**. Sleep-related breathing disorders in adults: recommendations for syndrome definition and measurement techniques in clinical research. *Sleep*, 1999: **22**:667–89.
19. **Steptoe A, Peacey V, Wardle J**. Sleep duration and health in young adults. *Arch Intern Med*, 2006; **166**:1689–92.
20. **Thorpy M**. Current concepts in the etiology, diagnosis and treatment of narcolepsy. 1389–9457. *Sleep Med*, 2001; **2**:5–17.
21. **Chaudhuri K R**. Nocturnal symptom complex in PD and its management. *Neurology*, 2003; **61**(Suppl 3):S17–23.
22. **Takegami M, Hayashino Y, Chin K**, et al. Simple four-variable screening tool for identification of patients with sleep-disordered breathing. *Sleep*, 2009; **32**:939–48.
23. **Romero E, Krakow B, Haynes P**, et al. Nocturia and snoring: predictive symptoms for obstructive sleep apnea. *Sleep Breath*, 2009 Oct 29 [Epub ahead of print].
24. **Pi-Sunyer X**. The medical risks of obesity. *Postgrad Med*, 2009; **121**:21–33.

1. Introduction

Table 5.2 AASM recommended protocol for the MWT. (Used with permission from [7])

Recommendations for the MWT protocol
(Developed from methods of Doghramji and colleagues, [43], modified by collective expert opinion using Rand/UCLA Appropriateness Method)

1. The 4-trial MWT 40-min protocol is recommended. The MWT consists of four trials performed at 2-h intervals, with the first trial beginning about 1.5–3 h after the patient's usual wake-up time. This usually equates to a first trial starting at 0900 or 1000 hours.
2. Performance of a PSG prior to MWT should be decided by the clinician based on clinical circumstances.
3. Based on the Rand/UCLA Appropriateness Method, no consensus was reached regarding the use of sleep logs prior to the MWT; there are instances, based on clinical judgment, when they may be indicated.
4. The room should be maximally insulated from external light. The light source should be positioned slightly behind the subject's head such that it is just out of his/her field of vision, and should deliver an illuminance of 0.10–0.13 lux at the corneal level (a 7.5 W night light can be used, placed 1 foot off the floor and 3 feet laterally removed from the subject's head). Room temperature should be set based on the patient's comfort level. The subject should be seated in bed, with the back and head supported by a headrest (bolster pillow) such that the neck is not uncomfortably flexed or extended.
5. The use of tobacco, caffeine and other medications by the patient before and during MWT should be addressed and decided upon by the sleep clinician before MWT. Drug screening may be indicated to ensure that sleepiness/wakefulness on the MWT is not influenced by substances other than medically prescribed drugs. Drug screening is usually performed on the morning of the MWT, but its timing and the circumstances of the testing may be modified by the clinician. A light breakfast is recommended at least 1 h prior to the first trial, and a light lunch is recommended immediately after the termination of the second noon trial.
6. Sleep technologists who perform the MWT should be experienced in conducting the test.
7. The conventional recording montage for the MWT includes central EEG (C3-A2, C4-A1) and occipital (O1-A2, O2-A1) derivations, left and right eye electrooculograms (EOGs), mental/submental electromyogram (EMG), and electrocardiogram (EKG).
8. Prior to each trial, the patient should be asked if they need to go to the bathroom or need other adjustments for comfort. Standard instructions for bio-calibrations (i.e. patient calibrations) prior to each trial include: (1) sit quietly with your eyes open for 30 s, (2) close both eyes for 30 s, (3) without moving your head, look to the right, then left, then right, then left, right and then left, (4) blink eyes slowly for 5 times, and (5) clench or grit your teeth tightly together.
9. Instructions to the patient consist of the following: "Please sit still and remain awake for as long as possible. Look directly ahead of you, and do not look directly at the light." Patients are not allowed to use extraordinary measures to stay awake such as slapping the face or singing.
10. Sleep onset is defined as the first epoch of greater than 15 s of cumulative sleep in a 30-s epoch.
11. Trials are ended after 40 min if no sleep occurs, or after unequivocal sleep, defined as three consecutive epochs of stage 1 sleep, or one epoch of any other stage of sleep.
12. The following data should be recorded: start and stop times for each trial, sleep latency, total sleep time, stages of sleep achieved for each trial, and the mean sleep latency (the arithmetic mean of the four trials).
13. Events that represent deviation from standard protocol or conditions should be documented by the sleep technologist for review by the sleep specialist.

Clinical use

The real clinical problem of most patients who complain of excessive sleepiness is not how quickly they fall asleep when they wish to fall asleep, but how difficult it is for them to remain awake when necessary. As a result, the MWT has become increasingly used to document success of treatment. The MWT is not used to diagnose narcolepsy, because it is terminated shortly after sleep onset so that REM onsets are rarely seen. Two treatment studies of modafinil at doses of 200 and 400 mg in 454 patients with narcolepsy found that the medication significantly improved MWT after both doses (5.3 min after placebo compared with 8.2 and 8.4 min after increasing medication) [19, 20]. In a review, Mitler summarized several narcolepsy treatment studies that used a variety of medications and showed that, while most treatments produced significant increases in latency on the MWT, those improvements were only 50–70% of normal MWT values [26].

Studies have examined MWT in patients with sleep apnea and after CPAP treatment [8, 44, 45]. Most studies used the MWT-40 protocol and one used a sham-CPAP control that did not show a statistically significant improvement [27]. Data are presented in Table 5.3.

The OSLER test

The OSLER test was developed in 1997 as a means of inferring a sleep onset (i.e. measuring sleepiness) without electroencephalographic measures by

5. Objective measures

Table 5.3 MWT in patients with Sleep Apnea and Controls (significant differences from control noted by*)

	OSA	Control	Pre-CPAP	CPAP
MWT-20	*11.0 ± 5.6 [44]	18.8 ± 3.3 [44]		
MWT-40	*23.2 ± 10.2 [45]	35.4 ± 6.8 [45]	*18.8 ± 9.9 [8]	26.3 ± 10 [8]
MWT-40			(placebo CPAP)14.4 ± 8.5 [27]	16.2±19.6 [27]

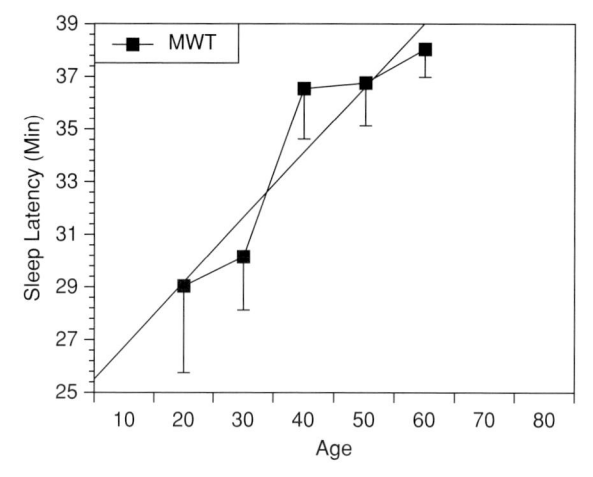

Figure 5.2 Mean and standard error for MWT as a function of age (modified and used with permission from [8]). A linear regression line is plotted to show significant changes with age.

tracking continuing behavioral responses to a light turning on with the assumption that consistent lack of responding, defined as missing seven consecutive light presentations, would correlate with sleep onset. As such, the test used a series of 40-min test periods, like the MWT, but required only a computer to turn on the light and record responses.

In the initial study, the OSLER test was validated against the MWT in a group of 10 patients newly diagnosed with sleep apnea and 10 controls [28]. In these two groups, latency as determined by the MWT was 7.3 and 38.1 min, respectively. Sleep latency based on the OSLER in the same groups was 10.5 and 39.8 min. These results have been replicated in at least two other studies that examined sleep apnea patients and normal individuals after a night of sleep deprivation [29, 30].

Methodology

This test was constructed to be analogous to the MWT in timing and presentation. The only difference is that the patient is provided with a switch to press in response to a light that was turned on automatically for one second every three seconds. The computer records responses, and the test continues until there are seven consecutive missed responses. At the seventh miss, the computer terminates the test and records the total time accumulated [29].

Normative data

Few published studies have used the OSLER, so there are few normal data. However, control groups from two published studies suggest that the mean value for controls around the age of 31 is 39.8 min and for controls around the age of 44 is 38.9 min [28, 29]. The test can be criticized because it is possible for a patient to appear sleepier by just not responding. However, it is also possible to criticize the MWT for a similar problem if a patient decides to try to fall asleep rather than following the test instruction of attempting to remain awake.

Clinical use

The OSLER was devised essentially as an MWT-40 test that did not require EEG monitoring or scoring. In a study in patients with sleep apnea, the OSLER result was 29.8 ± 8.5 min compared with a control value of 38.9 ± 2.3 min [29]. Values of 10.5 and 39.8 min for patients and controls were found in a second study [28].

Pupillography

It was noted as early as 1963 [31] that spontaneous oscillations in pupil size occurred in darkness during periods of sleepiness, and this finding was incorporated into tests of sleepiness [31, 32]. Several studies provided evidence to validate pupil measures by comparing them with other measures of sleepiness, such as subjective rating scales and the MSLT, during periods of sleep deprivation or in patients with disorders of excessive sleepiness. One recent study [33] compared results from a pupillary unrest index (PUI) with MSLT and subjective and objective performance measures in groups of young adults after one night of total sleep deprivation or normal sleep. When

1. Introduction

sleep deprivation values were compared with baseline values, moderate effect sizes were found for the change in subjective sleepiness and the MSLT (size effect, ES = .5–.6), and significant but smaller effect sizes were found for PUI (ES = .3) and reaction time lapses (ES = .2). When a principal components analysis was performed on the sleep deprivation data, the first factor loaded on the MSLT and pupil measures while subjective responses loaded on a second factor and reaction time on a third factor. Such results imply that the pupil response measures load on a similar, probably physiological dimension, with the MSLT. Another study presented correlations between PUI and latency to stage 1 on the MSLT in a small group of nine subjects who were not sleep-deprived and found a non-significant correlation of −.46 [34].

Methodology

In various studies, observations have been made as infrequently as once per day and as frequently as every 2 h throughout the day. In one fairly standard procedure [33], PUI was measured while subjects sat in a dark, quiet room for 11 min with their chin in a chin/headrest to allow them to stare at a dim red light on a computer screen. Subjects were observed, and, if they had an eye closure of more than 3 s, a soft click was presented to remind them to open their eyes. During the test, pupil diameter is continuously recorded and artifacts such as blinks removed. PUI is the integrated sum of slow movements of the pupil margin over time [35]. Greater movement (less stable) produces greater PUI. PUI has low values in alert subjects and values increase as sleepiness increases. The value should therefore have a negative correlation with MSLT.

Normative data

Standardized testing procedures and norms based upon standardized testing have not been developed for pupillography measures. In contrast to the other reported measures, sleep onset is not assessed, and subjects are actually aroused if necessary to keep their eyes open to perform the task.

Agreement of measures

Historically, sleepiness was viewed as a unitary measure. Therefore it would seem reasonable that these objective measures of sleepiness should be highly intercorrelated and, to the extent that they measure a latency to sleep onset, should return similar values. Published data for the MSLT reveal strong test–retest reliability. Correlations between different tests have not been as strong. Sangal et al. [6] performed the MSLT and 40-min MWT in 258 patients and found a correlation of $r = .41$. As indicated by the correlation, numerous patients were found who fell asleep quickly on the MSLT but not on the MWT, and a few patients were found with a similar latency on the two tests [6]. Poor correlations, between $r = .29$ and .30, have been found in other studies comparing the MSLT and the MWT as well [25,36]. Sangal and Sangal [36] looked at multiple measures of sleepiness by factor analysis and found a factor that loaded on both MSLT and MWT and another factor that loaded on information processing measures. Another study that compared MSLT with pupil responses, psychomotor performance and subjective responses [33] found that the MSLT loaded with the pupil measure in a separate factor from the performance measures with a third factor for the subjective measures. However, both of these studies were consistent in finding that the physiological measures of sleepiness loaded within the same factor rather than forming independent factors. Studies that have compared the MSLT with pupil measures have also found low and sometimes non-significant correlations between the two [34]. However, in one study that presented raw data (interpolated from a figure) from both the MWT-40 and the OSLER, the overall correlation including 10 normals and 10 sleep apnea patients was $r = .976$ ($p < .001$). When just the 10 patients with apnea were considered (almost all of the normals had 40 scores on the OSLER), the correlation was $r = .503$ ($p > .1$). These latter figures demonstrate how increasing variability in the sample by including both sleepy apnea patients and normals can have a large impact on correlation. Similar effects would hold by testing normal sleepers at baseline and after significant sleep deprivation.

Another means of examining the relationship between factors is to examine the results of the tests. It is instructive that means for the MSLT frequently are in the area of 10 min while means for the MWT in the similar-length 20-min version are in the area of 19 min in normal participants. Because the same sleep latency is measured in both tests, the implication is that simple procedural differences can result in large differences in measured sleep latency. What do those differences tell us about the tests? Can that information help in understanding why the measures are not highly correlated but still related? The MSLT was designed to be a "pure" test of sleepiness – subjects try to fall asleep in bed in a dark, quiet environment with minimal external arousing stimuli. The MWT alters that situation by propping patients up, turning on a dim light, and motivating participants to try to stay awake. Experiments have documented that the command to stay awake has a significant impact of about 4.5 min on sleep latency in a standard 20-min design [37] and 10.6–11.3 min in a 45-min design [25]. The latter study also showed that just being propped up in bed for the test increased sleep latency by 6.6–7.3 min. These observations coupled with the unusual observation that patients suffering from primary insomnia, which was defined by objectively reduced nocturnal sleep, had significantly longer latencies on the MSLT than control subjects in numerous studies [23], have led to the understanding that sleep tendency is more complex than originally thought. Sleep latency is heavily dependent upon the length of prior wakefulness, and this effect becomes overwhelming during periods of significant sleep deprivation. However, when prior wakefulness is low, as immediately after several nights of adequate sleep, sleep latency is more influenced by other factors. Numerous studies showing relationships between heart rate (or sympathetic activation) and sleep latency have suggested that sleep latency is determined by a combination of sleep factors (prior sleep and prior wake times) and arousal system factors (circadian arousal, trait level of arousal, and state arousal effects). The effects of circadian time have been appreciated for many years and are controlled by presentation of sleep latency tests at standard circadian times. The several findings of significantly increased MSLT times in patients with primary insomnia suggest that their sleep latency is also determined by their trait elevation in central nervous system activation [23]. This was additionally supported in normal young adults chosen to have characteristic short (versus long) latency on their MSLT who were also found to have significantly lower heart rate [38].

Finally, it is well known that sleep onset can be avoided by activation of the sympathetic nervous system (common manipulations are sitting up or standing up). Simple movement has been shown to have a large impact on momentary alertness [39]. However, even relatively small amounts of activity in proximity to MSLT observations can produce clinically significant effects – a 5-min walk prior to a nap observation significantly increased heart rate and sleep latency for at least 90 min (sleep latency was 13 min compared with 8.6 min in the control condition 90 min after the walk) [40]. Such findings suggest that sleep latency at a given point is determined by a summation of sleep system effects (Process S), circadian time, trait level of arousal, and state arousal effects. In a final experimental example of the interaction of these latter two arousal effects, groups of normal young adults or primary insomnia patients were given the MSLT on two separate days. On one day, subjects lay in bed and watched TV for 15 min prior to their MSLT. On the other day, subjects were allowed to walk around the hospital building for 5 min prior to their MSLT. Mean sleep latency for the normal subjects following the rest and walk conditions respectively was 6.7 and 13.0 min [41], while sleep latency for the insomnia patients for the respective conditions was 10.5 and 16.2 min [24]. These data suggest that trait arousal related to insomnia produced about a 3.2–3.8 increment in baseline sleep latency, while state arousal produced by the walk produced an additional 5.7–6.3 increase in sleep latency independent of group. For comparative purposes, the normal group also performed the sleep latency tests after a night with 4 h in bed, and their average latency in the rest condition was 5.2 min. These data indicated that the impact of both state and trait arousal on ability to fall asleep can be large enough to be clinically significant and enough to completely mask some sleep deprivation effects. Individual differences in underlying arousal could certainly help to explain the large variability usually found in sleep latency measures.

Summary

Several objective measures of sleep tendency have been commonly used for many years. The MSLT is supported by considerable reliability and validity data, but has been challenged by the observation that maintaining wakefulness may be a more relevant issue for many individuals than the ability to fall asleep quickly. Less research supports the OSLER and pupillography tests, but the OSLER, which attempts to measure sleep onset without traditional measurement of either performance or EEG, holds promise as a simpler but still time-consuming measure. Objective measurement of sleepiness is handicapped by the relatively low correlation between MSLT and MWT measures. The poor correlation suggests that sleep and wake are not a simple continuum. The tests measure more than a single sleep system and almost certainly reflect the summation of numerous sources of state and trait arousal in addition to the effects of circadian time, prior wakefulness and numerous underlying sleep and arousal pathologies. Further refinement of these measures will require additional understanding of the interplay between both sleep and arousal systems.

References

1. **Carskadon M A**, **Dement W C**. Sleepiness and sleep state on a 90-min schedule. *Psychophysiology*, 1977; **14**:127–33.
2. **Carskadon M A**, **Dement W C**. Effects of total sleep loss on sleep tendency. *Percept Mot Skill*, 1979; **48**:495–506.
3. **Richardson G S**, **Carskadon M A**, **Flagg W**, *et al*. Excessive daytime sleepiness in man: multiple sleep latency measurement in narcoleptic and control subjects. *Electroencephalogr Clin Neurophysiol*, 1978; **45**:621–27.
4. **Bonnet M H**, **Webb W B**. The return to sleep. *Biol Psychol*, 1979; **8**:225–33.
5. **Mitler M**, **Gujavarty K**, **Browman C P**. Maintenance of wakefulness test: a polysomnographic technique for evaluating treatment in patients with excessive somnolence. *Electroencephalogr Clin Neurophysiol*, 1982; **153**: 658–61.
6. **Sangal R B**, **Thomas L**, **Mitler M M**. Maintenance of wakefulness test (MWT) and multiple sleep latency test (MSLT) measure different abilities in patients with sleep disorders. *Chest*, 1992; **101**:898–902.
7. **Littner M**, **Kushida C**, **Wise M**, *et al*. Practice parameters for clinical use of the multiple sleep latency test and the maintenance of wakefulness test. *Sleep*, 2005; **28**:113–21.
8. **Arand D**, **Bonnet M**, **Hurwitz T**, *et al*. The clinical use of the MSLT and MWT. *Sleep*, 2005; **28**:123–44.
9. **Zwyghuizen-Doorenbos A**, **Roehrs T**, **Schaeffer M**, *et al*. Test-retest reliability of the MSLT. *Sleep*, 1988; **11**:562–65.
10. **Seidel W**, **Dement W C**. The Multiple Sleep Latency Test: test–retest reliability. *Sleep Res*, 1981; **10**:105.
11. **Drake C L**, **Rice M F**, **Roehrs T A**, *et al*. Scoring reliability of the multiple sleep latency test in a clinical population. *Sleep*, 2000; **23**:911–13.
12. **Chen L**, **Ho C K**, **Lam V K**, *et al*. Interrater and intrarater reliability in multiple sleep latency test. *J Clin Neurophysiol*, 2008; **25**:218–21.
13. **Rosenthal L**, **Roehrs T A**, **Rosen A**, *et al*. Level of sleepiness and total sleep time following various time in bed conditions. *Sleep*, 1993; **16**:226–32.
14. **Bonnet M H**. Performance and sleepiness as a function of frequency and placement of sleep disruption. *Psychophysiology*, 1986; **23**:263–71.
15. **Carskadon M A**, **Seidel W F**, **Greenblatt D J**, *et al*. Daytime carryover of triazolam and flurazepam in elderly insomniacs. *Sleep*, 1982; **5**:361–71.
16. **Bishop C**, **Roehrs T**, **Rosenthal L**, *et al*. Alerting effects of methylphenidate under basal and sleep-deprived conditions. *Exp Clin Psychopharmacol*, 1997; **5**:344–52.
17. **Punjabi N M**, **Bandeen-Roche K**, **Young T**. Predictors of objective sleep tendency in the general population. *Sleep*, 2003; **26**:678–83.
18. **Majer M**, **Jones J F**, **Unger E R**, *et al*. Perception versus polysomnographic assessment of sleep in CFS and non-fatigued control subjects: results from a population-based study. *BMC Neurol*, 2007; **7**:40.
19. **US Modafinil in Narcolepsy Multicenter Study Group**. Randomized trial of modafinil as a treatment for the excessive daytime somnolence of narcolepsy. *Neurology*, 2000; **54**:1166–75.
20. **US Modafinil in Narcolepsy Multicenter Study Group**. Randomized trial of modafanil for the treatment of pathological somnolence in narcolepsy. *Ann Neurology*, 1998; **43**:88–97.
21. **Mitler M M**, **Hajdukovic R**, **Erman M K**. Treatment of narcolepsy with methamphetamine. *Sleep*, 1993; **16**:306–17.
22. **George C F**, **Boudreau A C**, **Smiley A**. Comparison of simulated driving performance in narcolepsy and sleep apnea patients. *Sleep*, **19**: 711–17.
23. **Bonnet M H**, **Arand D L**. Hyperarousal and insomnia: state of the science. *Sleep Med Rev*, 2010; **14**:9–15.
24. **Bonnet M H**, **Arand D L**. Activity, arousal, and the MSLT in patients with insomnia. *Sleep*, 2000; **23**:205–12.
25. **Bonnet M H**, **Arand D L**. Arousal components which differentiate the MWT from the MSLT. *Sleep*, 2001; **24**:441–50.
26. **Mitler M M**, **Hajdukovic R**. Relative efficacy of drugs for the treatment of sleepiness in narcolepsy. *Sleep*, 1991; **14**:218–20.
27. **Engleman H**, **Kingshott R**, **Wraith P**, *et al*. Randomized placebo-controlled crossover trial of continuous positive airway pressure for mild sleep apnea/hypopnea syndrome. *Am J Respir Crit Care Med*, 1999; **159**:461–67.
28. **Bennett L S**, **Stradling J R**, **Davies R J**. A behavioural test to assess daytime sleepiness in obstructive sleep apnoea. *J Sleep Res*, 1997; **6**:142–45.
29. **Mazza S**, **Pepin JL**, **Deschaux C**, *et al*. Analysis of error profiles occurring during the OSLER test: A sensitive means of detecting fluctuations in vigilance in patients

with obstructive sleep apnea syndrome. *Am J Respir Crit Care Med* 2002; **166**(4): 474–78.

30. **Priest B**, **Brichard C**, **Aubert G**, *et al*. Microsleep during a simplified maintenance of wakefulness test. A validation study of the OSLER test. *Am J Respir Crit Care Med* 2001; **163**(7): 1619–25.

31. **Lowenstein O**, **Feinberg R**, **Loewenfeld I E**. Pupillary movements during acute and chronic fatigue: a new test for the objective evaluation of tiredness. *Invest Ophthalmol Vis Sci*, 1963; **2**:138–57.

32. **Wilhelm B**, **Wilhelm H**, **Ludtke H**, *et al*. Pupillographic assessment of sleepiness in sleep-deprived healthy subjects. *Sleep*, 1998; **21**:258–65.

33. **Franzen P L**, **Siegle G J**, **Buysse D J**. Relationships between affect, vigilance, and sleepiness following sleep deprivation. *J Sleep Res*, 2008; **17**:34–41.

34. **Danker-Hopfe H**, **Kraemer S**, **Dorn H**, *et al*. Time-of-day variations in different measures of sleepiness (MSLT, pupillography, and SSS) and their interrelations. *Psychophysiology*, 2001; **38**:828–35.

35. **Wilhelm B**, **Giedke H**, **Ludtke H**, *et al*. Daytime variations in central nervous system activation measured by a pupillographic sleepiness test. *J Sleep Res*, 2001; **10**:1–7.

36. **Sangal R B**, **Sangal J M**. Measurement of P300 and sleep characteristics in patients with hypersomnia: do P300 latencies, P300 amplitudes, and multiple sleep latency and maintenance of wakefulness tests measure different factors? *Clin Electroencephalogr*, 1997; **28**:179–84.

37. **Hartse K M**, **Roth T**, **Zorick F J**. Daytime sleepiness and daytime wakefulness: the effect of instruction. *Sleep*, 1982; **5**(Suppl 2):S107–18.

38. **Bonnet M H**, **Arand D L**. Performance and cardiovascular measures in normals with extreme MSLT and subjective sleepiness levels. *Sleep*, 2005; **28**: 681–89.

39. **Bonnet M H**, **Arand D L**. Level of arousal and the ability to maintain wakefulness. *J Sleep Res*, 1999; **8**:247–54.

40. **Bonnet M H**, **Arand D L**. Sleep latency testing as a time course measure of state arousal. *J Sleep Res*, 2005; **14**:387–92.

41. **Bonnet M H**, **Arand D L**. Sleepiness as measured by the MSLT varies as a function of preceding activity. *Sleep*, 1998; **21**:477–83.

42. **Carskadon M A**. Guidelines for the Multiple Sleep Latency Test (MSLT): a standard measure of sleepiness. *Sleep*, 1986; **9**:519–24.

43. **Doghramji K**, **Mitler M M**, **Sangal R B**, *et al*. A normative study of the maintenance of wakefulness test (MWT). *Electroencephalogr Clin Neurophysiol*, 1997; **103**:554–62.

44. **Browman C P**, **Mitler M M**. Hypersomnia and the perception of sleep–wake states: some preliminary findings. *Percept Mot Skills*, 1988; **66**:463–70.

45. **Hakkanen H**, **Summala H**, **Partinen M**, *et al*. Blink duration as an indicator of driver sleepiness in professional bus drivers. *Sleep*, 1999; **22**:798–802.

Section 1 Chapter 6

Introduction

Subjective measures of sleepiness

Christopher L. Drake

"There will be sleeping enough in the grave."

"For having lived long, I have experienced many instances of being obliged, by better information or fuller consideration, to change opinions, even on important subjects, which I once thought right but found to be otherwise."

"Early to bed and early to rise makes a man healthy, wealthy, and wise."
–Benjamin Franklin

Sleep deprivation has numerous harmful effects including death [1], as keenly illustrated by the following example quoted from an article in 1859 [2]:

A Chinese merchant had been convicted of murdering his wife, and was sentenced to die by being deprived of sleep. This painful mode of death was carried into execution under the following circumstances: – The condemned was placed in prison under the care of three of the police guard, who relieved each other every alternate hour, and who prevented the prisoner from falling asleep, night or day. He thus lived for nineteen days without enjoying any sleep. At the commencement of the eighth day his sufferings were so intense that he implored the authorities to grant him the blessed opportunity of being strangulated, guillotined, burned to death, drowned, garroted, shot, quartered, blown up with gunpowder, or put to death in any conceivable way which their humanity or ferocity could invent. This will give a slight idea of the horrors of death from want of sleep.

To keep from harm, our bodies homeostatically regulate sleep to approximately 8 h per night. The experience of sleepiness is the important homeostatic signal that helps one avoid a state of severe sleep deprivation. Thus, sleepiness serves a beneficial role to the human body. Without this signal, consumption of sleep would be delayed, leading to harmful effects. Thus, sleepiness is analogous to hunger or thirst, where an absence of these homeostatic signals may lead to severe dehydration or even starvation. However, as opposed to hunger and thirst, sleep does not require an object for its consumption. That is, one does not need an external object to satisfy the drive state. One consequence of the drive state of sleepiness is that it may engage the sleep system at inappropriate times, such as while driving, at work, or during other attention-demanding tasks. This can result in serious and often catastrophic consequences. Therefore, the sensation of sleepiness is an important factor influencing critical decision-making. Excessive sleepiness is also one of the most common and debilitating symptoms in terms of quality of life (e.g. job loss, poor school performance, and distressed social relationships) in patients with sleep disorders. The dimensions of sleepiness range from the tendency to fall asleep to the feeling state of sleepiness itself, and there have been suggestions that these aspects of sleepiness represent wholly different constructs. None the less, while the singularity of the construct of sleepiness has been debated, the complexities involved in its assessment are widely recognized.

This chapter will discuss subjective assays of sleepiness. For some readers, the term subjective infers a negative connotation. Terms such as self-report of sleepiness and introspective reports of sleepiness are a more accurate description of these scales. However, as the term subjective is commonly used, that will be the term used in this chapter. Also, differences between objective and subjective assays of sleepiness will be discussed. In that context it is important to not only think of their relative sensitivity to a variety of conditions, but rather the context in which each of these measures is more appropriate. Simply put, it is not which is better but rather how you use them appropriately. For example, an objective assay might be the assay of choice in evaluating the degree of sleepiness in a school bus

---

Sleepiness: Causes, Consequences and Treatment, ed. Michael J. Thorpy and Michel Billiard. Published by Cambridge University Press. © Cambridge University Press 2011.

driver, while a subjective assay may be more appropriate in determining the level of sleepiness seen in a large population of individuals.

History

Sleepiness as a focus of scientific inquiry dates back to ancient times as it occupied the interests of such philosophers as Aristotle, Hippocrates and other philosophers and scientists [3]. *The Cannon of Medicine*, a medical text published in 1025 and used for more than 700 years in Europe, devotes a chapter to sleep and wakefulness and points out "excessive sleepiness" (p. 280) as an adverse state, but the text fails to explain how the sleepiness state was measured and defined [4]. Few advances in the assessment of sleepiness were made until the nineteenth century, with the advent of scientific methods for the study of individual differences in psychology. Concurrently, the first sleep deprivation studies in humans were carried out by Patrick and Gilbert in 1896 showing effects on reaction time, memory, and attention [5]. Surprisingly, sleepiness was not assessed in that study, but informally inferred from the frequency and rapidity of unintentional sleep onsets during the experiment. Although it was recognized that sleepiness was an inordinate tendency to sleep, formalized assessments of *objective* sleepiness using sleep propensity were not developed until more than 70 years after Patrick and Gilbert's study (see Chapter 5 of this volume). Furthermore, standardized measures of *subjective* sleepiness were not even developed until the 1970s. Dement has stated, "…the phenomenon of sleepiness has been virtually ignored as an experimental variable by researchers for many years, even in studies of the consequences of experimental sleep deprivation" (p. 78) [6]. Therefore, prior to the 1970s, if the measurement of sleepiness was a topic of interest, it was typically determined by non-specific measures of mood/affect. Non-specificity is evidenced by the fact that areas of research used terms such as fatigue and vigor interchangeably with sleepiness and alertness.

As the number of human experiments devoted to sleep disorders increased during the twentieth century, researchers realized the necessity of developing objective measures to quantify sleepiness. Clinicians also recognized excessive sleepiness as a major complaint of patients with sleep disorders, and thus worked with researchers to develop measures used to quantify sleepiness and to employ these measures in specific studies of sleepiness and in sleep clinics. This increase in the scientific study of sleep fueled by the discovery of Rapid Eye Movement (REM) sleep and the advent of clinical sleep medicine brought about the first standardized scale, the Stanford Sleepiness Scale (SSS), for the measurement of sleepiness [7]. However, it was not until development of the Epworth Sleepiness Scale (ESS) in 1991 [8] that the standardized assessment of subjective sleepiness was widely used in clinical practice.

Subjective measurement of sleepiness is cost-effective, completion time is usually minimal, and measures are readily available and can usually be administered in a range of settings (clinic, laboratory, home, internet). Thus, validated subjective measures are the most widely used methods of assessing sleepiness. This chapter will review the psychometric properties, validation, and strengths and weaknesses of the most common measurement tools used for the subjective evaluation of sleepiness. The use of these instruments in both clinical practice and research settings will be covered. The chapter is not an exhaustive review of the available studies utilizing each of the measures covered, but rather serves as a conceptual and practical overview of the benefits and limitations of each tool. Importantly, differences between objective (laboratory) and subjective (self-report) measures of sleepiness will also be discussed.

Visual Analogue Scales (VAS)

One of the earliest means by which sleepiness was measured used subjective introspection, an in-depth description of one's own sensation of sleepiness. One significant limitation of this method is that the experience of sleepiness as well as the ability to introspectively describe a state varies from individual to individual. Therefore, such methods are often unreliable. Without strict operationalization of the construct under study, different emotional states brought about by sleep deprivation or disorders of excessive sleepiness (e.g. depressed mood, irritability, etc.) function as confounding variables and hinder the accurate assessment of sleepiness.

In order to account for these factors, standardized scales such as the Visual Analogue Scale (VAS) are utilized. A VAS scale comprises a 100-mm line with specific anchor points such as "extreme sleepiness" and "full alertness" on each end to denote a continuum of a distinct state. Subjects are asked to place a vertical

1. Introduction

mark on the line where they judge their current state to be. Degree of sleepiness is defined as the distance from the left anchor point to the subjects' mark. This operationalization of sleepiness provided a working assessment of the state under investigation and allowed researchers to standardize the quantification of sleepiness across time. Researchers have used combinations of several VAS scales in order to obtain a more global measure of sleepiness [9]. VAS measures of sleepiness continue to be widely used in research settings measuring the effects of pharmacological interventions, circadian variation, and other protocols where a simple indication of current level of sleepiness is needed and can be repeated indefinitely throughout an experiment to gain increased temporal resolution of state changes. The ease of use, availability (experimenters can devise their own scales), and repeatability of VAS scales make the VAS an ideal measure for use in studies investigating within-subject changes across time and in response to experimental manipulations.

There are, however, considerable limitations to utilizing the VAS in the assessment of sleepiness. First, although standardization is easily achieved within particular protocols and within a given laboratory, different investigators often use widely different terminology for anchor points which reduces the ability to compare results across studies. Comparisons between studies or even between individuals are also precluded by variations in each individual's perception of the terms used to anchor a given VAS measure of sleepiness. For example, judgment regarding the nature of the term "extremely sleepy" is not likely to be equal across subjects. Thus, it is difficult to collect reliable and generalizable normative data using the VAS – a fact which has prevented their widespread use in clinical settings where focus is on individual assessment, relative to normative values.

Profile of Mood States (POMS – Vigor)

One way to improve upon the VAS method of assessing subjective sleepiness is to develop scales which employ multiple terms describing the construct under study. This method reduces the inherent variability in the subject's interpretation of the terms chosen arbitrarily to serve as anchors in VAS measures of sleepiness. The POMS is a measure which evolved from the desire to utilize the varied descriptors of a given mood state to fully account for the between-subject differences in the perception of such a state. The POMS includes multiple items to minimize individual idiosyncrasies, thereby reducing error variance and allowing more accurate assessment. Indeed, normative data for the POMS were developed, and these norms became a major step in developing accurate cross-study comparisons of mood states including sleepiness.

The POMS comprises six mood scales (fatigue/inertia, vigor/activity, confusion/bewilderment, tension/anxiety, anger/hostility, depression/dejection), each containing approximately eight items [10]. While the POMS was developed as a mood checklist, the Vigor and Fatigue scales have been used to measure self-reported sleepiness [11]. Individual t-scores for each scale can be determined and compared to normative data. The POMS Vigor and Fatigue scales are sensitive to the effects of sleep deprivation [12], as well as in response to the alerting effects of caffeine and sedative effects of alcohol [13]. The POMS shares the strengths of the VAS – it can be measured repeatedly during a short period of time, and is easily administered and interpreted. However, it is not a scale specifically designed to measure sleepiness. Confounding effects of other mood states such as irritability, fatigue, and depression can be present for this measure, which limits its specificity for sleepiness particularly in clinical samples with high comorbidity.

Stanford Sleepiness Scale (SSS)

The increasing need for a more specific standardized and validated measure of sleepiness brought about the development of the Stanford Sleepiness Scale in 1972 [7]. This was the first measure to be specifically designed and validated with the intent of developing a state-of-the art, psychometrically sound method for the assessment of subjective sleepiness. Carskadon and Dement described sleepiness as "the physiological tendency for sleep to occur," [14] and Broughton described sleepiness as "the subjective feeling state of sleep need" [15]. Therefore, it is clear that sleepiness is a state with both a physiological/behavioral and psychological component. The biological need state is reflected in the behavior of falling asleep, and the experience of sleepiness is a warning signal that the need for sleep is accumulating. Thus, the SSS is a measure of the psychological experience of feeling sleepy. The SSS contains seven items, each containing several terms (Table 6.1). The use of multiple terms for each item attempts to capture the varied words individuals

6. Subjective measures

Table 6.1 Items from the Stanford Sleepiness Scale, Karolinska Sleepiness Scale, Epworth Sleepiness Scale, Pediatric Daytime Sleepiness Scale, and the Pediatric Sleep Questionnaire – Sleepiness Subscale

Stanford Sleepiness Scale

The SSS is a measure of alertness at time of administration. Only 1 item is selected.
1. Feeling active, vital, alert, or wide awake
2. Functioning at high levels, but not at peak; able to concentrate
3. Relaxed, awake, not at full alertness, responsive
4. A little foggy, not at peak, let down
5. Fogginess, beginning to lose interest in remaining awake, slowed down
6. Sleepiness, prefer to be lying down, fighting sleep, woozy
7. Almost in reverie, sleep onset soon, lost struggle to remain awake

Karolinska Sleepiness Scale

The KSS is a subject measure of sleepiness at a specific point in time. Only 1 item is selected.
1 = very alert
2
3 = alert
4
5 = neither sleepy nor alert
6
7 = sleepy but no effort to remain awake
8
9 = very sleepy, difficulty staying awake, fighting sleep

Epworth Sleepiness Scale

The ESS is a subjective measure of how likely the subject is to doze off in 8 situations. Rated from 0 to 3 for each item.
1. Sitting and reading
2. Watching TV
3. Sitting inactive in a public place
4. As a car passenger for an hour without a break
5. Lying down to rest in the afternoon
6. Sitting and talking to someone
7. Sitting quietly after lunch without alcohol
8. In a car while stopped for a few minutes in traffic

Pediatric Daytime Sleepiness Scale

The PDSS is a subjective measure of propensity for sleep in school-aged children. A total of 8 items are rated from 0 to 4 in each.
1. Falling asleep during class periods
2. Falling asleep while doing homework
3. Alertness during most of the day
4. Tired or grumpiness during the day
5. Trouble getting out of bed in morning
6. Falling asleep after waking up in morning
7. Needing someone to wake you up
8. Needing more sleep

Pediatric Sleep Questionnaire-Sleepiness Subscale

The PSQ-SS is a 4-item subjective measure of sleepiness in children that is administered to parents.
1. Does your child wake up feeling *unrefreshed* in the morning?
2. Does your child have a problem with sleepiness during the day?
3. Has a teacher or other supervisor commented that your child appears sleepy during the day?
4. Is it hard to wake your child up in the morning?

commonly use to convey the subjective state of sleepiness. The SSS has been shown to have high reliability [7], and studies have shown the SSS to be sensitive to circadian changes in sleepiness as well as to the effects of caffeine and bright light on sleepiness [16].

A criticism of the SSS is that within the 7 intervals appearing in the measure there are a total of 24 different descriptions concerning the state of the individual. A factor analysis of these 24 items has shown the presence of at least 2 different factors, one corresponding to energy or activation and another thought to reflect consciousness, sleepiness, and a loss of control over the ability to stay awake [17]. These factors are believed to be related to the subsets of vigor and fatigue, respectively, of the POMS. This finding suggests the SSS may reflect a more global measure of the subjective state, encompassing an undifferentiated measure of both sleepiness and fatigue, reducing its specificity for assessing sleepiness.

The SSS is useful in research paradigms, but it has significant limitations in clinical settings where general levels of sleepiness are of interest. Dement and colleagues found that the SSS often does not discriminate sleepiness in OSA patients prior to treatment and is not sensitive to treatment response [18]. A more recent study showed that the SSS does not differentiate severe from moderate OSA patients and that at several time points, patients with severe (mean respiratory disturbance index $= 70.2$) obstructive sleep apnea (OSA) rate themselves as less sleepy on the SSS relative to patients with mild to moderate severity (mean respiratory disturbance index $= 26.9$) [19]. Subjective measures of feeling state may also be easily influenced by transient factors such as activity level, posture, light, and motivation [14]. The issues noted above emphasize

1. Introduction

the importance of combining subjective with objective measures such as the gold standard Multiple Sleep Latency Test (MSLT) (see Chapter 5).

Karolinska Sleepiness Scale (KSS)

The KSS is similar to SSS in that it is a validated subjective measure that assesses sleepiness at a specific point in time in order to identify short-term changes in sleepiness over minutes to several hours [20]. The scale consists of nine statements from "very alert", to "very sleepy" (see Table 6.1). The KSS has been found to correlate well with EEG indices of sleepiness in normal subjects in a driving simulator during sleep deprivation [21]. In another driving simulator study, the KSS was strongly related to incident and accident risk within subjects [22]. Although the accuracy of individual predictions were variable, the study showed adjusted incident risk elevations occurred with scores above 7 and accident risk was elevated with scores above 8. It was estimated that accident risk would be reduced by approximately 96.5% if the KSS score were reduced from 9 to 7. While this was a simulator study in a well-controlled environment, the results suggest the possibility that the KSS may have some use in predicting actual accident risk, a possibility which remains to be tested. Despite the significant strengths of this measure, the KSS has some limitations. Similar to the SSS, the KSS has less utility in discrimination of sleepiness in sleep disorder patients, and is thus typically used in research studies where frequent repeated ratings of sleepiness are required to demonstrate treatment effects within subjects across time [23]. The KSS is also significantly affected by the context in which the sleepiness rating is performed. One study has shown that subjects report higher ratings of sleepiness after a reaction time task compared with ratings given following free activity [24]. As both conditions in this study were well controlled, this suggests that specific tasks may mask underlying sleepiness and that subjective sleepiness ratings may be particularly sensitive to such effects.

Subjective vs. objective measures

Objective measures of sleepiness have also been devised, but their correlation with subjective measures, while statistically significant, is low [25]. One reason may be that ceiling or floor effects, or restriction of range issues, interfered with accurate assessment of some physiological measures. That is, once a maximum (or minimum) score is reached on a given measure, increased sleepiness can no longer be detected even if present. This is an obvious psychometric limitation of some measures of sleepiness such as the MSLT (maximum sleep latency of 20 min). However, one of the most important reasons for the differences found between objective and subjective measures of sleepiness has been related to the concepts of manifest and physiological sleep tendency. Specifically, objective measures such as the MSLT are thought to reflect a direct measure of the underlying physiological tendency for sleep to occur, whereas subjective measures are reflections of feeling state which can change transiently in relation to numerous factors (i.e. motivation, activity, light, noise, room temperature, etc.). Situational components can play important roles in how sleepiness is manifested in an individual, but when present in a sleepy individual these situational factors mask underlying sleep tendency as opposed to reducing the physiological state of sleepiness. Similarly, non-activating situations do not cause sleepiness, but "unmask" the underlying state [14]. The conceptual difference lies in the assumption that objective measures of physiological sleep tendency are less influenced by transient alerting factors than subjective measures of sleepiness. Thus when certain masking factors such as physical activity are present, sleepy individuals may not feel or even appear sleepy.

As masking factors are removed, measures of manifest sleepiness such as the SSS become similar to measures of physiological sleepiness such as the MSLT. One study has shown that the concordance between subjective (VAS, SSS) and objective (MSLT) measures is enhanced significantly by standardizing the environment in which subjective sleepiness is measured. This is achieved by having individuals sit quietly with eyes closed for 1 min before a sleepiness rating is obtained [26]. This effect is similar to that found with the KSS, where sleepiness ratings were reduced simply by removing the masking effects of activity. However, a smaller study did not find such an effect [27]. In that study, within-subject correlations between subjective (SSS) and objective sleepiness (MSLT) were high ($r = -.65$), while between-subject correlations at any given time point were near zero ($r = -0.05$ to 0.02). These data suggest (1) that it is variation between different individuals' reference point for their subjective feeling state of sleepiness that is one of the greatest contributors to the subjective/objective discrepancy, and (2) that it follows that when measurements are taken over time, variation in sleepiness assessed with subjective measures does accurately reflect the change seen in objective measures of sleepiness. This suggests that objective and subjective measures of sleepiness are measuring the same unitary construct, but that individual differences and methodological approach can obscure their parallelism.

If one accepts the assumption that both subjective and objective measures of sleepiness are aimed at measuring a similar construct, then one way to address the discrepancies is to devise a method of subjectively assessing sleepiness that is less dependent upon the feeling state. This can be done by linking the measure directly to sleep tendency in a variety of situations, including sedentary ones. Although the majority of subjective measures do not reflect sleep tendency, one subjective measure, the Epworth Sleepiness Scale (ESS), addresses this issue by focusing items on a specific behavior (i.e. the propensity to doze off) in a set of commonly experienced, mostly sedentary, situations.

Epworth Sleepiness Scale

Because descriptors of personal experiences such as "sleepiness" or "alertness" do not have openly available referents (they use an internal frame of reference rather than an external one), the ESS was designed to measure the subjective estimate of the behavioral tendency to fall asleep in various situations rather than a judgment of feeling state. The ESS is the most widely used measure of subjective sleepiness, particularly with respect to the identification of the severity of sleepiness in patients with sleep disorders. Developed and validated by Johns in 1991, the eight-item ESS has several advantages over other subjective measures [8]. The most important of these is that it is an attempt to more closely reflect sleep tendency/sleep propensity by requiring individuals to rate the likelihood of dozing (never to high chance) in a variety of common situations (mostly sedentary) where sleepiness may be "unmasked" (Table 6.1). Each item (i.e. situation) can vary from 0 (would never doze) to 3 (high chance of dozing). The total score is a sum of these items and ranges from 0 to 24. A total score >10 is used to indicate sleepiness [8]. The ESS measures a unitary construct, has high internal consistency (Chronbach's alpha = 0.88), high 5-month test–retest reliability in normal samples ($r = 0.82$) and is easily administered within a few minutes [28]. Although the reliability of the ESS in clinical samples has been ques-

Table 6.2 Epworth Sleepiness Scale means for selected clinical samples

Patient sample	ESS score: mean±SD	Reference
Normal sleepers ($N = 72$)	4.6 ± 2.8	[49]
Medical students ($N = 172$)	10.7 ±4.03	[50]
Moderate OSA (RDI 34.8 ± 9.4) ($N = 41$)	13.0±4.7	[51]
Severe OSA (RDI 56.6 ± 5.9) ($N = 41$)	16.2±3.3	[51]
Narcolepsy ($N = 124$)	20.1±3.6†	[52]
RLS ($N = 41$)	6.5±4.9	[53]
Periodic Limb Movement Disorder ($N = 592$)	9.1±4.1	[54]
Insomnia ($N = 57$)	10.6±4.4	[55]
Idiopathic hypersomnia ($N = 85$)	17.0±7.0^	[56]
MDD ($N = 100$)	10.0±5.6	[57]
Fibromyalgia with hypersomnolence ($N = 16$)	15.0±4.0	[58]
Parkinson's ($N = 89$)	10.5±5.1*†	[59]

MDD, major depressive disorder.
† Pooled standard deviation from groups was used.
* Subject's in these studies were on medication for the primary disorder.
^ Median ESS score was reported.

tioned [29], this measure has been shown to detect the effects of treatment in patients with sleep disorders [30]. In a study examining the multidimensional nature of subjective sleepiness, factor analyses of two separate samples determined that the ESS measures a component of sleepiness very different from the VAS, SSS and POMS and is likely more reflective of sleep propensity [31].

The epidemiological data regarding this measure in the general population have been extensively studied (see Chapter 1). The ESS can differentiate the degree of sleepiness between a number of normal and clinical samples [8]. Because of its ease of use and popularity, this measure of sleepiness has the largest amount of normative data relative to other measures. Table 6.2 provides selected references showing mean ESS scores for a range of commonly encountered disorders of excessive sleepiness. The clinical data showing that few individuals score at the maximum (24) or minimum (0) of the ESS suggest minimal ceiling or floor effects on this measure (see Table 6.2).

1. Introduction

The ESS was intended to reflect sleep propensity over various situations. However, studies in patients have shown low or non-significant relationships between the ESS and objective sleep propensity measures such as the MSLT [32]. Some researchers have suggested that because the ESS quantifies sleep propensity in multiple situations, the results more accurately reflect sleep propensity in the real world. However, this speculation does not fit with data showing the MSLT is a stronger predictor of verified automotive crashes than the ESS [33]. In fact, the concept of a representative real world is a bit artificial. For example, the chance of falling asleep in a conversation at 2 in the morning in a quiet room is different from the chance of falling asleep in a conversation walking on a crowded street at 10 a.m. Several other reasons for the subjective-objective discrepancy are likely. For example, the ESS reflects a component of judgment in that response options are graded from no chance (of dozing) through slight, moderate, and high. The subjective judgments of these gradations are not likely to be equal across all patients and this introduces measurement error when comparing between individuals. Moreover, the situations identified and the degree and frequency with which each is experienced by a given patient (i.e. differing commute times, frequency of lying to rest in the afternoon) also vary widely. This introduces additional unwanted variance when compared to a standardized situation. The presence of ceiling and/or floor effects present in some objective measures of sleepiness may also contribute to the discrepancy between the ESS and objective measures.

Another limitation of subjective measures which can increase the likelihood of false negatives (reporting no sleep tendency when actually sleepy) is that the degree and chronicity of sleepiness experienced by an individual can reduce the accuracy of one's subjective judgment. When sleep loss is experienced rapidly, as is the case following a full night of sleep loss, individuals are able to easily detect increases in sleepiness. In contrast, when sleep is restricted to 6 h per night for several nights, physiological indications of increased sleepiness are present and deterioration in cognitive performance occurs [12], but sleepiness is not detected by subjective measures (Figure 6.1). Similar effects are also seen when examining performance-based measures of sleepiness [34]. These effects demonstrating a reduced ability to detect sleepiness can also occur in patients when moderate amounts of sleep loss occur over years or even decades. Indeed, patients often report themselves to be alert while showing objective signs of sleepiness [18]. This probably accounts for the common clinical observation in OSA patients where following the initial treatment night, individuals describe how unaware of their sleepiness they were prior to treatment. Thus, over time many chronically sleepy patients lose their frame of reference for what it means to be fully alert. Alternatively, there is the possibility that there are physiological adaptive mechanisms which counteract sleepiness when present over the long term – a type of upregulation of the sleepiness system. This type of upregulation is not uncommon with many physiological systems.

Clinical assessment/clinical judgment

The primary advantages of using standardized subjective measures in the clinical context are usefulness in quick screening of patients (need to work-up), estimation of severity of sleepiness relative to norms (need to treat), and in the accurate evaluation of treatment response and follow-up (treatment adjustment). Clinical judgment should not be used in place of standardized assessment, but rather to reduce the limitations inherent in such measures. Although the situations described in the ESS are common, they are not always relevant for a given patient. Some patients may be frequent passengers in a car while for others this may be a rare occurrence. Other items such as watching TV or reading may produce similar limitations of assessment in certain patients. With situational measures aimed at identifying behaviors indicative of excessive sleepiness, not endorsing a particular item may simply mean that the patient does not regularly or ever engage in such behavior. It is the clinician's responsibility to assess this potential limitation in each patient while retaining the value of the normative data available. If the clinician is aware, for example, of a patient falling asleep at the wheel, and the ESS score is well below 10, there still remains an obvious case for intervention despite the lack of ESS evidence. Conversely, a patient with a severe ESS score may have misinterpreted instructions; the assessment may be confounded by a fatigue-related disorder, cultural differences in the response to items, or masking effects. Indeed, large studies have demonstrated that racial/ethnic differences are present in subjective measures of sleepiness [35].

Patients commonly use terms such as "fatigue", "tiredness" and numerous other descriptors to convey

6. Subjective measures

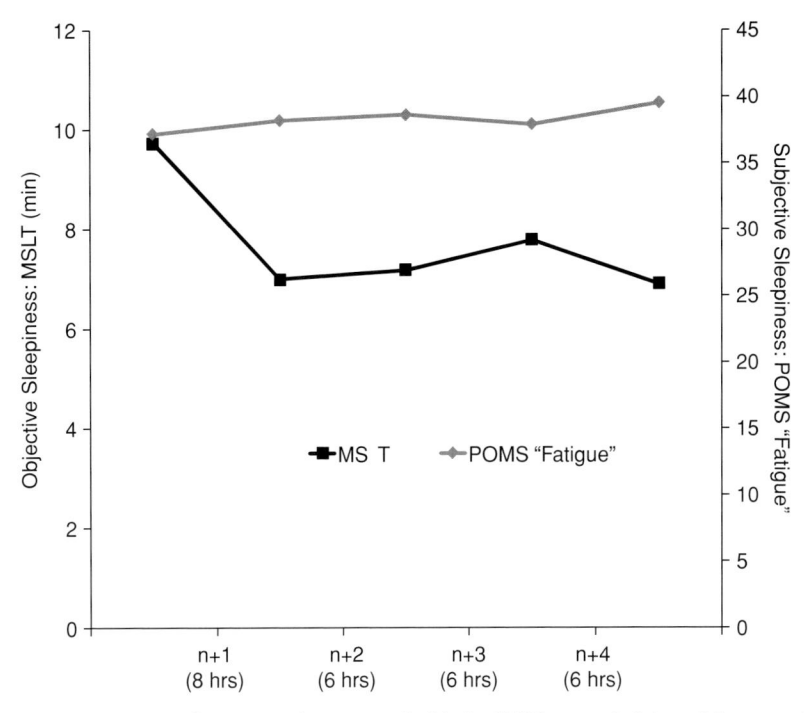

Figure 6.1 POMS "fatigue" scale compared with the MSLT across 4 nights of sleep restriction (6 h).
Data were obtained from a study comparing rapid to slow sleep loss where physiological measures of sleepiness, cognitive performance (memory and psychomotor functioning), and subjective ratings of sleepiness were obtained several times per day during rapid (total sleep loss) moderate (4 h per night) and slow (6 h per night) sleep loss. The same subjects completed each of the conditions controlling for potential individual differences in sleep need. During the 4-h sleep restriction condition, subjects were able to detect increasing sleepiness which was also present on the MSLT (data not shown). Starting after 1 night of sleep restricted to 6 h the MSLT showed a significant decline (increased sleepiness) while subjective sleepiness as assessed by the POMS did not change across the 4-night restriction period, indicating an inability of subjects to detect physiological sleepiness. These data also suggest that *desensitization* of subjective sleepiness is more likely to occur when sleep is lost slowly (reductions of only 1–2 h per night).

the feeling state of sleepiness. The extensive number of terms used to describe sleepiness, and the knowledge that patients may exaggerate or minimize symptoms by falsifying responses to circumvent or elicit treatment, emphasizes the need for standardized assessment. Nonetheless, quantification of sleepiness and combining such measures with excellent history-taking and sound clinical judgment is paramount. For example, the subjective experience of sleepiness involves a constellation of physical and mental symptoms (sleeping in the waiting room, nodding, yawning, eye rubbing, heaviness in the limbs, disruptions of thought, attention, and memory processes, etc.), and these may be differentially experienced by patients and conspicuously absent from standardized questionnaires. In such cases, inquiring about additional sleepiness-related experiences, such as dozing off while driving or at work, improves the ability to identify sleepiness and minimize false negatives. As most individuals attribute their sleepiness to external variables (warm room, boring conversation, dull book, etc.), asking the patient what makes you feel sleepy is often helpful. In addition, the data reviewed regarding the objective–subjective discrepancies show that if standardized assessments are utilized, they may be most informative when assayed across time within a given patient to identify the effects of treatment or reveal other temporal changes in disease state.

One of the most challenging problems in the assessment of subjective sleepiness is differentiating it from feeling fatigue [25]. Although these are separate constructs, patients often confuse sleepiness with fatigue and the terms are often used interchangeably by patients, clinicians, and researchers. Indeed, the study of sleepiness in transportation is commonly and inappropriately described as "fatigue" research. If these descriptors are not differentiated by experts in the field, one can likewise expect limited distinctions by patients. A useful approach to clinically determining if a patient with a presentation of "fatigue" is truly sleepy is to inquire about their tendency to sleep in any sedentary situations they have been specifically exposed to recently. Patients with mental, depression, or muscle-related fatigue – *without sleepiness* – will often respond that sedentary situations improve or attenuate their symptoms. In contrast, patients with excessive sleepiness typically report that sedentary situations exacerbate their symptoms of "fatigue" and find it difficult to stay awake. This is analogous to the *unmasking* of physiological sleep tendency.

People with insomnia often endorse subjective feelings of sleepiness (see Chapter 16). However, there are numerous studies demonstrating an absence of objective sleepiness in people with insomnia. Although individuals with primary insomnia experience hyperarousal and are not sleepy on objective measures, large community-based samples have shown that people with insomnia report higher levels of sleepiness compared to people without insomnia as assessed by the ESS [36]. Thus, it remains possible this reflects differences in primary and comorbid insomnia, with the latter more likely to show signs of sleepiness. However, it seems more parsimonious that subjective measures of sleepiness are more likely to reflect the additional experience of fatigue commonly endorsed by insomnia patients [37]. A potential advantage of the ESS in the clinical setting is that false positives induced by other states such as fatigue may be somewhat less likely with the Epworth relative to mood/judgment-based measures because specific situations related to sleep propensity are assessed rather than a subjective feeling state. A study in 283 sleep disorder patients supports this possibility, as the ESS measure of subjective sleepiness was only weakly correlated with a validated subjective measure of fatigue ($r = .18$) despite high reports of fatigue in the sample [38].

Subjective sleepiness in children

Children present with a variety of sleep disorders associated with excessive sleepiness. Similar to adults, the most common cause of excessive sleepiness in this population is insufficient sleep, particularly as sleep requirements are higher for children. In contrast to adults, however, children with excessive sleepiness may show symptoms of hyperactivity rather than complaints of sleepiness or fatigue. Thus, the use of standardized measures is of considerable importance in pediatric populations. The ESS has been modified for use in children by omitting mention of alcohol from item 7 and indicating that the individual is a passenger in the car for item 8 [39], but measures specifically designed for this age group have also been developed. Space limitations prevent a comprehensive review of subjective sleepiness in children in the present chapter (see [40] for a review, and Chapter 24); however, the most commonly used measures of subjective sleepiness (self-report and parents' report) for this population are reviewed below.

School Sleep Habits Survey (sleepiness scale)

One of the first sleepiness scales to be developed for use in children is a subscale of the larger School Sleep Habits Survey [41,42]. The sleepiness scale is a 10-item measure which inquires about the struggle to stay awake or actually falling asleep in a number of common situations experienced by adolescents (e.g. in school, watching television). This scale is completed by adolescents themselves and has been shown to be elevated in those with reduced total sleep time as well as those with a weekend delay in bedtimes.

Pediatric Sleep Questionnaire, Sleepiness Subscale (PSQ-SS)

The PSQ-SS is a four-item parent-completed questionnaire that can be used to measure subjective sleepiness in children [43]. This is a subscale of a larger 22-item sleep questionnaire, the PSQ. To our knowledge this is the only pediatric sleepiness scale that has been validated against the MSLT in children [44]. However, similar to adults, the correlations between measures were low in a sample of children scheduled for adenotonsillectomy for suspected sleep-disordered breathing ($r = -0.23, p = .006$).

Pediatric Daytime Sleepiness Scale (PDSS)

The Pediatric Daytime Sleepiness Scale (PDSS) is a validated self-report measure of sleepiness specifically designed for use in school-aged children and can be completed in a few minutes [45]. Similar to the ESS, this measure was designed to reflect the general propensity for sleep in a variety of situations. This eight-item scale has excellent psychometric properties and normative data are available. Internal consistency (i.e. reliability) for each of two split-half samples was 0.80 and 0.81. The sum of the final eight items make up the total scale score (item 3 is reversed). The PDSS has been translated into several languages and data from multinational samples have been collected [46]. This measure is sensitive to variations in habitual sleep duration [45]. The PDSS is elevated in adolescents with narcolepsy and is sensitive to the effects of treatment with sodium oxybate [47]. Data for samples reflecting sleep-disordered breathing have also been collected and the PDSS total score has been validated against known risk factors for sleep apnea in more than 2800 middle-school/high-school students [46]. In addition, adverse school outcomes (poor grades) have also been measured and show an association with PDSS scores, an effect which has been replicated in multiple samples [45,46]. Importantly, for every one point increase in sleepiness as measured by the PDSS, a 5% increase in the risk of course failure for both math and literature has been demonstrated [46].

Conclusions and future directions

The advantages of self-report measures of sleepiness include their low cost, ease and speed of administration, simple interpretation, and wide availability. Their limitations include increased measurement error, susceptibility to transient masking effects, discordance with objective measures, limited sensitivity and specificity for detecting sleepiness in sleep disorders including insomnia, and susceptibility to being confused with other mood states such as fatigue and depression. Important aspects of each of these strengths and limitations are present to varying degrees depending on the measure of subjective sleepiness used. The most widely used measure of sleepiness, the ESS, may be most useful for the evaluation and treatment of sleep disorders, whereas the use of the older but effective VAS is practical and useful in a variety of research contexts where serial measurement of sleepiness is required.

Due to frequent low concordance of self-report with objective measurement of sleepiness, even effective self-report measures are not likely to supplant the objective measurement of sleepiness in clinical or research settings in the near future. However, the continued development of subjective measures which more closely reflect objective indices of sleepiness is an important aim for future research. Subjective and objective measures of sleepiness differ in important ways, and one question is the degree to which each may be independently related to specific types of functional outcomes. For example, it appears that objective measures of sleepiness such as the MSLT are better predictors of accident risk relative to subjective measures of sleepiness; however, subjective sleepiness may be a more useful indicator of poor quality of life or therapy-seeking. Subjective sleepiness is also critical as it is often the initial symptom of underlying sleep pathology, and a major presenting complaint that clinicians must understand and address. As patients may minimize symptoms, in cases where subjective measures indicate a low level of sleepiness, but disease severity suggests a high potential for accident risk, objective measurement of sleepiness should be obtained. Thus, both subjective and objective measures are important to assess and their potential independent contributions in research settings and in the context of patient evaluations is certainly worthy of further study. Individuals differ in the degree to which they tolerate and mask sleepiness and studies of these factors as well as the desensitization of subjective sleepiness over time are important areas for future study. More work is also needed on potential cultural and racial differences in subjective sleepiness and in relation to specific types of measurement. It has been shown that subjective sleepiness is accompanied by EEG changes including selective slowing of specific frequency bands. Thus, the possibility that sleepiness is at times a form of sleep and may be an important restorative process should also be investigated in controlled studies. Finally, a recent study has shown that the subjective rating of sleepiness is in part genetically determined, with a 38% heritability estimate, further demonstrating that subjective sleepiness is a state with valuable biological underpinnings that are likely important for the survival and success of our species [48].

Acknowledgments

The author would like to thank Elise Fazio, Fan Zhang, and Drs. Thomas Roth and Timothy Roehrs for their helpful comments on this manuscript.

References

1. **Everson C A**, **Bergmann B M**, **Rechtschaffen A**. Sleep deprivation in the rat: III. Total sleep deprivation. *Sleep*, 1989; **12**:13–21.

2. **Bemiss S M**, **Benson J W**. Death from want of sleep. *Semi-Monthly Med News*, 1859; **1**:54.

3. **Kryger M H**. History of sleep medicine and physiology. In: Kryger M, Ed. *Atlas of Clinical Sleep Medicine*. Philadelphia: Saunders, 2010: 8–19.

4. **Avicenna**. *The Cannon of Medicine*. Chicago: KAZI, 1999 [1025].

5. **Patrick G T W**, **Gilbert J A**. Studies from the psychological laboratory of the University of Iowa: on the effects of loss of sleep. *Psychol Rev*, 1896; **3**:469–83.

6. **Dement W C**. *Sleep and Dreams* (1st Ed.). Stanford: REM Productions, 1993.

7. **Hoddes E**, **Zarcone V**, **Smythe H**, *et al*. Quantification of sleepiness: a new approach. *Psychophysiology*, 1973; **10**:431–36.

8. **Johns M W**. A new method for measuring daytime sleepiness: the Epworth sleepiness scale. *Sleep*, 1991; **14**:540–45.

9. **Monk T H**. A Visual Analogue Scale technique to measure global vigor and affect. *Psychiatry Res*, 1989; **27**:89–99.

10. **McNair D M**, **Lorr M**, **Droppleman L F**. *Manual Profile of Mood States*. Educational & Industrial testing service, 1971.

11. **Reynolds C F**, 3rd, **Kupfer D J**, **Hoch C C**, *et al*. Sleep deprivation in healthy elderly men and women: effects on mood and on sleep during recovery. *Sleep*, 1986; **9**:492–501.

12. **Drake C L**, **Roehrs T A**, **Burduvali E**, *et al*. Effects of rapid versus slow accumulation of eight hours of sleep loss. *Psychophysiology*, 2001; **38**:979–87.

13. **Drake C L**, **Roehrs T**, **Turner L**, *et al*. Caffeine reversal of ethanol effects on the multiple sleep latency test, memory, and psychomotor performance. *Neuropsychopharmacology*, 2003; **28**:371–78.

14. **Carskadon M A**, **Dement W C**. The multiple sleep latency test: what does it measure? *Sleep*, 1982; **5**(Suppl 2):S67–72.

15. **Broughton R J**. Sleep attacks, naps and sleepiness in medical sleep disorders. In: Dinges D, Broughton RJ, Eds. *Sleep and Alertness: Chronobiological, Behavioural and Medical Aspects of Napping*. New York, NY: Raven Press, 1989: 267–98.

16. **Wright K P**, Jr., **Badia P**, **Myers B L**, *et al*. Combination of bright light and caffeine as a countermeasure for impaired alertness and performance during extended sleep deprivation. *J Sleep Res*, 1997; **6**:26–35.

17. **MacLean A W**, **Fekken G C**, **Saskin P**, *et al*. Psychometric evaluation of the Stanford Sleepiness Scale. *J Sleep Res*, 1992; **1**:35–39.

18. **Dement W C**, **Carskadon M A**, **Richardson G**. Excessive daytime sleepiness in the sleep apnea syndrome. In: Guilleminault C, Dement WC, Eds. *Sleep Apnea Syndromes: Proceedings*. New York, NY: Liss, 1978: 23–46.

19. **Sauter C**, **Asenbaum S**, **Popovic R**, *et al*. Excessive daytime sleepiness in patients suffering from different levels of obstructive sleep apnoea syndrome. *J Sleep Res*, 2000; **9**:293–301.

20. **Akerstedt T**, **Gillberg M**. Subjective and objective sleepiness in the active individual. *Int J Neurosci*, 1990; **52**:29–37.

21. **Horne JA**, **Baulk SD**. Awareness of sleepiness when driving. *Psychophysiology*, 2004; **41**:161–65.

22. **Ingre M**, **Akerstedt T**, **Peters B**, *et al*. Subjective sleepiness and accident risk avoiding the ecological fallacy. *J Sleep Res*, 2006; **15**:142–48.

23. **Czeisler CA**, **Walsh JK**, **Wesnes KA**, *et al*. Armodafinil for treatment of excessive sleepiness associated with shift work disorder: a randomized controlled study. *Mayo Clin Proc*, 2009; **84**:958–72.

24. **Akerstedt T**, **Kecklund G**, **Axelsson J**. Effects of context on sleepiness self-ratings during repeated partial sleep deprivation. *Chronobiol Int*, 2008; **25**:271–78.

25. **Watson N F**, **Jacobsen C**, **Goldberg J**, *et al*. Subjective and objective sleepiness in monozygotic twins discordant for chronic fatigue syndrome. *Sleep*, 2004; **27**:973–77.

26. **Yang C M**, **Lin F W**, **Spielman A J**. A standard procedure enhances the correlation between subjective and objective measures of sleepiness. *Sleep*, 2004; **27**:329–32.

27. **Short M**, **Lack L**, **Wright H**. Does subjective sleepiness predict objective sleep propensity? *Sleep*, 2010; **33**:123–29.

28. **Johns M W**. Reliability and factor analysis of the Epworth Sleepiness Scale. *Sleep*, 1992; **15**:376–81.

29. **Nguyen A T**, **Baltzan M A**, **Small D**, *et al*. Clinical reproducibility of the Epworth Sleepiness Scale. *J Clin Sleep Med*, 2006; **2**:170–74.

30. **Black J E**, **Hirshkowitz M**. Modafinil for treatment of residual excessive sleepiness in nasal continuous positive airway pressure-treated obstructive sleep apnea/hypopnea syndrome. *Sleep*, 2005; **28**:464–71.

31. **Pilcher J J**, **Pury C L**, **Muth E R**. Assessing subjective daytime sleepiness: an internal state versus behavior approach. *Behav Med* 2003; **29**:60–67.

32. **Chervin R D**, **Aldrich M S**, **Pickett R**, *et al*. Comparison of the results of the Epworth Sleepiness Scale and the Multiple Sleep Latency Test. *J Psychosom Res*, 1997; **42**:145–55.

33. **Drake C L**, **Roehrs T**, **Breslau N**, *et al*. The 10-year risk of verified motor vehicle crashes in relation to physiologic sleepiness. *Sleep*, 2010; **33**:745–52.

34. **Van Dongen H P**, **Maislin G**, **Mullington J M**, *et al*. The cumulative cost of additional wakefulness: dose–response effects on neurobehavioral functions and sleep physiology from chronic sleep restriction and total sleep deprivation. *Sleep*, 2003; **26**: 117–26.

35. **Gander P H**, **Marshall N S**, **Harris R**, *et al*. The Epworth Sleepiness Scale: influence of age, ethnicity, and socioeconomic deprivation. Epworth Sleepiness scores of adults in New Zealand. *Sleep*, 2005; **28**:249–53.

36. **Sanford S D**, **Lichstein K L**, **Durrence H H**, *et al*. The influence of age, gender, ethnicity, and insomnia on Epworth sleepiness scores: a normative US population. *Sleep Med*, 2006; **7**:319–26.

37. **Moul D E**, **Nofzinger E A**, **Pilkonis P A**, *et al*. Symptom reports in severe chronic insomnia. *Sleep*, 2002; **25**:553–63.

38. **Hossain J L**, **Ahmad P**, **Reinish L W**, *et al*. Subjective fatigue and subjective sleepiness: two independent consequences of sleep disorders? *J Sleep Res*, 2005; **14**:245–53.

39. **Melendres M C**, **Lutz J M**, **Rubin E D**, *et al*. Daytime sleepiness and hyperactivity in children with suspected sleep-disordered breathing. *Pediatrics*, 2004; **114**:768–75.

40. **Fallone G**, **Owens J A**, **Deane J**. Sleepiness in children and adolescents: clinical implications. *Sleep Med Rev*, 2002; **6**:287–306.

41. **Wolfson A R**, **Carskadon M A**. Sleep schedules and daytime functioning in adolescents. *Child Dev*, 1998; **69**:875–87.

42. **Wolfson A R**, **Carskadon M A**, **Acebo C**, *et al*. Evidence for the validity of a sleep habits survey for adolescents. *Sleep*, 2003; **26**:213–16.

43. **Chervin R D**, **Hedger K**, **Dillon J E**, *et al*. Pediatric sleep questionnaire (PSQ): validity and reliability of scales for sleep-disordered breathing, snoring, sleepiness, and behavioral problems 1. *Sleep Med*, 2000; **1**:21–32.

44. **Chervin R D**, **Weatherly R A**, **Ruzicka D L**, *et al*. Subjective sleepiness and polysomnographic correlates in children scheduled for adenotonsillectomy vs other surgical care. *Sleep*, 2006; **29**:495–503.

45. **Drake C**, **Nickel C**, **Burduvali E**, *et al*. The pediatric daytime sleepiness scale (PDSS): sleep habits and school outcomes in middle-school children. *Sleep*, 2003; **26**:455–58.

46. **Perez-Chada D**, **Perez-Lloret S**, **Videla A J**, *et al*. Sleep disordered breathing and daytime sleepiness are associated with poor academic performance in teenagers. A study using the Pediatric Daytime Sleepiness Scale (PDSS). *Sleep*, 2007; **30**:1698–703.

47. **Huang Y S**, **Guilleminault C**. Narcolepsy: action of two gamma-aminobutyric acid type B agonists, baclofen and sodium oxybate. *Pediatr Neurol*, 2009; **41**:9–16.

48. **Watson N F**, **Goldberg J**, **Arguelles L**, *et al*. Genetic and environmental influences on insomnia, daytime sleepiness, and obesity in twins. *Sleep*, 2006; **29**:645–49.

49. **Johns M**, **Hocking B**. Daytime sleepiness and sleep habits of Australian workers. *Sleep*, 1997; **20**:844–49.

50. **Rodrigues R N**, **Viegas C A**, **Abreu E S A A**, *et al*. Daytime sleepiness and academic performance in medical students. *Arq Neuropsiquiatr*, 2002; **60**:6–11.

51. **Johns M W**. Daytime sleepiness, snoring, and obstructive sleep apnea. The Epworth Sleepiness Scale. *Chest*, 1993; **103**:30–36.

52. **Chen S Y**, **Clift S J**, **Dahlitz M J**, *et al*. Treatment in the narcoleptic syndrome: self assessment of the action of dexamphetamine and clomipramine. *J Sleep Res*, 1995; **4**:113–18.

53. **Jama L**, **Hirvonen K**, **Partinen M**, *et al*. A dose-ranging study of pramipexole for the symptomatic treatment of restless legs syndrome: polysomnographic evaluation of periodic leg movements and sleep disturbance. *Sleep Med*, 2009; **10**:630–36.

54. **Scofield H**, **Roth T**, **Drake C**. Periodic limb movements during sleep: population prevalence, clinical correlates, and racial differences. *Sleep*, 2008;**31**:1221–27.

55. **Means M K**, **Lichstein K L**, **Epperson M T**, *et al*. Relaxation therapy for insomnia: nighttime and day-time effects. *Behav Res Ther*, 2000; **38**:665–78.

56. **Ali M**, **Auger R**, **Slocumb N L**, *et al*. Idiopathic hypersomnia: clinical features and response to treatment. *J Clin Sleep Med*, 2009; **5**:562–68.

57. **Gaspar-Barba E**, **Calati R**, **Cruz-Fuentes C S**, *et al*. Depressive symptomatology is influenced by chronotypes. *J Affect Disord*, 2009; **119**:100–06.

58. **Sarzi-Puttini P**, **Rizzi M**, **Andreoli A**, *et al*. Hypersomnolence in fibromyalgia syndrome. *Clin Exp Rheumatol*, 2002; **20**:69–72.

59. **Gjerstad M D**, **Alves G**, **Wentzel-Larsen T**, *et al*. Excessive daytime sleepiness in Parkinson disease: is it the drugs or the disease? *Neurology*, 2006; **67**:853–58.

1. Introduction

vulnerable to sleepiness because of their dependence on the PFC.

Another complication arising from the available literature on executive functioning in the context of sleepiness is the heterogeneity of tasks that have been used for performance testing. Any given executive functions performance task is likely to tap multiple executive-type cognitive processes [44]. Moreover, non-executive cognitive processes such as stimulus encoding and motor response are also involved in task performance, and may contribute critically to the effect of sleepiness on task performance (the "task impurity" problem [45]). For example, performance degradation on a Sternberg working memory task after 51 h of total sleep deprivation was shown to be associated with delays in non-executive cognitive processes, whereas the executive functions processes of working memory scanning efficiency and resistance to proactive interference remained intact [46] (see Figure 7.5). Thus, the impact of sleepiness on executive functions performance tasks may be attributable to non-executive aspects of the tasks, and not the executive components that the tasks are claimed to assay.

An understudied facet of executive functioning performance in sleepy individuals is the role of mood and affect. Decision-making, an important aspect of executive functioning, often involves emotional processing and bias [47]. The emotional states of individuals can affect their decision-making in helpful or harmful ways depending on the situation. It has been found that negative affect can lead to more risk-taking behaviors, whereas positive affect can lead to more risk-averse behaviors [48]. Sleepiness has the potential to alter emotional states [49] and bias the interpretation of the emotional context of a situation, and may thereby influence decision-making [11]. The implications for real-world operational situations could be profound. For instance, in policing and military operations, risky decisions with potentially costly consequences are made in emotionally charged circumstances, often under conditions of sleep restriction; and sleepiness has at least anecdotally been implicated in police decision errors with deadly outcomes [50].

Learning and memory

Poor memory is a common complaint of people who do not obtain adequate sleep. Learning and long-term memory have been found experimentally to be linked to sleep [51]. Long-term memory is under-

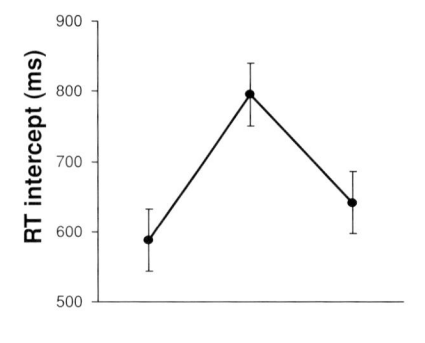

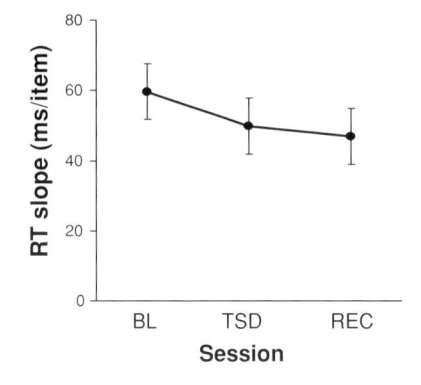

Figure 7.5 Performance degradation on a Sternberg task during sleep deprivation is attributable to non-executive cognitive processes. In the Sternberg task [80], subjects are shown a set of items to be held in working memory, and then a probe item. They respond by indicating whether or not the probe item was in the memory set. The number of items in the memory set is varied across trials, and the linear relationship between the number of items and subjects' reaction times (RT) is analyzed. The top panel shows the intercept of this relationship, which measures non-executive cognitive processes involved in performing the task. The bottom panel shows the slope of the linear relationship, which measures a process of executive functioning referred to as working memory scanning efficiency. Means±standard errors are shown for 12 healthy adults tested in a laboratory during baseline (BL), after 51 h of total sleep deprivation (TSD), and following two nights of recovery sleep (REC). Only the non-executive cognitive processes involved in performing the Sternberg task were adversely affected (delayed) by sleepiness induced by sleep deprivation. Figure adapted from Tucker et al. [46], with permission.

stood to evolve over three primary stages of processing: encoding, consolidation, and recall and recognition. Research on memory in the context of sleepiness has focused mostly on these three stages. Other stages of long-term memory processing, including association, reactivation and reconsolidation, have received scant experimental attention in sleep and sleepiness research and are therefore not discussed here.

Memory encoding, or the conversion of sensory input into a neural representation, appears to be adversely affected by lack of prior sleep [52]. The ability

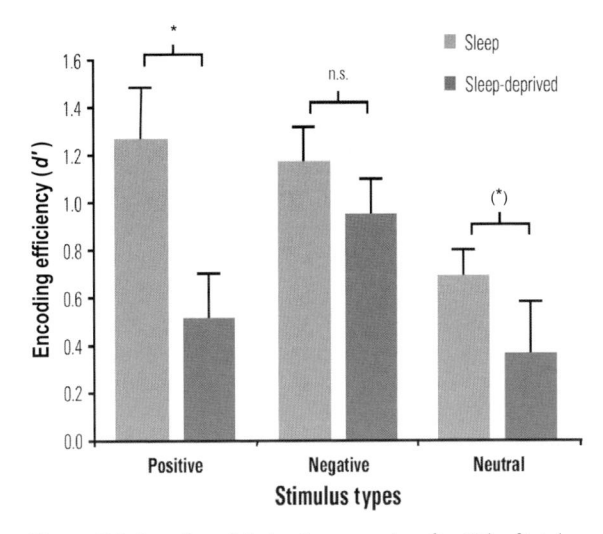

Figure 7.6 Encoding of declarative memories after 38 h of total sleep deprivation, compared to baseline, by emotional valence (positive, negative and neutral). Means and standard errors (error bars) are shown for 36 subjects. At baseline, encoding efficiency as measured with d' (average recognition level) was higher for positive and negative emotional memories than for non-emotional memories. After sleep deprivation, relative to baseline, memory encoding was significantly impaired for positive stimuli (with a trend toward significance for neutral stimuli), but not for negative stimuli. Figure adapted from figure 4 in the monograph "Neurocognitive, executive, and behavioral impairment in sleep/wake disorders: mechanisms, interindividual differences, and ongoing management" (Simon Jr R, Thorpy M, Van Dongen H P A, Walker M), after Walker and Stickgold [52], with permission. *$P<0.01$; (*)$P<0.08$; n.s., non-significant.

to encode verbal [42, 46] and visual [53] information has been found to be impaired by experimentally induced sleep loss. Neuroimaging studies have further revealed that during encoding of episodic (declarative autobiographical) information, significant reduction in activation of the hippocampus – a region known to be critical for learning new episodic memories – is observed after one night of sleep deprivation, associated with a decline in encoding ability [54]. The findings suggest that adequate sleep prior to learning is needed for the proper functioning of brain regions involved in encoding new memories. However, negative emotional stimuli seem to be relatively resistant to encoding impairment from prior sleep loss, as compared to positive stimuli [52, 55] (see Figure 7.6). As a consequence, sleep insufficiency may produce a negative learning bias, which may have implications for downstream processes, including decision-making (see above). This may also help to explain the higher rates of comorbid mood disorder in patients with sleep disorders, such as OSA [56].

Sleep *after* the encoding process is also believed to be important for memory formation. Following the encoding of new input, a set of complex processes occurs in the brain, which enhances and stabilizes the initial memory trace. This consolidation process involves reprocessing of memory traces, which facilitates later recall of the information. Sleep is one mechanism that allows for neuronal restructuring and memory consolidation [52]. Sleep may even facilitate gaining non-obvious insights from previously acquired information, such as a hidden pattern in the correct responses of a cognitive task [57]. Conversely, deprivation of sleep has been repeatedly documented to disrupt the consolidation of procedural memory (i.e. memory for motor tasks and perceptual skills). For example, total or partial sleep deprivation has been reported to impair retention of motor adaptation tasks, motor sequence learning, and visual textural learning [58]. These effects are typically modest in magnitude, but it is possible that chronic sleep insufficiency would result in substantial procedural memory deficiency over time.

There is less clarity about the ability to consolidate declarative (fact) information, rather than procedural information, in the face of sleepiness. Patients suffering from sleepiness as a consequence of chronic insomnia have been reported to display impairments in the consolidation of declarative memories [59]. However, whether this observation implies that sleep is an active promoter of declarative memory consolidation is not firmly established. Sleep may also confer passive benefits for consolidation, such as blocking external stimuli that could otherwise interfere with the memory trace [60]. Nonetheless, regardless of the explanation, adequate sleep after learning appears to be no less important for successful memory formation than adequate sleep before learning.

For discussing the effects of sleepiness on the final stage of memory, recall and recognition, it is important to distinguish recognition from free recall. As a case in point, in the rested state, free recall of episodic memory is believed to be associated with the PFC, whereas recognition of episodic memory relies on the medial temporal regions and the thalamus [61]. Perhaps due to the difference in underlying neural pathways, recall of declarative information under conditions of sleep deprivation is often shown to be impaired, whereas recognition memory appears to be less vulnerable to sleepiness [20, 62]. For instance, recall, but not recognition, of temporal memory (i.e. the ability to

1. Introduction

remember when an event occurred) [63, 64] and verbal items [65] has been shown to be impaired by prior sleep loss. For procedural memory, it is not a-priori clear how recall and recognition should be defined, beyond how the procedural task is carried out. Therefore, whereas procedural learning is significantly impaired in sleep-deprived subjects [66] and OSA patients [67], it is difficult to attribute that impairment unequivocally to a specific memory stage.

The difficulty of linking observed impairments in task performance to the recall and recognition stage of memory is not only encountered in procedural memory, but also in declarative memory. The reason is that problems with recall and recognition may also be due to prior difficulties encoding or consolidating the information. Patient populations are typically as sleepy and impaired during encoding and consolidation of memories as they are during recall or recognition, making it difficult to differentiate the source(s) of reported memory problems. In OSA patients, common verbal memory recall deficits (e.g. not recalling names and phone numbers [67, 68]) could be related to OSA-associated morphological changes within the hippocampus [69], possibly resulting from long-term intermittent hypoxia [70].

Whether or not sleepiness affects memory recall and recognition directly, there is little doubt that sleepiness interferes with the normal sequence of encoding, consolidation and recall, and as such may lead to long-term memory impairment and forgetfulness. This may have far-reaching consequences early in life – neurocognitive abilities and academic performance are lower in school children that have poor sleep quality and/or quantity and experience daytime sleepiness compared to those that do not [71]. This has prompted some regions in the USA to delay school start times to allow adolescents to sleep longer, which has had a positive influence on academic performance [72].

Despite the growing literature asserting a critical role for sleep in learning and memory, the effects of sleepiness on the underlying mechanisms are still relatively poorly understood. Significant deficits in encoding following sleep loss have been reported for memory tasks [52, 53, 55]; however, whether performance impairment on these tasks can be attributed solely to deficits in encoding – as distinct from recall – has not been convincingly demonstrated. Several brain regions activated during performance of memory tasks overlap those associated with attentional processes [73]. For instance, an fMRI study revealed increased functional connectivity between the hippocampus and vigilance networks of the thalamus and brainstem during sleep deprivation relative to baseline [55], which could be interpreted as evidence of an elevated need for attentional control on learning when sleepy. This raises the interesting possibility that deficits in memory formation in the face of sleepiness may be due to failure to direct attention to the information to be learned, rather than in memory encoding or consolidation processes per se. Likewise, performance tasks used to test the quality of memory formation following sleep deprivation may show reduced recall rates because of sleepiness-based attentional deficits impeding performance on such tasks, instead of genuine memory deficits.

Other methodological issues present additional potential confounds in the sleep-related literature on learning and memory. For example, motor sequence learning has been shown to improve after sleep, suggesting a sleep-specific memory benefit – but when time of day, practice effects and build-up of fatigue across the day were controlled for, no sleep-related learning enhancement remained [74]. Methodologically more rigorous studies are needed to better understand the effects of sleep and sleepiness on long-term memory.

Conclusion

Sleepiness has wide-ranging adverse consequences for attention and vigilance, executive functioning, and learning and memory. The available evidence is most extensive for sleepiness induced by sleep deprivation and by OSA, and more sporadic and mixed for sleepiness associated with insomnia [75] and other sleep disorders [20]. Importantly, the effects of sleepiness are not homogeneous across and within different cognitive domains [62]. Furthermore, there appear to be remarkable inconsistencies in the published literature in this area. This issue has been broadly overlooked or misinterpreted as a mere side-effect of differences among cognitive performance assays in sensitivity to sleepiness. It is true that sensitivity/specificity, signal-to-noise-ratio and other psychometric properties of cognitive tasks – as well as a variety of confounding factors such as task difficulty, practice effects and speed/accuracy trade-off [6] – play an important role in task responsiveness to varying levels of sleepiness. Yet, ignoring all inter-task variability in sleepiness effects on this basis would disregard potentially insightful information about the neurobiological mechanisms underlying sleepiness and cognition.

The heterogeneity of the cognitive effects of sleepiness is at least partly due to the "task impurity" problem [45], which refers to the intertwined involvement of multiple cognitive processes during performance of a task. Sleepiness may affect these cognitive processes differentially, so that the effects of sleepiness depend on the ensemble of cognitive processes required to perform the task at hand. However, changes in the individual cognitive processes typically cannot be distinguished in overall task performance, leaving their influence on performance differences between tasks difficult to trace. Cognitive tasks designed specifically to tease apart the effects of sleepiness on distinct cognitive processes are gradually being introduced into sleep research to address this problem [46, 76] (e.g. see Figure 7.5). These efforts contribute to the development of a theoretical framework for understanding the effects of sleepiness on cognitive performance and its underlying mechanisms, which one day will allow us to make precise predictions about the impact of sleepiness on specific cognitive performance tasks in the laboratory and, ultimately, about the occurrence of errors, incidents and accidents due to sleepiness in the real world [77–79].

References

1. **Yerkes R M**, **Dodson J D**. The relation of strength of stimulus to rapidity of habit formation. *J Comp Neurol Psychol*, 1908; **18**:459–82.
2. **Patrick G T W**, **Gilbert J A**. Studies from the psychological laboratory of the University of Iowa: on the effects of loss of sleep. *Psych Rev*, 1896; **3**:469–83.
3. **Monk T H**, **Carrier J**. Speed of mental processing in the middle of the night. *Sleep*, 1997; **20**:399–401.
4. **Durmer J S**, **Dinges D F**. Neurocognitive consequences of sleep deprivation. *Semin Neurol*, 2005; **25**:117–29.
5. **Young P T**. *Motivation of Behavior*. London: Wiley, 1936.
6. **Van Dongen H P A**, **Dinges D F**. Circadian rhythms in sleepiness, alertness, and performance. In: Kryger M H, Roth T, Dement W C, Eds. *Principles and Practice of Sleep Medicine* (4th Ed.). Philadelphia, PA: Elsevier Saunders, 2005: 435–43.
7. **Van Dongen H P A**, **Vitellaro K M**, **Dinges D F**. Individual differences in adult human sleep and wakefulness: leitmotif for a research agenda. *Sleep*, 2005; **28**:479–96.
8. **Balkin T**, **Bliese P**, **Belenky G**, et al. Comparative utility of instruments for monitoring sleepiness-related performance decrements in the operational environment. *J Sleep Res*. 2004; **13**:219–27.
9. **Lim J**, **Dinges D F**. Sleep deprivation and vigilant attention. *Ann NY Acad Sci*, 2008; **1129**:305–22.
10. **Harrison Y**, **Horne J A**, **Rothwell A**. Prefrontal neuropsychological effects of sleep deprivation in young adults – a model for healthy aging? *Sleep*, 2000; **23**:1067–73.
11. **Harrison Y**, **Horne J A**. The impact of sleep deprivation on decision making: a review. *J Exp Psych A*, 2000; **6**:236–49.
12. **Jones K**, **Harrison Y**. Frontal lobe function, sleep loss and fragmented sleep. *Sleep Med Rev*, 2001; **5**:463–75.
13. **Doran S M**, **Van Dongen H P A**, **Dinges D F**. Sustained attention performance during sleep deprivation: evidence of state instability. *Arch Ital Biol*, 2001; **139**:253–67.
14. **Williams H**, **Lubin A**, **Goodnow J**. Impaired performance with acute sleep loss. *Psych Monogr Gen Appl*, 1959; **73**:1–23.
15. **Dinges DF**, **Mallis M**, **Maislin G**, et al. Evaluation of techniques for ocular measurement as an index of fatigue and as a basis for alertness management. *Technical report DOT HS 808 762*. Washington, DC: US Department of Transportation, 1998.
16. **Wierwille W W**, **Ellsworth L A**. Evaluation of driver drowsiness by trained raters. *Accid Anal Prev*, 1994; **26**:571–81.
17. **Cajochen C**, **Khalsa S B**, **Wyatt J K**, et al. EEG and ocular correlates of circadian melatonin phase and human performance decrements during sleep loss. *Am J Physiol*, 1999; **277**:R640–49.
18. **Howard M**, **Gora J**, **Swann P**, **Pierce R**. Alpha and theta activity and slow eye closure are related to driving performance in professional drivers. *Sleep*, 2002; **25**:A148.
19. **Dinges D F**, **Kribbs N B**. Performing while sleepy: effects of experimentally-induced sleepiness. In: Monk T H, Ed. *Sleep, Sleepiness and Performance*. Oxford: John Wiley & Sons, 1991: 97–128.
20. **Fulda S**, **Schulz H**. Cognitive dysfunction in sleep disorders. *Sleep Med Rev*, 2001; **5**:423–45.
21. **Horne J A**, **Pettitt A N**. High incentive effects on vigilance performance during 72 hours of total sleep deprivation. *Acta Psychol*, 1985; **58**:123–39.
22. **Drummond S P A**, **Bischoff-Grethe A**, **Dinges D F**, et al. The neural basis of the psychomotor vigilance task. *Sleep*, 2005; **28**:1059–68.

23. **Chee M W L**, **Tan J C**, **Zheng H**, *et al*. Lapsing during sleep deprivation is associated with distributed changes in brain activation. *J Neurosci*, 2008; **28**:5519–28.

24. **Bills A G**. Blocking: a new principle of mental fatigue. *Am J Psych*, 1931; **43**:230.

25. **Van Dongen H P A**, **Belenky G**. Alertness level. In: Binder M D, Hirokawa N, Windhorst U, Eds. *Encyclopedia of Neuroscience*. Berlin: Springer, 2008: 75–77.

26. **Koslowsky M**, **Babkoff H**. Meta-analysis of the relationship between total sleep deprivation and performance. *Chronobiol Int*, 1992; **9**:132–36.

27. **Van Dongen H P A**, **Belenky G**, **Krueger J M**. Investigating the temporal dynamics and underlying mechanisms of cognitive fatigue. In: Ackerman PL, Ed. *Cognitive Fatigue*. Washington, DC: American Psychological Association; in press.

28. **Krueger J M**, **Rector D M**, **Roy S**, *et al*. Sleep as a fundamental property of neuronal assemblies. *Nat Rev Neurosci*, 2008; **9**:910–19.

29. **Filley C M**. Clinical neurology and executive function. *Semin Speech Lang*, 2002; **21**:95–108.

30. **Horne J**. Neuroscience. Images of lost sleep. *Nature*, 2000; **403**: 605–06.

31. **Tinguely G**, **Finelli L A**, **Landolt H P**, *et al*. Functional EEG topography in sleep and waking: state-dependent and state-independent features. *NeuroImage*, 2006; **32**:283–92.

32. **Thomas M**, **Sing H**, **Belenky G**, *et al*. Neural basis of alertness and cognitive performance impairments during sleepiness. I. Effects of 24 h of sleep deprivation on waking human regional brain activity. *J Sleep Res*, 2000; **9**:335–52.

33. **Wu J C**, **Gillin J C**, **Buchsbaum M S**, *et al*. Frontal lobe metabolic decreases with sleep deprivation not totally reversed by recovery sleep. *Neuropsychopharmacology*, 2006; **31**:2783–92.

34. **Nilsson J P**, **Söderström M**, **Karlsson A U**, *et al*. Less effective executive functioning after one night's sleep deprivation. *J Sleep Res*, 2005; **14**:1–6.

35. **Pace-Schott E F**, **Hutcherson C A**, **Bemporad B**, *et al*. Failure to find executive function deficits following one night's total sleep deprivation in university students under naturalistic conditions. *Behav Sleep Med*, 2009; **7**:136–63.

36. **Venkatraman V**, **Chuah Y**, **Huettel S**, *et al*. Sleep deprivation elevates expectation of gains and attenuates response to losses following risky decisions. *Sleep*, 2007; **30**:603–09.

37. **Beebe D W**, **Gozal D**. Obstructive sleep apnea and the prefrontal cortex: towards a comprehensive model linking nocturnal upper airway obstruction to daytime cognitive and behavioral deficits. *J Sleep Res*, 2002; **11**:1–16.

38. **Macey P M**, **Kumar R**, **Woo M A**, *et al*. Brain structural changes in obstructive sleep apnea. *Sleep*, 2008; **31**:967–77.

39. **Chee M W L**, **Choo W C**. Functional imaging of working memory after 24 hours of total sleep deprivation. *J Neurosci*, 2004; **24**:4560–67.

40. **Chee M**, **Chuah L**, **Venkatraman V**, *et al*. Functional imaging of working memory following normal sleep and after 24 and 35 h of sleep deprivation: correlations of fronto-parietal activation with performance. *NeuroImage*, 2006; **31**:419–28.

41. **Drummond S P A**, **Brown G G**. The effects of total sleep deprivation on cerebral responses to cognitive performance. *Neuropsychopharmacology*, 2001; **25**:S68–73.

42. **Habeck C**, **Rakitin B C**, **Moeller J**, *et al*. An event-related fMRI study of the neurobehavioral impact of sleep deprivation on performance of a delayed-match-to-sample task. *Cog Brain Res*, 2004; **18**:306–21.

43. **Van Dongen, H P A**. Brain activation patterns and individual differences in working memory impairment during sleep deprivation. *Sleep*, 2005; **28**:386–88.

44. **Pennington B F**, **Ozonoff S**. Executive functions and developmental psychopathology. *J Child Psychol Psychiatry*, 1996; **37**:51–87.

45. **Phillips L**. Do "frontal tests" measure executive functions? Issues of assessment and evidence from fluency tests. In: Rabbit P, Ed. *Methodology of Frontal and Executive Function*. Hove: Psychology Press, 1997: 191–213.

46. **Tucker A M**, **Whitney P**, **Belenky G**, *et al*. Effects of sleep deprivation on dissociated components of executive functioning. *Sleep*, 2010; **33**:47–57.

47. **Bechara A**, **Damasio A R**. The somatic marker hypothesis: a neural theory of economic decision. *Games Econ Behav*, 2005; **52**:336–72.

48. **Isen A M**, **Patrick R**. The effect of positive feelings on risk taking: when the chips are down. *Org Behav Human Decision Processes*, 1983; **31**:194–202.

49. **Pilcher J J**, **Huffcutt A I**. Effects of sleep deprivation on performance: a meta-analysis. *Sleep*, 1996; **19**:318–26.

50. **Vila B**. Impact of long work hours on police officers and the communities they serve. *Am J Ind Med*, 2006; **49**:972–80.

51. **Maquet P**. The role of sleep in learning and memory. *Science*, 2001; **294**:1048–52.

52. **Walker M**, **Stickgold R**. Sleep, memory, and plasticity. *Ann Rev Psych*, 2006; **57**:139–66.

53. **Chee M**, **Chuah L**. Functional neuroimaging and behavioural correlates of capacity decline in visual short-term memory after sleep deprivation. *Proc Natl Acad Sci* USA, 2007; **104**:9487–92.

54. **Yoo S**, **Hu P**, **Gujar N**, *et al*. A deficit in the ability to form new human memories without sleep. *Nat Neurosci*, 2007; **10**:385–92.

55. **Yoo S**, **Gujar N**, **Hu P**, *et al*. The human emotional brain without sleep – a prefrontal amygdala disconnect. *Curr Biol*, 2007; **17**:R877–78.

56. **Benca R M**, **Obermeyer W H**, **Thisted R A**, **Gillin J C**. Sleep and psychiatric disorders. a meta-analysis. *Arch Gen Psychiatry*, 1992; **49**:651–68.

57. **Wagner U**, **Gais S**, **Haider H**, *et al*. Sleep inspires insight. *Nature*, 2004; **427**:352–55.

58. **Stickgold R**. Sleep-dependent memory consolidation. *Nature*, 2005; **437**:1272–78.

59. **Backhaus J**, **Junghanns K**, **Born J**, *et al*. Impaired declarative memory consolidation during sleep in patients with primary insomnia: influence of sleep architecture and nocturnal cortisol release. *Biol Psychiatry*, 2006; **60**:1324–30.

60. **Ellenbogen J M**, **Hulbert J C**, **Jiang Y**, *et al*. The sleeping brain's influence on verbal memory: boosting resistance to interference. *PLoS ONE*, 2009; **4**:e4117.

61. **Hwang D Y**, **Golby A J**. The brain basis for episodic memory: insights from functional MRI, intracranial EEG, and patients with epilepsy. *Epilepsy Behav*, 2006; **8**:115–26.

62. **Alhola P**, **Polo-Kantola P**. Sleep deprivation: impact on cognitive performance. *Neuropsych Disease Treat*, 2007; **3**:553–67.

63. **Morris G**, **Williams H**, **Lubin A**. Misperception and disorientation during sleep. *Arch Gen Psychiatry*, 1960; **2**:247–54.

64. **Harrison Y**, **Horne J A**. Sleep loss and temporal memory. *Q J Exp Psych A*, 2000; **53**:271–79.

65. **Drummond S P A**, **Brown G**, **Gillin C**, *et al*. Altered brain response to verbal learning following sleep deprivation. *Nature*, 2000; **403**:655–57.

66. **Smith C**. Sleep states and memory processes in humans: procedural versus declarative memory systems. *Sleep Med Rev*, 2001; **5**:491–506.

67. **Naegele B**, **Launois S**, **Mazza S**, *et al*. Which memory processes are affected in patients with obstructive sleep apnea? An evaluation of 3 types of memory. *Sleep*, 2006; **29**:533–44.

68. **Salorio C F**, **White D A**, **Piccirillo J**, *et al*. Learning, memory, and executive control in individuals with obstructive sleep apnea syndrome. *J Clin Exp Neuropsych*, 2002; **24**:93–100.

69. **Morrell M J**, **McRobbie D W**, **Quest R A**, *et al*. Changes in brain morphology associated with obstructive sleep apnea. *Sleep Med*, 2003; **4**:451–54.

70. **Gozal D**, **Daniel J M**, **Dohanich G P**. Behavioral and anatomical correlates of chronic episodic hypoxia during sleep in the rat. *J Neurosci*, 2001; **21**:2442–50.

71. **Curcio G**, **Ferrara M**, **De Gennaro L**. Sleep loss, learning capacity and academic performance. *Sleep Med Rev*, 2006; **10**:323–37.

72. **Wahlstrom K**. Changing times: findings from the first longitudinal study of later high school start times. *NASSP Bull*, 2002; **86**:3–21.

73. **Cabeza R**, **Dolcos F**, **Prince S E**, *et al*. Attention-related activity during episodic memory retrieval: a cross-function fMRI study. *Neuropsychologia*, 2003; **41**:390–99.

74. **Rickard T**, **Cai D**, **Rieth C**, *et al*. Sleep does not enhance motor sequence learning. *J Exp Psych*, 2008; **34**:834–42.

75. **Varkevisser M**, **Kerkhof G A**. Chronic insomnia and performance in a 24-h constant routine study. *J Sleep Res*, 2005; **14**:49–59.

76. **Ratcliff R**, **Van Dongen H P A**. Sleep deprivation affects multiple distinct cognitive processes. *Psychon Bull Rev*, 2009; **16**:742–51.

77. **Leger D**. The cost of sleep-related accidents: a report for the National Commission of Sleep Disorders Research. *Sleep*, 1994; **17**:84–93.

78. **George C**, **Smiley A**. Sleep apnea & automobile accidents. *Sleep*, 1999; **22**:790–95.

79. **Lindberg E N**, **Carter T**, **Gislason T**, **Janson C**. Role of snoring and daytime sleepiness in occupational accidents. *Am J Respir Crit Care Med*, 2001; **164**:2031–35.

80. **Sternberg S**. High-speed scanning in human memory. *Science*, 1966; **153**:652–54.

Section 1 Chapter 8

Introduction

Motor vehicle driving and excessive sleepiness

Anna Anund and Göran Kecklund

Sleep-related crashes

This chapter starts with a section about traffic fatalities and injuries as a public health problem and driver sleepiness involvement in crashes, followed by a section of determinants of sleepiness. Finally, there is a section of countermeasures against sleepiness.

According to WHO data [1], deaths from road traffic injuries account for around 25% of all deaths from injury. Worldwide, the number of people killed in road traffic crashes each year is estimated at almost 1.2 million, while the number injured could be as high as 50 million. Injuries including deaths represent 12% of the global burden of disease, the third most important cause of overall mortality, and the main cause of death among people aged 1–40 years. Worldwide, injuries including deaths are dominated by those due to road crashes. The total number of road traffic injuries in the world, including deaths, are forecast to rise by approximately 65% between the years 2000 and 2020 [1]. However, the tendency in the majority of the developed countries is a decrease in number of deaths and severe injuries during the last years.

In Europe, road traffic accidents are a major public health issue, claiming about 127 000 lives per year and about 2.4 million injured people. Road traffic accidents are the leading cause of death among young people in Europe and are predicted to increase in countries with low or medium income as they become more highly motorized [2].

Prevention of road crashes is a major priority in most countries. Prevention requires a clear understanding of the causes of crashes. There is no single theory accepted by the traffic research community that explains driver behavior and the relation to events resulting in injuries and deaths in traffic [3]. One approach to understand the causes of traffic injuries is based on analysis of crash data. Haddon developed a matrix [4], which includes the contributions of human, vehicle/equipment and environmental factors (both physical and socio economical) behind the injuries including fatal crashes, focusing on the pre-crash, crash and post-crash phases. The major component in crash causation is the "human factor" (as opposed to mechanical failure, weather conditions), involved in around 90% of the crashes.

There are several important causes of road accidents that need to be taken into account in the future to reduce deaths and injuries in traffic, such as temporary driver impairments such as distraction, reduced attention, and sleepiness. This chapter deals with driver sleepiness [5]. In the literature of driver sleepiness, terms such as fatigue, sleepiness and drowsiness are used interchangeably. Sleepiness is operationally defined as a physiological drive to sleep. This is the latent, fundamental type of sleepiness that in some cases can be masked by surrounding factors and result in manifest sleepiness. From a driving point of view, sleepiness can be seen as the lack of ability to maintain a wake state of attention without the aid of the surroundings/situation.

For a long time, sleepiness-related crashes have attracted no official or public interest, since the incidence has been considered very low. Figures have varied between 1 and 3% [6]. At the same time, studies that specifically focused on sleepy driving estimate that between 10 and 30% of crashes involve sleepiness [5, 7]. In an unpublished but recently performed representative and large questionnaire study in Sweden (sample size = 11 000 in the age group 18–84; response rate = 60.4%) in Sweden (from 2009), 30% of drivers in the 18–24 age range reported severe sleepiness or falling asleep while driving during the past 12 months

---

Sleepiness: Causes, Consequences and Treatment, ed. Michael J. Thorpy and Michel Billiard. Published by Cambridge University Press. © Cambridge University Press 2011.

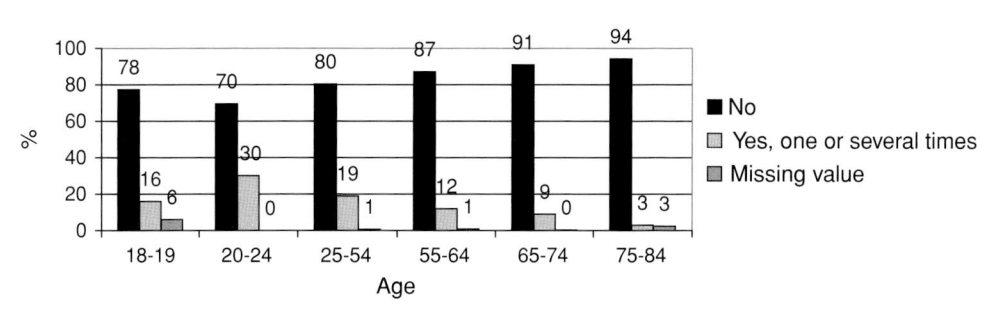

8. Motor vehicle driving and excessive sleepiness

Figure 8.1 Question: During the past 12 months have you experienced severe sleepiness or felt asleep when driving? *Source*: National questionnaire in Sweden 2009. The study was carried out by the Swedish Road Administration.

(see Figure 8.1). The prevalence of sleepy driving declined with increasing age.

In field studies with long-term video recording of the driver and the traffic situation [8], sleepiness was found to be the major cause of self-caused crashes/near crashes. The National Transportation Safety Board (US) has pointed out that sleepiness while driving is one of the most important factors contributing to road crashes, and there is a widespread scientific consensus on this estimate [5]. Recently, it was also shown that sleepiness may be a stronger cause of road crashes than alcohol and that the two factors interact in a dramatic way [9].

The discrepancy between scientific data and official statistics is very likely due to the lack of adequate methodological tools for estimating the cause of the crash, and lack of standardized official reporting procedures. Hence, most official registers still do not systematically collect relevant information on driver sleepiness/fatigue in crashes. Exceptions, however, are the Canadian police force and some of the US states. Apparently, there is a need for raising traffic research activities to also include sleepiness/fatigue.

Determinants of sleepiness

In order to understand and prevent sleep-related crashes it is necessary to describe how physiology and behavior change during sleepy driving and what is the precipitating cause of the impaired behavior involved in a crash.

Indicators of sleepiness

The physiological and behavioral changes of sleepiness are discussed in a general sense in other chapters. Many of those measurements are applicable also in relation to sleepy driving. However, some measurements/indicators are unique to driving, or need at least to be modified for driving. Finding relevant measurements which describe changes in driving behavior caused by sleepiness is difficult. One reason, suggested by Brown 40 years ago [10], was that normal driving is a task with a high degree of automation. Therefore, a sleepy driver may manage rather simple driving fairly well, despite the general functional capacity being clearly deteriorated. Thus, during simple and automated driving negative effects of sleepiness on driving performance will be difficult to observe. However, certain critical situations, which probably seldom occur, may be more vulnerable to sleepiness. Driving during such situations is more likely to show impairment, even with moderate sleepiness, than routine driving tasks (relying on highly automated skills). One should keep in mind that our knowledge of the interaction between the driving scenario and the sleepiness level is very limited and most of the research involves simple driving without introducing more complex and difficult situations. However, in a driving simulator it has been shown that a night of prior sleep loss increases the levels of established indicators of sleepiness behind the wheel even if the driving situation required frequent interactions with other cars on the road. However, blink duration (mean and variability) was shorter during overtaking compared to other situations even when going home after a night shift [11].

An objective way of measuring sleepiness is through driving parameters associated with performance impairment during sleepy driving. Commonly used measurements of driver sleepiness both in

83

1. Introduction

simulators and during naturalistic driving are measurements related to variability of the lateral position and involuntarily lane departures [12], which increases as the driver becomes sleepy. Lateral position is easily measured in simulators, but is more difficult to track on real roads due to sensor limitations. A measurement based on already existing sensors is the steering wheel reversal rate. However, this is a measurement not easily computed, since it requires an identification of the maximum and minimum in the signal. A variety of thresholds have been used showing different results. Speed deviations (from the posted limit) have also shown some relation with sleep loss [13], but may also be influenced by many other factors. Many of the variables referred to above have been tested in support systems for drivers in order to warn of impending danger due to high levels of sleepiness [14].

The measurement of brain waves has been another variable of choice when sleepiness at the wheel is investigated. Spectral analysis of the EEG seems to dominate the sleepy driver studies in this sense. However, the spectral content of the EEG does not involve a definition of sleep, which would be helpful in making estimates of sleep in the evaluation of results. Another methodological problem is that the EEG signal often contains a lot of noise, mainly due to movements. Thus, removal of noise due to artifacts may cause quite large data loss which makes it unfeasible for an automated sleepiness detection and warning system. Results from simulator studies show that, among the physiological parameters, increased frequency in the alpha and theta bands of the EEG seem to be parameters of interest [15], but also parameters based on blink behavior [16]. In particular, eye blink duration is sensitive to variations in alertness and involves increased eye-lid closure duration [17], or slow rolling eye movements when driving [18].

It is also argued that a combined scoring of EOG and EEG measurement is a promising method for estimating physiological sleepiness under conditions of driving. One way of scoring this is the so-called Karolinska Drowsiness Score (KDS) [19]. The KDS is based on a classification performed in two-second epochs that yield continuous measurements (0–100%, in steps of 10%, out of each 20- or 30-s epoch). A driving simulator study showed that at KDS level 30% (meaning sleepiness signs 30% of the time within a given time frame) the risk of lane departure was 2.6 times higher; at KDS 40% the risk of lane departure is more than 6 times higher [20]. The relation between KDS and variability of blink duration shows that at KDS 30% the variability has changed from 0.04 to 0.07 s.

Simulator studies and driving on real roads

Most studies are carried out using simple driving simulators and with a relatively boring and monotonous scenario without other vehicles on the road that may require actions [7, 15]. The effect of time on task has been proven to be task-dependent in comparisons of a simple vigilance task with a monotonous driving task in a simulator [21]. It could be hypothesized that this would also be true if the simple scenario in a simulator was compared with a more complex one. In many countries the traffic law forbids sleepy driving, which makes it difficult to carry out experimental sleep deprivation studies on real roads. Philip *et al.* [12] concluded in a comparative study that sleepiness can be studied equally well in real and simulated driving conditions. The effects are the same, except that the simulator will show more frequent line crossings and road departures compared to the real environment. One explanation for this could be the difference in complexity in the driving scenario. On the one hand, a more complex scenario will also be more sensitive and vulnerable to sleep loss. A complex scenario may also be more stimulating and activating compared to monotonous driving. Thus, it is difficult to predict how the driving scenario will affect sleepiness and vice versa. In addition, naturalistic driving often includes both monotonous driving and more complex situations characterized by higher traffic intensity and more active driving. It may also be that sleep deprivation impairs driving performance for complex driving tasks, e.g. the distance to cars one has to follow can decrease (with increased risk of collision with an oncoming vehicle) and unsafe overtaking can occur more frequently. Clearly, a driving simulator suffers from weaknesses in comparison to real-life driving; for example, the lack of a real safety risk is a disadvantage. However, there seem to be no studies investigating to what extent a simulator study leads to erroneous conclusions compared to what would have been found in real-life studies. Still, the simulator provides the opportunity to monitor the driver without any risk, all the way to sleep onset and actual lane departure. The simulator also offers total control over environmental conditions, which increases the possibility of drawing reliable conclusions. The simulator also permits cost-efficient use of research subjects and other resources, making larger and more representative samples possible. Future studies will need to be carried out in real driving situations to verify key implications resulting from simulator studies.

Another observation in previous research is that there are very few studies that have attempted to describe the detailed physiological and behavioral changes that immediately precede *an event* of interest, that is, a crash or a lane departure (defined as a two wheels outside the road). Such detailed information can be recorded in well-controlled simulator studies. In simulators it is possible to obtain data on what precedes dangerous driving, e.g. whether there is a clear sleepiness event in the pre-incident phase, as well as providing a deeper understanding of the relation between sleepiness and near-crash incidents, which sometimes would lead to a crash. One wonders, for example, if sleep intrusions in the waking EEG, long eye closure durations, or lane drifting appear immediately before a crash. What are the dynamics of sleepiness indicators; is the sleepiness attack abrupt and rapid, or does it develop slowly? Is the driver aware of the sleepiness level? The latter is suggested by Reyner and Horne [22]. The same group also indirectly shows that driving incidents, in a simulator, occur at high levels of alpha plus theta activity, but they do not explicitly describe the changes in physiology leading to an incident or a crash.

Risk groups and individual differences

In the previous section, the main causes of sleepiness were discussed in a general sense. Here we focus on what is known about the specific causes of sleep-related crashes or, at least, of sleepiness at the wheel.

Sleep pathology is a well-known risk factor for sleep-related crashes. Thus, many studies show that obstructive sleep apnea syndrome (OSAS) and narcolepsy [23] are associated with increased levels of road crashes. It has also been shown that drivers with untreated sleep apnea have an increased risk of lane departures, and there have been several international consensus documents establishing the importance of obstructive sleep apnea as an important factor behind road crashes [24]. However, treatment of the sleep disorder, such as CPAP for OSAS, significantly reduces the crash risk as well as sleepiness during driving [25]. Although transient insomnia seems to increase the risk for sleep-related crashes [6], there is a lack of studies on motor vehicle crashes and chronic insomnia. There are a few cross-sectional studies where insomniacs have been compared with good sleepers; however, the results are not consistent [25].

Work hours and sleep habits seem to be equally important factors. Barger *et al.* found that extended work shifts (>24 h often during on-call work) among interns were associated with a higher risk (odds ratio: 2.3, 95% CI: 1.6–3.3) for a motor vehicle crash [26]. They also found a higher risk for falling asleep at the wheel if the interns had worked 5 or more extended work shifts during a month. Many studies show that night driving increases crash risk several fold (5–6 times) [27]. Night shift work is also associated with increased reported sleepiness [28], and studies have shown that train drivers [18], truck drivers [28, 29], and others, show clear intrusions of sleep-like EEG patterns when working at night. The latter has also been demonstrated in a truck simulator [19]. Also, driving home after a night shift is associated with at least a doubling of the risk of a crash [30]. If driving performance or physiological indicators of sleepiness are taken into account [31], it was seen that driving home from the night shift are associated with an increased number of incidents (two wheels outside the lane marking, increased from 2.4 to 7.6 times). There was also a decreased time to first crash, increased lateral deviation (from 18 to 43 cm), increased eye closure duration (0.102 to 0.143 s), and increased subjective sleepiness. This holds true even if the scenario is more complex with interactions with other vehicles [11]. The reason for the crash risk associated with the post-night shift commute is, most likely, the combination of driving close to the circadian low (around 0400h–0500h) and an extended time awake (often awake since the previous morning and without any nap),as has been demonstrated in many laboratory studies [32]. The total effect on road crash risk of the circadian low, prior time awake, and prior amount of sleep has recently been demonstrated [9]. The results show a strong capacity to predict crash risk. The sleepiness effects during the morning commute are in line with the epidemiological studies that have demonstrated an increased crash risk in shift workers travelling home after a night shift [6, 30]. They are also in line with a number of studies that demonstrate increased risks of road crashes in connection with early morning driving [33, 34]. Observations on strong effects of reduced sleep on sleepiness have been made in many simulator studies of sleep loss, daytime

1. Introduction

driving, for lateral variability [15], or eye closure durations [16].

The crash risk is also higher with increased duration of driving [35]. However, the effects are confounded with other factors such as time of day, time awake, and prior sleep, which often covary with the duration of driving. Results from simulator studies show pronounced time-on-task effects on sleepiness [15, 36]. A crash study showed increased risk of truck crashes with time at the wheel [35]. However, in this type of study it is likely that there are strong effects of time of day as well as effects of circadian rhythm, since driving time spans durations from a few hours up to 10–15 h. Whether real driving is as sensitive to time on task as simulator driving is not known. However, Kecklund and Åkerstedt found in a field study on truck drivers that physiological sleepiness correlated positively with work shift duration during long-distance night driving [29]. In one study no effect on involuntary line crossing was seen during 10 h of highway driving on the day [37]. However, breaks occurred every second hour, which may have maintained alertness. The same group did show pronounced effects when 2, 4, and 8 h of night driving, without breaks, were compared [37]. This was the first study of real-life sleepy driving that controlled for prior amount of sleep, prior time awake, and circadian rhythm.

Sleep duration would be expected to be related to increased crash risk but very few studies exist. A study by Connor *et al.* showed that sleep <5 h was associated with a doubling of the crash risk [33]. With respect to simulator studies of sleepy driving, virtually all seem to have been based on manipulation of prior sleep – total or partial sleep deprivation [15].

The risk of sleepiness-related crashes is strongly related to individual differences. Young drivers, for example, are more frequently involved in road crashes [34, 38]. Young drivers (18–24 years) had a 5–10-times higher risk of being involved in a traffic crash late at night than older drivers. Age differences in driving performance have been observed in earlier studies [39]. These studies suggested that young drivers are more susceptible to sleepiness than older drivers. The reasons are not clearly established as to why young drivers show an excess risk of having a crash late at night, but factors related to self-confidence, risk-taking and drug use have been suggested [40]. The increased night time risk for young drivers may also be related to increased exposure of car driving during this time of the day. Another very likely reason is

sleepiness. It has been a hypothesis that young drivers more easily fall asleep/nod off in sleepy situations and in connection with sleep loss than do older drivers [27, 41]. However, very few studies have studied age effects in connection with night driving. In a recent simulator study [20, 42], it was shown that young drivers (18–24 years of age) were more sleepy while driving at night compared to drivers 55–64 years of age. In a review focusing on adolescents' driving risks, it was concluded that one major cause that contributed significantly to an increased driving risk in teens is sleep deprivation and the consequences of insufficient sleep (sleepiness, lapses in attention, susceptibility to aggression, and negative synergy with alcohol) [43]. One additional explanation for an increased risk is the adolescent brain maturation that indicates that essential parts of the brain regulating emotions (prefrontal cortex) are not fully developed until the adolescent is above 18 years old.

Closely related to age is the age of the driving licence. Individuals with a recently obtained license are involved in a disproportionately high number of crashes [44].

Countermeasures

Considering the central role of sleepiness in crash causation, knowledge of the use of countermeasures is an important issue. One may structure countermeasures in three levels according to Michon, i.e. strategic, tactical and operative levels [3], as shown in Table 8.1.

With respect to the strategic level countermeasures, obviously one should avoid night driving, and make sure sufficient amounts of sleep have been obtained before driving. Here, for example, Fatigue Management Programs and work scheduling for professional drivers play a major role [45]. In most countries there are hours of service (HOS) regulations. However, those do not take into account the underlying problems (circadian and sleep/wake pattern). In a review of theories, it was argued that the most promising solutions would be to shift from a focus on HOS regulations to a Safety Management System (SMS) in which fatigue is one component [45]. The suggested theoretical framework was represented using Reason's hazard control framework and regarded a fatigue-related incident or crash as the final segment in a causal chain of events or error trajectory. The model precedes the fatigue-related incident for which the hazard and the control are identified on

Table 8.1 Examples of countermeasures at a pre-crash level according to the Michon model [3]

Strategic	Tactical	Operative
Fatigue management systems	Driver support system (feedback – warning)	Rumble strips
Hours of service regulations	Road signs	Driver support systems (warning and intervention)
Information/education	Parking areas	Campaigns targeted to increased awareness of alertness-enhancing activities that can be carried out during rest
Strategies for planning	Route guidance to parking areas	
Fit for duty test		
Enforcement/control		

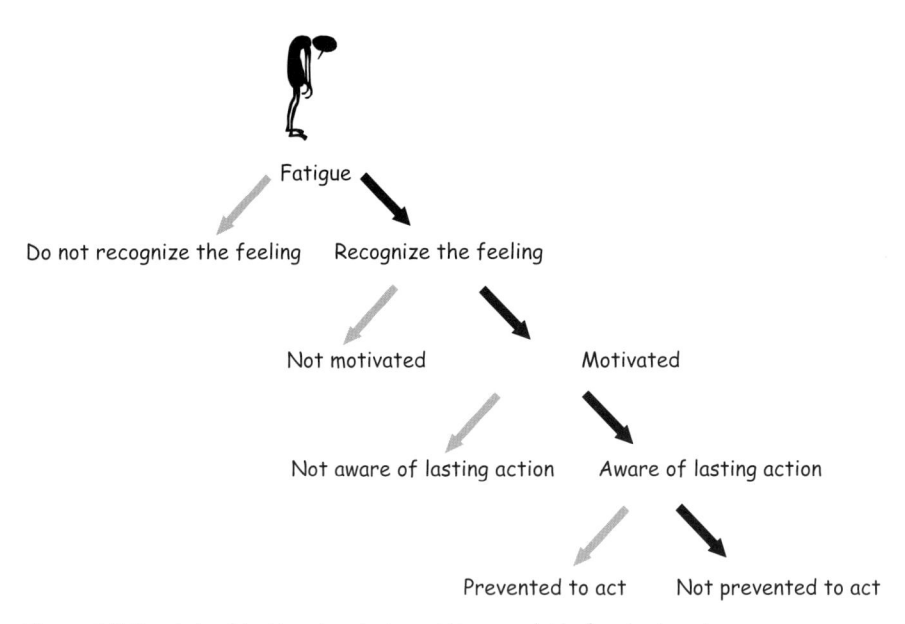

Figure 8.2 The chain of decisions in order to avoid increased risk of crash when sleepy.

four suggested levels (sleep opportunity/actual sleep obtained/behavior symptoms/fatigue-related errors).

During the drive, there are critical decisions a driver needs to take in order to avoid the risk of a sleep-related crash. First of all, the driver has to recognize the sensation of sleepiness. In the next step, the driver must be motivated to take corrective actions, and have knowledge of which countermeasures are effective and lasting. Finally, the driving circumstances should allow the driver to act according to an effective strategy, as shown in Figure 8.2.

The driver's preference for a countermeasure will not only influence the motivation to do something about it, but also the probability of choosing an effective countermeasure. It appears that actions such as opening a window, turning on the radio, or taking a break are common [46]. However, laboratory studies indicate that these three suggested countermeasures, including exercise during the break, do not improve long-term alertness [36]. Horne and Reyner have demonstrated that caffeine and taking a brief nap (<30 min) significantly reduce driving impairments, subjective sleepiness and electroencephalographic (EEG) indications of drowsiness [36]. The dramatic alerting effects of these behaviors have also been demonstrated repeatedly in laboratory studies with other performance measurements [47]. Bright lights suppress melatonin, which peaks at the late night hours, and increase alertness [48]. However, it may be difficult to administer bright light in the car without impairing other aspects of vision.

Apart from the interest in understanding what countermeasures are used, one also needs to know whether the use of countermeasures differs between different driver groups. Inappropriate use of countermeasures may be related to long-term risk of crash. This type of knowledge may aid in identifying vulnerable groups that do not know how to handle sleepiness while driving. Age is probably such a factor because of its close relation to crash risk and risk behavior, the group in focus being young drivers [49]. Gender is another factor, with greater risk attached to males [27]. One may also hypothesize that experience of drowsy driving and sleep-related crashes, shift work, and being a professional driver may influence the use of countermeasures, since these characteristics may be associated with a greater awareness of the dangers of sleepy driving. Higher education and old age may also be associated with greater insights of sleepy driving and how to handle it. When it comes to differences in countermeasures between driver groups, reported by the drivers themselves, it has been shown that counteracting sleepiness with a nap (a presumably efficient method) is practised by those with experience of sleep-related crashes or of driving during severe sleepiness, as well as by professional drivers, males and drivers aged 46–64 years, and the most endorsed means of information to the driver about sleepiness was in-car monitoring of driving performance [46]. The increase in preference for efficient countermeasures with increasing age is interesting from the standpoint of the lower risk of sleepiness-related crashes in higher age groups [34, 38]. Also, being male was associated with a preference for a nap. The reason for this is not immediately obvious. Interestingly, having disturbed sleep, being a snorer or being a shift worker were not related to identifying a nap as important, despite the fact that such individuals should have ample experience of sleepiness [25].

Apart from driver-initiated countermeasures one may also consider various types of information to the driver about fatigue risks in driving. Information in the media could be one such way. Public campaigns along the roads may be another. Information in connection with the annual vehicle safety inspection may be a third. In addition, there has been considerable development in the area of driver support systems, focused on feedback on hazardous driving in terms of impaired lateral control [14], or focused on the physiological state of the individual sleepiness [50]. More recently, researchers have shown the need for a combination of indicators based on driver and driving behavior [51]. Several car manufacturers provide technological driver support systems that are supposed to detect and warn against driver sleepiness. However, as far as we know, there are no independent studies demonstrating the effectiveness of such systems. Since driver support systems are associated with sizeable investments by society and/or manufacturers, it would be of interest to investigate the attitude among end-users towards such countermeasures, as well as to study whether background factors are related to such attitudes. Thus, the sleepiness detection and warning systems should be seen as a fall-back safety aid, in particular since one may assume that the performance of the technological systems may differ between individuals. A questionnaire study showed that the most accepted sign of driver sleepiness was feedback of driving performance [46]. This is similar to what has been found in a field study on truck drivers [17]. Another more systematic public intervention approach, not based on individual preferences, is the so-called "rumble strip". A rumble strip refers to a narrow band of built-in unevenness in the road surface, normally placed close to the edge line and/or at the center line. The purpose is to cause vibrations or noise when a vehicle wheel makes contact with the rumble strip. The rumble strip may be profiled (raised) above the road surface or milled into the road surface (see Figure 8.3).

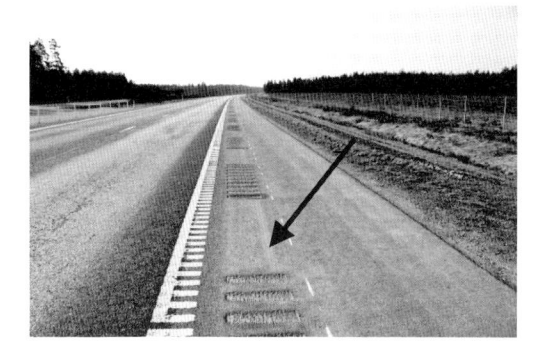

Figure 8.3 Rumble strip milled into the road surface at the shoulder. (See color plate section).

Rumble strips have been systematically evaluated in several studies, and the introduction of rumble strips at the center line has reduced crashes by approximately 15% and the effect of rumble strips at the shoulder is even more positive (40–50%) [52, 53]. While the reason for this may be a redirection of attention in alert-distracted drivers, it seems likely that an alerting effect in a sleepy driver may also be as important. In a driving simulator study it has been shown that a sleepy driver leaving the lane and hitting the rumble strip will be awakened and show improved driving behavior [54]. However, the results also showed that the sleepiness sign returned 5 min after the rumble strip was hit. The study concluded that various aspects of sleepiness are increased before hitting a rumble strip and that the effect is very short.

Conclusion and future work

Driver sleepiness is a common cause for traffic crashes and results in severe injuries and fatalities. During the last decade the knowledge of how to measure sleepy driving, its consequences (i.e. impaired driving performance), and how one should combat driver sleepiness has increased considerably. However, there are still gaps in knowledge, for example, related to individual differences in vulnerability to sleepy driving. Another critical area is related to how to persuade sleepy drivers to stop for a nap and/or caffeine intake. There is also a need for research that evaluates how drivers respond to the use of (technological) driver support system, and this is an important target for future field operational tests (such as the 100-car study) [8].

In order to reduce driver sleepiness, a holistic approach may be a promising strategy that takes technological, organizational and individual factors into account. Combating driver sleepiness is not only a question of developing technological driver support systems. It is likely that "soft" countermeasures are equally important and that sleepy driving should be counteracted on the strategic, tactical and operative level. Evidence-based fatigue management programs are a key factor in this approach and should reassure that professional drivers have the rosters, tools and knowledge to maintain high alertness and safe driving. To achieve this goal, the drivers need, for example, education and training focusing on the acceptance and knowledge of the risk of driving under sleepiness, information along the roadside to remind the drivers of the risks associated with driver sleepiness, and rumble strips at the shoulders and in the center of the road in case of an involuntary lane departure. Finally, it is important that the organizational and individual factors are evaluated with respect to operational sleepiness and crash risk, i.e. in order to demonstrate whether it is an effective safety-enhancing strategy. Last but not least a common definition to classify sleep related crashes is needed. A definition that includes not only sleepiness but also insufficient sleep.

References

1. **Peden M, McGee K, Sharma G**. *The Injury Chart Book: A Graphical Overview of the Global Burden of Injuries*. Geneva: WHO, 2002.
2. **Racioppi F, Eriksson L, Tingvall C**, et al. *Preventing Road Traffic Injury: A Public Health Perspective for Europe*. Copenhagen: World Health Organization, Europe, 2004.
3. **Michon J**. A critical view of driver behaviour models: what do we know, what should we do? In: Evans L, Schwing R, Eds. *Human Behaviour and Traffic Safety*. New York, NY: Plenum Press, 1985: 485–520.
4. **Haddon W J**. A logical framework for categorizing highway safety phenomena and activity. *J Trauma*, 1972; **12**:193–207.
5. **Åkerstedt T**. Consensus statement: fatigue and accidents in transport operations. *J Sleep Res*, 2000; **9**:395.
6. **Stutts J, Wilkins J, Osberg S**, et al. Driver risk factors for sleep-related crashes. *Accid Anal Prev*, 2003; **35**:321–31.
7. **Horne J, Reyner L**. Sleep related vehicle accidents. *BMJ*, 1995; **310**:565–67.
8. **Dingus T, Neale V, Klauer S**, et al. The development of a naturalistic data collection system to perform critical incident analysis: an investigation of safety and fatigue issues in long-haul trucking. *Accid Anal Prev*, 2006, **38**:1127–36.
9. **Åkerstedt T, Connor J, Gray A**, et al. Predicting road crashes from a mathematical model of alertness regulation – The Sleep/Wake Predictor. *Accid Anal Prev*, 2008; **40**:1480–85.
10. **Brown I D**. Measuring the "spare mental capacity" of car drivers by subsidiary auditory task. *Ergonomics*, 1962; **5**:247–50.
11. **Anund A, Kecklund G, Tapani A**, et al. The effects of driving situation on sleepiness indicators after sleep loss: a driving simulator study. *Ind Health*, 2009; **47**:1–9.
12. **Philip P, Sagaspe P, Taillard J**, et al. Fatigue, sleepiness, and performance in simulated versus real driving conditions. *Sleep*, 2005; **28**:1511–16.
13. **Arnedt J, Wilde G, Munt P**, et al. How do prolonged wakefulness and alcohol compare in the decrements they produce on a simulated driving task? *Accid Anal Prev*, 2001; **33**:337–44.

14. **Dinges D**, **Mallis M**. Managing fatigue by drowsiness detection: can technological promises be realized. In: Hartley L, Ed. *Managing Fatigue in Transportation*. Oxford: Pergamon Press, 1998: 209–29.

15. **Åkerstedt T**, **Ingre M**, **Kecklund G**, *et al*. Reactions of sleepiness indicators to partial sleep deprivation, time of day and time on task in a driving simulator – the DROWSI project. *J Sleep Res*, 2010; **19**:298–309.

16. **Wierwille W**, **Ellsworth L**. Evaluation of driver drowsiness by trained raters. *Accid Anal Prev*, 1994; **26**:571–81.

17. **Dinges D**, **Maislin G**, **Brewster R**, *et al*. Pilot test of fatigue management technologies. US Transportation Research Record; 2005. Report No.: Issue 1922.

18. **Torsvall L**, **Åkerstedt T**. Sleepiness on the job: continuously measured EEG changes in train drivers. *Electroencephalogr Clin Neurophysiol*, 1987; **66**:502–11.

19. **Gillberg M**, **Kecklund G**, **Åkerstedt T**. Sleepiness and performance of professional drivers in a truck simulator – comparisons between day and night driving. *J Sleep Res*, 1996; **5**:12–15.

20. **Anund A**, **Kecklund G**, **Peters B**, *et al*. Driver impairment during night and the relation with physiological sleepiness. *Scand J Work Environ Health*, 2008; **34**:142–50.

21. **Richter S**, **Marsalek K**, **Glatz C**, *et al*. Task-dependent differences in subjective fatigue scores. *J Sleep Res*, 2005; **14**:393–400.

22. **Reyner L A**, **Horne J A**. Falling asleep whilst driving: are drivers aware of prior sleepiness? *Int J Legal Med*, 1998; **111**:120–23.

23. **Terán-Santos J**, **Jimnénez-Gómez A**, **Cordero-Guevara J**. The association between sleep apnea and the risk of traffic accidents. *N Engl J Med*, 1999; **240**:847–51.

24. **Alonderis A**, **Barbé F**, **Bonsignore M**, *et al*. Medico-legal implications of sleep apnoea syndrome: driving license regulations in Europe. *Sleep Med*, 2008; **9**:362–75.

25. **Philip P**, **Akerstedt T**. Transport and industrial safety, how are they affected by sleepiness and sleep restriction? *Sleep Med Rev*, 2006; **10**:347–56.

26. **Barger L**, **Cade B**, **Ayas N**, *et al*. Extended work shifts and the risk of motor vehicle crashes among interns. *N Engl J Med*, 2005; **352**:125–34.

27. **Åkerstedt T**, **Kecklund G**. Age, gender and early morning highway accidents. *J Sleep Res*, 2001; **10**:105–10.

28. **Mitler M**, **Miller J**, **Lipsitz J**, *et al*. The sleep of long-haul truck drivers. *N Engl J Med*, 1997; **337**:755–61.

29. **Kecklund G**, **Åkerstedt T**. Sleepiness in long distance truck driving: an ambulatory EEG study of night driving. *Ergonomics*, 1993; **36**:1007–17.

30. **Gold D R**, **Rogacz S**, **Bock N**, *et al*. Rotating shift work, sleep, and accidents related to sleepiness in hospital nurses. *Am J Publ Health*, 1992; **82**:1011–14.

31. **Åkerstedt T**, **Peters B**, **Anund A**, *et al*. Impaired alertness and performance driving home from the night shift: a driving simulator study. *J Sleep Res*, 2005; **14**:17–20.

32. **Dijk D**, **Czeisler C**. Contribution of the circadian pacemaker and the sleep homeostat to sleep propensity, sleep structure, electroencephalographic slow waves, and sleep spindle activity in humans. *J Neurosci*, 1995; **15**:3526–38.

33. **Connor J**, **Norton R**, **Ameratunga S**, *et al*. Driver sleepiness and risk of serious injury to car occupants: population based case control study. *BMJ*, 2002; **324**:1125.

34. **Åkerstedt T**, **Kecklund G**, **Hörte L**. Night driving, season, and risk of highway accidents. *Sleep*, 2001; **24**:401–06.

35. **Hamelin P**. Lorry driver's time habits in work and their involvement in traffic accidents. *Ergonomics*, 1987; **30**:1323–33.

36. **Horne J A**, **Reyner L A**. Counteracting driver sleepiness: effects of napping, caffeine and placebo. *Psychophysiology*, 1996; **33**:306–09.

37. **Sagaspe P**, **Taillard J**, **Akerstedt T**, *et al*. Extended driving impairs nocturnal driving performances. *PLoS ONE*, 2008; **3**:e3493.

38. **Pack A I**, **Pack A M**, **Rodgman E**, *et al*. Characteristics of crashes attributed to the driver having fallen asleep. *Accid Anal Prev*, 1995; **27**:769–75.

39. **Campagne A**, **Pebayle T**, **Muzet A**. Correlation between driving errors and vigilance level: influence of the driver's age. *Physiol Behav*, 2004; **80**:515–24.

40. **Gregersen N**, **Bjurulf P**. Young novice drivers: towards a model of their accident involvement. *Accid Anal Prev*, 1996; **28**:229–41.

41. **Sagaspe P**, **Taillard J**, **Chaumet G**, *et al*. Aging and nocturnal driving: better with coffee or a nap? A randomized study. *Sleep*, 2007; **30**:1808–13.

42. **Lowden A**, **Anund A**, **Kecklund G**, *et al*. Wakefulness in young and elderly subjects driving at night in a car simulator. *Accid Anal Prev*, 2009; **41**:1001–07.

43. **Dahl R**. Biological, developmental, and neurobehavioral factors relevant to adolescent driving risks. *Am J Prev Med*, 2008; **35**:278–84.

44. **Laapotti S**, **Keskinen E**. Differences in fatal loss-of-control accidents between young male and female drivers. *Accid Anal Prev*, 1998; **30**:435–42.

45. **Dawson D**, **McCulloch K**. Managing fatigue: it's about sleep. *Sleep*, 2005; **9**:365–80.
46. **Anund A**, **Kecklund G**, **Peters B**, *et al*. Driver sleepiness and individual differences in preferences for countermeasures. *J Sleep Res*, 2008; **17**:16–22.
47. **Tietzel A**, **Lack L**. The recuperative value of brief and ultra-brief naps on alertness and cognitive performance. *J Sleep Res*, 2002; **11**:213–18.
48. **Lowden A**, **Holmbäck U**, **Åkerstedt T**, *et al*. Performance and sleepiness during a 24 h awake in constant conditions are affected by diet. *Biol Psychol*, 2004: **65**:251–63.
49. **Galvan A**, **Hare T**, **Voss H**, *et al*. Risk-taking and the adolescent brain: who is at risk? *Dev Sci*, 2007; **10**:F8–14.
50. **Wierwille W**, **Ellsworth L**, **Wreggit S**, *et al*. Research on vehicle based driver status/performance monitoring: development, validation, and refinement of algorithms for detection of driver drowsiness; 1994. Report No.: DOT HS 808.
51. **Liu C**, **Hosking S**, **Lenné M**. Predicting driver drowsiness using vehicle measures: recent insights and future challenges. *J Sleep Res*, 2009; **40**:239–45.
52. **Mahoney R**, **Porter R**, **Donnell D**, *et al*. *Evaluation of Centerline Rumble Strips on Lateral Vehicle Placement and Speed on Two-lane Highways*. Harrisburg, PA: Pennsylvania Department of Transportation, 2003.
53. **Persaud B**, **Retting R**, **Lyon C**. *Crash Reduction Following Installation of Centreline Rumble Strips on Rural Two-Lane Roads*. Toronto, Canada: Ryerson University, 2003.
54. **Anund A**, **Kecklund G**, **Vadeby A**, *et al*. The alerting effect of hitting a rumble strip – a simulator study. *Accid Anal Prev*, 2008; **40**:1970–76.

Section 1
Chapter 9

Introduction

Medico-legal consequences of excessive sleepiness

Charles F. P. George

Background

Sleepiness is both an objective and subjective phenomenon. As a subjective sensation, it is associated with a number of behaviors such as yawning, stretching, or rubbing the eyes. Subjective sleepiness can often be transiently overcome under certain conditions of stress or motivation. However, as intrinsic sleepiness increases, there will be periods where vigilance becomes unstable despite motivation. In these conditions, intrinsic sleepiness becomes manifest and results in important implications for personal safety and public health. The potential for this is widespread, as highlighted in the Maastricht Cohort Study of "Fatigue at Work" [1]. This prospective cohort study of employees from a wide range of companies and organizations found that fatigue and need for recovery were independent risk factors for being injured in an occupational incident. These results were not limited to the transportation industries, but also included agriculture, public utilities, construction, general industry, and hotel and restaurant sectors. Regardless of the situation or etiology, when sleepiness is manifest and gives rise to impairments in vigilance and/or performance, such excessive sleepiness can lead to accidents and important legal consequences.

This chapter will deal specifically with situations where such legal consequences have occurred or have the potential to occur. It reviews relevant case law on liability for injuries associated with sleep disorders or sleepiness. It covers possible liability of drivers, employers and physicians. Although many of the cases do not directly involve the physician, it does highlight the potential of impacting on any individual doctor–patient relationship, and physicians need to be aware in this constantly evolving area of medicine.

Liability for injuries caused by drowsiness or falling asleep

According to the US National Highway Traffic Safety Administration, there may be as many as 100 000 crashes from driver fatigue each year, with an estimated 1550 deaths, 71 000 people injured, causing $12.5 billion economic losses. Although there are clear risk factors for drowsy driving and certain characteristics of sleepiness-related crashes, it is often still difficult to attribute crashes directly to sleepiness. As such, these estimates likely underestimate the magnitude of the problem.

Anyone operating a motor vehicle has a duty to operate such vehicle in a safe manner. This applies to all drivers, although the potential for loss is arguably greater in commercial vehicle drivers. With respect to sleepiness, a driver with a sleep disorder or extreme sleepiness from whatever cause is at risk for a sleepiness-related accident. If that individual does not take measures to reduce this risk, then they may be guilty of dangerous driving and liable for the consequences of falling asleep while driving a motor vehicle. This presupposes, however, that the individual is aware of the risk or had any perception of sleepiness of drowsiness before the accident.

In the case of *Regina v. Hundal* [2], the Supreme Court of Canada dealt with the issue of dangerous driving. Prior to that, the courts had wrestled with what is required of drivers as they exercise their licensed privilege to drive on Canadian highways. The courts stated:

Although an objective test must be applied to the offence of dangerous driving, it will remain open to the accused to raise a reasonable doubt that a reasonable person would have been aware of the risks of

---

Sleepiness: Causes, Consequences and Treatment, ed. Michael J. Thorpy and Michel Billiard. Published by Cambridge University Press. © Cambridge University Press 2011.

the accused's conduct. The test must be applied with some measure of flexibility. That is to say the objective test should not be applied in a vacuum but rather in the context of the events surrounding the incident.

There will be occasions when the manner of driving viewed objectively will clearly be dangerous, yet the accused should not be convicted. Take, for example, a driver who, without prior warning, suffers a totally unexpected heart attack, epileptic seizure or detached retina. As a result of the sudden onset of a disease or physical disability the manner of driving would be dangerous, yet those circumstances could provide a complete defence despite the objective demonstration of dangerous driving. Similarly, a driver who, in the absence of any warning or knowledge of its possible effects, takes a prescribed medication which suddenly and unexpectedly affects the driver in such a way that the manner of driving was dangerous to the public, could still establish a good defence to the charge although it had been objectively established. These examples, and there may well be others, serve to illustrate the aim and purpose of the modified objective test. It is to enable a court to take into account the sudden and unexpected onset of disease and similar human frailties as well as the objective demonstration of dangerous driving."

With respect to sleepiness, the key point is whether or not the subject is actually aware of their drowsiness or can be aware that they did or may have fallen asleep just prior to an accident. This is often problematic, since a drowsy driver may have no recollection of having fallen asleep. Reyner and Horne looked at awareness of sleepiness before an accident in 28 healthy young adults who drove for 2 h in the afternoon in an interactive real-car simulator incorporating a dull and monotonous roadway [3]. All were experienced drivers and were restricted to 5 h of sleep the night before. Lane drifting, as is found with drowsy driving, was subdivided into minor and major incidents, where the latter was indicative of actually falling asleep. A distinction was made between the subjective perceptions of sleepiness and the likelihood of falling asleep, which drivers reported separately. Increasing sleepiness was closely associated with an increase in the number of incidents. Major incidents were usually preceded by self-awareness of sleepiness well beforehand and typically, subjects reached the stage of fighting sleep when these incidents happened. The perceived likelihood of falling asleep was highly correlated with increasing sleepiness, although some subjects failed to appreciate that extreme sleepiness is accompanied by a high likelihood of falling asleep.

Most courts hold that the driver who fell asleep bears the burden of presenting evidence that (s)he was not culpable in order to avoid criminal and/or civil liability. Courts often will consider several circumstances in determining whether continued driving when sleepy constitutes disregard of the safety of others. These include: (a) the duration of sleep in the period preceding the accident; (b) the duration of driving before the accident, i.e. was the driving long enough to become fatigued; and (c) whether the driver had any warning of drowsiness or dizziness (i.e. whether he or she had warning symptoms of sleep).

A driver is not guilty of reckless or careless driving by reason of what he does when asleep; but he can be convicted of careless (or reckless) driving if he falls asleep at the wheel, on the theory that he was guilty of the offense not at the moment when the crash occurred, but at the prior moment when he should have realized that he was sleepy and should have stopped driving.

This was highlighted in *R v. Gill* [4], a case of a university student driving home from studying for year-end exams. Following an exam, the defendant had socialized, studied and napped until 6:00 the next morning, and began driving home at about 6:00 a.m. She failed to notice a highway diversion barricade and struck and killed a tow truck operator assisting at the scene of a previous accident. In finding the driver guilty of dangerous driving, the court noted:

A reasonable driver, knowing that they had stayed awake for 24 hours and had already fallen asleep as a consequence, unexpectedly, during that time period, and feeling the need to take action while driving to prevent the onset of sleep, such as turning up a radio (or some other folk myth like opening windows for a blast of fresh air), is expected by law to exercise a standard of care by not driving until the impairment has been corrected.

While almost all jurisdictions in the USA would charge a person for causing a fatality during a sleep-related motor vehicle crash, the state of New Jersey is the only one to enact legislation dealing with sleep-related accidents. The specific statute [5] states:

…Criminal homicide constitutes vehicular homicide when it is caused by driving a vehicle or vessel recklessly. 1[For the purposes of this section, driving a vehicle or vessel while knowingly fatigued shall constitute recklessness. "Fatigued" as used in this section means having been without sleep for a period in excess of 24 consecutive hours.] Proof that the defendant fell asleep while driving or was driving after having been without sleep for a period in excess of 24 consecutive hours [shall] may give rise to an inference that the defendant was driving recklessly.

1. Introduction

The law is named after Maggie McDonnell, a 20-year-old college student from Gloucester County who died in July 1997 when another car swerved across three lanes and struck her vehicle head on. The other driver admitted he fell asleep at the wheel after 30 h without sleep and was acquitted of vehicular homicide and fined $200 for reckless driving. With the passage of "Maggie's Law", a conviction results in a second-degree crime and penalties can range as high as 10 years in prison and a $100 000 fine. Violation of the law applies to operators of boats as well as car drivers.

One of the most dramatic sleepiness-related accidents is the Selby (UK) train disaster [6]. A sleep-deprived driver went over an embankment onto a railway track where his vehicle was struck by a freight train, which derailed and caused the derailment of a second (passenger) train traveling in the opposite direction. The driver was tried on 10 counts of causing death by dangerous driving, found guilty, and sentenced to five years' imprisonment.

Employer liability for injuries caused by drowsiness or falling asleep

Employers are liable to employees under workers' compensation statutes for all injuries occurring within the scope of employment, regardless of cause. That said, courts would not hold employers liable in cases of employee misconduct (i.e. if it is clear that the employee was willfully negligent in continuing to drive when tired) [7]. Employers may also be liable to third parties injured by employees who drove negligently while acting within the scope of employment.

Commercial vehicle drivers cover large annual mileages, many on major highways and often at times when sleepiness is most prevalent. Such drivers are at risk for motor vehicle crashes as highlighted in a number of studies. A UK study of 996 heavy goods vehicle (HGV) drivers investigated the relationship between HGV drivers' accidents, daytime sleepiness (measured using the Epworth Sleepiness Scale) and other relevant physical characteristics [8]. Subjects drove an average of 69 700 miles annually (SD 36 120), and had a mean score on the Epworth daytime sleepiness scale of 5.65 (SD 3.31). Accident liability increased with increasing scores on the Epworth daytime sleepiness scale.

Drivers employed at bus depots within 30 miles of Edinburgh were given a sleep questionnaire [9]. One thousand, eight hundred and fifty-four drivers were approached, and 677 (37%; 25 female) completed questionnaires with a 97% response rate among the 456 given directly to drivers by the researcher. Twenty percent of the responding drivers (133/677) reported an Epworth sleepiness score >10. Eight percent of drivers reported falling asleep at the wheel at least once per month, and 7% having an accident, and 18% a near-miss accident due to sleepiness while working. This study shows a concerning high rate of sleepiness and sleep-related accidents among bus drivers.

If the injury occurs within the scope of employment, then an employer may be liable to an employee or to a third party for any injuries sustained in a sleep-related occupational accident or motor vehicle crash. Determining whether an injury occurred in the scope of employment can be difficult, however, as demonstrated by the case of Mayes V. Goodyear Tire & Rubber Co.[10]. An employee fell asleep while driving home in a company truck, causing a serious crash and injuring others. Because the employee had a load of tires to deliver on the way home, was available via pager 24 h per day, had no restrictions from using the employer's truck for personal business, and had received workers' compensation payments for the injuries sustained in the crash, the court found that the crash occurred within the scope of employment. However, this decision was subsequently overturned by the Supreme Court of Texas.

There are many examples of sleepiness and accidents due to work schedule-derived sleepiness. As a result, many jurisdictions now have hours of service (HOS) restrictions. Still, these may be ignored by employers, and employees can feel pressured to comply with the employers' demands.

The case of *Campbell v. James Gordon Hitchcock* highlights this and the risks of fatigue in the long-haul trucking industry [11]. The case involves an accident involving two articulated trucks where one of the drivers was killed. Long-haul truck drivers need to counter fatigue by taking sufficient rest-stops. In this case the Company failed to ensure that its employed drivers had sufficient opportunity for rest. On the contrary, the drivers employed by the Company worked to set delivery and pick-up times. The deceased was under pressure to deliver his final load at a particular time and this prevented him from taking urgently needed sleep. Moreover, the Company did not monitor its drivers' log-books, nor was there any evidence that the Company monitored rest periods in any way.

In 1989, the grounding of the oil tanker *Exxon Valdez* resulted in one of the most devastating human-caused environmental disasters ever to occur at sea. The US National Transportation Safety Board concluded that, among other factors, sleepiness and fatigue were responsible in that the third mate failed to properly maneuver the vessel, possibly due to fatigue and excessive workload, and that the captain failed to provide navigation watch and was sleeping below (alcohol likely involved). Moreover, the Exxon Shipping Company failed to supervise the captain and provide a rested and sufficient crew for the *Exxon Valdez* [12].

Physician liability

Physicians have a duty of care to accurately diagnose and treat patients. Those with expertise in sleep disorders are expected to recognize and diagnose subjects with sleep apnea or other sleep disorders affecting daytime function. Physicians should inquire about excessive sleepiness or other symptoms of sleep apnea in any patient who drives, but especially in patients who are commercial vehicle drivers (e.g. bus, truck, etc.) (Table 9.1). Moreover, physicians may have a duty to advise patients not to drive while under the influence of prescribed drugs, while undergoing medical treatment, or suffering from conditions that might impede driving ability.

However, physicians do not necessarily have a duty to protect third parties for a patient's actions resulting from or influenced by their sleep disorder or its treatment.

In *Calwell v. Hassan*, a doctor was treating a patient for daytime drowsiness and began a treatment regimen, but the patient did not follow up with appointments [13]. After leaving for work one day, she fell asleep while driving, injuring two bicyclists. The bicyclists brought an action against the physician, alleging that he negligently treated the patient for her sleep disorder and failed to warn her not to drive. The state supreme court found that the physician did not owe a duty to the bicyclists to protect them from his patient's actions. The court observed that, as a general rule, a person has no duty to control the conduct of a third person to prevent harm to others in the absence of a special relationship. According to the court, the only basis for imposing such a special relationship in this case was under the theory that the physician's actions created a risk of harm to the bicyclists. However, the court found that the patient was already aware of the disorder at the time she sought treatment; moreover,

Table 9.1 Screening recommendation for commercial drivers with possible or probable sleep apnea*

Medically fit to drive:
- No positive findings suggesting sleep apnea (see In-Service factors below)
- Documented compliance with CPAP – driver with known OSA

Conditional medically fit to drive (3 month maximum) but in-service evaluation required
- High pre-test probability of OSA
  ○ Subjective: snoring, witnessed apneas, daytime sleepiness
  ○ Objective:
    1. Two or more of the following: (a) BMI ≥ 35 kg or > 40 cm (b) neck circumference > 16 inches (women) or 17 inches or > 43 cm (men); (c) hypertension (new, uncontrolled or on 2+ medication)
    2. 2. ESS >10
    3. Unknown compliance with therapy for known sleep disorder
    4. OSA (AHI 5–29) but not sleepy (ESS < 11) and no history of motor vehicle accidents or hypertension on <2 medications

Not medically fit to drive – immediately out-of-service and evaluation required
- Sleeping in examination or waiting room or confessed excessive sleepiness
- Motor vehicle accident attributed to sleepiness
- ESS ≥ 16 or FOSQ < 18
- AHI >30
- Untreated OSA (non-compliant, treatment not tolerated or results unknown)

* Adapted from the Joint Task Force of the American College of Chest Physicians, American College of Occupational and Environmental Medicine, and the National Sleep Foundation.
Abbreviations: AHI, apnea–hypopnea index; BMI, body mass index; CPAP, continuous positive airway pressure; ESS, Epworth Sleepiness Scale; FOSQ, Functional Outcomes of Sleep Questionnaire; OSA, obstructive sleep apnea.

the patient admitted to knowing that she should have stopped driving when she felt drowsy. Thus, the doctor had no duty to protect the patient from what she already knew.

As observed in this case, a fundamental rule of actionable negligence is that such negligence must be based on a breach of duty. Without a duty there can be no breach to support the claims of plaintiffs. Whether or not a duty exists is a question of law which will vary between jurisdictions.

For example, in many Canadian provinces, there are laws which create a statutory duty for physicians to report certain medical conditions. In Ontario, the relevant Highway traffic act states [14]:

203. (1) Every legally qualified medical practitioner shall report to the Registrar the name, address and clinical condition of every person sixteen years of age or over attending upon the medical practitioner for medical services who, in the opinion of the medical practitioner, is suffering from a condition that may make it dangerous for the person to operate a motor vehicle.

(2) No action shall be brought against a qualified medical practitioner for complying with this section.

(3) The report referred to in subsection (1) is privileged for the information of the Registrar only and shall not be open for public inspection, and the report is inadmissible in evidence for any purpose in any trial except to prove compliance with subsection (1)

The burden of making a mandatory report in subsection (1) is alleviated by the legal protection against litigation which is guaranteed by subsection (2). The physician is also provided some flexibility in judging which patients and conditions are making it dangerous to operate a motor vehicle. However, physicians need to be aware of their relevant local laws since ignorance of the law provides no legal defense. This was clearly outlined in the Ontario case of *Spillane v. Wasserman* [15].

A patient suffering from epilepsy drove for a living as a local courier. He was treated for epilepsy, and some time after his condition was stable and well controlled, he stopped returning for medical follow-up. Subsequently, he decided he no longer needed his anticonvulsants and discontinued treatment. Sometime thereafter he had a generalized seizure while driving and killed a cyclist. The family of the deceased brought legal action against the driver, and also against the family physician and neurologist who had been involved in the patient's care. The evidence at trial established that the doctors were both aware – or should have been aware – that the defendant suffered nocturnal and daytime seizures on a fairly regular basis. The trial judge further concluded that the doctors failed to run blood tests on a routine basis to confirm control and compliance of prescribed drugs.

The court held that the physician was held liable for failure to report under the statute, as well as failure to follow the minimum College of Physicians and Surgeons of Ontario and Canadian Medical Association standards. Further, it was held to be insufficient to state that the patient was "a normal compliant patient because he did not fit the pattern of a noncompliant one". As a result, the court held the physicians 40% liable for the damages in negligence (physician's liability subsequently reduced to 5% on appeal).

Although this case deals specifically with epilepsy, one could easily substitute the diagnosis of obstructive sleep apnea for epilepsy, the discontinuation of CPAP treatment for stopping anticonvulsant therapy and the ensuing daytime sleepiness (instead of seizure) resulting in a fatal accident.

At all times a physician should advise any sleep apnea patient that driving while sleepy is very dangerous. It is advisable to put the warning in writing, as this will reinforce the seriousness of the warning and reduces (but may not eliminate) the risk of legal liability.

Many physicians will be asked to provide medical examinations to qualify a commercial vehicle driver for their operators license. This activity is likely to increase based on the recent Statement From the Joint Task Force of the American College of Chest Physicians, American College of Occupational and Environmental Medicine, and the National Sleep Foundation [16]. In addition, the Federal Motor Carrier Safety Administration have been reviewing their medical fitness guidelines with respect to sleep apnea and sleepiness. If adopted, it will put more pressure on patients and physicians to rapidly and accurately diagnose and treat sleep disorders. This could create new situations of liability risk for physicians.

Summary

The legal consequences of excessive sleepiness may impact patients, their physicians, and the public at large. Individuals with daytime sleepiness and/or known or suspected sleep disorders need to take precautions at work or when driving to ensure that they do not pose a risk to themselves or others. Physicians and healthcare workers need to be aware of the accident risks associated with sleep disorders and the legal implications around this in their particular jurisdiction. Laws regarding impaired drivers vary widely and practitioners should consult an attorney about applicable laws and regulations. With increasing awareness of the effects of sleepiness on performance, employers are taking a greater role in identifying at-risk employees and incorporating safe work practices in the workplace. The development of new guidelines and medical standards in the transportation industry will eventually impact on physicians, employers and drivers alike. Legislators must continue to work with practitioners and scientists to balance adequate protection of the public interest with individual rights.

References

1. **Swaen G M H**, **van Amelsvoort L P G M**, **Bültmann U**, *et al*. Fatigue as a risk factor for being injured in an occupational accident: results from the Maastricht Cohort Study. *Occup Environ Med*, 2003; **60**(Suppl I):i88–92.
2. **Regina v. Hundal** (1993) 79 C.C.C. (3d) 97 S.C.C.
3. **Reyner L A**, **Horne J A**. Falling asleep whilst driving: are drivers aware of prior sleepiness? *Int J Legal Med*, 1998; **111**:120–23.
4. **R v. Gill** 2005 BCPC 0665.
5. **N.J.S.2C**:11–5 2003.
6. **GNER v. Hart** [2003] EWHC 2450 (QB).
7. **Schoof v. Byrd**, 415 P.2d 384 (Kan. 1966); Estate of Coe v. Willmes Trucking, L.L.C., 689 N.W.2d 318 (Neb. 2004).
8. **Maycock, G.** Sleepiness and driving: the experience of heavy goods vehicle drivers in the UK. *J Sleep Res*, 1997; **6**:238–44.
9. **Vennelle M**, **Engleman H M**, **Douglas N J**. Sleepiness and sleep-related accidents in commercial bus drivers. *Sleep Breath*, 2009Jul 9. [Epub ahead of print]PMID: 19588178.
10. **Mayes v. Goodyear** Tire & Rubber Co., 144 S.W.3d 50 (Tex. App. 2004).
11. **Inspector Campbell v James Gordon Hitchcock** [2004] NSWIRComm 87.
12. **Exxon Shipping Company**, *et al*. v. Grant Baker, *et al*. 554 U.S. 128 S.Ct. 2605.
13. **Calwell v. Hassan**, 925 P.2d 422 (Kan. 1996).
14. **Ontario Highway Traffic Act**, R.S.O. 1990, c. H.8.
15. **Spillane v. Wasserman** (1992), 42 C.C.L.T. (2d) 267 (Gen Div.; affirmed (1998), 41 C.C.L.T. (2d) 292 (C.A.).
16. **Hartenbaum N**, **Collop N**, **Rosen I**, *et al*. Sleep apnea and commercial motor vehicle operators: Statement from the Joint Task Force of the American College of Chest Physicians, American College of Occupational and Environmental Medicine, and the National Sleep Foundation. *J Occup Environ Med*, 2006; S1–37.

Section 2 Chapter 10

Sleep Disorders and Excessive Sleepiness

Sleep deprivation: biomarkers for identifying and predicting individual differences in response to sleep loss

Namni Goel and David F. Dinges

Overview

Insufficient sleep is common, affecting 20–40% of adults, and resulting from sleep disorders, medical conditions, work demands, stress/emotional distress, and social/domestic responsibilities. It produces significant social, financial and health-related costs, and it has increasingly become a major public health concern as population studies worldwide have found that reduced sleep duration is associated with increased risks of obesity, morbidity, and mortality. It is well established that sleep loss causes fatigue and sleepiness, as well as errors and accidents that are due to its adverse neurobehavioral effects on alertness, mood, and cognitive functions. However, recent evidence reveals that there are substantial, trait-like (phenotypic) differences among individuals in the extent to which they experience such neurobehavioral deficits when either acutely or chronically sleep-deprived; thus far, such differences are not explained by subjects' baseline functioning or a number of other potential predictors including prior sleep history. Common genetic variations involved in sleep–wake, circadian, and cognitive regulation may underlie these large phenotypic differences in neurobehavioral vulnerability to sleep deprivation and may thus serve as biomarkers. Beyond genetic variants, neuroimaging techniques may produce brain markers to predict such differential vulnerability. Determination of biomarkers of differential neurobehavioral vulnerability to sleep loss will help inform public policies pertaining to the need for adequate sleep; help identify who is most in need of prevention of sleep debt and in need of countermeasures for sleep loss; and further understanding and management of vulnerability to excessive sleepiness due to common sleep and medical disorders. This chapter summarizes trait-like (phenotypic) individual differences in neurobehavioral vulnerability to sleep deprivation, and current promising efforts to identify objective and biological markers of such differences.

Sleep deprivation: prevalence and risks

Adequate sleep is vital for healthy neurobehavioral functioning [1]. Insufficient sleep occurs in millions of individuals who have medical conditions that disrupt sleep (e.g. untreated or ineffectively treated sleep apnea; certain types of insomnia; restless legs syndrome and periodic limb movements; circadian rhythm sleep disorders such as shift work sleep disorder and delayed sleep phase type; disorders that produce nocturnal pain, nocturia, or otherwise fragment sleep consolidation or increase premature awakenings). Demographic factors such as being a non-Hispanic African-American, and lifestyle factors such as having children less than 2 years of age or working long hours, are also associated with sleep curtailment [e.g. 2–4].

It is estimated that 20–40% of the adult US population sleep less than 7 h per night [5] – the minimum sleep duration that we and other researchers have found in large-scale laboratory experiments necessary to prevent cumulative deterioration in performance on a range of cognitive tasks [6, 7]. The proportion of people curtailing their sleep due to lifestyle is increasing [5], and is likely higher than surveys indicate, since physiological sleep duration is one hour or more below self-reported sleep duration [8, 9]. In certain subgroups – such as night shift workers, hospital nurses [10], physicians in training [11], and adolescents [12] – inadequate sleep is highly prevalent, chronic, and

---

Sleepiness: Causes, Consequences and Treatment, ed. Michael J. Thorpy and Michel Billiard. Published by Cambridge University Press. © Cambridge University Press 2011.

associated with increased risks of behavioral morbidity, suggesting pervasive deleterious effects and highlighting the critical need for interventions that reduce the negative impact of sleep deprivation.

Sleep loss, including chronic partial sleep deprivation (PSD) – a condition associated with a wide range of serious health consequences and experienced by millions of people on a consecutive and daily basis – can result from medical conditions, sleep disorders, work demands, stress/emotional distress, and social/domestic responsibilities [5]. It is associated with significant social, financial and health-related costs, in large part because it produces impaired cognitive performance due to increasing sleep propensity and instability of waking neurobehavioral functions [5]. Sleep loss has increasingly become a major public health concern as population studies worldwide have found reduced sleep duration (less than 7 h) associated with increased risks of obesity, morbidity, and mortality [e.g. 4, 13, 14]. In addition to a wide range of behavioral risks associated with inadequate sleep, more than 50 population-based studies have found reduced sleep duration (less than 7 h per night) to be a risk factor for obesity, cardiovascular disease and diabetes, and mortality [e.g. 4, 13, 14]. It remains unknown whether the association between short sleep and morbidity and mortality is causal. However, for the majority of people, sleep reduction directly causes significant risks via increased fatigue and sleep propensity, and via deficits in mood and neurocognitive functions including vigilant and executive attention, cognitive speed and working memory, and executive functions [5, 15]. Moreover, insufficient sleep also increases the risk of motor vehicle crashes [16, 17], and workplace errors and accidents [18, 19], which have been estimated to cost between $43 and $56 billion annually [15].

Stable trait-like individual differences in response to sleep deprivation

Although it is common for people – including sleep experts – to speak of the effects of sleep loss as occurring equally in all individuals, it has been known for some time that this is categorically not the case [20–22]. As a group of otherwise healthy individuals undergo either acute total sleep deprivation (TSD) for a night, or repeated nights of chronic PSD, the changes in sleepiness and other sensitive neurobehavioral measures not only reveal a mean change over time, but also an ever-greater standard deviation over time [20, 21]. This proportionality between the mean and standard deviation indicates that although the average (and median) neurobehavioral response to sleep loss is increasing over time, some individuals are experiencing much more sleepiness and neurobehavioral instability than others. The longstanding assumption that this inter-subject variance in response to sleep loss was primarily random error variance was called into question by the results of the first systematic experimental effort to replicate these individual responses to sleep deprivation [23, 24].

In the past 100 years, only two experiments repeated TSD in a small number of healthy adults [25, 26]. These studies anecdotally noted that there were large, consistent interindividual differences in performance deficits. Our laboratory was the first to experimentally establish that subjects undergoing acute TSD – in which no sleep is obtained – show differential vulnerability to sleep loss, demonstrating robust interindividual (trait-like, phenotypic) differences in response to the same laboratory conditions, as measured by various physiological and subjective sleep measures and neurobehavioral tasks sensitive to sleep loss [e.g. 22, 27]. The intraclass correlation coefficients (ICCs) – which express the proportion of variance in the data explained by systematic interindividual variability – revealed that stable (trait-like) responses accounted for 58 and 68% of the overall variance in psychomotor vigilance test (PVT) lapses (greater than 500 ms reaction times) between multiple sleep-deprivation exposures in the same subjects [6, 23, 24, 27]. Thus, individuals who showed high PVT lapse rates during TSD after one exposure also showed high lapse rates during a second exposure; similarly, those with low PVT lapse rates during one exposure showed low PVT lapse rates during a second exposure. Most importantly, because these high ICCs were found when the subjects were exposed to TSD 2–3 times under markedly different conditions (e.g. high versus low stimulation [23]; 6-h versus 12-h sleep time per night [22]), the marked differences in cognitive vulnerability to sleep deprivation are considered phenotypic.[1] Figure 10.1

[1.] A phenotype has the following characteristics: (1) it is an observed trait or characteristic of an organism (e.g., morphology, development, behavior); (2) it is a characteristic that can be made visible by some technical procedure; (3) it is a product of genotypes, but is also influenced by extragenetic

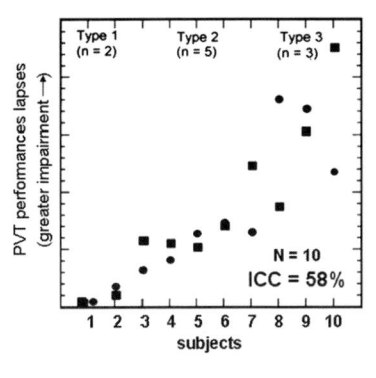

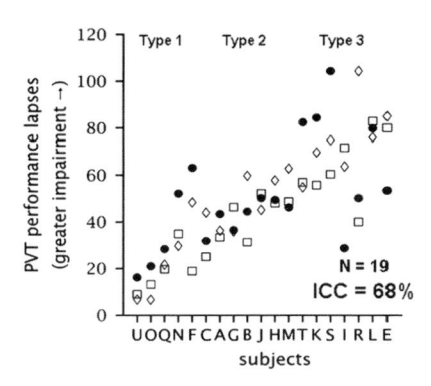

Figure 10.1 The **left panel** shows mean psychomotor vigilance test (PVT) performance lapses per test bout after acute total sleep deprivation (TSD) from an initial experiment on 10 healthy adults studied during two separate acute TSD periods (circles versus squares) that differed by the degree of activity and social stimulation [data from 23, 24]. The intraclass correlation (ICC), which expresses the proportion of variance explained by systematic interindividual variability, was 58% between the two experiments. The **right panel** shows results of a second experiment from our laboratory in which 19 adults underwent (in randomized order) 3 nights of acute TSD on 3 separate occasions, 2 of which followed a week of sleep extension of 12 h time in bed (squares: first exposure to TSD following sleep extension; diamonds: second exposure to TSD following sleep extension), and one of which (solid circles) involved a prior week of chronic PSD (6 h time in bed). Despite markedly different sleep histories, the ICC revealed that 68% of the variance in PVT lapsing during acute TSD was stable (trait-like) among subjects [data from 22]. Thus, both experiments confirmed that differential cognitive vulnerability to acute TSD was a major source of variance, and that some subjects consistently had few lapses of attention in response to sleep loss (i.e. Type 1 responders), while others showed large increases in lapsing (Type 3 responders), and some were in the intermediate lapse range (Type 2 responders). Thus, PVT performance deficits from acute TSD varied significantly among individuals and were stable within individuals. Importantly, these stable individual differences in responses to sleep deprivation were not merely a result of variations in sleep history or other factors. Rather, they were a result of trait-like differential vulnerability to impairment from sleep loss.

shows data demonstrating the stability of the trait-like (phenotypic) differences in PVT lapses of attention to one night of acute TSD in these protocols, and highlights the fact that while some individuals are highly vulnerable to cognitive performance deficits when sleep-deprived (Type 3), others show remarkable levels of cognitive resistance to sleep loss (Type 1), and others show intermediate responses (Type 2; [27]).

Other laboratories have confirmed our findings of large, stable (trait-like) differences in cognitive responses to acute TSD [e.g. 28, 29]. Notably, such differences have not (yet) been accounted for by demographic factors (age, sex, IQ), by baseline functioning, by circadian chronotype, or by sleep need; moreover, psychometric scales have not reliably identified cognitively vulnerable individuals [6, 22, 24]. Our group [6, 30] and others [31] have found similar differential vulnerability to chronic PSD, in which sleep is restricted to 3–7 h time in bed per night.

Such phenotypic differences in vulnerability to the neurobehavioral effects of sleep loss explain a relatively common observation of field studies and clinical populations. For example, a major field study of long-haul truck drivers observed that only 14% of long-haul truck drivers accounted for 54% of drowsy-driving episodes [32]. It has been reported that approximately 10% of night and rotating shift workers suffer Shift Work Disorder (SWD), which involves severe nighttime sleepiness on the job [33, 34]. Phenotypic vulnerability to sleepiness would also explain why correlations between sleep apnea severity measured by respiratory disturbance index/apnea–hypopnea index (RDI/AHI) and excessive daytime sleepiness (EDS) are often low, and why some patients remain sleepy after using CPAP for greater than 7 h per night [35].

At present, it remains unknown whether the same individuals vulnerable to the adverse effects of chronic PSD are also cognitively vulnerable to acute TSD. The few reports comparing responses to both acute TSD and chronic PSD have used small sample sizes (number of subjects ranging from 9 to 13) and limited assessments [6, 36, 37]. Moreover, only one of these studies has systematically studied the same subjects in both acute TSD and chronic PSD [36].

Finding phenotypes of differential cognitive vulnerabilities to sleep loss will help identify persons who are prone to fatigue and excessive sleepiness [38], who

or environmental factors. In addition, phenotypic variation (due to underlying heritable genetic variation) is a fundamental prerequisite for evolution by natural selection.

are at risk for cognitive deficits and behavioral morbidity from sleep loss [6], and who therefore need to prevent or mitigate sleep deprivation through lifestyle choices and effective interventions and countermeasures. Such identification may also permit a greater utilization of personnel and resources in work and operational settings. Thus, identifying those individuals at greatest risk for experiencing the adverse effects of inadequate sleep is of critical importance.

Biomarkers of differential vulnerability to sleep loss

Candidate genes associated with individual differences in vulnerability to sleep deprivation

The stable, trait-like interindividual differences observed in response to acute TSD – with intraclass correlation coefficients accounting for 58–92% of the variance in neurobehavioral measures [22, 27] – point to an underlying genetic component. Until recently, however, the genetic basis of such differential vulnerability to sleep loss in normal healthy subjects has received little attention [15]. Available data suggest that common genetic variations (polymorphisms) involved in sleep–wake, circadian, and cognitive regulation may underlie symptomatic aspects of these large interindividual differences in neurobehavioral vulnerability to sleep deprivation in healthy adults [15, 39].

PERIOD3 VNTR polymorphism: differential role of a circadian gene in response to acute TSD and chronic PSD

Two related publications reported on the role of the variable number tandem repeat (VNTR) polymorphism of the circadian gene *PERIOD3* (*PER3*) in response to TSD. *PER3* is characterized by a 54-nucleotide coding region motif repeating in 4 or 5 units and shows similar allelic frequencies in African Americans and Caucasians. Compared with the 4-repeat allele ($PER3^{4/4}$; $N = 14$), the longer, 5-repeat allele ($PER3^{5/5}$; $N = 10$) was associated with worse cognitive performance during sleep loss and with higher sleep propensity including slow-wave activity (SWA) in the sleep EEG – a putative marker of sleep homeostasis – before and after TSD [40]. A subsequent report on the same subjects clarified that the $PER3^{5/5}$ performance deficits were found only on specific executive function tests, and only at 2–4 h following the melatonin circadian rhythm peak, from approximately 6 to 8 am [41]. Such performance differences were hypothesized to be mediated by sleep homeostasis [40, 41]. Although the work on *PER3* VNTR variants and cognitive responses to TSD is important, replication of such data are necessary to consider this polymorphism as a biomarker of cognitive vulnerability to sleep loss.

Moreover, the aforementioned *PER3* findings may not generalize to responses to chronic PSD. We recently evaluated whether the *PER3* VNTR polymorphism contributed to cumulative neurobehavioral deficits and sleep homeostatic responses during chronic PSD in $PER3^{4/4}$, $PER3^{4/5}$ and $PER3^{5/5}$ healthy adults [30]. As shown in Figure 10.2, the $PER3^{4/4}$, $PER3^{4/5}$ and $PER3^{5/5}$ genotypes demonstrated large but equivalent cumulative increases in sleepiness and cumulative decreases in cognitive performance and physiological alertness, across five nights of chronic sleep restriction to 4 h per night. Such effects were accompanied by increasing daily inter-subject variability in all genotypes (see Figure 10.2). During chronic PSD, $PER3^{5/5}$ subjects had slightly but reliably elevated sleep homeostatic pressure as measured by non-REM slow-wave energy (NREM SWE) compared with $PER3^{4/4}$ subjects (see Figure 10.3). In contrast to published data in TSD paradigms, the *PER3* VNTR variants did not differ on baseline sleep measures or in their physiological sleepiness, cognitive, executive functioning or subjective responses to chronic PSD. Thus, the *PER3* VNTR polymorphism is not a genetic marker of differential vulnerability to the cumulative neurobehavioral effects of chronic PSD. It remains possible, however, that the $PER3^{5/5}$ genotype may contribute to differential neurobehavioral vulnerability to acute TSD because it involves wakefulness at a specific circadian time in the early morning hours (6–8 am), when subjects in our study were asleep [30].

COMT polymorphism: role of a cognitive gene in differential vulnerability to TSD

The Val158Met polymorphism of the *catechol*-O-*Methyltransferase* (*COMT*) gene modulates cortical dopaminergic catabolism and has been reported to predict prefrontal cortex functioning and cognitive performance in healthy subjects [42, 43]. In acute

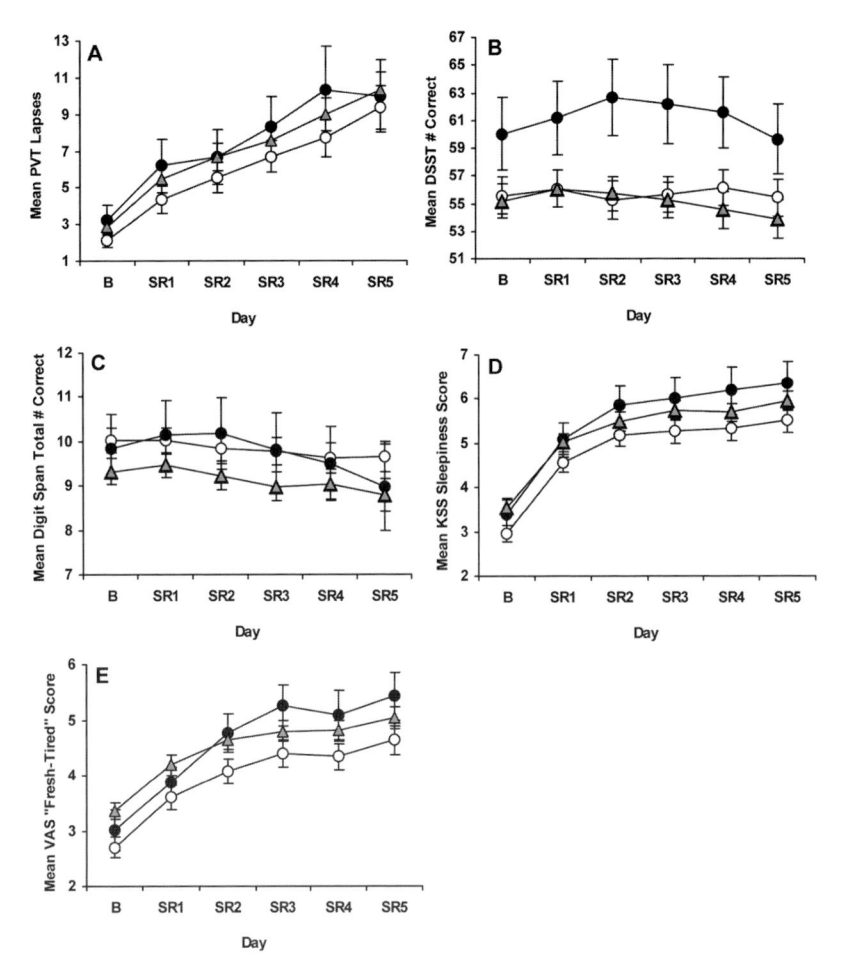

Figure 10.2 This figure shows neurobehavioral performance at baseline and during chronic partial sleep deprivation for the *PER3* groups. Mean (± SEM) (**A**) PVT lapses (>500 ms reaction times) per trial, (**B**) total number correct per trial on the Digit Symbol Substitution Task (DSST) and (**C**) Digit Span (DS) task, and scores per trial on the (**D**) Karolinska Sleepiness scale (KSS) and (**E**) "Fresh–Tired" visual analog scale (VAS) at baseline (B) and each partial sleep deprivation/restriction night (SR1-SR5) for *PER3*$^{4/4}$ (open circles), *PER3*$^{4/5}$ (gray triangles) and *PER3*$^{5/5}$ (closed circles) subjects. Although all genotypes showed increased PVT lapses and variability across chronic PSD, there were no differential responses in lapses nor did one genotype show more lapses than the other groups at baseline or during chronic PSD. *PER3*$^{5/5}$ subjects had better cognitive throughput than their *PER3*$^{4/4}$ counterparts, as indicated by significantly higher DSST scores across days; there were no differential changes in DSST scores across chronic PSD or significant changes across days. For all groups, DS total correct scores significantly decreased, and KSS and VAS scores significantly increased across chronic PSD, but there were no differential changes or group differences in these measures during chronic PSD. (Reprinted with permission from Goel N, Banks S, Mignot E, et al. PER3 polymorphism predicts cumulative sleep homeostatic but not neurobehavioral changes to chronic partial sleep deprivation. PLoS ONE 2009; 4: e5874.)

TSD, the *COMT* Val158Met polymorphism has been found to predict interindividual differences in brain alpha (α) oscillations [43]. It has also been shown to modulate the efficacy of the wake-promoting drug modafinil on waking function, but neither this *COMT* genotype nor modafinil has been shown to affect sleep-deprivation-induced changes in recovery sleep [42]. We are currently investigating whether the *COMT* Val158Met polymorphism contributes to cumulative neurobehavioral deficits and sleep homeostatic responses during chronic PSD in Met/Met, and Val/Val healthy adults.

*DQB1*0602* allele predicts interindividual differences in physiological sleep structure, sleepiness and fatigue

The human leukocyte antigen (HLA) *DQB1*0602* allele is closely associated with narcolepsy, a neurological sleep disorder characterized by excessive

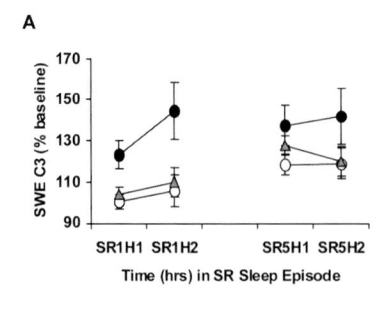

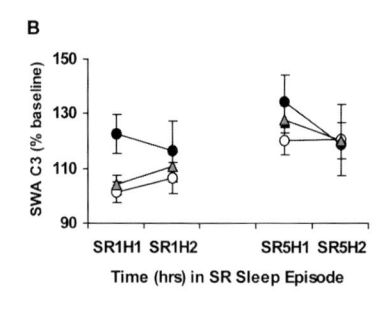

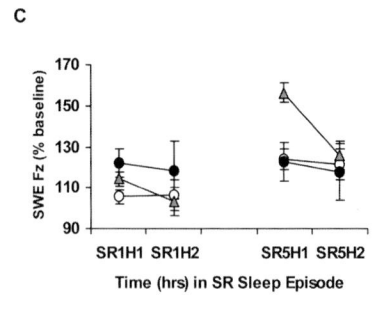

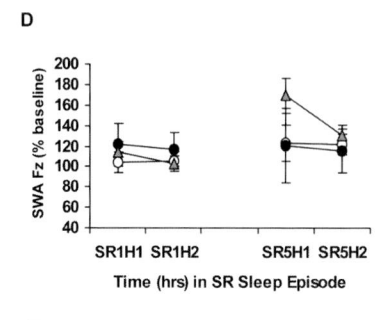

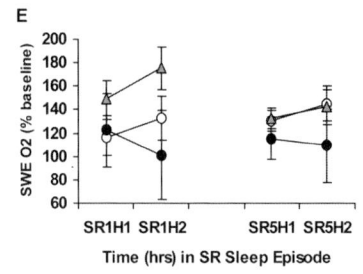

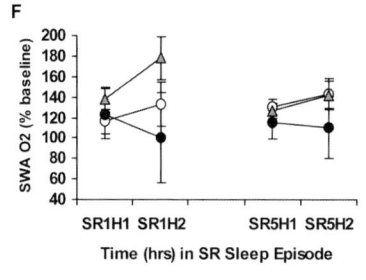

Figure 10.3 This figure shows slow-wave energy and slow-wave activity during chronic partial sleep deprivation for the *PER3* genotypes. Mean (±SEM) hourly slow-wave energy (SWE) and slow-wave activity (SWA) as a percentage of baseline at the same corresponding hour derived from the C3 (**A**, **B**), Fz (**C**, **D**) or O2 (**E**, **F**) channels at partial sleep deprivation/restriction night 1 (SR1) and partial sleep deprivation/restriction night 5 (SR5) for hour 1 (H1) and hour 2 (H2) in *PER3*$^{4/4}$ (open circles), *PER3*$^{4/5}$ (gray triangles) and *PER3*$^{5/5}$ (closed circles) subjects. SWE derived from C3 (but not from Fz or O2) was significantly higher during chronic PSD in *PER3*$^{5/5}$ compared with *PER3*$^{4/4}$ and *PER3*$^{4/5}$ subjects. (Reprinted with permission from Goel N, Banks S, Mignot E, et al. PER3 polymorphism predicts cumulative sleep homeostatic but not neurobehavioral changes to chronic partial sleep deprivation. *PLoS ONE* 2009; 4: e5874.)

daytime sleepiness, fragmented sleep, and shortened REM latency [44]. We investigated the sleep homeostatic responses, fatigue and sleepiness responses, and cognitive deficits as a result of chronic PSD in healthy sleepers positive and negative for *DQB1*0602*, as a potential novel marker of differential vulnerability to chronic PSD [45]. During baseline, although *DQB1*0602*-positive subjects were significantly sleepier and more fatigued by self-report, they showed greater sleep fragmentation, and decreased sleep homeostatic pressure and differentially sharper declines during the night, measured by non-REM electroencephalographic slow-wave energy (NREM EEG SWE) [45]. During chronic PSD, despite SWE elevation comparable to *DQB1*0602*-negative subjects, *DQB1*0602*-positive subjects were sleepier and showed more fragmented sleep. Moreover, they showed differentially greater reductions in REM latency and smaller reductions in stage 2 sleep and differentially greater increases in fatigue. Both groups demonstrated comparable cumulative decreases in cognitive performance and increases in physiological sleepiness to chronic PSD, and did not differ on executive function tasks [45].

*DQB1*0602* positivity in a healthy population represents a continuum of some sleep–wake features of narcolepsy. *DQB1*0602* was associated with interindividual differences in sleep homeostasis, physiological sleep, sleepiness and fatigue – but not in cognitive measures – during baseline and chronic PSD. Thus, *DQB1*0602* may signify a genetic biomarker for predicting individual differences in both basal and sleep loss conditions. The influence of the *DQB1*0602* allele on sleep homeostatic and neurobehavioral responses has not been examined in healthy subjects undergoing acute TSD.

Adenosine-related candidate genes: role for individual differences and response to total sleep deprivation

Other studies have investigated the role of select adenosine-related candidate genes in individual differences and in response to acute total sleep deprivation. Rétey et al. [46] found that the 22G→A polymorphism of the adenosine deaminase gene (*ADA*) was associated with enhanced slow-wave sleep (SWS) and NREM SWA, contributing to interindividual variability in baseline sleep; however, this study did not test responses to sleep deprivation. The c.1083T > C polymorphism of the adenosine A2A receptor gene (*ADORA2A*) has been related to objective and subjective differences in the effects of caffeine on NREM sleep after TSD [47], and has been associated with individual differences in baseline EEG during sleep and wakefulness [46]. While promising, replication of these data in independent samples is needed; in addition, the role of these genetic variants in response to chronic PSD has not yet been established.

Future considerations for genetic biomarkers of differential vulnerability to sleep loss

Because of reported differences in behavioral, sleep homeostatic and physiological responses to chronic PSD and acute TSD [6, 36, 37], it is possible that specific candidate genes play different roles in the degree of vulnerability and/or resilience to the neurobehavioral and homeostatic effects of acute TSD and chronic PSD. In support of this possibility, and as reviewed above, we found that the *PERIOD3* VNTR polymorphism related to individual differences in sleep homeostatic (i.e. NREM SWE) but not neurobehavioral responses to chronic PSD [30]. Future studies are needed to explore this avenue of research and to determine predictors of those individuals most vulnerable to the neurobehavioral effects of both types of sleep loss.

To date, with the exception of our recent studies, which employed a total of 129 subjects [30, 45] all candidate gene studies involving sleep physiological and neurobehavioral variables have employed small sample sizes ($N = 14–24$) and have only examined homozygotic individuals [40–43, 46, 47]. Larger sample sizes and assessment of phenotype–genotype relationships in both homozygous and heterozygous individuals are needed to definitively determine whether such candidate genes involved in regulation of sleep–wake, circadian and cognitive functions are associated with interindividual neurobehavioral responses to sleep loss across an entire population. This is particularly the case, given that individuals are necessarily categorized into different genotypes, reducing sample sizes in each subgroup. Thus, future candidate gene studies must consistently use sample sizes in the hundreds, rather than tens, to detect statistically reliable differences across genotypes. In addition, as noted above, replication of findings in independent samples is needed to determine whether findings are genuine and are not due to chance.

Neuroimaging and individual differences in cognitive vulnerability to sleep deprivation

Although there are many published neuroimaging [functional magnetic resonance imaging (fMRI), positron emission tomography (PET)] studies on the effects of sleep deprivation on brain activity in healthy adults [15], few studies have examined the relationship between brain activity and differential behavioral performance deficits following sleep deprivation. Only four neuroimaging studies have been published on this topic, and all of these studies have employed blood oxygenation level-dependent functional magnetic resonance imaging (BOLD fMRI) in small study samples. In one study, 33 healthy young men, including 10 sleep-deprivation resistant and 10 sleep-deprivation vulnerable subjects were scanned during performance of the Sternberg Working Memory Task (SWMT) after a normal night of sleep and following 30 h of sleep deprivation [48]. The sleep-deprivation resistant group showed significantly more activation than the vulnerable group during rested baseline and after sleep deprivation. Sleep deprivation significantly decreased the activation level (BOLD signal changes) and the number of activated voxels in frontal and parietal regions in the vulnerable group, but not in the resistant group. In another study, 10 military pilots were scanned during SWMT performance and compared to 10 vulnerable and 10 resistant non-pilot subjects [49]. BOLD activation in the pilots resembled that of resistant rather than vulnerable non-pilot subjects. In the pilot group, the amount of global activation during SWMT positively correlated ($r = 0.777$) with average flight performance during 37 h of continuous wakefulness. In a third study, 26 healthy subjects were scanned during performance of working memory tasks after normal sleep, and at 24 and 35 h of sleep deprivation [50]. Greater activation in the frontal and parietal regions after normal sleep was associated with reduced performance declines during sleep deprivation.

Collectively, the findings of these early neuroimaging studies of differential vulnerability to sleep deprivation suggest that cognitive resistance may be associated with greater activity preservation during sleep deprivation (lower activity decreases from baseline to sleep deprivation or greater pre-existing activity at baseline before sleep deprivation). By contrast, results from a fourth study showed that reduced activation in the right prefrontal cortex after normal sleep was associated with better performance after sleep deprivation [51]. This finding suggests that cognitive vulnerability may be associated with the failure to engage additional activity in alternative (not pre-occupied) neural resources when demand increases. One recent study found that 27 healthy subjects stratified according to homozygosity for the aforementioned *PER3* VNTR genotype ($N = 15$ $PER3^{4/4}$ subjects, $N = 12$ $PER3^{5/5}$ subjects) showed markedly different cerebral blood flow profiles (using BOLD fMRI) and corresponding differences in vulnerability of executive function performance in response to TSD [52].

Much larger sample sizes and newer imaging techniques that allow absolute quantification of signal changes, that are not task dependent, and that can assay sleep deprivation-induced neural activity changes over periods greater than a few minutes (such as arterial spin labeling, ASL, MRI) are needed to more fully characterize the neural mechanisms mediating trait-like differential vulnerability to sleep deprivation in normal healthy individuals, to dissociate the effects of sleep deprivation on resting neural activity and on task activation, and to examine the relationship of the neural mechanisms mediating trait-like differential vulnerability to sleep deprivation with selective candidate genes.

Conclusions

The impairing effects of sleep loss on neurobehavioral functions are the most well-established and conspicuous consequences of sleep deprivation. They include fatigue and sleepiness and unstable wakefulness; deficits in attention, working memory and executive functions; reduced mood-affect regulation; and increased accidents and injuries [5, 15]. However, there are substantial differences among people in the extent to which they experience such deficits when sleep deprived.

In recent years – since our group originally identified such stable, trait-like (phenotypic) neurobehavioral vulnerability to sleep loss – there has been a growing search for biomarkers of this cognitive vulnerability, in an effort to identify this large and critical source of variance in human neurobehavioral responses to sleep deprivation. Indeed, recent seminal findings employing candidate gene and neuroimaging techniques suggest the efforts are feasible. Identifying who is more likely to suffer neurobehavioral impairments from sleep loss would significantly improve prevention of sleep deprivation and mitigation of its behavioral morbidity, and further our understanding and management of vulnerability to excessive sleepiness due to common sleep and medical disorders (e.g. sleep apnea, certain insomnias, affective disorders, medical conditions involving pain, shift work sleep disorder).

Acknowledgments

This chapter was supported by NIH NR004281 and CTRC UL1RR024134, and by the National Space Biomedical Research Institute through NASA NCC 9–58. This project also received support from a grant from the Institute for Translational Medicine and Therapeutics' (ITMAT) Transdisciplinary Program in Translational Medicine and Therapeutics. The project described was supported in part by Grant Number UL1RR024134 from the National Center for Research Resources. The content is solely the responsibility of the authors and does not necessarily represent the official views of the National Center for Research Resources or the National Institutes of Health.

References

1. **Meerlo P**, **Mistlberger R E**, **Jacobs B L**, et al. New neurons in the adult brain: the role of sleep and consequences of sleep loss. *Sleep Med Rev*, 2009; **13**:187–94.

2. **Basner M**, **Dinges D F**. Dubious bargain: trading sleep for Leno and Letterman. *Sleep*, 2009; **32**:747–52.

3. **Basner M**, **Fomberstein K M**, **Razavi F M**, et al. American Time Use Survey: sleep time and its relationship to waking activities. *Sleep*, 2007; **30**:1085–95.

4. **Krueger P M**, **Friedman E M**. Sleep duration in the United States: a cross-sectional population-based study. *Am J Epidemiol*, 2009; **169**:1052–63.

5. **Banks S**, **Dinges D F**. Behavioral and physiological consequences of sleep restriction in humans. *J Clin Sleep Med*, 2007; **3**:519–28.

6. **Van Dongen H P A**, **Maislin G**, **Mullington J M**, et al. The cumulative cost of additional wakefulness: dose–response effects on neurobehavioral functions and sleep physiology from chronic sleep restriction and total sleep deprivation. *Sleep*, 2003; **26**:117–26.

7. **Belenky G**, **Wesensten N J**, **Thorne D R**, et al. Patterns of performance degradation and restoration during sleep restriction and subsequent recovery: a sleep–dose response study. *J Sleep Res*, 2003; **12**:1–12.

8. **Silva G E**, **Goodwin J L**, **Sherrill D L**, et al. Relationship between reported and measured sleep times: the Sleep Heart Health Study (SHHS). *J Clin Sleep Med*, 2007; **3**:622–30.

9. **Lauderdale D S**, **Knutson K L**, **Yan L L**, et al. Self-reported and measured sleep duration: how similar are they? *Epidemiology*, 2008; **19**:838–45.

10. **Rogers A E**, **Hwang W-T**, **Scott L D**, et al. The working hours of hospital staff nurses and patient safety. *Health Aff*, 2004; **23**:202–12.

11. **Ayas N T**, **Barger L K**, **Cade B E**, et al. Extended work duration and the risk of self-reported percutaneous injuries in interns. *JAMA*, 2006; **296**:1055–62.

12. **Roberts R E**, **Roberts C R**, **Duong H T**. Sleepless in adolescence: prospective data on sleep deprivation, health and functioning. *J Adolesc*, 2009; **32**:1045–57.

13. **Ferrie J E**, **Shipley M J**, **Cappuccio F P**, et al. A prospective study of change in sleep duration: associations with mortality in the Whitehall II cohort. *Sleep*, 2007; **30**:1659–66.

14. **Cappuccio F P**, **Taggart F M**, **Kandala N-B**, et al. Meta-analysis of short duration and obesity in children and adults. *Sleep*, 2008; **31**:619–26.

15. **Goel N**, **Rao H**, **Durmer J S**, et al. Neurocognitive consequences of sleep deprivation. *Semin Neurol*, 2009; **29**:320–39.

16. **Horne J A**, **Reyner L**. Vehicle accidents related to sleep: a review. *Occup Environ Med*, 1999; **56**:289–94.

17. **Barger L K**, **Cade B E**, **Ayas N T**, et al. Extended work shifts and the risk of motor vehicle crashes among interns. *N Engl J Med*, 2005; **352**:125–34.

18. **Dinges D F**. An overview of sleepiness and accidents. *J Sleep Res*, 1995; **4**:4–11.

19. **Landrigan C P**, **Rothschild J M**, **Cronin J W**, et al. Effect of reducing interns' work hours on serious medical errors in intensive care units. *N Engl J Med*, 2004; **351**:1838–48.

20. **Dinges D F**, **Kribbs N B**. Performing while sleepy: effects of experimentally-induced sleepiness. In: Monk T H, Ed. *Sleep, Sleepiness and Performance*. Chichester: John Wiley and Sons, 1991: 97–128.

21. **Doran S M**, **Van Dongen H P A**, **Dinges D F**. Sustained attention performance during sleep deprivation: evidence of state instability. *Arch Ital Biol*, 2001; **139**:253–67.

22. **Van Dongen H P A**, **Baynard M D**, **Maislin G**, et al. Systematic interindividual differences in neurobehavioral impairment from sleep loss: evidence of trait-like differential vulnerability. *Sleep*, 2004; **27**:423–33.

23. **Dijkman M**, **Sachs N**, **Levine E**, et al. Effects of reduced stimulation on neurobehavioral alertness depend on circadian phase during human sleep deprivation. *Sleep Res*, 1997; **26**:265.

24. **Van Dongen H P A**, **Dijkman M V**, **Maislin G**, et al. Phenotypic aspect of vigilance decrement during sleep deprivation. *Physiologist*, 1999; **42**:A-5.

25. **Wilkinson R T**. Interaction of lack of sleep with knowledge of results, repeated testing, and individual differences. *J Exp Psychol*, 1961; **62**:263–71.

26. **Webb W B**, **Levy C M**. Effects of spaced and repeated total sleep deprivation. *Ergonomics*, 1984; **27**:45–58.

27. **Van Dongen H P**, **Maislin G**, **Dinges D F**. Dealing with interindividual differences in the temporal dynamics of fatigue and performance: importance and techniques. *Aviat Space Environ Med*, 2004; **75**:A147–54.

28. **Leproult R**, **Colecchia E F**, **Berardi A M**, et al. Individual differences in subjective and objective alertness during sleep deprivation are stable and unrelated. *Am J Physiol Regulat Integr Comp Physiol*, 2003; **284**:R280–90.

29. **Frey D J**, **Badia P**, **Wright K P** Jr. Inter- and intra-individual variability in performance near the circadian nadir during sleep deprivation. *J Sleep Res*, 2004; **13**:305–15.

30. **Goel N**, **Banks S**, **Mignot E**, et al. PER3 polymorphism predicts cumulative sleep homeostatic but not neurobehavioral changes to chronic partial sleep deprivation. *PLoS ONE*, 2009; **4**:e5874.

31. **Bliese P D**, **Wesensten N J**, **Balkin T J**. Age and individual variability in performance during sleep restriction. *J Sleep Res*, 2006; **15**:376–85.

32. **Mitler M M**, **Miller J C**, **Lipsitz J J**, et al. The sleep of long-haul truck drivers. *N Engl J Med*, 1997; **337**:755–61.

33. **Drake C L**, **Roehrs T**, **Richardson G**, *et al*. Shift work sleep disorder: prevalence and consequences beyond that of symptomatic day workers. *Sleep*, 2004; **27**:1453–62.

34. **Czeisler C A**, **Walsh J K**, **Roth T**, *et al*. Modafinil for excessive sleepiness associated with shift-work sleep disorder. *N Engl J Med*, 2005; **353**:476–86.

35. **Weaver T E**, **Maislin G**, **Dinges D F**, *et al*. Relationship between hours of CPAP use and achieving normal levels of sleepiness and daily functioning. *Sleep*, 2007; **30**:711–19.

36. **Drake C L**, **Roehrs T A**, **Burduvali E**, *et al*. Effects of rapid versus slow accumulation of eight hours of sleep loss. *Psychophysiology*, 2001; **38**:979–87.

37. **Rowland L M**, **Thomas M L**, **Thorne D R**, *et al*. Oculomotor responses during partial and total sleep deprivation. *Aviat Space Environ Med*, 2005; **76**:C104–13.

38. **Roehrs T**, **Timms V**, **Zwyghuizen-Doorenbos A**, *et al*. Sleep extension in sleepy and alert normals. *Sleep*, 1989; **12**:449–57.

39. **Landolt H P**. Genotype-dependent differences in sleep, vigilance, and response to stimulants. *Curr Pharm Des*, 2008; **14**:3396–407.

40. **Viola A U**, **Archer S N**, **James L M**, *et al*. PER3 polymorphism predicts sleep structure and waking performance. *Curr Biol*, 2007; **17**:613–18.

41. **Groeger J A**, **Viola A U**, **Lo J C**, *et al*. Early morning executive functioning during sleep deprivation is compromised by a PERIOD3 polymorphism. *Sleep*, 2008; **31**:1159–67.

42. **Bodenmann S**, **Xu S**, **Luhmann U**, *et al*. Pharmacogenetics of modafinil after sleep loss: catechol-O-methyltransferase genotype modulates waking functions but not recovery sleep. *Clin Pharmacol Ther*, 2009; **85**:296–304.

43. **Bodenmann S**, **Rusterholz T**, **Dürr R**, *et al*. The functional Val158Met polymorphism of *COMT* predicts interindividual differences in brain α oscillations in young men. *J Neurosci*, 2009; **29**:10 855–62.

44. **Dauvilliers Y**, **Tafti M**. Molecular genetics and treatment of narcolepsy. *Ann Med*, 2006; **38**:252–62.

45. **Goel N**, **Banks S**, **Mignot E**, *et al*. HLA DQB1 *0602 allele predicts interindividual differences in physiological sleep structure, sleepiness and fatigue during baseline and chronic partial sleep deprivation. *Neurology*, 2010, **75**: 1509–19.

46. **Rétey J V**, **Adam M**, **Honegger E**, *et al*. A functional genetic variation of adenosine deaminase affects the duration and intensity of deep sleep in humans. *Proc Natl Acad Sci USA*, 2005; **102**:15676–81.

47. **Rétey J V**, **Adam M**, **Khatami R**, *et al*. A genetic variation in the adenosine A(2A) receptor gene (*ADORA2A*) contributes to individual sensitivity to caffeine effects on sleep. *Clin Pharmacol Ther*, 2007; **81**:692–98.

48. **Mu Q**, **Nahas Z**, **Johnson K A**, *et al*. Decreased brain activation during a working memory task at rested baseline is associated with vulnerability to sleep deprivation. *Sleep*, 2005b; **28**:433–46.

49. **Caldwell J A**, **Mu Q**, **Smith J K**, *et al*. Are individual differences in fatigue vulnerability related to baseline differences in cortical activation? *Behav Neurosci*, 2005; **119**:694–707.

50. **Chee M W**, **Chuah L Y**, **Venkatraman V**, *et al*. Functional imaging of working memory following normal sleep and after 24 and 35 h of sleep deprivation: correlations of fronto-parietal activation with performance. *NeuroImage*, 2006; **31**:419–28.

51. **Chuah Y M L**, **Venkatraman V**, **Dinges D F**, *et al*. The neural basis of inter-individual variability in inhibitory efficiency following sleep deprivation. *J Neurosci*, 2006; **26**:7156–62.

52. **Vandewalle G**, **Archer S N**, **Wuillaume C**, *et al*. Functional magnetic resonance imaging-assessed brain responses during an executive task depend on interaction of sleep homeostasis, circadian phase, and PER3 genotype. *J Neurosci*, 2009; **29**:7948–56.

Section 2, Chapter 11

Sleep Disorders and Excessive Sleepiness

Narcolepsy

Astrid van der Heide and Gert Jan Lammers

Introduction

Narcolepsy is best characterized as a disorder of the regulation of sleep and wakefulness, resulting in a variety of symptoms such as excessive daytime sleepiness (EDS), cataplexy, hypnagogic hallucinations, sleep paralysis, and disturbed nocturnal sleep. According to the current classification of sleep disorders [1], narcolepsy can be divided into narcolepsy with and without cataplexy. Narcolepsy with cataplexy is considered to be a homogeneous disease entity, a "morbus sui generis", of which the pathophysiological hallmark is a disturbed hypocretin transmission. Narcolepsy without cataplexy may be no more than a heterogeneous group of disorders characterized by EDS in combination with abnormal expressions of REM sleep on polysomnography (PSG). Whether the PSG findings in question are at all specific is debatable; there are indications that chronic sleep deprivation in otherwise healthy individuals may be enough to cause the PSG abnormalities. At any rate, most cases of narcolepsy without cataplexy do not develop cataplexy later on, so it is not simply an early stage of narcolepsy with cataplexy.

This chapter focuses on narcolepsy with cataplexy, or, from now on, "narcolepsy" for short. "Narcolepsy without cataplexy" will be discussed in the sections on pathophysiology and differential diagnosis.

Epidemiology

Narcolepsy is relatively rare, with an estimated prevalence of 25–50 per 100 000 and an estimated incidence of 0.74 per 100 000 person years [2, 3]. The latency of about 10 years between the occurrence of the first symptoms and the diagnosis emphasizes the trend towards late detection, and possibly also to failed detection. However, this latency tends to become shorter.

Men and women seem to be affected at equal rates, although one paper reported a higher incidence in men [2, 4]. The disease may start at any age, but starts most often during adolescence. There is a small second peak in the age at onset around 35 years of age [5]. Life expectancy of narcolepsy patients does not differ from that of the general population.

Clinical features

EDS

EDS is the leading symptom of narcolepsy. It is invariably present in all patients and is usually the first symptom [6]. It typically develops over weeks to months, but may also start more acutely. EDS is relentlessly present daily. It is characterized both by an inability to stay awake, and in the majority of patients by an almost continuous feeling of sleepiness dependent upon the level of activity. Monotonous activities such as watching television, reading, attending a meeting or being a passenger in a car increase the feeling of sleepiness and greatly increase the chance of a sleep attack. Conversely, intense physical or mental activity decreases sleepiness and prevents sleep attacks. In more severe cases, sleep attacks may also occur when patients are more active, such as during dinner, while walking, or even when riding a bicycle. Sleep attacks tend to be short, usually less than 20 min, and refreshing for some time. The number of attacks may vary from 1 to over 10 each day, depending on the severity of the narcolepsy and the circumstances. EDS does not just cause restrictions and embarrassment, but also carries an increased risk of traffic accidents or other accidents, such as with machinery.

Sleepiness: Causes, Consequences and Treatment, ed. Michael J. Thorpy and Michel Billiard. Published by Cambridge University Press. © Cambridge University Press 2011.

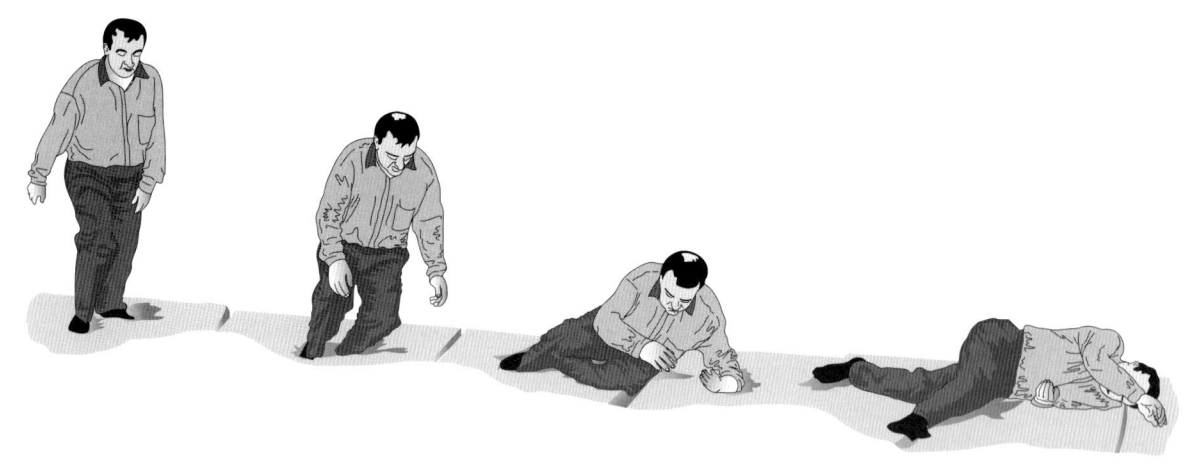

Figure 11.1 Photographs showing a complete cataplectic attack; note that it takes several seconds for the attack to build up.

EDS is typically accompanied by a pronounced difficulty to concentrate and to sustain attention, leading to an impaired performance. This expression of EDS may even cause more problems in interpersonal relationships than the sleep attacks. A subject seemingly awake but unable to perform will receive less compassion than one who is not able to perform because they are clearly asleep.

It is not hard to imagine that the described consequences of EDS severely reduce the quality of life.

Cataplexy

Cataplexy is characterized by a sudden bilateral loss of muscle tone, with preserved consciousness, elicited by emotions. All striated muscles can be involved. Notable exceptions are extrinsic eye muscles and muscles involved in respiration. Cataplexy may be "complete", indicating complete loss of activity of all muscle groups (Figure 11.1). In most cases it is partial, only affecting control over the knees, face and neck. Sometimes, attacks may be so subtle that they are only recognized by experienced observers. Occasionally not even patients themselves are aware of subtle attacks. Patients notice partial attacks as their knees "giving way" or sagging of the head or jaw. Muscle twitches and jerky movements may be part of the attack. Complete attacks may cause falls. Since it takes several seconds for a complete attack to build up, most patients are able to take countermeasures, such as sitting down. In the long term, most patients learn "tricks" to prevent or abort attacks.

Cataplexy is most often provoked by an emotional trigger. Rather than the actual emotion, its anticipation may trigger an attack. Common examples are not being able to tell the punchline of a joke and not being able to score a goal during soccer because the opportunity to do so triggers an attack. Mirth is the most typical trigger, which usually involves laughing out loud; smiling does not usually trigger an attack. Another common trigger is an unexpected meeting with an acquaintance. Anger can also provoke attacks. For such events to actually trigger an attack, a certain mind set seems to be important, which is difficult to define. A degree of relaxation or comfort with the situation may be a prerequisite, as uncomfortable or stressful situations such as medical consultations prevent their occurrence.

The frequency of attacks varies widely from dozens a day to less than once a month. Most attacks last seconds to half a minute, sometimes up to two minutes, but only rarely longer. Partial attacks tend to be shorter, the majority even less than 10 s. Occasionally it is difficult to establish the duration of an individual attack, especially when the trigger remains present for minutes. In such a situation, repeated attacks may occur, giving the impression of a very long-lasting single attack. The frequency, severity, and how well patients cope with attacks determine the impact on the quality of life. Patients may avoid situations in which cataplexy may occur; they may stop themselves laughing out loud, stop visiting comedy shows, or even avoid social contacts in general.

Although cataplexy is the only truly specific feature of narcolepsy, it is the first symptom to appear in less than 10% of cases [7]. Usually it appears shortly after EDS has started, but it may appear months to years afterwards. One result of this is that patients may seem to have narcolepsy without cataplexy initially, while a follow-up reveals this patient to have the start of narcolepsy with cataplexy.

Hypnagogic hallucinations

Hypnagogic hallucinations (HH) are very vivid, dreamlike experiences that occur during the transition from wakening to sleep. Originally "hypnopompic hallucinations" was used to mean their occurrence during waking, but "hypnagogic" is now commonly used for the transition in either direction. The content of the hallucinations varies, but in general they are extremely unpleasant and frightening. In 85% of the hallucinations multiple senses are simultaneously involved: visual, auditory, and tactile [8]. HH are typically "pasted" over the actual environment, i.e. the room in which they are. Examples are that someone they know seems to enter that room, or patients may hallucinate that they are undergoing surgery without anesthesia in their own bed. Often, HH appear so realistic that patients have difficulty telling them apart from real events after waking up. Sometimes confirmation by others is even needed to tell the difference. Usually narcolepsy patients recognize the events as not being real, which helps distinguish HH from hallucinations in a psychiatric context. Their occurrence during the transition between wakefulness and sleep also helps the diagnosis, as hallucinations in psychiatric disorders can occur at any moment. There is no reason to think that HH point towards a psychotic disorder: psychotic disorders do not occur more often in narcolepsy than in the general population [8].

HH are not specific for narcolepsy with cataplexy, since they are also present in the general population and in other sleep disorders [9]. However, the prevalence, and probably also the frequency, are higher in narcolepsy.

Sleep paralysis

Sleep paralysis is the inability to move at awakening or when falling asleep while being subjectively awake and conscious. The paralysis may be complete, so patients are unable to raise as much as a little finger. Attacks last up to several minutes. Sleep paralysis has similarities with both cataplexy and HH: the timing resembles that of HH, whereas the pattern of affected muscles resembles that of complete attacks of cataplexy. Sleep paralysis may occur simultaneously with HH.

Sleep paralysis occurs as a symptom on its own and is therefore not specific for narcolepsy [10].

Disturbed nocturnal sleep

Sleep latency in narcolepsy is typically very short: patients usually fall asleep as soon as they lie down and their head touches the pillow. They do not stay asleep, however, which is reflected in frequent awakening. Most awakenings are brief but some last for more than one hour. The total duration of nocturnal sleep is by and large comparable to the situation before they developed narcolepsy [11]. In a minority of cases, nocturnal sleep time increases temporarily or structurally. Remarkably there is no clear correlation between the severity of EDS and the extent of disturbed nocturnal sleep.

Associated symptoms

The previously mentioned features are the classical core symptoms of narcolepsy. However, there are some other features frequently present that may, at least in part, be related to the inability to sustain attention. One of them is automatic behavior: the performance of a semi-purposeful, inadequate daytime activity. For instance, a patient may continue to write in a state of drowsiness, resulting in illegible handwriting, or drive to a certain place by car without knowing how and why they did so. Memory complaints occur frequently, for which there might be explanations other than temporary lapses in attention.

A final symptom, not directly related to impaired sustained attention, is obesity. About 30% of patients have a BMI of at least 30 kg/m^2, compared to 12.5% of the Dutch population [12]. Obesity may be explained in part by decreased activity or increased caloric intake, but, since it typically occurs in hypocretin-deficient patients, may be a direct consequence of hypocretin deficiency.

Comorbidity

EDS in narcolepsy can be accompanied by the feeling of being short of energy or fatigued. However, this is a qualitatively different complaint and it is of importance to differentiate between them. Fatigue can be present in numerous conditions of which sleep disorders are only a small part.

Table 11.1 ICSD-2 diagnostic criteria of narcolepsy with cataplexy

A. The patient has a complaint of excessive daytime sleepiness occurring almost daily for at least three months.
B. A definite history of cataplexy, defined as sudden and transient episodes of loss of motor tone triggered by emotions, is present.
C. The diagnosis of narcolepsy with cataplexy should, whenever possible, be confirmed by nocturnal polysomnography followed by an MSLT; the mean sleep latency on MSLT is less than or equal to 8 min and two or more SOREMPs are observed following sufficient nocturnal sleep (minimum 6 h) during the night prior to the test. Alternatively, hypocretin-1 levels in the CSF are less than or equal to 110 pg/ml or one-third of mean control values.
D. The hypersomnia is not better explained by another sleep disorder or neurological disorder, mental disorder, medication use, or substance use disorder.

Table 11.2 ICSD-2 diagnostic criteria of narcolepsy due to medical condition

A. The patient has a complaint of excessive daytime sleepiness occurring almost daily for at least three months.
B. One of the following is present:
   1. A definite history of cataplexy, defined as sudden and transient episodes of loss of muscle tone (muscle weakness) triggered by emotion, is present.
   2. If cataplexy is not present or is very atypical, polysomnographic monitoring performed over the patient's habitual sleep period followed by an MSLT must demonstrate a mean sleep latency on the MSLT of less than 8 min with two or more SOREMPs, despite sufficient nocturnal sleep prior to the test (minimum 6 h).
   3. Hypocretin-1 levels in the CSF are less than 110 pg/ml (or 30% of mean control values), provided the patient is not comatose.
C. A significant underlying medical or neurological disorder accounts for the daytime sleepiness.
D. The hypersomnia is not better explained by another sleep disorder, mental disorder, medication use, or substance use disorder.

Sleep apnea and parasomnias are frequently present, but at an unknown frequency. One recent study reported the presence of obstructive sleep apnea (OSA) in 25% of the patients with narcolepsy [13]. Periodic limb movements in sleep (PLMS) have been described in up to two-thirds of the subjects with narcolepsy [14], although its contribution to the impaired quality of sleep and EDS is doubted. REM sleep behavior disorder (RBD) has a significantly higher prevalence compared to the general population, affecting 12–36% of the patients [15].

Since depression may cause complaints of EDS and lack of energy, and neurophysiological abnormalities that may resemble narcolepsy, it can be difficult to diagnose depression as a comorbid disorder. Nevertheless, depression is considered to have a higher prevalence in narcoleptics than in the general population; 5–30% of the patients are reported to fulfill the criteria for depression [16].

Diagnosis

Narcolepsy with cataplexy is diagnosed according to the criteria of the International Classification of Sleep Disorders (ICSD-2) (Table 11.1) [1]. The presence of EDS and cataplexy, both of which must be evaluated by careful history-taking, is required, and should be confirmed with polysomnographical studies including a multiple sleep latency test (MSLT) and / or hypocretin-1 measurement in the CSF.

During history-taking, it must be kept in mind that many patients will have read information about narcolepsy before consultation, so physicians have to distinguish between real complaints and interpretations.

Hypocretin measurement

The sensitivity of low or absent hypocretin-1 levels in the CSF of patients suffering from narcolepsy with cataplexy is about 90% [17]. Specificity is even higher. As the sensitivity and the specificity of the MSLT are, respectively, 71.5 and 66% [18], hypocretin-1 measurement is more reliable for the confirmation of narcolepsy with cataplexy. In atypical cases, such as those who are suffering from a familial form or those who are HLA-negative, hypocretin-1 is less often low or undetectable. They make up the majority of the 10% of patients who have normal levels.

The currently available commercial kit for the hypocretin-1 RIA has a large interassay variation and therefore reference samples must always be included. Many centers use reference samples from Stanford and convert their values to the Stanford values. For these labs, levels below 110 pg/ml are diagnostic for narcolepsy.

Differential diagnosis

EDS in combination with cataplexy is pathognomonic for narcolepsy with cataplexy. If a patient presents with these features, the only relevant question is whether it concerns the idiopathic form or "Narcolepsy due to medical condition" (Table 11.2).

Table 11.3 ICSD-2 diagnostic criteria of narcolepsy without cataplexy

A. The patient has a complaint of excessive daytime sleepiness occurring almost daily for at least three months.
B. Typical cataplexy is not present, although doubtful or atypical cataplexy-like episodes may be reported.
C. The diagnosis of narcolepsy without cataplexy must be confirmed by nocturnal polysomnography followed by an MSLT. In narcolepsy without cataplexy, the mean sleep latency on MSLT is less than or equal to 8 min and two or more SOREMPs are observed following sufficient nocturnal sleep (minimum 6 h) during the night prior to the test.
D. The hypersomnia is not better explained by another sleep disorder or neurological disorder, mental disorder, medication use, or substance use disorder.

Table 11.4 Differential diagnosis for EDS and cataplexy

Excessive daytime sleepiness	Cataplexy
Behaviorally induced insufficient sleep	*Isolated cataplexy*
Sleep apnea syndrome	Niemann–Pick disease
Periodic Limb Movement Disorder	Prader–Willi syndrome
Idiopathic hypersomnia	Norrie disease
Recurrent hypersomnia	Secondary to diencephalic tumors
Drug intoxication/withdrawal	*Familial cataplexy*
Circadian rhythm disorders	Coffin–Lowry syndrome
Thalamic infarction	*Non-cataplectic attacks*
Metabolic encephalopathy	Startle syndromes
Depression	Drop attacks
Fatigue	Atonic/gelastic seizures
Malingering	Psychogenic
	Malingering

In the absence of cataplexy the diagnosis is more difficult, but can be made if patients meet the PSG criteria (Table 11.3). However, it has been demonstrated that the clinical as well as the MSLT findings can be induced by chronic sleep deprivation [19]. In those cases, a low or undetectable hypocretin-1 level can prove the diagnosis. Yet it has to be borne in mind that hypocretin-1 concentrations will only be decreased in about 10% of the subjects with narcolepsy without cataplexy [17]. In HLA-negative subjects an even lower percentage is found. In case of doubt, the patient should always be advised to resign to a regular sleep–wake rhythm, which allows enough time spent in bed to obtain a sufficient amount of nocturnal sleep. Only if complaints remain after applying such a schedule should pharmacological treatment be considered.

From a clinical point of view, the differentiation from idiopathic hypersomnia (IH) may also be difficult, particularly IH without long sleep time. In these cases the MSLT will sort them out by the presence of fewer than two SOREMPs. Moreover, hypocretin-1 levels are always normal in IH [17].

The differential diagnoses of EDS and cataplexy are summarized in Table 11.4.

Pathophysiology

The hypocretin (orexin) system

The hypocretin system includes two peptides, hypocretin 1 and 2, and two receptors, receptors 1 and 2. The peptides were independently discovered by two groups [20, 21], which explains why orexin-A and -B are synonymous with hypocretin-1 and -2, respectively. Both hypocretin peptides are cleaved from a common precursor (preprohypocretin) and have a different receptor affinity profile. Hypocretin-1 has equal affinity for both receptors, while hypocretin-2 preferentially binds to the hypocretin receptor-2.

Hypocretins are produced by a small number of neurons located in the dorsolateral hypothalamus, centered around the fornix and adjacent areas. Although the hypocretin cell bodies lie in a small area, their axons project throughout the whole neuraxis, except the cerebellum (Figure 11.2).

The discovery that monogenetic forms of narcolepsy in dogs were caused by mutations in the hypocretin receptor-2 gene, and the report that hypocretin knockout mice develop narcolepsy led to exciting new insights into the pathophysiology of human narcolepsy [22, 23]. Hypocretin deficiency turned out to be the hallmark of human narcolepsy with cataplexy. The first study pointing in this direction was a blinded controlled study in which hypocretin-1 concentrations were measured in the CSF [24]. Hypocretin-1 was undetectable in the majority of patients, in contrast to stable concentrations far exceeding the detection limit that were found in control subjects. Follow-up studies in large numbers of patients have confirmed this finding. To date, measurement of hypocretin-2 in CSF has failed, probably because it is very unstable in the CSF, in contrast to hypocretin-1. Since both hypocretin-1 and -2 are derived from the common precursor

2. Sleep Disorders and Excessive Sleepiness

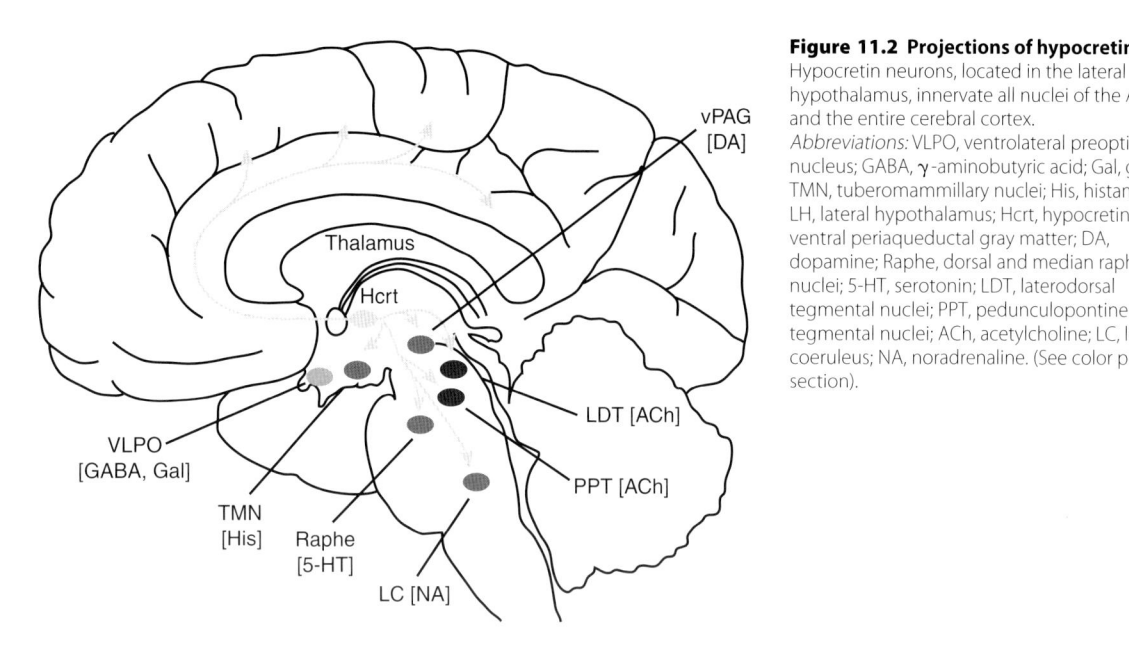

Figure 11.2 Projections of hypocretin.
Hypocretin neurons, located in the lateral hypothalamus, innervate all nuclei of the AAS and the entire cerebral cortex.
Abbreviations: VLPO, ventrolateral preoptic nucleus; GABA, γ-aminobutyric acid; Gal, galanin; TMN, tuberomammillary nuclei; His, histamine; LH, lateral hypothalamus; Hcrt, hypocretin; vPAG, ventral periaqueductal gray matter; DA, dopamine; Raphe, dorsal and median raphe nuclei; 5-HT, serotonin; LDT, laterodorsal tegmental nuclei; PPT, pedunculopontine tegmental nuclei; ACh, acetylcholine; LC, locus coeruleus; NA, noradrenaline. (See color plate section).

preprohypocretin, it seems probable that hypocretin-2 is low or absent in narcolepsy with cataplexy as well. This assumption is supported by subsequently performed post-mortem brain studies that indicated an almost complete selective loss of hypocretin cells in the hypothalamus of patients who suffered from narcolepsy with cataplexy [25]. It is currently presumed that narcoleptic symptoms start to occur when the majority of the hypocretin cells have disappeared, and the severity of symptoms and the occurrence of cataplexy may be determined by the number of degenerated cells. Direct evidence for this theory has not yet been found, but is based on recent studies that found a 90% neuron loss in narcolepsy with cataplexy compared to a 33% neuron loss in patients without cataplexy [26, 27].

"Sleep switch"

To understand the pathophysiology of narcolepsy it is essential to understand the current concept of the normal regulation of sleep and wakefulness [28, 29].

The main nuclei for the promotion of wakefulness and sleep are located in the hypothalamus and the reticular formation of the mesencephalon and pons, concerning the dorsal and median raphe nuclei (Raphe), the locus coeruleus (LC), the ventral periaqueductal gray matter (vPAG) and the pedunculopontine and laterodorsal tegmental nuclei (PPT/LDT) (Figure 11.3). Besides projections to the thalamic intralaminar nuclei and the hypothalamus, these nuclei project diffusely to the cortex of the entire hemisphere. Together with the tuberomammillary nuclei (TMN), located in the hypothalamus, these previously mentioned nuclei and their branches are called the ascending arousal system (AAS). The ascending arousal system plays a crucial role in the regulation of wakefulness and comprises two pathways with:

1. *Cholinergic branch* – the PPT/LDT project to the thalamic reticular nucleus via thalamic relay neurons and activate the cerebral cortex.
2. *Monoaminergic branch* – the LC, dorsal and median raphe nuclei (DR), TMN and vPAG project diffusely to the cortex of the entire hemisphere.

During wakefulness, both the cholinergic and monoaminergic branches are active, and their activity is augmented by the hypocretin neurons from the lateral hypothalamus.

The AAS is influenced by many other systems, one of them being the ventrolateral preoptic nucleus (VLPO), located in the hypothalamus (Figure 11.4). Activity of the VLPO facilitates sleep. The phase of the diurnal rhythm of the biological clock and the duration of previous wake are major determinants of the activity of the VPLO. During NREM sleep the wake-promoting cholinergic and monoaminergic nuclei are all inhibited by the VLPO. During REM sleep only

Figure 11.3 Ascending arousal system (AAS). The AAS comprises two pathways: (1) *Monoaminergic branch (red)*; the locus coeruleus (LC), dorsal and median raphe nuclei (Raphe), tuberomammillary nuclei (TMN) and ventral periaqueductal gray matter (vPAG) project diffusely to the cortex of the entire hemisphere. This pathway receives also contribution from peptidergic neurons in the lateral hypothalamus (LH) containing hypocretin (Hcrt). (2) *Cholinergic branch (blue)*; the pedunculopontine and laterodorsal tegmental nuclei (PPT, LDT), project to the thalamic reticular nucleus via thalamic relay neurons and activate the cerebral cortex. *Abbreviations:* VLPO, ventrolateral preoptic nucleus; GABA, γ-aminobutyric acid; Gal, galanin; His, histamine; DA, dopamine; 5-HT, serotonin; ACh, acetylcholine; NA, noradrenalin. (See color plate section).

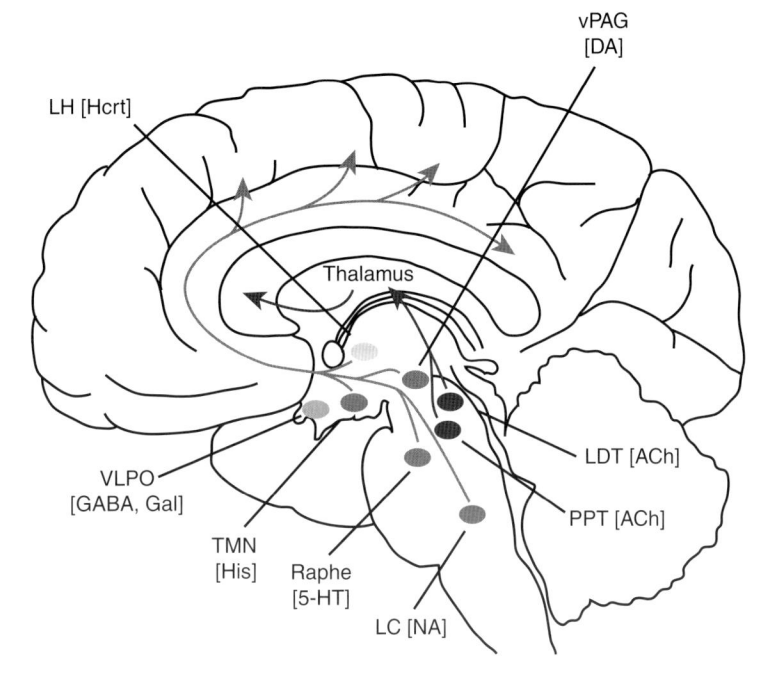

Figure 11.4 Projections of the ventrolateral preoptic nucleus (VLPO). The VLPO has projections to the nuclei of both the monoaminergic branch (red) and the cholinergic branch (blue).
Abbreviations: GABA, γ-aminobutyric acid; Gal, galanin; TMN, tuberomammillary nuclei; His, histamine; vPAG, ventral periaqueductal gray matter; DA, dopamine; Raphe, dorsal and median raphe nuclei; 5-HT, serotonin; LDT, laterodorsal tegmental nuclei; PPT, pedunculopontine tegmental nuclei; ACh, acetylcholine; LC, locus coeruleus; NA, noradrenalin. (See color plate section).

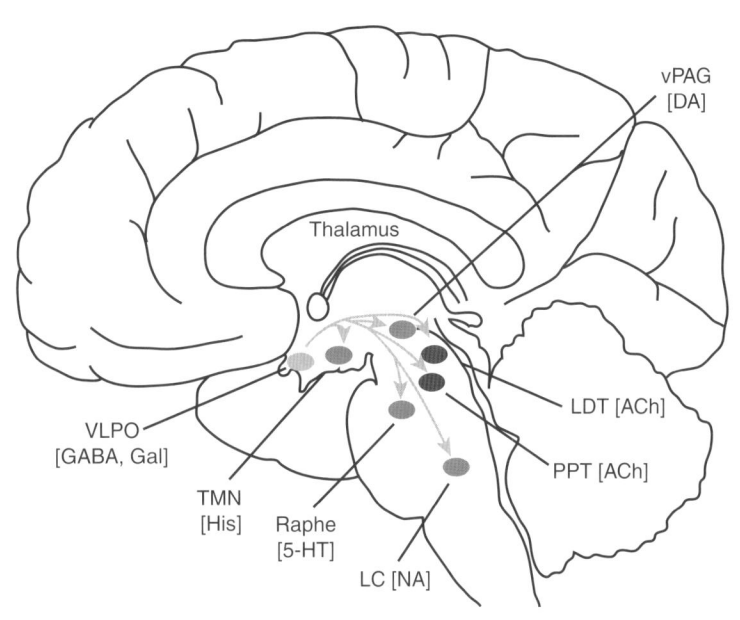

the monoaminergic nuclei are inhibited, whereas the cholinergic nuclei are even more active than during wakefulness.

Not only has the VLPO an inhibitory function on the monoaminergic nuclei, the monoaminergic nuclei also inhibit the VLPO, resulting in a reciprocal inhibition. Such a circuit resembles a "flip-flop switch" (Figure 11.5), a term used by electrical engineers. By analogy, the circuitry regulating sleep and wakefulness is called the "sleep-switch" [28, 29].

The two sides of a flip-flop circuit, by each strongly inhibiting the other, create a feedback loop with a self-reinforcing firing pattern resulting in two possible states. It prevents the occurrence of intermediate states: if there is a transition, it is abrupt and complete. Therefore, the "sleep-switch" allows only two

Pharmacological treatment

A variety of substances may be used in the treatment of narcolepsy. This observation indicates that there is not one drug that is efficacious in all. As most drugs predominantly act on either excessive daytime sleepiness (EDS) or cataplexy, combinations are often needed to control both symptoms. The only available drug that may improve all major symptoms of narcolepsy is sodium oxybate (SO). Nevertheless, combinations of SO with, for example, stimulants may have a synergetic effect for the amelioration of EDS, and may therefore be preferred over monotherapy with SO.

What should be borne in mind when making a choice for a certain drug or combinations of drugs in an individual patient, and how can its efficacy be evaluated?

- The expectation and goal of a treatment are of major importance in the judgment of the efficacy. Sleepiness will never be completely alleviated in any patient, whereas cataplexy may completely disappear in some. Long-term improvement of nocturnal sleep is only reached with SO. Patients must be made aware of this, and this knowledge must guide physicians in trying new drugs or combinations of drugs and in deciding on the right balance between efficacy and side effects.
- Ideally, drug efficacy should be assessed with a generally accepted, objective test to quantify the severity and the individual impact of a symptom. Unfortunately, there is no such test for narcolepsy as a whole, or for its constituent symptoms. Sleepiness can be assessed with a variety of subjective and objective tests, but none of them is generally accepted as a valid indicator of daytime functioning. In fact, it is uncertain if either the impaired concentration while awake or sleeping during daytime is the more invalidating symptom. In case of the first, vigilance tests are more appropriate than sleep tests [42]. Nocturnal sleep, cataplexy, HH and sleep paralysis all present similar assessment problems. Cataplexy cannot be simply quantified, as its severity depends on many features: frequency, duration, the number of muscles involved, as well as behavioral consequences, such as avoidance of situations in which attacks may occur.
- In the absence of objective tests, history-taking is the main instrument to evaluate efficacy and the occurrence of side-effects.
- The interpretation of pharmacological trials is hampered by the lack of well-designed studies of older drugs, and a shortage of studies comparing different substances. Moreover, strict inclusion and exclusion criteria prevent the results of large trials being applicable for all patients.
- Individual differences in efficacy, side-effects and tolerability appear large. Knowledge about efficacy of a drug as assessed in groups is therefore of relative importance for individuals.
- Pharmacokinetic aspects, i.e. short- and fast-acting versus slow- and long-acting, may be more important than the expected efficacy.

Treatment of EDS

Stimulants are the mainstay of the treatment of EDS [43, 44]. These include dextroamphetamine (5–60 mg/day), methamphetamine (10–50 mg/day), methylphenidate (10–60 mg/day), and mazindol (1–6 mg/day). Side-effects and tolerance are the major drawbacks in the use of stimulants. The most important side-effects include irritability, agitation, headache and peripheral sympathetic stimulation. These are usually dose related. Although addiction does not seem to be a problem in narcoleptics [45], some patients tend to increase their dosage because they prefer high alertness. Tolerance develops in about a third of the patients [45, 46]. Mazindol has been withdrawn in most countries due to observed uncommon, but severe, side-effects in related drugs that suppress appetite, in particular fenfluramines. The side-effects were pulmonary hypertension and valvular regurgitation [47]. As some patients respond better to mazindol than to any other drug it may still be considered, provided that treatment is closely monitored.

Modafinil (100–400 mg/day) is usually grouped with the stimulants, but is chemically unrelated to amphetamine. The efficacy is probably equal to that of the stimulants, although direct comparisons are lacking. The clinical impression is that all the described side-effects of stimulants, and also tolerance, may occur during treatment with modafinil, but, in general, less frequently and less severely. More specific side-effects of modafinil are headache and nausea; however, they usually disappear after 2–3 weeks of treatment.

Long-acting agents (modafinil, dexamphetamine, methamphetamine, methylphenidate controlled release) are generally better tolerated than the short-acting agents (methylphenidate). The quick- and short-acting agents can be used to good effect when "targeted" at social events or difficult periods during the day. For this reason, combinations of stimulants may be tailored to the circumstances. Unfortunately, there are no studies assessing the advantages or disadvantages of combinations of stimulants.

Recent studies with sodium oxybate (SO), the sodium salt of gamma-hydroxybutyrate, have shown that it is effective in reducing EDS. The usual starting dose is 2.25 g twice a night. The dose must be gradually increased, keeping in mind that the optimal daytime effects are reached after weeks. A relevant improvement of EDS is in most patients achieved with higher dosages (6–9 g/night). The effect on EDS of higher doses is similar to that of modafinil, and side-effects, if present, are usually mild [48]. The combination of both therapies is even more effective. The most frequent side-effect is nausea, and the most disabling are enuresis and sleep walking. Lowering the dose may solve these problems. Weight loss may occur [49].

In follow-up studies there is no indication that tolerance develops, and abrupt cessation does not induce rebound cataplexy. However, long-term clinical experience shows that a substantial proportion of patients may develop tolerance for the sleep-promoting effects, although efficacy for the other symptoms remains.

SO should not be used in conjunction with other sedatives or alcohol. If patients have consumed alcohol in the evening, they should omit one or both doses afterwards. In patients with comorbid OSAS, treatment should be closely monitored, since SO may worsen OSAS. Cotreatment with CPAP may be indicated [50].

Unfortunately, there is concern for misuse. Although potential threats related to misuse may result in hesitation in patients to take, and in physicians to prescribe, the substance, it is important to realize that when the drug is used properly, it is safe, and bears no risk for dependence [51].

Caffeine may alleviate sleepiness, but has a weak effect: the alerting effect of six cups of strong coffee is comparable with that of 5 mg of dexamphetamine [45, 46]. Selegiline and brofaromine may alleviate EDS as well [44].

Treatment of REM sleep dissociation phenomena

Most studies concerning the treatment of the REM dissociation phenomena focused on cataplexy. Amelioration of cataplexy is generally associated with improvement of hypnagogic hallucinations and sleep paralysis. SO and tricyclic antidepressants are the most effective treatments. The different tricyclic antidepressants all inhibit the reuptake of norepinephrine and serotonin and are potent REM sleep inhibitors. The most commonly used ones are imipramine (10–100 mg/day), and clomipramine (10–150 mg/day) [4, 43, 44]. Very low doses, up to 20 mg, may sometimes be remarkably effective. Most authors consider clomipramine to be the treatment of choice [52]. Some patients even experience improvement of EDS when treated with clomipramine. Tolerance may occur. As with stimulants, side-effects, and to a lesser extent tolerance, are a major drawback. Side-effects are largely due to the anticholinergic properties; the most frequently reported are a dry mouth, increased sweating, sexual dysfunction (impotence, delayed orgasm, erection and ejaculation dysfunction), weight gain, tachycardia, constipation, blurred vision, and urinary retention. These are severe enough to lead to dose reductions or stopping its use. However, in some patients, very low doses may be very effective without causing significant side-effects. Tricyclic antidepressants should never be stopped abruptly because of the risk of severe aggravation of cataplexy, which may even lead to a status cataplecticus.

Many alternative antidepressants have been studied, especially selective serotonin reuptake inhibitors (SSRIs), and more selective noradrenergic reuptake inhibitors such as fluoxetine, zimelidine, viloxazine, femoxitine, fluvoxamine and paroxetine in a relative higher dosage than the tricyclics [4, 44, 53]. All these substances appear to have anti-cataplectic properties and less (disabling) side-effects compared to the tricyclics. These substances seem to act mainly via less selective desmethyl metabolites, which are potent adrenergic uptake inhibitors [54].

During recent years, venlafaxine and atomoxetine have become very popular in the treatment of cataplexy, although there are no randomized placebo-controlled studies available. In the authors' experience, venlafaxine is not clearly superior. Atomoxetine, however, has occasionally been shown to be effective when the others have failed [55].

SO is the best-studied drug and is a very potent inhibitor of cataplexy [56]. It has never been compared to any antidepressant so it is difficult to know whether it is really more effective. However, the relatively mild side-effect profile makes it a more favorable drug, even independent of the beneficial effect of SO on the other symptoms.

Other alternatives, less well-studied and probably less potent, are mazindol, selegiline, and brofaromine. They may, just like SO, have a combined impact on sleepiness as well as on REM dissociation phenomena.

Theoretically, several drugs may be expected to aggravate cataplexy, but the only one for which this is reliably documented is prazosin, an alpha 1 antagonist used to treat hypertension.

Treatment of the disturbed nocturnal sleep

Disturbed nocturnal sleep can be a major complaint of patients. Unfortunately, treatment options are limited, as SO is the only drug with a proven long-term effect on nocturnal sleep [57]. Short-term beneficial effects of benzodiazepines have been described [58]. Although nocturnal sleep may (temporarily) be improved with benzodiazepines, improvement of EDS is not the rule.

Treatment of associated symptoms/disorders

Obesity is an associated symptom, for which there is no treatment other than for any obese person.

Fatigue or lack of energy may occasionally improve during treatment with stimulants or SO. There is no other therapy with a proven effect for this complaint.

Sleep apnea is more prevalent in narcolepsy patients. However, treatment does not usually improve the EDS, and compliance to CPAP and other treatments is a problem. Whether there is an indication for treatment is controversial [13]. Treatment with SO may facilitate the acceptance of CPAP treatment. However, since SO may worsen the course of sleep apnea, it is important in these cases that patients are compliant [50].

Treatment of periodic limb movements must be considered if there is coexistent RLS, otherwise only in very severe cases.

Treatment for RBD is rarely indicated; in those cases, clonazepam and melatonin can be considered.

Recommendations for the initiation of pharmacological treatment

Pharmacological treatment is supplementary to behavioral advice and should be tailored individually. The recommendations given below should therefore only be considered as a guide to initiate pharmacotherapy.

For patients who predominantly suffer from EDS, modafinil is a good first choice. If EDS is relatively mild or mostly situation-based, methylphenidate as "on demand" treatment may be a good alternative. If modafinil monotherapy is not sufficient to reach a satisfactory situation, combination therapy with SO or methylphenidate can be considered. Women of childbearing age who use low-dose ethinyloestradiol (30 µg) contraceptives should be advised to switch to a compound with a higher ethinyloestradiol content before the start of modafinil.

Patients with full-blown symptomatology, or who predominantly suffer from cataplexy and/or disturbed nocturnal sleep, are good candidates for first-line SO treatment. In case of comorbid OSAS, the therapy must be closely monitored and a combination of CPAP and SO may be considered. If residual EDS complaints remain, the addition of modafinil or methylphenidate may be indicated. If cataplexy is not completely controlled, a very low dose (10 mg) of clomipramine can be added.

Future pharmacological treatments

Symptomatic therapies

- Armodafinil is the *r*-enantiomer of modafinil and has shown to be effective in narcolepsy patients. There are no studies that compare its efficacy with modafinil. The drug is available in the US but not in most European countries [43].
- Several histamine-3 receptor antagonists are currently being studied for the treatment of EDS. A published pilot study showed encouraging results [59].

Immune-based therapy

- Particularly intravenous immunoglobulins (IVIg). These therapies are given close to disease onset and are supposed to modulate the presumed, but not proven, autoimmune process leading to the hypocretin deficiency. A beneficial effect in particular on cataplexy has been claimed [60]. Note, however, that studies were small and not blinded, that possible spontaneous severity fluctuations may have influenced outcome, and that the placebo effect may be large [61].

Potential hypocretin-based therapies

- Hypocretin agonists: very attractive from a theoretical point of view. None are as yet available.
- Cell transplantation might potentially provide a cure [62]. However, at present the techniques need to be improved and there is the potential problem of an immune reaction to the graft in view of the autoimmune hypothesis of narcolepsy.
- Gene therapy is promising, but has potentially dangerous side-effects. There is no appropriate vector yet.

References

1. **American Academy of Sleep Medicine**. *International Classification of Sleep Disorders, Diagnostic and Coding Manual.* (2nd Ed.) Westchester, IL: American Academy of Sleep Medicine, 2005.
2. **Silber M H, Krahn L E, Olson E J**, et al. The epidemiology of narcolepsy in Olmsted County, Minnesota: a population-based study. *Sleep*, 2002; **25**:197–202.
3. **Longstreth W T**, Jr., **Koepsell T D, Ton T G**, et al. The epidemiology of narcolepsy. *Sleep*, 2007; **30**:13–26.
4. **Overeem S, Mignot E, van Dijk J G**, et al. Narcolepsy: clinical features, new pathophysiologic insights, and future perspectives. *J Clin Neurophysiol*, 2001; **18**:78–105.
5. **Dauvilliers Y, Montplaisir J, Molinari N**, et al. Age at onset of narcolepsy in two large populations of patients in France and Quebec. *Neurology*, 2001; **57**:2029–33.
6. **Dauvilliers Y, Arnulf I, Mignot E**. Narcolepsy with cataplexy. *Lancet*, 2007; **369**:499–511.
7. **Guilleminault C**. Cataplexy. In: Guilleminault C, Dement W C and Passouant P., Eds. *Narcolepsy*. New York, NY: Spectrum, 1976: 125–44.
8. **Fortuyn H A, Lappenschaar G A, Nienhuis F J**, et al. Psychotic symptoms in narcolepsy: phenomenology and a comparison with schizophrenia. *Gen Hosp Psychiatry*, 2009; **31**:146–54.
9. **Ohayon M M, Priest R G, Zulley J**, et al. Prevalence of narcolepsy symptomatology and diagnosis in the European general population. *Neurology*, 2002; **58**:1826–33.
10. **Ohayon M M**. From wakefulness to excessive sleepiness: what we know and still need to know. *Sleep Med Rev*, 2008; **12**:129–41.
11. **Broughton R, Dunham W, Newman J**, et al. Ambulatory 24 hour sleep–wake monitoring in narcolepsy–cataplexy compared to matched controls. *Electroencephalogr Clin Neurophysiol*, 1988; **70**:473–81.
12. **Kok S W, Overeem S, Visscher T L**, et al. Hypocretin deficiency in narcoleptic humans is associated with abdominal obesity. *Obes Res*, 2003; **11**:1147–54.
13. **Sansa G, Iranzo A, Santamaria J**. Obstructive sleep apnea in narcolepsy. *Sleep Med*, 2010; **11**:93–95.
14. **Dauvilliers Y, Pennestri M H, Petit D**, et al. Periodic leg movements during sleep and wakefulness in narcolepsy. *J Sleep Res*, 2007; **16**:333–39.
15. **Nightingale S, Orgill J C, Ebrahim I O**, et al. The association between narcolepsy and REM behavior disorder (RBD). *Sleep Med*, 2005; **6**:253–58.
16. **Broughton R, Ghanem Q, Hishikawa Y**, et al. Life effects of narcolepsy in 180 patients from North America, Asia and Europe compared to matched controls. *Can J Neurol Sci*, 1981; **8**:299–304.
17. **Mignot E, Lammers G J, Ripley B**, et al. The role of cerebrospinal fluid hypocretin measurement in the diagnosis of narcolepsy and other hypersomnias. *Arch Neurol*, 2002; **59**:1553–62.
18. **Arand D, Bonnet M, Hurwitz T**, et al. The clinical use of the MSLT and MWT. *Sleep*, 2005; **28**:123–44.
19. **Marti I, Valko P O, Khatami R**, et al. Multiple sleep latency measures in narcolepsy and behaviourally induced insufficient sleep syndrome. *Sleep Med*, 2009; **10**:1146–50.
20. **Sakurai T, Amemiya A, Ishii M**, et al. Orexins and orexin receptors: a family of hypothalamic neuropeptides and G protein-coupled receptors that regulate feeding behavior. *Cell*, 1998; **92**:573–85.
21. **de Lecea L, Kilduff T S, Peyron C**, et al. The hypocretins: hypothalamus-specific peptides with neuroexcitatory activity. *Proc Natl Acad Sci U S A*, 1998; **95**:322–27.
22. **Lin L, Faraco J, Li R**, et al. The sleep disorder canine narcolepsy is caused by a mutation in the hypocretin (orexin) receptor 2 gene. *Cell*, 1999; **98**:365–76.
23. **Chemelli R M, Willie J T, Sinton C M**, et al. Narcolepsy in orexin knockout mice: molecular genetics of sleep regulation. *Cell*, 1999; **98**:437–51.
24. **Nishino S, Ripley B, Overeem S**, et al. Hypocretin (orexin) deficiency in human narcolepsy. *Lancet*, 2000; **355**:39–40.
25. **Thannickal T C, Siegel J M, Nienhuis R**, et al. Pattern of hypocretin (orexin) soma and axon loss, and gliosis,

in human narcolepsy. *Brain Pathol*, 2003; **13**:340–51.

26. **Thannickal T C**, **Moore R Y**, **Nienhuis R**, *et al*. Reduced number of hypocretin neurons in human narcolepsy. *Neuron*, 2000; **27**:469–74.

27. **Thannickal T C**, **Nienhuis R**, **Siegel J M**. Localized loss of hypocretin (orexin) cells in narcolepsy without cataplexy. *Sleep*, 2009; **32**:993–98.

28. **Saper C B**, **Chou T C**, **Scammell T E**. The sleep switch: hypothalamic control of sleep and wakefulness. *Trends Neurosci*, 2001; **24**:726–31.

29. **Saper C B**, **Scammell T E**, **Lu J**. Hypothalamic regulation of sleep and circadian rhythms. *Nature*, 2005; **437**:1257–63.

30. **Broughton R**, **Valley V**, **Aguirre M**, *et al*. Excessive daytime sleepiness and the pathophysiology of narcolepsy–cataplexy: a laboratory perspective. *Sleep*, 1986; **9**:205–15.

31. **Peyron C**, **Faraco J**, **Rogers W**, *et al*. A mutation in a case of early onset narcolepsy and a generalized absence of hypocretin peptides in human narcoleptic brains. *Nat Med*, 2000; **6**:991–97.

32. **Mignot E**. Genetic and familial aspects of narcolepsy. *Neurology*, 1998; **50**:S16–22.

33. **Lin L**, **Hungs M**, **Mignot E**. Narcolepsy and the HLA region. *J Neuroimmunol*, 2001; **117**:9–20.

34. **Overeem S**, **Black J L, III**, **Lammers G J**. Narcolepsy: immunological aspects. *Sleep Med Rev*, 2008; **12**:95–107.

35. **Tanaka S**, **Honda Y**, **Inoue Y**, *et al*. Detection of autoantibodies against hypocretin, hcrtrl, and hcrtr2 in narcolepsy: anti-Hcrt system antibody in narcolepsy. *Sleep*, 2006; **29**:633–38.

36. **Black J L, III**, **Silber M H**, **Krahn L E**, *et al*. Studies of humoral immunity to preprohypocretin in human leukocyte antigen DQB1*0602-positive narcoleptic subjects with cataplexy. *Biol Psychiatry*, 2005; **58**:504–09.

37. **Black J L, III**, **Silber M H**, **Krahn L E**, *et al*. Analysis of hypocretin (orexin) antibodies in patients with narcolepsy. *Sleep*, 2005; **28**:427–31.

38. **Cvetkovic V**, **Bayer L**, **Dorsaz S**, *et al*. Tribbles homolog 2 as an autoantigen in human narcolepsy. *J Clin Invest*, 2010; **120**:713–19.

39. **Hallmayer J**, **Faraco J**, **Lin L**, *et al*. Narcolepsy is strongly associated with the T-cell receptor alpha locus. *Nat Genet*, 2009; **41**:708–11.

40. **Mullington J**, **Broughton R**. Scheduled naps in the management of daytime sleepiness in narcolepsy–cataplexy. *Sleep*, 1993; **16**:444–56.

41. **Bruck D**, **Armstrong S**, **Coleman G**. Sleepiness after glucose in narcolepsy. *J Sleep Res*, 1994; **3**:171–79.

42. **Fronczek R**, **Middelkoop H A**, **van Dijk J G**, *et al*. Focusing on vigilance instead of sleepiness in the assessment of narcolepsy: high sensitivity of the Sustained Attention to Response Task (SART). *Sleep*, 2006; **29**:187–91.

43. **Wise M S**, **Arand D L**, **Auger R R**, *et al*. Treatment of narcolepsy and other hypersomnias of central origin. *Sleep*, 2007; **30**:1712–27.

44. **Billiard M**, **Bassetti C**, **Dauvilliers Y**, *et al*. EFNS guidelines on management of narcolepsy. *Eur J Neurol*, 2006; **13**:1035–48.

45. **Parkes J D**, **Dahlitz M**. Amphetamine prescription. *Sleep*, 1993; **16**:201–03.

46. **Mitler M M**, **Aldrich M S**, **Koob G F**, *et al*. Narcolepsy and its treatment with stimulants. ASDA standards of practice. *Sleep*, 1994; **17**:352–71.

47. **Ryan D H**, **Bray G A**, **Helmcke F**, *et al*. Serial echocardiographic and clinical evaluation of valvular regurgitation before, during, and after treatment with fenfluramine or dexfenfluramine and mazindol or phentermine. *Obes Res*, 1999; **7**:313–22.

48. **Black J**, **Houghton W C**. Sodium oxybate improves excessive daytime sleepiness in narcolepsy. *Sleep*, 2006; **29**:939–46.

49. **Husain A M**, **Ristanovic R K**, **Bogan R K**. Weight loss in narcolepsy patients treated with sodium oxybate. *Sleep Med*, 2009; **10**:661–63.

50. **Feldman N T**. Clinical perspective: monitoring sodium oxybate-treated narcolepsy patients for the development of sleep-disordered breathing. *Sleep Breath*, 2010; **14**:77–79.

51. **Lammers G J**, **Bassetti C**, **Billiard M**, *et al*. Sodium oxybate is an effective and safe treatment for narcolepsy. *Sleep Med*, 2010; **11**:105–06.

52. **Parkes D**. Introduction to the mechanism of action of different treatments of narcolepsy. *Sleep*, 1994; **17**:S93–96.

53. **Nishino S**, **Mignot E**. Pharmacological aspects of human and canine narcolepsy. *Prog Neurobiol*, 1997; **52**:27–78.

54. **Nishino S**, **Arrigoni J**, **Shelton J**, *et al*. Desmethyl metabolites of serotonergic uptake inhibitors are more potent for suppressing canine cataplexy than their parent compounds. *Sleep*, 1993; **16**:706–12.

55. **Niederhofer H**. Atomoxetine also effective in patients suffering from narcolepsy? *Sleep*, 2005; **28**:1189.

56. **U.S. Xyrem Multicenter Study Group**. Sodium oxybate demonstrates long-term efficacy for the treatment of cataplexy in patients with narcolepsy. *Sleep Med*, 2004; **5**:119–23.

57. **U.S. Xyrem Multicenter Study Group**. A 12-month, open-label, multicenter extension trial of orally

administered sodium oxybate for the treatment of narcolepsy. *Sleep*, 2003; **26**:31–35.

58. **Thorpy M J**, **Snyder M**, **Aloe F S**, *et al*. Short-term triazolam use improves nocturnal sleep of narcoleptics. *Sleep*, 1992; **15**:212–16.

59. **Lin J S**, **Dauvilliers Y**, **Arnulf I**, *et al*. An inverse agonist of the histamine H(3) receptor improves wakefulness in narcolepsy: studies in orexin−/− mice and patients. *Neurobiol Dis*, 2008; **30**:74–83.

60. **Dauvilliers Y**. Follow-up of four narcolepsy patients treated with intravenous immunoglobulins. *Ann Neurol*, 2006; **60**:153.

61. **Fronczek R**, **Verschuuren J**, **Lammers G J**. Response to intravenous immunoglobulins and placebo in a patient with narcolepsy with cataplexy. *J Neurol*, 2007; **254**:1607–08.

62. **Arias-Carrion O**, **Murillo-Rodriguez E**. Cell transplantation: a future therapy for narcolepsy? *CNS Neurol Disord Drug Targets*, 2009; **8**:309–14.

Section 2 Sleep Disorders and Excessive Sleepiness
Chapter 12
Idiopathic hypersomnia

Michel Billiard

Introduction

In contrast to narcolepsy first described in 1877 [1] and 1880 [2], and to the Kleine–Levin syndrome first described in 1925 [3], the identification of idiopathic hypersomnia is much more recent [4]. Yet there is little interest taken in it, especially if one considers the number of entries on Pubmed as of December 2009: 3178 for narcolepsy, 237 for the exceptional Kleine–Levin syndrome and only 169 for idiopathic hypersomnia. This may be due to its less striking clinical features, e.g. excessive sleep without accompanying symptoms such as cataplexy or compulsive eating and hypersexuality, to the absence of characteristic electrophysiological or biological markers and to the very limited insight into its pathophysiology. In addition, all efforts to clarify demographics, pathophysiology and treatment have been hampered by the nosological uncertainty on the borders of idiopathic hypersomnia. Although the ICSD-2 has improved the characterization of the condition in defining idiopathic hypersomnia with and without long sleep time, many issues are still pending [5]. This chapter provides an overview of idiopathic hypersomnia together with a discussion on the nosological limits of the condition.

Historical background

The word idiopathic hypersomnia was coined by Bedrich Roth in 1976 [4], but the development of the concept dates back to 20 years earlier when the same author published a paper entitled "Spankova opilost a spankova obrna" [Sleep drunkenness and sleep paralysis] [6], followed one year later by a masterbook, "Narkolepsie a Hypersomnia, S. Hlediska Fysiologie Spanku" [Narcolepsy and hypersomnia from the aspect of physiology of sleep] [7]. In these two publications, Roth described carefully the symptom of sleep drunkenness and distinguished two forms of it: one sporadic, occurring once or a few times in a subject's lifetime, when being artificially woken out of deep sleep; and one persistent, occurring day after day on awakening, forming an independent group among the various forms of functional hypersomnia. In his first classification of hypersomnias published in the above-referred book, Roth distinguished narcolepsy (155 cases) and hypersomnia (93 cases) and within hypersomnia, functional hypersomnia (50 cases), organic hypersomnia (29 cases) and independent post-dormital drunkenness (14 cases), later referred to as idiopathic hypersomnia [7]. In 1972, a special paper on 58 cases of hypersomnia with sleep drunkenness was published [8], and finally, in 1976, a paper entitled "Narcolepsy and hypersomnia: review and classification of 642 personally observed cases" [4]. This classification included 368 cases of narcolepsy and 274 cases of hypersomnia. Hypersomnia was divided into symptomatic hypersomnia (61 cases) and functional hypersomnia (213 cases); functional hypersomnia divided into functional hypersomnia with a short cycle (191 cases) and functional hypersomnia with a long cycle (22 cases); functional hypersomnia with a short cycle divided into idiopathic hypersomnia monosymptomatic form (71 cases), idiopathic hypersomnia polysymptomatic form (103 cases), neurotic hypersomnia (5 cases) and hypersomnia with disorders of breathing during sleep (12 cases). In 1979, the Diagnostic Classification of Sleep and Arousal Disorders referred to idiopathic CNS hypersomnolence as one of the disorders of excessive somnolence [9], and in 1990, the International Classification of Sleep Disorders (ICSD) referred to idiopathic hypersomnia as one of the intrinsic sleep disorders [10]. Both classifications ignored the division of idiopathic hypersomnia into two forms, as suggested by Roth

Sleepiness: Causes, Consequences and Treatment, ed. Michael J. Thorpy and Michel Billiard. Published by Cambridge University Press. © Cambridge University Press 2011.

[4]. In 1997, Bassetti and Aldrich proposed to distinguish three forms of idiopathic hypersomnia: "classic" idiopathic hypersomnia, referring to patients who tended to have sleepiness that was not overwhelming, to take long unrefreshing naps up to 4 h, to have prolonged nighttime sleep and to have difficult awakening; "narcoleptic"-like hypersomnia, referring to patients who tended to have overwhelming excessive daytime sleepiness, to take short refreshing naps and to awaken without difficulties; and "mixed" idiopathic hypersomnia, referring to patients who had clinical features intermediate between the two other groups [11]. In 1998, Billiard et al. suggested to come back to Roth's initial distinction and used the terms of complete and incomplete forms of idiopathic hypersomnia [12]. Eventually, the latest International Classification of Sleep Disorders (2nd edition) confirmed the distinction of two forms of idiopathic hypersomnia and used a new wording of idiopathic hypersomnia with long sleep time and idiopathic hypersomnia without long sleep time [13].

Demographics

Due to nosological uncertainty, prevalence studies of idiopathic hypersomnia have not been conducted so far. If one considers large series of patients from different sleep disorders centers, the ratio of idiopathic hypersomnias to narcolepsies varies from a maximum of 47.2% to a minimum of 5.0%, average 30%, likely due to a failure to strictly adhere to ICSD-2 diagnostic criteria (Table 12.1) [4, 7, 11, 12, 14–25]. In some of these studies the number of patients with narcolepsy with and without cataplexy and the number of patients with and without long sleep time is detailed: the number of narcolepsy with cataplexy patients is consistently greater than the number of narcolepsy without cataplexy patients, whereas the number of idiopathic hypersomnia with long sleep time patients is only slightly greater than the number of idiopathic hypersomnia without long sleep time patients [4, 7, 12, 14, 23].

A female predominance has been reported in some series [18]. The age of onset varies from childhood to young adulthood and in some patients the symptoms may have been present since birth [26]. In contrast to narcolepsy, specifying the age of onset within a year is often difficult due to the progressive nature of occurrence.

Clinical features

The two forms of idiopathic hypersomnia require separate descriptions.

Idiopathic hypersomnia with long sleep time is remarkable for three symptoms: a complaint of more or less constant excessive daytime sleepiness and unwanted nap(s), generally not more than one or two per day, of longer duration and less irresistible than in narcolepsy, and non-refreshing irrespective of their duration; night sleep is abnormally prolonged; morning or nap awakening is laborious. In the morning, patients do not awaken to the ringing of a clock and often rely on their family members who must use vigorous and repeated procedures to wake them up. Even then, some patients are unable to begin any task, remain confused, unable to react adequately to external stimuli, a state referred to as "sleep drunkenness". Associated symptoms are sometimes observed suggesting an autonomic nervous system dysfunction, such as fainting episodes, lightheadedness on standing, orthostatic hypotension, headache, and cold hands and feet. Cataplexy is never present, but hypnagogic hallucinations and sleep paralysis may be present [11, 18].

Idiopathic hypersomnia without long sleep time is much less characteristic. It manifests itself as an isolated excessive daytime sleepiness. According to subjective data, unwanted daytime sleep episodes are more frequent, more irresistible and more refreshing than in the form with long sleep time; closer to those of narcolepsy. Abnormally long sleep time and difficulty in awakening do not belong to this form.

Diagnostic procedures

The diagnosis of idiopathic hypersomnia with long sleep time is mainly based on clinical features and on the absence of associated symptoms such as snoring or cataplexy. However, polysomnography and the multiple sleep latency test (MSLT) are indispensable to rule out other conditions. The ICSD-2 provides a set of clinical and polysomnographic diagnostic criteria [13]:

A. The patient has a complaint of excessive daytime sleepiness occurring almost daily for at least three months.
B. The patient has prolonged nocturnal sleep (more than 10 h) documented by interview, actigraphy, or sleep logs. Waking up in the morning or at the end of naps is almost always laborious.

difficulty on awakening and in some cases sleep drunkenness. Moreover, mean sleep latency on the MSLT may be normal or almost normal [24]. Thus one may question the limit between long sleeper and idiopathic hypersomnia with long sleep time. However, normal long sleepers neither complain about sleep drunkenness, nor about difficulty on awakening, and do not report excessive daytime sleepiness as long as they obtain the usual amount of sleep they normally need.

As for idiopathic hypersomnia without long sleep time and narcolepsy without cataplexy, their current distinction is not based on clinical features but on the number of SOREMPs on the MSLT, less than two in the former and two or more in the latter, a rather arbitrary and subtle criterion. Conversely, the two disorders seem to be quite similar in terms of clinical features, and a recent paper comparing narcolepsy with cataplexy patients, narcolepsy without cataplexy HLA-positive patients, narcolepsy without cataplexy HLA-negative patients, and idiopathic hypersomnia without long sleep time patients, did not find differences between the two latter groups in terms of mean sleep latency on the MSLT and ESS score before and after treatment with stimulants [33]. Moreover, 15–20% of narcolepsy with cataplexy patients have a positive family history of relatives presenting isolated repeated episodes of naps or lapses into sleep, most often negative for DQB1*0602, very similar to idiopathic hypersomnia without cataplexy patients [34, 35]. Finally, in a recent study on health-related quality of life in drug-naive patients with narcolepsy with cataplexy, narcolepsy without cataplexy, and idiopathic hypersomnia without long sleep time, the magnitude of impairment of quality of life was not different among the three disease categories [36]. Consequently, idiopathic hypersomnia without long sleep time is quite similar to narcolepsy without cataplexy and it may actually belong to the spectrum of narcolepsy (Table 12.2).

Obviously further studies comparing narcolepsy with cataplexy, narcolepsy without cataplexy, idiopathic hypersomnia without long sleep time and idiopathic hypersomnia with long sleep time are necessary before any final statement can be made.

Clinical variant

A recent paper has reported two cases of patients who met the ICSD-2 diagnostic criteria of idiopathic hypersomnia with long sleep time and who had latent hypothyroidism, namely normal thyroid hormones

Table 12.2 Clinical spectra of narcolepsy and idiopathic hypersomnia, according to ICSD-2 (top of the table) and proposed (bottom of the table). SOREMPs, sleep onset REM episodes.

ICSD-2 spectra

	Narcolepsy		Idiopathic hypersomnia	
w/ cataplexy	w/o cataplexy		w/o LST	w/ LST
two or more SOREMPs	two or more SOREMPs		fewer than two SOREMPs	fewer than two SOREMPs

Suggested spectra

	Narcolepsy			Idiopathic hypersomnia
w/ cataplexy	w/o cataplexy	w/o cataplexy		w/ LST
two or more SOREMPs	two or more SOREMPs	fewer than two SOREMPs		fewer than two SOREMPs

(normal fT3 and fT4 levels) and increased thyroid-stimulating hormone (TSH) together with absent myxoedema, tachycardia or bradycardia, in whom levothyroxin was effective for hypersomnia [37].

Differential diagnosis

Idiopathic hypersomnia is frequently overdiagnosed due to a persistent tendency to label as such hypersomnias that do not fit the criteria of either sleep-disordered breathing or narcolepsy.

Narcolepsy with cataplexy is clearly different from idiopathic hypersomnia with or without long sleep time. On the other hand, as already pointed out, narcolepsy without cataplexy is not very different from idiopathic hypersomnia without long sleep time except for the presence of two or more sleep onset REM periods on the MSLT.

Sleep-disordered breathing, especially the upper airway resistance syndrome, should be considered when polysomnography shows repetitive short alpha electroencephalographic arousals lasting 3–14 s. In practice, as mentioned above, sleep fragmentation should be directed towards additional polysomnography with nasal pressure cannula or pulse transit time measurement.

Hypersomnia not due to substance or known medical condition is often similar in its presentation to idiopathic hypersomnia with long sleep time. These subjects tend to complain about intractable daytime sleepiness. They usually rank very high on the Epworth Sleepiness Scale (ESS). However, night sleep is often poor. Polysomnography shows frequent awakenings and, most often, MSLT does not demonstrate an abnormally short mean sleep latency. Positive diagnosis may be relatively easy in the case of bipolar type II disorder (recurrent major depressive episodes with hypomanic episodes) [38], but much more difficult in the case of dysthymic disorder, conversion or undifferentiated somatoform disorder. Indeed patients are intensely focused on their hypersomnia, and psychiatric symptoms do not necessarily reveal themselves at first interview.

Post-traumatic hypersomnia may mimic idiopathic hypersomnia with long sleep time. Past medical history including an initial coma after head traumatism and CT or MRI showing focal abnormalities are revealing [39, 40].

Hypersomnia following a viral infection such as pneumonia, infectious mononucleosis or Guillain–Barré syndrome usually develops within weeks or months after the infection, with the subject complaining of residual fatigue and extremely long sleep. Prognosis is favorable, but recovery may take months or years [41].

Chronic fatigue syndrome is characterized by persistent or relapsing fatigue that does not resolve with sleep or rest. The disabling fatigue is accompanied by joint and muscle pain, headache, poor concentration, impaired short-term memory, disturbed sleep, recurrent subjective feverish feelings, and sore throat [42]. Polysomnography shows reduced sleep efficiency and may include alpha-intrusion into sleep EEG.

Insufficient sleep syndrome is associated with excessive daytime sleepiness, impaired concentration and lowered energy level. A detailed history of the subject's current sleep schedule is needed for the diagnosis [43] or even an actigraphic recording if the history is inconclusive.

A long sleeper is an individual who consistently sleeps more in 24 h than the conventional amount of sleep for his or her age group. The main difference with idiopathic hypersomnia is that there is no complaint of daytime sleepiness or difficulty in awakening as long as sufficient sleep is obtained to fulfill the increased sleep need. If an MSLT is performed, no evidence of pathological sleepiness is present, assuming that the patient has obtained the usual sleep amount he needs for several nights before the procedure [13].

Predisposing factors

Idiopathic hypersomnia with long sleep time is remarkable for 27–40% of probands reporting family members affected with the same symptoms [26, 44–46]. An autosomal-dominant mode of inheritance has been discussed [45]. Having reached the point when phenotypic features of idiopathic hypersomnia, particularly idiopathic hypersomnia with long sleep time, are well characterized, it is certainly timely to develop genetic studies of different types. Twin studies comparing the similarities between monozygotic and dizygotic twins would allow the determination of the impact of genetic factors versus environmental factors in the development of the sleep disorder. In addition, in an attempt to localize the gene(s) likely to be responsible for idiopathic hypersomnia with long sleep time, two types of approaches may be envisaged. First, linkage analysis in multiplex families, to test the likelihood of the cosegregation of a genetic marker and of the disease. The other strategy is that of candidate genes; the known physiology of a gene raising questions as to its possible implication in idiopathic hypersomnia with long sleep time.

Pathophysiology

In contrast with narcolepsy, there is no available natural model of idiopathic hypersomnia. This limits an experimental approach. Almost 40 years ago, Petitjean and Jouvet reported hypersomnia with a proportional increase of NREM and REM sleep suggestive of idiopathic hypersomnia with long sleep time, after destruction of norepinephrine neurons of the rostral third of the locus coeruleus complex or of the norepinephrine bundle at the level of the isthmus in the cat [47]. Unfortunately this experimental approach has not been pursued.

In humans, the few neurochemical studies conducted in idiopathic hypersomnia patients have not distinguished patients with idiopathic hypersomnia with long sleep time from patients without, and none of them has been replicated. Montplaisir et al. found that dopamine and indoleacetic acid, a tryptophane metabolite, were decreased in the CSF of both idiopathic hypersomniac and narcoleptic patients [48]. Faull et al. did not find any difference in the mean CSF concentrations of monoamine metabolites, 3,4-dihydroxy phenylacetic acid (DOPAC); 3-methoxy-4-hydroxyphenyl-ethyleneglycol (MHPG); homovanillic acid (HVA); and 5-hydroxyindoleacetic acid (5-HIAA) in narcoleptic and idiopathic hypersomnia patients and in control subjects [49]. However, a later reanalysis of the results of this study using principal component analysis showed that all four monoamine metabolites were highly intercorrelated in normal volunteers [50]. In contrast, HVA and DOPAC, the dopamine (DA) metabolites, did not correlate with the other two metabolites in narcoleptic patients, and MHPG, the norepinephrine (NE) metabolite, did not correlate with the other three metabolites in the idiopathic hypersomnia patients. According to these results, a malfunction of the DA system in narcolepsy and a malfunction of the NE system in idiopathic hypersomnia were hypothesized. Much more recently, two studies have shed further light on the possible neurochemical basis of idiopathic hypersomnia. Kanbayashi *et al.* reported that histamine levels were low in patients with narcolepsy and in patients with idiopathic hypersomnia, whereas they were relatively normal in obstructive sleep apnea–hypopnea patients, hence the hypothesis that low histamine levels may be specific to hypersomnias of central origin [51]. If histamine levels are low in both conditions, it remains to be explained why narcoleptic patients have an abnormal propensity to fall asleep and idiopathic hypersomnia with long sleep time patients an inability to wake up. Another recent study, published as an abstract, has reopened the issue of dopaminergic transmission in idiopathic hypersomnia [52]. Using positron emission tomography in seven untreated patients with idiopathic hypersomnia, the authors have shown an increased dopamine-receptor availability in the putamen and nucleus caudatus, suggesting the existence of a dysfunctional dopamine transmission in idiopathic hypersomnia. One of the most recent striking findings in the neurophysiology of wakefulness has been the discovery of the role of hypocretin [53]. In narcolepsy with cataplexy patients, the hypocretin-1 subtype is deficient in about 90% of cases [54, 55]. However, the same neuropeptide is at a normal level in the CSF of idiopathic hypersomnia patients, in favor of another mechanism [22, 28–30].

Another perspective has been the study of the homeostatic and circadian aspects of sleep–wake regulation. A dysregulation of the homeostatic and circadian process of sleep has been hypothesized in idiopathic hypersomnia with long sleep time patients [56]. In line with this hypothesis, a higher sleep spindle density has been documented during the second half of the night in 11 patients with idiopathic hypersomnia (all reporting a sleep time longer than 8 h) in comparison with controls [57] and in two patients with idiopathic hypersomnia with long sleep time [56], suggesting an altered NREM sleep homeostasis. In addition, a disturbed circadian rhythm has been hypothesized on the basis of a phase delay in the rhythm of melatonin and cortisol secretion in 15 patients suffering from idiopathic hypersomnia with long sleep time [58].

Treatment

Despite a different type of sleepiness, at least in the case of idiopathic hypersomnia with long sleep time, the pharmacological options for idiopathic hypersomnia have mirrored the development of treatments of excessive daytime sleepiness in narcolepsy. Stimulants, amphetamine and methylphenidate have been the basic treatment of idiopathic hypersomnia, in most cases with only partial relief. Since the second half of the 1990s, modafinil has been considered as the first-line treatment for idiopathic hypersomnia, although its effects are not fully satisfactory. According to an open-label study comparing sleep diary data before and after treatment in 15 idiopathic hypersomnia patients, excessive daytime sleepiness and unwanted sleep episodes decreased significantly ($p<0.05$ and $p<0.01$) [59]. On the other hand, in a follow-up study conducted in 54 idiopathic hypersomnia patients put on modafinil (mean dose 400 mg), only 39 remained on modafinil alone and 24 of these (44.4% of the total sample) had sustained benefit over a mean follow-up period of 3.8 years [26]. Randomized, double-blind, placebo-controlled clinical trials have never been conducted. Anecdotally, an improvement in half of 10 idiopathic hypersomnia patients treated with melatonin (2 mg of slow release at bed time) has been reported [60]. As for sodium oxybate, now extensively used in the treatment of narcolepsy, it has not yet been used in idiopathic hypersomnia. Finally, in contrast with narcolepsy, behavioral treatment in the form of daytime nap(s) is not beneficial and the prolongation of sleep times suggested by Roth does not bring relief in the long term.

Conclusion

In contrast with narcolepsy with or without cataplexy, characterized by an abnormal propensity to fall asleep, idiopathic hypersomnia with long sleep time is remarkable for an inability to terminate sleep. This difficulty in awakening is often resistant to stimulants used in narcolepsy. Up to now, no consistent hypothesis has been found to explain this abnormality. On the other hand, idiopathic hypersomnia without long sleep time seems quite similar to narcolepsy without cataplexy, to the extent that a single test, the multiple sleep latency test, allows separation of the two conditions on the basis of an arbitrary polygraphic cut off. Further research is highly necessary both to specify the limits of idiopathic hypersomnia with and without long sleep time and to investigate their predisposing factors and pathophysiology.

References

1. **Westphal C**. Eigentümliche mit Einschlafen verbundene Anfälle. *Arch Gen Psychiatr Nervenkr*, 1877; **7**:631–65.
2. **Gelineau J**. De la narcolepsie. *Gaz des Hôp (Paris)*, 1880; **55**, 626–28; 635–37.
3. **Kleine W**. Periodische Schlafsucht. *Mschr Psychiat Neurol*, 1925; **57**:285–320.
4. **Roth B**. Narcolepsy and hypersomnia: review and classification of 642 personally observed cases. *Schweiz Arch Neurol Neurochir Psychiat*, 1976; **119**:31–41.
5. **Billiard M**. Diagnosis of narcolepsy and idiopathic hypersomnia. An update based on the international classification of sleep disorders, 2nd edition. *Sleep Med Rev*, 2007; **11**:377–88.
6. **Roth B**. Spankova opilost a spánkova óbrna. *Ceskoslovenska Neurol*, 1956; **19**:48–58.
7. **Roth B**. *Narkolepsie a Hypersomnie S. Hlediska Fysiologie Spanku*. Praha: Statni Zdravonické Nakladatelstvi, 1957.
8. **Roth B, Nevsimalova S, Rechtschaffen A**. Hypersomnia with sleep drunkenness. *Arch Gen Psychiat*, 1972; **26**:456–62.
9. **Association of Sleep Disorders Centers**. Diagnostic Classification of Sleep and Arousal Disorders, First edition, prepared by the Sleep Disorders Classification Committee, HP. Roffwarg, Chairman. *Sleep*, 1979; **2**:1–137.
10. **ICSD**. *International Classification of Sleep Disorders: Diagnostic and Coding Manual*. Diagnostic Classification Steering Committee. Thorpy M J, Chairman. Rochester, MN: American Sleep Disorders Association, 1990.
11. **Bassetti C, Aldrich M S**. Idiopathic hypersomnia. A series of 42 patients. *Brain* 1997; **120**:1423–35.
12. **Billiard M, Merle C, Carlander B**, et al. Idiopathic hypersomnia. *Psychiatr Clin Neurosci* 1998; **52**:125–29.
13. **American Academy of Sleep Medicine**. *International Classification of Sleep Disorders. Diagnostic and Coding Manual* (2nd Ed). Westchester, IL: American Academy of Sleep Medicine, 2005.
14. **Nevsimalova-Bruhova S**. On the problem of heredity in hypersomnia, narcolepsy and dissociated sleep disturbances. *Acta Univ Carol Med (Praha)*, 1973; **18**:109–60.
15. **Van Den Hoed J, Kraemer H, Guilleminault C**, et al. Disorders of excessive daytime somnolence: polygraphic and clinical data for 100 patients. *Sleep*, 1981; **4**:23–37.
16. **Coleman R M, Roffwarg H P, Kennedy S J**, et al. Sleep–wake disorders based on a polysomnographic diagnosis. A national cooperative study. *JAMA*, 1982; **247**:997–1003.
17. **Baker T L, Guilleminault C, Nino-Murcia G**, et al. Comparative polysomnographic study of narcolepsy and idiopathic central nervous system hypersomnia. *Sleep*, 1986; **9**:232–42.
18. **Aldrich M S**. The clinical spectrum of narcolepsy and idiopathic hypersomnia. *Neurology*, 1996; **46**:393–401.
19. **Bruck D, Parkes J D**. A comparison of idiopathic hypersomnia and narcolepsy using self report measures and sleep diary data. *J Neurol Neurosurg Psychiatry*, 1996; **60**:576–78.
20. **Vignatelli L, d'Alessandro R, Mosconi P**, et al. Health-related quality of life in Italian patients with narcolepsy: the SF-36 health survey. *Sleep Med*, 2004; **5**:467–75.
21. **Heier M S, Evsiukova T, Vilming S**, et al. CSF hypocretin-1 levels and clinal profiles in narcolepsy and idiopathic CNS hypersomnia in Norway. *Sleep*, 2007; **30**:969–73.
22. **Kanbayashi T, Inoue Y, Chgiba S**, et al. CSF hypocretin-1 (orexin-A) concentrations in narcolepsy with and without cataplexy and idiopathic hypersomnia. *J Sleep Res*, 2002; **11**:91–93.
23. **Vernet C, Arnulf I**. Idiopathic hypersomnia with and without long sleep time: a controlled series of 75 patients. *Sleep*, 2009; **32**:753–59.
24. **Vernet C, Arnulf I**. Narcolepsy with long sleep time: a specific entity? *Sleep*, 2009; **32**:1229–35.
25. **Dauvilliers Y, Paquereau J, Bastuji H**, et al. Psychological health in central hypersomnias: the French Harmony Study. *J Neurol Neurosurg Psychiatry*, 2009; **80**:636–41.
26. **Anderson K N, Pilsworth S, Sharples L D**, et al. Idiopathic hypersomnia: a study of 77 cases. *Sleep*, 2007; **30**:1274–81.
27. **Sangal R B, Sangal J M**. P300 latency: abnormal in sleep apnea with somnolence and idiopathic

hypersomnia, but normal in narcolepsy. *Clin Electroencephalogr*, 1995; **26**:146–53.

28. **Mignot E**, **Lammers G J**, **Ripley B**, et al. The role of cerebrospinal fluid hypocretin in the diagnosis of narcolepsy and other hypersomnias. *Arch Neurol*, 2002; **59**:1553–62.

29. **Bassetti C**, **Gugger M**, **Bischof M**, et al. The narcoleptic borderland: a multimodal diagnostic approach including cerebrospinal fluid levels of hypocretin-1 (orexin). *Sleep Med*, 2003; **4**:7–12.

30. **Dauvilliers Y**, **Baumann C R**, **Carlander B**, et al. CSF hypocretin-1 levels in narcolepsy, Kleine–Levin syndrome, and other hypersomnias and neurological conditions. *J Neurol Neurosurg Psychiatry*, 2003; **74**:1667–73.

31. **Broughton R**, **Nevsimalova S**, **Roth B**. The socioeconomic effects (including work, education, recreation and accidents) of idiopathic hypersomnia. *Sleep Res*, 1978; **7**:217.

32. **Billiard M**. Narcolepsy and idiopathic hypersomnia. In: Léger D, Pandi-Perumal S R, Eds. *Sleep Disordes: their Impact on Public Health*. Abingdon: Informa Healthcare, 2007:225–34.

33. **Sasai T**, **Inoue Y**, **Komada Y**, et al. Comparison of clinical characteristics among narcolepsy with and without cataplexy and idiopathic hypersomnia without long sleep time focusing on HLA-DRB1(7)1501/DQB1(7)0602 finding. *Sleep Med*, 2009; **10**:961–66.

34. **Billiard M**, **Pasquié-Magnetto V**, **Heckman M**, et al. Family studies in narcolepsy. *Sleep*, 1994; **17**:S54–59.

35. **Mignot E**. Genetic and familial aspects of narcolepsy. *Neurology*, 1998; **50**(Suppl 1):S16–22.

36. **Ozaki A**, **Inoue Y**, **Nakajima T** et al. Health-related quality of life among drug-naïve patients with narcolepsy with cataplexy, narcolepsy without cataplexy, and idiopathic hypersomnia without long sleep time. *J Clin Sleep Med*, 2008; **4**:572–78.

37. **Shinno H**, **Inami Y**, **Inagaki T**, et al. Successful treatment with levothyroxine for idiopathic hypersomnia patients with subclinical hypothyroidism. *Gen Hosp Psychiat*, 2009; **31**: 190–93.

38. **Nofzinger E A**, **Thase M E**, **Reynolds C F** III, et al. Hypersomnia in bipolar depression: a comparison with narcolepsy using the multiple sleep latency test. *Am J Psychiatry*, 1991; **148**:1177–81.

39. **Guilleminault C**, **Faull K F**, **Miles L**, et al. Post-traumatic excessive daytime sleepiness. A review of 20 patients. *Neurology*, 1980; **33**:1584–89.

40. **Rao V**, **Rollings P**. Sleep disturbances following traumatic brain injury. *Curr Treat Opt Neurol*, 2002; **4**:77–82.

41. **Guilleminault C**, **Mondini S**. Infectious mononucleosis and excessive daytime sleepiness. A long-term follow-up study. *Arch Inter Med*, 1986; **146**:1333–35.

42. **Fukuda D**, **Strauss S E**, **Hickie I**, et al. The chronic fatigue syndrome: comprehensive approach to its definition and study. *Ann Int Med*, 1994; **121**:953–59.

43. **Roehrs T**, **Zorick F**, **Sicklesteel J**, et al. Excessive daytime sleepiness associated with insufficient sleep. *Sleep*, 1983; **6**:319–25.

44. **Billiard M**, **Dauvilliers Y**. Idiopathic hypersomnia. *Sleep Med Rev*, 2001; **5**:351–60.

45. **Nevsimalova-Bruhova S**, **Roth B**. Heredofamilial aspects of narcolepsy and hypersomnia. *Schweiz Arch Neurol Neurochir Psychiat*, 1972; **110**:45–54.

46. **Roth B**. Idiopathic hypersomnia. In: Roth B, Ed. *Narcolepsy and Hypersomnia*. Basel: Karger, 1980:207–27.

47. **Petitjean F**, **Jouvet M**. Hypersomnie et augmentation de l'acide 5-hydroxy-indoleacétique cérébral par lésion isthmique chez le chat. *C R séances Soc Biol (Lyon)*, 1970; **164**:2288–93.

48. **Montplaisir J**, **de Champlain J**, **Young S N**, et al. Narcolepsy and idiopathic hypersomnia: biogenic amines and related compounds in CSF. *Neurology*, 1982; **32**:1299–302.

49. **Faull K F**, **Guilleminault C**, **Berger P A**, et al. Cerebrospinal fluid monoamine metabolites in narcolepsy and hypersomnia. *Ann Neurol*, 1983; **13**:258–63.

50. **Faull K F**, **Thiemann S**, **King R J**, et al. Monoamine interactions in narcolepsy and hypersomnia: a preliminary report. *Sleep*, 1986; **9**:246–49.

51. **Kanbayashi T**, **Kodama T**, **Kondo H**, et al. CSF histamine contents in narcolepsy, idiopathic hypersomnia and obstructive sleep apnea syndrome. *Sleep*, 2009; **32**:175–80.

52. **Bassetti C L**, **Khatami R**, **Poryazova R**, et al. Idiopathic hypersomnia: a dopaminergic disorder. *Sleep*, 2009; **32**:A248–49 (abstract suppl).

53. **Mühlethaler M**. Potential mechanisms of the wake-promoting action of hypocretin/orexin. In Bassetti C L, Billiard M, Mignot E, Eds. *Narcolepsy and Hypersomnia*. New York, NY: Informa Healthcare, 2007:347–54.

54. **Nishino S**, **Ripley B**, **Overeem S**, et al. Hypocretin (orexin) deficiency in human narcolepsy. *Lancet*, 2000; **355**:39–40.

55. **Nishino S**, **Ripley B**, **Overeem S**, et al. Low CSF hypocretin (orexin) and altered energy homeostasis in human narcolepsy. *Ann Neurol*, 2001; **50**:381–88.

56. **Billiard M**, **Rondouin G**, **Espa F**, *et al.* Pathophysiology of idiopathic hypersomnia. *Rev Neurol (Paris)*, 2001; **157**:5S101–06.

57. **Boeve A**, **Culebras A**, **Moore J T**, *et al.* Relationship between sleep spindles and hypersomnia. *Sleep*, 1994; **17**:449–55.

58. **Nevsimalova S**, **Blazejova K**, **Illnerova H**, *et al.* A contribution to pathophysiology of idiopathic hypersomnia. In: Ambler Z, Nevsimalova S, Kadanza Z, Rossini P M, Eds. *Clinical Neurophysiology at the Beginning of the 21st Century* (supplement to Clinical Neurophysiology), 2000; 53:366–70.

59. **Bastuji H**, **Jouvet M**. Successful treatment of idiopathic hypersomnia and narcolepsy with modafinil. *Prog NeuroPsychopharmacol and Biol. Psychiat*, 1988; **12**:695–700.

60. **Montplaisir J**, **Fantini L**. Idiopathic hypersomnia: a diagnostic dilemma. *Sleep Med Rev*, 2001; **5**:361–62.

Section 2 Chapter 13

Sleep Disorders and Excessive Sleepiness

Kleine–Levin syndrome

Isabelle Arnulf

Summary

Kleine–Levin syndrome (KLS) is a rare neurological disorder (1–2 cases per million inhabitants) primarily affecting young subjects. It is characterized by relapsing-remitting episodes of hypersomnia in association with cognitive and behavioral disturbances. Case reports, small series, meta-analysis and recent large, prospective studies are consistent with a homogeneous, genuine disease entity. Patients are mostly male (68–78%) and adolescents (81%), with mean onset at 15 years (range 4–82 years). The first episode is triggered by an infection in 72% of patients. Patients experience an average of 7–19 episodes of 10–13 days each, relapsing every 3.5 months. Episodes recur more quickly in patients with childhood onset. The median disease course is 8–14 years, with longer course in men, in patients with hypersexuality, and when age of onset is after 20. During episodes, all patients have hypersomnia (with sleep lasting 15–21 h per day), cognitive impairment (apathy, confusion, slowness, amnesia) and a specific feeling of derealization (dreamy state, altered perception). Less frequently, patients experience hyperphagia (66%), hypersexuality (53%, principally men) and depressed mood (53%, predominantly women). Patients are remarkably similar to controls between episodes regarding sleep, vigilance, mood, and eating attitude, but may have increased body mass index. Structural brain imaging, evaluation of the cerebrospinal fluid and serological inflammatory markers are unremarkable. EEG slowing is notable in 70% of cases during episodes, without epileptic activity. Sleep structure varies from hypersomnia with initial decrease in slow-wave sleep then in REM sleep, to hypoarousal with low sleep efficiency. The brain scintigraphy may show hypoperfusion, mostly focused on the thalamic, hypothalamic and fronto-temporal areas, especially when contrasted to images obtained between episodes. Newly identified factors include increased birth and developmental problems, Jewish heritage and genetics (5% multiplex families, suggesting autosomal recessive transmission). The association of KLS with HLA-DRB1*201, found in a small series, is not replicated in a larger independent sample. There is no increased family history for neuropsychiatric disorders. Some stimulants (amantadine, but more rarely modafinil or amphetamine) and mood stabilizers (mostly lithium) have a marginal efficacy. In the 10% KLS cases secondary to various genetic, inflammatory, vascular or paraneoplasic conditions, patients are older, have more frequent and longer episodes, but their clinical symptoms, disease course and treatment response are similar to primary cases. The most promising findings are the familial clustering and a potential Jewish founder effect, supporting a role for genetic susceptibility factors. KLS is a puzzling and disabling disease. Until its cause well is identified, disease management should be primarily supportive and educational.

Case report

B is a 16-year-old boy, with no previous medical history. He is an eleventh-grade student with excellent performances, fond of sports, with a girlfriend and good social contacts. During the February vacations, his parents took him to the West Indies for a week of sea, beach and sun. But when he arrived on the island, he felt exhausted (possibly jet-lagged), with a mild headache. He stayed in his room, in the dark, sleeping continuously during the week. He ate only when asked to, mechanically. The local physician could not identify any abnormalities, and the family concluded

---

Sleepiness: Causes, Consequences and Treatment, ed. Michael J. Thorpy and Michel Billiard. Published by Cambridge University Press. © Cambridge University Press 2011.

he might have had a local virus, and needed to rest after a hard semester. Back at home, when he was awake, he stood in front of the TV watching new movies, and felt like he could foretell what the actors were about to say. He progressively felt better after 10 days, reported 2 days of difficulty falling asleep, and then was able to go back to school. He vaguely remembered having travelled, but was not sure if it had been a dream or not. He had good grades during the next semester, until June. Two days before the Literature exam, he again felt exhausted during school, and came home to sleep. His parents tried to wake him. To their great surprise, they were insulted by their usually well-bred son. They took him with difficulty to the physician's, but in the waiting room, when B saw another lady waiting, he said inappropriately, speaking loudly: "How fat she is, this lady there!" He barely answered the physician, and was sent to the emergency department. After he had normal results on various tests (MRI, EEG, lumbar puncture, toxic and alcohol in the urine), he was sent to the psychiatric hospital. This 1.80-m-high athletic man cried and did not want his mother to leave him alone there. After a few days, he told his mother that he felt like he was about to die. His parents signed a waiver to allow him to leave. He got better after 10 days while sleeping continuously in the dark, waking up only for voiding and eating automatically, and not showering. When he went to the kitchen, he took and ate several boxes of cookies and potato chips. He could not stand the noise of the vacuum in his room, and stopped using his cell phone and computer games (which was remarkably different from normal...). After his parents called a neurologist, he was sent to our department during an asymptomatic period. He was perfectly normal after this second episode in all aspects of physical and mental health (cognition, mood, sleep, sociability). We explained the diagnosis of Kleine–Levin syndrome, and suggested trying amantadine in case of a new episode and to evaluate the frequency of the episodes before instituting a preventive therapy. His parents stayed at home alternatively when he was ill. Afterwards, he had similar 7–14-day-long episodes in July, September and November (twice needing sublingual bromazepam on the ninth day, as he suddenly experienced a day-long acute depression and panic), so we prescribed valproate in December for 6 months. As he had four episodes in the next six months, we stopped the valproate. When we saw him during an episode, his head was drooping, with an exhausted face, answering slowly but correctly, even for calculations. The time to end the Stroop test had doubled compared to his previous performance. He cried and refused to finish the other tests. During the 24-h sleep monitoring, he did not sleep that much, but oscillated continuously between a quiet wake in alpha rhythm, and sleep stage N1. Notably, he wanted his mother to lay with him in the hospital bed. The episodes spaced progressively, from seven in the first year to three in the second and third years, then two and none the last year. B attended a summer school, obtained help for disabled students, and succeeded to integrate at a prestigious University of Economics in Paris. He had a single, late relapse 5 years after KLS onset, after he got drunk one evening.

Epidemiology

The exact prevalence of KLS is unknown, but it is considered a very rare disease. In France, as a national reference center with no social restriction for being taken in charge, and a large amount of information given to colleagues and available on the Internet, we receive 8–10 new cases per year, which (if the duration is around 14 years, and the population is 60 million) suggests a higher estimate of 2.3 cases/million. The female: male sex ratio varies from 1:3 to 1:4. The majority of patients are teenagers at KLS onset, but there are rare cases beginning around 9 years of age [1], or after 35 years of age [2, 3]. The syndrome has been reported worldwide, in Europe, America, Asia, Australia and Africa. As it is more frequent in Israel [1, 4], and in American Jews [5], a founding effect is suspected. Although familial risk is low (1% per first-degree relative), there are 5% multiplex families (with brother and sister, parent and child, and cousins) [6–10], leading to an estimate of an 800- to 4000-fold increased risk in first-degree relatives [5].

Clinical symptoms

The diagnosis criteria for KLS are shown in Table 13.1 [11]. The first episode usually begins within a few hours, with patients becoming extremely tired, generally after an identifiable triggering event, such as a banal infection in most cases, alcohol intake (alone or combined with sleep deprivation), or a head trauma. The symptomatic periods involve hypersomnia, and cognitive, behavioral and psychological problems (when awake), and last from two days to several weeks. They alternate with long (e.g. months) periods with normal sleep, cognition, mood and behavior. An

Table 13.1 Diagnosis criteria for recurrent hypersomnia and KLS [11]

A. Recurrent hypersomnia
1. The patient experiences recurrent episodes of excessive sleepiness of 2 days' to 4 weeks' duration.
2. Episodes recur at least once a year.
3. The patient has normal alertness, cognitive functioning and behavior between attacks.
4. The hypersomnia is not better explained by another sleep disorder, medical or neurological disorder, mental disorder, medication use, or substance use disorder.

B. Kleine–Levin syndrome
In addition to all criteria listed in A, the hypersomnia should be clearly associated with at least one of these symptoms:
1. Megaphagia.
2. Hypersexuality.
3. Abnormal behavior such as irritability, aggression or odd behavior.
4. Cognitive abnormalities such as feeling of unreality, confusion and hallucination.

example of the frequency of the episodes within one year is shown in Figure 13.1.

Hypersomnia

KLS belongs to periodic hypersomnia. The affected teenagers experience a sudden extreme fatigue and a need to rest, retire in their room and sleep for 15–24 h a day, for one to several weeks. The average time asleep per 24 h was 17.9 ± 3.6 h, with a minimum of 14.7 ± 4.8 h and a maximum of 21.3 ± 2.5 h in a prospective series of 108 patients. They remain arousable, however, but look exhausted and irritable when prevented from resuming sleep. The long sleep episodes may occur night and day, with no clear circadian rhythms, and possible awakening during the night. Most of them experience intense dreaming and hypnagogic hallucinations (50%), while sleep paralysis is uncommon. After several episodes, they may not sleep that much, but still need to stay inactive and in the dark in their room. At the end of an episode, many patients have one to several days of insomnia: "All I want to do is stay awake and get things done that I was unable to while in the episode," reports a patient. Typically, the sleep and vigilance are normal between the episodes, when monitored and on questionnaires.

Cognitive impairment

Patients report difficulties (and lack of desire) in communicating, speaking, reading, concentrating, deciding, memorizing, performing two tasks simultaneously, coordinating movement and orientating in time and space. However, the confusion is mild, in contrast with a major apathy, and patients remain able to count and answer complex questions, but with a slowness that contrasts with their previous cognition. "I have trouble forming thoughts into words. I respond mostly with grunts, groans and other such caveman sounds, which my family has learned to interpret," said one. A guitar player could play solo but not duo with her husband on the piano during an episode. Perception is altered in most if not all patients, resulting in a striking feeling of derealization. Seeing, hearing, smelling, tasting, feeling cold/hot and pain could be "wrong": "Part of the time, the environment felt 'flat,' 2-dimensional, but figure-ground"; "Things seemed hazy, foggy before the onset of an episode"; "I broke my foot once in the beginning of an episode and didn't understand when it happened or that I had broken it". As many as 81% of patients feel like they are in a dream, a feeling called "derealization"(Figure 13.2), "almost as if what you do doesn't have a consequence". This led one patient to "try to do something to get a normal reaction i.e. break a cup to see if it would break to reassure me things were normal." After the episode, only 13% had a complete recollection of what happened: "I have to have everything confirmed because I thought I 'dreamt' it"; "it seems more like a movie that is cut up, so scenes are missing and the picture quality is horrible."

Behavioral problems

The most demonstrative behavioral disorders in KLS patients are hyperphagia and hypersexuality. They are, however, inconsistent, while hypersomnia and cognitive problems are not. Two-thirds of patients eat more, sometimes compulsively, eating more sweets and snacks than usual: "I would not eat for 10–14 hours then would eat 4 or 5 Peanut Butter and Jelly – without even chewing very fast, then would start to fall sleep again with the last piece of food still in my mouth." The other patients eat rather less: they sleep all the time and are called to the family table, where they eat mechanically. Boys are more often hypersexual than girls (58% vs. 35%), with more frequent masturbation, and inappropriate sexual behaviors: "He masturbates frenetically, with very frequent sexual intercourse with his fiancée at the hospital, in his room, hidden from the nurses". Repetitive behaviors are frequent. Around one-third of patients sing sing-song, pace, tap, snap fingers, listen to the same music or watch the same video in a continuous loop. Some patients are in a regressive behavior such as skipping all the time,

Figure 13.1 Days with symptoms are circled by the mother of a 15-year-old girl with KLS.

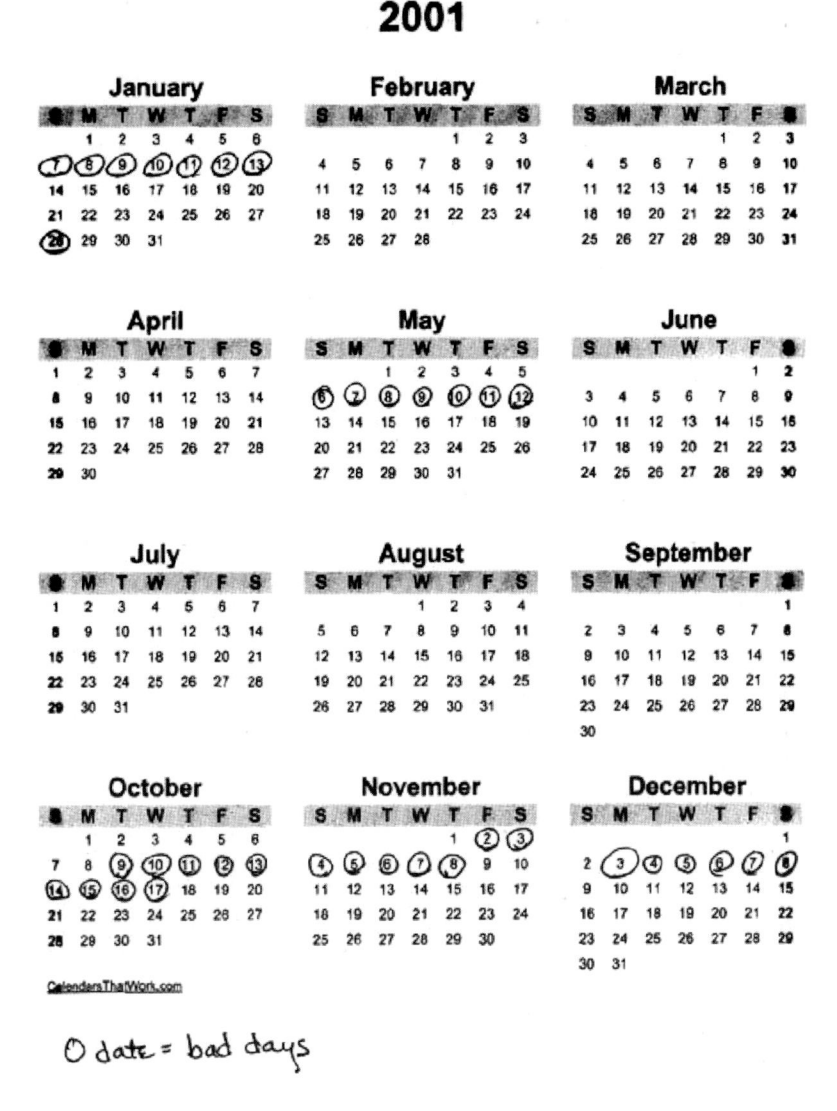

playing with one's fingers. Three-quarters of them neglect their hygiene during an episode.

Psychological troubles

Flattened affect and sad mood (with rare cases of suicidal attempts) are more prevalent in women than in men. Decreased mood may last for only a day (often close to the end of an episode), with teenagers crying and feeling as if the disease would never end. In rare cases, the sad mood overshoots the sleep episode. Most commonly, the termination of an episode is characterized by logorrhea, excitation and insomnia, for one or two days, as if patients try to catch up on the lost time. Anxiety can be high, especially when the patient is suddenly left in an unfamiliar environment such as the hospital. A regressive behavior is reported by some parents, with teenagers speaking with a child-like voice, and using childish words. On the contrary, some young patients become rude, and aggressive, especially when prevented from resting or sleeping. A child beat his grandmother [12], an adult patient beat his dog [13], another child bit his father, a teenager spat in the face in his physician [14], one threw stones and was caught by the police [15], while a teenager had such an anger outburst at school that the police evacuated the classroom [16]. In one-third of patients, mild, short-lasting hallucinations and delusions are

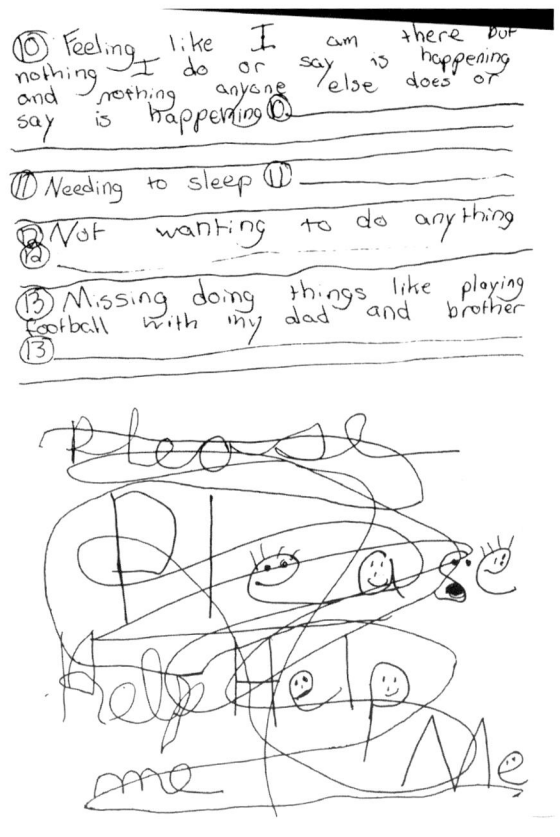

⑩ Feeling like I am there but nothing I do or say is happening and nothing anyone else does or say is happening ⑩.

⑪ Needing to sleep ⑪

⑫ Not wanting to do anything ⑫

⑬ Missing doing things like playing football with my dad and brother ⑬

Figure 13.2 Symptoms as described by a 14-year-old girl during a KLS episode. Note how she describes derealization (item 10).

described. All these psychological symptoms contrast dramatically with the usual behavior and psychological profile of the teenager.

Vegetative symptoms

Headache, photophobia, and phonophobia are frequent. The face of the teenager during the episode is usually peculiar, with a tired face, an empty gaze, and possibly flushing. Patients may void less often (e.g. only once a day), and have, in rare cases, a urine retention. Other autonomic signs are exceptional. They include abnormally high or low blood pressure [17, 18], bradycardia or tachycardia [2], and ataxic respiration [19].

Clinical forms

Despite KLS being a rare disease, it is possible to observe various forms of the disease. Contrarily to ancient small series, the full-blown KLS does not mandatorily include the "hypersomnia + megaphagia + hypersexuality" triad (which is present in only 45% patients), but rather the "hypersomnia + confusion + apathy + derealization" tetrad, which is found in 100% of patients [5].

Benign vs. severe forms

In our experience, there are some mild, benign forms of KLS, with teenagers experiencing one-week symptomatic periods two to three times a year. In contrast, some patients experience 7–10-day episodes every month, while others have very long-lasting (e.g. 3–6 months) episodes, suffering from an altered cognition, apathy, abnormal behavior and sleep cycling on a rhythm greater than 24 h. Eventually, some patients may experience 40–80 episodes with no evidence of cure, and possibly a long-term alteration of attention or mood. When KLS starts after 20 years of age, the chance of spontaneous disappearance of the disease is much lower. All in all, the former concept of a benign disease that spontaneously disappears should now be challenged.

Primary vs. secondary forms

We defined secondary KLS as when neurological symptoms are present prior to KLS onset and persist between episodes. In 18 patients, KLS-like symptoms have been observed in association with stroke or post-traumatic brain hematoma ($n=5$), genetic or developmental diseases ($n=6$, including mosaicism, Prader-Willi [9], Asperger's syndrome [20], mental retardation), multiple sclerosis [21], hydrocephalus [22], paraneoplasia in the context of a carcinoma of the cervix utero [23], an autoimmune encephalitis [24], or a severe infectious encephalitis ($n=3$) [25, 26]. The disease begins later in patients with secondary than primary KLS, but does not, however, last longer. Patients with secondary KLS experience more frequent and longer episodes, but with similar cardinal symptoms [27]. The neurological signs observed between the episodes are various, with very few commonalities between patients.

Menstruation-linked hypersomnia

Hypersomnia associated with behavioral, cognitive and mood problems associated with menstruation (just before or at time of) have been reported under the name of menstruation-linked hypersomnia [28], as a disease even rarer than KLS. Note that Dr. Kleine had already included a woman with episodes occurring in association with menstruation in his first series of periodic hypersomnia [29]. We fail to see any clinical differences between women with KLS (who can have episodes occurring more frequently before menstruations) and the few cases with menstruation-linked hypersomnia that we have seen. The main difference would rather be in terms of treatment, as a total blockade of the sexual hormones may reduce the number of episodes in these women.

Disease course and complications

Episodes duration and frequency

The episodes follow an unpredictable course. They last a mean of 13 days, but short "aborted" episodes lasting 1–2 days (generally during a weekend) may occur between long episodes. On the other hand, very long (3–4 months) episodes are observed in rare but otherwise typical KLS cases [7]. During a given episode, the hypersomnia is generally marked during the first days, and changes towards less sleep and more apathy and altered cognition at the end of the episode. After several episodes, the symptoms may change, with episodes containing less sleep and more apathy and altered cognition. The mean interval between episodes is 5.7 months, with ranges of 0.5–66 months. Episodes recur more frequently in patients with childhood onset.

Disease duration

In our prospective series of 108 patients, the disease lasts a median of 13.6 ± 4.3 years. Thus, it is common to say to the patient and family that the disease will disappear (in most cases) after 30 years of age. Male sex and the presence of hypersexuality predicts longer disease duration. When KLS starts after 20 years of age, it is not possible to calculate the disease course, as more than 50% of the patients are not cured after 25 years with KLS, suggesting that the disease is more fixed in the adult-onset form [5]. In the meta-analysis of 186 KLS cases in the literature, we observed that patients with numerous episodes during the first year of the disease had shorter course [27].

Complications

The disease is generally considered as benign, as most subjects are normal between the episodes. However, the episodes are sudden, possibly during school or university tests (as they may be triggered by sleep deprivation and stress), impacting on the professional career of the patients, and sometimes those of their parents. During the episode, the behavioral disorders (mostly the lack of politeness, the overtly, inappropriate sexual behavior, and in rare cases major aggressiveness with rage) of the patient may be embarrassing and sometimes dangerous for the family [12]. As patients are mostly irritable when prevented from sleeping or resting, and when transferred to a novel environment, safe advice is to keep them at home under the supervision of their parents, rather than taking them to the hospital. Major behavioral problems, including rage, could require a short hospitalization in a safe psychiatric department. We are aware of a few cases having had a road accident while driving in an episode (one fatal). Rarely, patients may have some vegetative problems, including urine retention and cardiac arrhythmia. One patient was so agitated during an episode that she broke a bone and later died from a fat embolism [24]. Another ate so quickly during an episode with megaphagia that he died from an aspiration pneumonia [30]. The patient may be frustrated during an episode (generally close to the end of it), cry and experience an acutely depressive mood, with rare suicidal ideation [31, 32]. Some rare patients may have long-term changes in mood, due to difficulty in adjusting to the disease. Patients who eat a lot can gain 5–7 kg in a week, leading to skin scars. Between episodes, patients may remain overweight [5]. Some authors report subclinical long-term memory impairment in a few KLS patients during the episodes [33–37].

Differential diagnosis

Interview

The diagnosis of KLS is clinical, as there are no biological or physiological markers yet. It is mostly obtained by a close interview with the parents. They live with their child and can notice subtle behavior differences that are missed by a physician who has not met the child previously. They usually describe a teenager suddenly different from before, "closed in his bubble," during a few days, and progressively coming back to reality. An open description of the symptoms, with questions about the behavior of the teenager towards sleep, food, showering and personal hygiene, use of cell phone and video games, seeing or not their usual friends is informative. The patients themselves describe well the derealization feelings, but are less informative for other features, because they do not have a clear memory of the episode, or are ashamed and annoyed to evoke what they have done during the episode.

Non-psychiatric diagnoses

As the disease is exceptional and not known from many practitioners, several more common diseases are usually evoked first. When brought to the emergency department during the first episodes, before the KLS diagnosis is performed, most patients undergo the classical tests in case of sudden confusion and behavioral changes in teenagers. It includes checking for alcohol intake, drug and illegal substance intake, having a brain morphological imaging (mostly an MRI) for ruling out tumors, inflammatory disease, multiple sclerosis, stroke, looking with an EEG at a temporal status epilepticus, performing serum levels of ammoniac for ornithin carnityl transferase deficiency (but gastric signs are more prominent than in KLS), tests for intermittent porphyria and Lyme disease, and frequently a spinal tap looking for encephalitis. All these tests are usually normal in KLS, although a few, non-specific EEG sharp waves may be observed. Among these tests, the EEG is probably the most helpful, as it can document localized or generalized background slowing in up to 70% of patients during an episode. Several symptoms, such as food utilization, verbal perseverations, withdrawal and de-inhibition behavior, are reminiscent of frontal lobe syndrome, while the association of megaphagia and hypersexuality has also been described in the syndrome of Kluver–Bucy associated with bitemporal lesions, and in orbito-frontal lesions. Idiopathic stupor is a rare differential diagnosis of KLS, usually occurring in middle-aged subjects, with stuporous episodes lasting no more than 48 h.

Psychiatric diagnoses

The most difficult differential diagnoses are psychiatric disorders (psychosis and depression), hence many patients are sent to the psychiatric department before the diagnosis of KLS is made. The main differences between KLS with psychotic symptoms and psychotic disorders are the sudden aspect of delusion and hallucinations in KLS, the absence of long-term adhesion to the belief, the presence of associated neurological symptoms (mainly slowness, confusion, amnesia, and hypersomnia), and the abrupt cessation of the psychotic symptoms. The recurrence of symptoms after one to several months without psychosis is also characteristic of KLS. The difference between KLS with mood changes and a depressive disorder is how suddenly the symptoms come and then go, in a previously happy teenager, and the association with cognitive and behavioral symptoms. A teenager sleeping more than 20 h a day is also not common in depressive disorders, even when they are severe. Also, an abnormal EEG, with slow waves when awake, is suggestive that the disorder is not psychiatric but neurological. What can make the picture less clear in some rare cases is the occasional persistence of a sad mood between some episodes, especially as a difficulty in adjusting to the disease.

Brain imaging, neurophysiology, biological markers and neuropathology

Brain imaging

Morphological brain imaging (computerized tomography scan, magnetic resonance imaging) is normal, except for unspecific variants of the norms. In 50% of patients, functional brain imaging (single photo-emission tomography) can document some temporal hypoperfusion between the episodes, as compared to normative SPECT [18, 38, 39]. This suggests that there are some functional abnormalities persisting between the episodes in a small subset of patients. When SPECT are performed during an episode, subtracted to the images obtained between the episode, and repositioned on a brain MRI, some areas are clearly hypoperfused: mostly the thalamus, but also, with variations between patients, the hypothalamus, temporal and frontal areas [40]. A striking illustration is shown in Figure 13.3 [41]. In a single case studied with magnetic resonance spectroscopy, there was a decrease in the concentration of glutamate in the thalamus during the episode.

Electroencephalography

A quarter of patients have a normal EEG during episodes. In 70% of the patients, a non-specific diffuse slowing of background EEG activity, such as the alpha frequency band being slowed toward 7–8 Hz, is observed [42, 43]. Less frequently, low-frequency, high-amplitude waves (delta or theta) occur

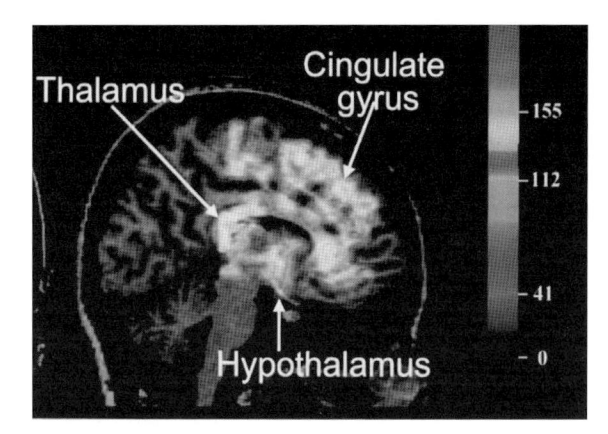

Figure 13.3 Brain scintigraphy during vs. after an episode, coregistered to MRI. Thalamic, hypothalamic, cingulate and frontal area are hypoactivated (in yellow and red) during the episode. Figure reproduced with the authorization of the *Sleep* journal [41]. (See color plate section).

in isolation or in sequence, mainly in the bilateral temporal or temporo-frontal areas, paralleling the SPECT findings.

Sleep monitoring

In our experience, sleep monitoring is not very useful for the diagnosis of KLS: it may be difficult to organize sleep monitoring during the first days of an episode; the sleep duration and structure depend on the time when the test is performed; most patients cannot commit to the multiple sleep latency test procedure (which can contain short sleep onset latencies and sleep onset REM periods, transiently resembling narcolepsy in one-third to one-sixth of patients); and they may stay in bed for hours in a generalized hypoarousal, with a diffuse alpha EEG rhythm that is difficult to score as wakefulness and alternate with fragmented sleep stages N1–N2. An example of 24-h sleep monitoring in an 18-year-old patient at the beginning of a KLS episode is shown in Figure 13.4. When systematically analyzing the literature, the mean total sleep time was 445 ± 122 min during the night ($n = 19$; Stage 1: $6 \pm 4\%$; Stage 2: $56 \pm 9\%$; Stage 3–4: $19 \pm 11\%$; REM sleep: $19 \pm 6\%$) and 838 ± 288 min ($n = 10$) on a 24-h basis. Night sleep lasted 568 ± 204 min during an episode and 384 ± 59 min between, in a series of 14 patients studied in Israel [44]. In a series of 18 patients monitored over 24 h while in an episode, the total sleep duration was 701 ± 270 min [9]. In a series of 17 patients in Taiwan, when night time sleep was monitored before the end of the first half of the symptomatic period, an important reduction in slow-wave sleep was always present with progressive return to normal during the second half despite persistence of clinical symptoms [45]. REM sleep remained normal in the first half of the episode but decreased in the second half.

Biological markers

There is no biological marker of KLS yet. Serum biology is typically normal during and between the episode, including inflammation markers and white cells. We found normal C-reactive protein levels in 108 patients with KLS, compared to 108 controls [5]. The agents responsible for this first infection, when it triggers KLS, are rarely identified, and include Epstein–Barr virus, varicella virus, Asian influenza virus, enterovirus, and streptococcus. The hormonal pituitary axis is normal, except for a few inconsistent abnormalities [46–48]. Leptin levels are also normal [5].

As young age of onset, recurrence, and presence of inflammatory lesions in the brain may suggest that KLS is an autoimmune disease, the human leukocyte antigen class II genotypes were studied in 30 European KLS trios, and in 108 American KLS trios. There was a two-times more frequent DRB1*0301–DQB1*0201 and DRB1*0701–DQB1*0202 genotype in European KLS patients [9], an association which was not replicated in the larger American study [5].

CSF white cell count and protein count are normal in patients, ruling out an infectious meningitis. There was no oligoclonal secretion of antibodies (as in multiple sclerosis, another remittent neurological disease), in the CSF of four patients with KLS. The cerebrospinal levels of hypocretin are within normal ranges [7, 49, 50].

Neuropathology

The examination of brain has been performed after the death of four patients (with primary, $n = 2$ and secondary KLS, $n = 2$) [19, 23, 24, 30]. The cortex was intact in three patients, while a patient with KLS secondary to a paraneoplastic syndrome had perivascular infiltrates in the amygdala and temporal lobe. There were intense signs of inflammatory encephalitis within the thalamus and hypothalamus in two patients (abundant infiltrates of inflammatory cells, perivascular lympho-monocyte infiltrate, microglial proliferation), mild inflammation in one patient and none in the last patient (only mildly depigmented substantia nigra and locus coeruleus).

Management and treatment

After making the right diagnosis (which is perceived as beneficial for the patients and their family), most families enquire about the behavior to adopt toward the sick patient. Our suggestions are displayed in Table 13.2. Many drug trials have been disappointing in KLS. However, a few drugs may help to manage the symptoms during the episodes, and to prevent the recurrence of episodes when used between episodes. During the episodes, the usual stimulants (modafinil, methylphenidate, amphetamine) are rarely beneficial against the severe hypersomnia, and may at best unmask the other, disagreeable cognitive and behavioral symptoms. Amantadine, which is also an antiviral, may curiously help to abort episodes when given from the first day. When psychotic symptoms are prolonged and prominent, risperidone is more helpful than other neuroleptics. In case of major anxiety, benzodiazepine may help the patients. The episodes are usually too short to require and benefit from antidepressant drugs. When the episodes are frequent (i.e. occurring 4–12 times/year), a daily prevention by lithium may be tried [27]. There is no explanation of how this drug helps in KLS, and especially no link (personal and familial) with bipolar disease [5]. This treatment has a narrow therapeutic window, and requires frequent blood test to obtain a serum lithium level between 0.8 and 1.2 mEq/L. The benefit (25–50%)/risk ratio should be re-evaluated every six months. The antiepileptics seem less efficacious in our experience (and when looking at all published cases and at our series). When the episodes are timely associated with menstruations, a blockade

Table 13.2 Suggested management of a patient with KLS

1. Obtain a detailed history from the parents or spouse.
2. Check for normal brain imaging, EEG, and psychiatric examination out of an episode.
3. During the episodes, recommend the patient to stay at home, under family supervision. This attitude limits the fear for novelty, the risk of embarrassing public behaviors, and is safer for the patient.
4. Firmly recommend not driving a car or a motorbike during an episode, as sleepiness, automatism and altered perception expose to a high risk of road accident.
5. The family should regularly check during an episode if the patient drinks and eats enough (in case of reduced eating/drinking) or not too much (in case of megaphagia), urinates at least once a day (in case of urine retention), and has no suicidal ideas.
6. Between episodes, keep regular sleep/wake schedules, avoid alcohol and contact with infectious subjects.
7. Try, at least once, amantadine at the beginning of an episode, as it can abort an episode.
8. During an episode, in case of intense anxious symptoms, use sublingual bromazepam. If delusions or behavioral disturbances are severe enough to justify a neuroleptic treatment, consider a very short treatment with risperidone.
9. If episodes are short and frequent (e.g. lasting one week every 1–3 months), consider using prolonged-release lithium (in order to obtain a serum lithium level between 0.8 and 1.2 mEql). Re-evaluate the benefit/risk ratio every 6 months.

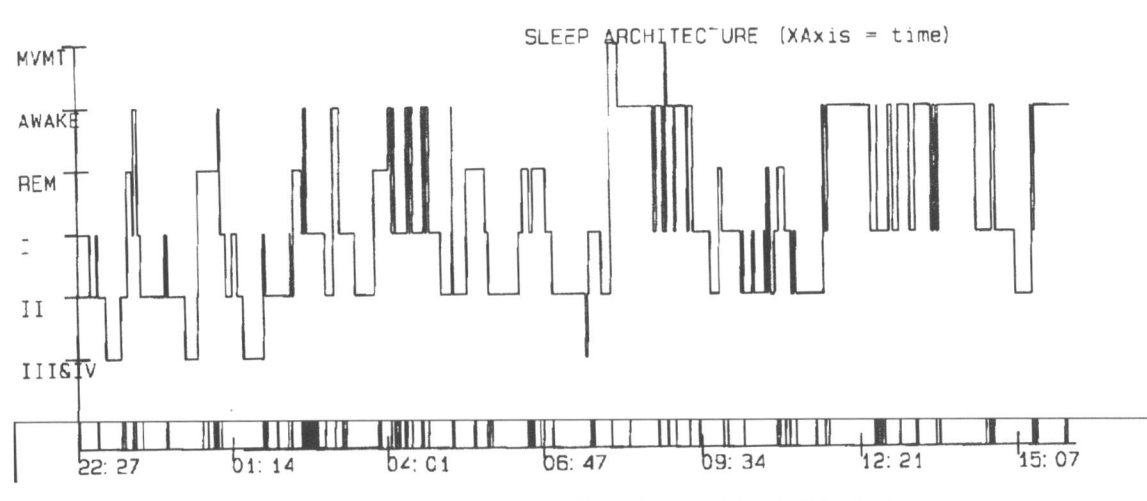

Figure 13.4 Long-term sleep monitoring in an 18-year-old woman during the second day of a KLS episode.

of the hypophysis axis with high doses of oestro-progestative may be tried. Antidepressants are devoid of prophylactic effects in KLS.

Conclusion

KLS is an intriguing, severe, homogeneous disease, known for more than a century, with no obvious cause or treatment. Recent methods of investigation such as SPECT indicate that the brain dysfunction could be larger than expected, and would encompass both cortical and subcortical (and especially thalamus and hypothalamus) areas. In addition, persistent post-KLS memory and SPECT defects recently observed in a few cases raise the possibility of long-term brain damage in a disease which was assumed to be benign. The finding of a possible Jewish predisposition, occasional familial clustering, and association with infectious triggering factors suggest that KLS is due to environmental factors acting on a vulnerable genetic background. This general picture and the fluctuating symptoms in KLS are consistent with the possibility of an autoimmune mediation of the disorder.

Acknowledgments

We thank the Kleine–Levin Foundation (Boston, USA) who allowed us to start working on this disease. The French KLS cohort research program is financed by the national grant PHRC 070138.

References

1. **Kesler A**, **Gadoth N**, **Vainstein G**, et al. Kleine Levin syndrome (KLS) in young females. *Sleep*, 2000; **23**:563–67.
2. **Hegarty A**, **Merriam A E**. Autonomic events in Kleine–Levin syndrome. *Am J Psychiatry*, 1990; **147**:951–52.
3. **Manni R**, **Martinetti M**, **Ratti M T**, et al. Electrophysiological and immunogenetic findings in recurrent monosymptomatic-type hypersomnia: a study of two unrelated Italian cases. *Acta Neurol Scand*, 1993; **88**:293–95.
4. **Lavie P**, **Gadoth N**, **Gordon C R**, et al. Sleep patterns in Kleine–Levin syndrome. *Electroencephalogr Clin Neurophysiol*, 1979; **47**:369–71.
5. **Arnulf I**, **Lin L**, **Gadoth N**, et al. Kleine–Levin syndrome: a systematic study of 108 patients. *Ann Neurol*, 2008; **63**:482–93.
6. **Thacore V R**, **Ahmed M**, **Oswald I**. The EEG in a case of periodic hypersomnia. *Electroencephalogr Clin Neurophysiol*, 1969; **27**:605–06.
7. **Katz J D**, **Ropper A H**. Familial Kleine–Levin syndrome: two siblings with unusually long hypersomnic spells. *Arch Neurol*, 2002; **59**:1959–61.
8. **Janicki S**, **Franco K**, **Zarko R**. A case report of Kleine–Levin syndrome in an adolescent girl. *Psychosomatics*, 2001; **42**:350–52.
9. **Dauvilliers Y**, **Mayer G**, **Lecendreux M**, et al. Kleine–Levin syndrome: an autoimmune hypothesis based on clinical and genetic analyses. *Neurology*, 2002; **59**:1739–45.
10. **Bahammam A**, **Gadelrab M**, **Owais S**, et al. Clinical characteristics and HLA typing of a family with Kleine–Levin syndrome. *Sleep Med*, 2008; **9**:575–78.
11. **American Academy of Sleep Medicine**. *The International Classification of Sleep Disorders – Revised*. Hauri P, Ed. Chicago, IL: AASM, 2005.
12. **Powers P S**, **Gunderman R**. Kleine–Levin syndrome associated with fire setting. *Am J Dis Child*, 1978; **132**:786–89.
13. **Yassa R**, **Nair N P**. The Kleine–Levine syndrome – a variant? *J Clin Psychiatry*, 1978; **39**:254–59.
14. **Mukaddes N M**, **Kora M E**, **Bilge S**. Carbamazepine for Kleine–Levin syndrome. *J Am Acad Child Adolesc Psychiatry*, 1999; **38**:791–92.
15. **Prabhakaran N**, **Murthy G K**, **Mallya U L**. A case of Kleine–Levin syndrome in India. *Br J Psychiatry*, 1970; **117**:517–19.
16. **Crumley F E**. Valproic acid for Kleine–Levin syndrome. *J Am Acad Child Adolesc Psychiatry*, 1997; **36**:868–69.
17. **Critchley M**. Periodic hypersomnia and megaphagia in adolescent males. *Brain*, 1962; **85**:627–56.
18. **Portilla P**, **Durand E**, **Chalvon A**, et al. [SPECT-identified hypoperfusion of the left temporomesial structures in a Kleine–Levin syndrome]. *Rev Neurol (Paris)*, 2002; **158**:593–95.
19. **Koerber R K**, **Torkelson R**, **Haven G**, et al. Increased cerebrospinal fluid 5-hydroxytryptamine and 5-hydroxyindoleacetic acid in Kleine–Levin syndrome. *Neurology*, 1984; **34**:1597–600.
20. **Berthier M L**, **Santamaria J**, **Encabo H**, et al. Recurrent hypersomnia in two adolescent males with Asperger's syndrome. *J Am Acad Child Adolesc Psychiatry*, 1992; **31**:735–38.
21. **Testa S**, **Opportuno A**, **Gallo P**, et al. A case of multiple sclerosis with an onset mimicking the Kleine–Levin syndrome. *Ital J Neurol Sci* 1987; **8**:151–55.
22. **Lobzin V S**, **Shamrei R K**, **Churilov Iu K**. [Pathophysiologic mechanisms of periodic sleep and the Kleine–Levin syndrome]. *Zh Nevropatol Psikhiatr Im S S Korsakova*, 1973; **73**:1719–24.

23. **Takrani L B**, **Cronin D**. Kleine–Levin syndrome in a female patient. *Can Psychiatr Assoc J*, 1976; **21**: 315–18.

24. **Fenzi F**, **Simonati A**, **Crosato F**, *et al*. Clinical features of Kleine–Levin syndrome with localized encephalitis. *Neuropediatrics*, 1993; **24**:292–95.

25. **Merriam A E**. Kleine–Levin syndrome following acute viral encephalitis. *Biol Psychiatry*, 1986; **21**:1301–04.

26. **Persson T**, **Olsson L**, **Ortman E**. The Kleine–Levin syndrome: report of a case and discussion. *Behav Neuropsychiatry*, 1969; **1**:4–6.

27. **Arnulf I**, **Zeitzer J M**, **File J**, *et al*. Kleine–Levin syndrome: a systematic review of 186 cases in the literature. *Brain*, 2005; **128**:2763–76.

28. **Billiard M**, **Guilleminault C**, **Dement W C**. A menstruation-linked periodic hypersomnia. Kleine–Levin syndrome or new clinical entity? *Neurology*, 1975; **25**:436–43.

29. **Kleine W**. Periodische Schlafsucht. *Monatsschrr Psychiatrie Neurologie*, 1925; **57**:285–320.

30. **Carpenter S**, **Yassa R**, **Ochs R**. A pathologic basis for Kleine–Levin syndrome. *Arch Neurol*, 1982; **39**: 25–28.

31. **Gallinek A**. The Kleine–Levin syndrome: hypersomnia, bulimia, and abnormal mental states. *World Neurol*, 1962; **3**:235–43.

32. **Vlach V**. Periodical somnolence, bulimia and mental changes (Kleine–Levin Syndrome). *Cesk Neurol*, 1962; **25**:401–05.

33. **Smolik P**, **Roth B**. Kleine–Levin syndrome ethiopathogenesis and treatment. *Acta Univ Carol Med Monogr*, 1988; **128**:5–94.

34. **Sagar R S**, **Khandelwal S K**, **Gupta S**. Interepisodic morbidity in Kleine–Levin syndrome. *Br J Psychiatry*, 1990; **157**:139–41.

35. **Masi G**, **Favilla L**, **Millepiedi S**. The Kleine–Levin syndrome as a neuropsychiatric disorder: a case report. *Psychiatry*, 2000; **63**:93–100.

36. **Landtblom A M**, **Dige N**, **Schwerdt K**, *et al*. Short-term memory dysfunction in Kleine–Levin syndrome. *Acta Neurol Scand*, 2003; **108**:363–67.

37. **Engström M**, **Vigren P**, **Karlsson T**, *et al*. Working memory in 8 Kleine–Levin syndrome patients: an fMRI study. *Sleep*, 2009; **32**:681–88.

38. **Landtblom A M**, **Dige N**, **Schwerdt K**, *et al*. A case of Kleine–Levin syndrome examined with SPECT and neuropsychological testing. *Acta Neurol Scand*, 2002; **105**:318–21.

39. **Lu M L**, **Liu H C**, **Chen C H**, *et al*. Kleine–Levin syndrome and psychosis: observation from an unusual case. *Neuropsychiatry Neuropsychol Behav Neurol*, 2000; **13**:140–42.

40. **Huang Y S**, **Guilleminault C**, **Kao P F**, *et al*. SPECT findings in the Kleine–Levin syndrome. *Sleep*, 2005; **28**:955–60.

41. **Hong S B**, **Joo E Y**, **Tae W S**, *et al*. Episodic diencephalic hypoperfusion in Kleine–Levin syndrome. *Sleep*, 2006; **29**:1091–93.

42. **Vollmer R**, **Toifl K**, **Kothbauer P**, *et al*. [EEG- and biochemical findings in Kleine–Levin syndrome. A case report (author's transl)]. *Nervenarzt*, 1981; **52**:211–18.

43. **Papacostas S S**, **Hadjivasilis V**. The Kleine Levin syndrome. Report of a case and review of the literature. *Eur Psychiatry*, 2000; **15**:231–35.

44. **Gadoth N**, **Kesler A**, **Vainstein G**, *et al*. Clinical and polysomnographic characteristics of 34 patients with Kleine–Levin syndrome. *J Sleep Res*, 2001; **10**:337–41.

45. **Huang Y**, **Lin Y**, **Guilleminault C**. Polysomnography in Kleine–Levin syndrome. *Neurology*, 2008; **70**:795–801.

46. **Chesson A L Jr.**, **Levine S N**, **Kong L S**, *et al*. Neuroendocrine evaluation in Kleine–Levin syndrome: evidence of reduced dopaminergic tone during periods of hypersomnolence. *Sleep*, 1991; **14**:226–32.

47. **Mayer G**, **Leonhard E**, **Krieg J**, *et al*. Endocrinological and polysomnographic findings in Kleine–Levin syndrome: no evidence for hypothalamic and circadian dysfunction. *Sleep*, 1998; **21**:278–84.

48. **Malhotra S**, **Das M K**, **Gupta N**, *et al*. A clinical study of Kleine–Levin syndrome with evidence for hypothalamic–pituitary axis dysfunction. *Biol Psychiatry*, 1997; **42**:299–301.

49. **Mignot E**, **Lammers G J**, **Ripley B**, *et al*. The role of cerebrospinal fluid hypocretin measurement in the diagnosis of narcolepsy and other hypersomnias. *Arch Neurol*, 2002; **59**:1553–62.

50. **Dauvilliers Y**, **Baumann C R**, **Carlander B**, *et al*. CSF hypocretin-1 levels in narcolepsy, Kleine–Levin syndrome, and other hypersomnias and neurological conditions. *J Neurol Neurosurg Psychiatry*, 2003; **74**:1667–73.

Section 2 Chapter 14

Sleep Disorders and Excessive Sleepiness

Menstrual-related hypersomnia

Fiona C. Baker

Introduction

This chapter reviews what is known about menstrual-related hypersomnia, a rare disorder of recurrent hypersomnia that is temporally linked with menses. In light of the rareness of cases of menstrual hypersomnia, the chapter also discusses the influence of the menstrual cycle on levels of daytime sleepiness in women during normal cycles and in those with premenstrual syndrome.

During a normal ovulatory menstrual cycle, which lasts about 28 days, there are cyclical changes in reproductive hormones coordinated through the central nervous system (CNS). Estrogen levels are low during the pre-ovulatory follicular phase and peak just before ovulation, which occurs about 14 days after the onset of menses. During the post-ovulation luteal phase, progesterone and estrogen levels are maintained at relatively high levels, being secreted by the corpus luteum [1]. During the last few days of the cycle (premenstrual or late-luteal phase), as hormone levels decline, as well as during menses, when hormone levels are low, women are most likely to experience negative somatic and mood-related symptoms.

Menstrual-related hypersomnia

History

Menstrual-related hypersomnia is characterized by excessive daytime sleepiness that begins a few days before the onset of menstrual flow and disappears shortly after menstruation begins. Hypersomnia related to the menstrual cycle was first proposed as a clinical disorder distinct from Kleine–Levin syndrome in 1975 by Billiard and others [2]. "Premenstrual hypersomnia", as it was originally termed, was proposed as a sleep disorder in the International Classification of Sleep Disorders (ICSD) under the category of "menstrual-associated sleep disorder" [3]. Also included under this category were premenstrual insomnia and menopausal insomnia.

As a general category a menstrual-associated sleep disorder was defined as, "a disorder of unknown cause, characterized by a complaint of either insomnia or excessive sleepiness, that is temporally related to the menses or the menopause" [3]. In the more recent second edition of the ICSD [4], menstrual-related hypersomnia was classified as a type of recurrent hypersomnia, along with Kleine–Levin syndrome. Kleine–Levin syndrome is characterized by recurrent episodes of hypersomnia, frequently associated with cognitive disturbances, compulsive eating behavior and hypersexuality [5]. There is at least a 2:1 male:female ratio for Kleine–Levin syndrome [5]. The specific relationship of hypersomnia with the menstrual cycle distinguishes menstrual-related hypersomnia from Kleine–Levin syndrome.

Clinical findings

There are few case studies published of menstrual-related hypersomnia and the prevalence of the disorder in the general female population is unknown. Two out of 235 consecutive patients referred over a five-year period to the Stanford Sleep Clinic with a complaint of excessive daytime sleepiness were diagnosed with periodic hypersomnia associated with menstruation (later termed menstrual-related hypersomnia) [6]. Both of these patients were adolescents. Based on these and other case studies published or presented in conference proceedings [7, 8], it appears that menstrual-related hypersomnia affects mainly adolescents (as is the case with Kleine–Levin syndrome), although there

---

Sleepiness: Causes, Consequences and Treatment, ed. Michael J. Thorpy and Michel Billiard. Published by Cambridge University Press. © Cambridge University Press 2011.

is one case report of a 42-year-old woman with the disorder [9]. The duration of the disease is unknown.

Patients with menstrual-related hypersomnia present with discrete intervals of hypersomnia beginning before menses and abating a few days after the onset of menses. The periods of hypersomnia may be preceded by or associated with changes in behavior, such as increased irritability or aggression [2, 8]. Patients show extreme hypersomnia, sleeping almost continuously for a period of up to 8 days, with marked reduction in frequency of micturition and lack of interest in eating or drinking. Plasma levels of follicle stimulating hormone (FSH), luteinizing hormone (LH), estradiol, and progesterone all appear to be within normal ranges and indicate normal ovulatory menstrual cycles [2, 8]. Other accounts of hypersomnia in relation to the menstrual cycle are reported in the literature [10–14], but it is unclear if these are cases of Kleine–Levin syndrome or menstrual-related hypersomnia. For example, Papy et al. [14] reported a case study of an adolescent girl with periods of hypersomnia (and hyperphagia) that occurred 5–6 days *after* rather than before menstruation.

Laboratory investigations

Characteristics of the waking and sleep electroencephalogram (EEG) in menstrual-related hypersomnia have been published for only two patients [2, 8]. Continuous polysomnographic recordings were made over a period of 24–60 h in one patient (13 years of age) during a period of hypersomnia and again when asymptomatic [2]. During hypersomnia, total nighttime sleep was increased by about 2 h but the organization of sleep appeared normal. The patient had one morning nap, consisting mainly of Stage 1 and Stage 2 sleep, whereas an afternoon nap contained a large percentage of slow-wave sleep (27%). She slept for almost 14.5 h within a 24-h period of hypersomnia, as compared to about 10 h when asymptomatic. The increased total sleep time consisted mostly of stage 2 sleep, with essentially no change in slow-wave sleep [2]. Sleep spindles, K-complexes, high-amplitude slow waves, and rapid eye movements are preserved during sleep in episodes of hypersomnia in these patients [2, 8]. During a period of hypersomnia, the waking EEG is characterized by greater amounts of slow theta activity (4–8 Hz) compared with an asymptomatic period [2, 8]. Recently, another case study of an adolescent patient with menstrual-related hypersomnia was presented in conference proceedings [7]. The patient, who experienced 5–6 days of hypersomnia before the onset of menstruation, also showed large amounts of theta activity in the waking EEG during hypersomnia episodes (B. Andreica, personal communication, 21 December 2009). Power density in the theta (4–8 Hz) band of the waking EEG has been shown to increase across periods of sustained wakefulness and correlates negatively with subjective alertness levels [15, 16]. These EEG findings during waking periods in patients with menstrual-related hypersomnia, therefore, compliment subjective reports of apathy and inactivity [2, 8].

Pathology

The pathophysiology of menstrual-related hypersomnia is unknown. Evidence indicates that ovulation is necessary for hypersomnia episodes to appear in affected individuals. Hypersomnia episodes were associated with ovulatory but not anovulatory cycles, as monitored with basal temperature measurements, in one patient [8], and prevention of ovulation with oral contraceptive treatment effectively alleviates the hypersomnia [7, 8].

It has been hypothesized that progesterone could trigger hypersomniac episodes in patients with menstrual-related hypersomnia [2]. Progesterone has a sedating effect, inducing sleep when administered intravenously in supraphysiological doses to humans [17]. It is thought that the sedating effect of progesterone may be mediated through progesterone metabolites acting on the γ-aminobutyric acid (GABA) receptor rather than via actions on intracellular progesterone receptors [18]. Progesterone administered to rats reduces sleep onset latency, decreases wakefulness after sleep onset, and increases EEG activity in the spindle and higher frequencies [19], similar to the effects of benzodiazepines, which are agonistic modulators of the $GABA_A$ receptor [20]. However, periods of hypersomnia in patients with menstrual-related hypersomnia occur in the late-luteal (premenstrual) phase when progesterone levels are declining and plasma levels of progesterone are normal in patients, arguing against the direct involvement of progesterone. However, exposure to progesterone during the luteal phase after ovulation may still be necessary for the development of hypersomnia, possibly exerting a priming effect. Also, the magnitude of change or sensitivity to progesterone rather than absolute levels of progesterone may be crucial for the development of hypersomnia in these patients.

Another candidate that has been proposed to be involved in the etiology of menstrual-related hypersomnia is prolactin [9]. Bamford [9] described a 42-year-old patient with complaints of excessive sleepiness beginning in the week before each menstrual period and resolving with menstruation. Subsequently, she developed secondary amenorrhea due to hypothalamic–pituitary dysfunction but she continued to have hypersomnia episodes, although each episode lasted only a few hours instead of days and occurred every few days to weeks. These brief periods of hypersomnia were associated with marked elevations in plasma prolactin levels relative to periods of alertness. High levels of prolactin in patients with prolactinoma are associated with an elevated percentage of slow-wave sleep [21], although there are no reports of excessive daytime sleepiness in these patients. Given the role of dopamine in inhibiting prolactin release from the pituitary [22], it has been hypothesized that the elevation of prolactin coincident with hypersomnia implicates a disturbance of dopaminergic and possibly other monoamineric pathways in menstrual-related hypersomnia [9]. There are a few caveats in this case study. The patient was taking several medications, including metoclopramide, a dopamine antagonist that is associated with elevated prolactin levels, and her hormone profile was not obtained in association with hypersomnia periods linked with her menstrual cycle but rather when she was amenorrheic. Prolactin levels measured every other day across a menstrual cycle in an adolescent girl with menstrual-related hypersomnia were normal [8], indicating that elevated prolactin is not evident in all cases of menstrual-related hypersomnia.

Other possible factors that could be evaluated as being potentially involved in the etiology of menstrual-related hypersomnia include sleep-promoting inflammatory cytokines, prostaglandins, and monoamines. One case study found evidence of abnormal serotonin turnover based on measurement of 5-hydroxyindolacetic acid, a serotonin metabolite, in cerebrospinal fluid in a patient with menstrual-related hypersomnia [2], but more direct quantification of serotonin turnover in the brain is needed to confirm this result. Estrogen positively modulates serotonergic raphe neurons, the norepinephrine network and its hypothalamic targets [23]. Since monoamines are critically involved in sleep regulation, hypersomnia could occur if responses of monoamine pathways to estrogen fluctuations in the brain are altered in patients with menstrual-related hypersomnia.

Alternatively, menstrual-related hypersomnia may be an autoimmune disease, as has been hypothesized for Kleine–Levin syndrome [24]. The frequency of a particular allele of the human leukocyte antigen (HLA-DQB1*0201) is significantly increased in patients with Kleine–Levin syndrome compared with controls [24]. A patient with menstrual-related hypersomnia, on whom HLA-DQB1 genotyping was performed, also carried the HLA-DQB1*0201 allele [24].

Management

Adolescent cases of menstrual-related hypersomnia have been successfully treated with oral contraceptive pills, containing estradiol and a progestin [7, 8], or with estrogen alone [2]. In these cases, treatment successfully abolished the hypersomnia. Treatment of hypersomnia in one patient (42 years of age) with combined estrogen/progestin contraceptive pills was unsuccessful [9], suggesting that the etiology of the hypersomnia may have differed compared with adolescent cases. This patient was prescribed methylphenidate to alleviate her symptoms.

Summary

Menstrual-related hypersomnia is an extremely rare disorder that manifests predominantly during adolescence. Investigation of more patients with menstrual-related hypersomnia is needed to understand the etiology of the disorder and may also shed light on the interaction between the reproductive and sleep regulatory systems in healthy women.

Sleepiness in association with the normal menstrual cycle and in women with premenstrual syndrome

While the extreme hypersomnia in association with the menstrual cycle described above is very rare, many women experience increased feelings of sleepiness and fatigue around the time of menstruation, as discussed in the following section.

Subjective reports

Associated with normal menstrual cycles, women commonly report increased levels of lethargy and fatigue in the few days leading up to and during menstruation [25]. They also may have greater levels of sleepiness, as measured with the Stanford Sleepiness Scale (SSS) [26], daytime in the late-luteal (premenstrual) phase relative to the follicular phase [27]. Few studies have investigated these symptoms in any detail. Manber and Bootzin [28] analyzed sleep and daytime diaries of 32 women between the ages of 27 and 51 years. Self-reported levels of daytime sleepiness were significantly correlated with a premenstrual index; women with more severe premenstrual symptoms reported higher levels of sleepiness.

Women with severe premenstrual syndrome (PMS) have greater levels of daytime sleepiness, based on scores on the SSS, in the symptomatic luteal and menstruation phases compared with the symptom-free follicular phase of the menstrual cycle [29]. Two recent studies used the SSS in addition to a subjective alertness scale to investigate daytime sleepiness and alertness in women with significant premenstrual symptoms compared to women with minimal symptoms [30, 31]. Similar to earlier studies, women with significant premenstrual symptoms were sleepier and less alert than women with minimal symptoms in the late-luteal phase and compared with their own symptom-free follicular phase. Women with PMS also report higher levels of fatigue [30], which is distinct from sleepiness [32], and an inability to concentrate [29] in the late-luteal phase than the follicular phase, and compared with controls. Between 3 and 8% of women report disabling symptoms during the late-luteal phase that are predominantly psychological which qualify them for a diagnosis of premenstrual dysphoric disorder (PMDD) as defined in the *Diagnostic and Statistical Manual of Mental Disorders* (DSM-IV) [33]. Sleep complaints (insomnia or hypersomnia) is listed as one of the defining criteria in the DSM-IV for a diagnosis of PMDD. Based on daily ratings of symptoms, we have found that hypersomnia is reported as "severe" during the late-luteal phase and/or during the first couple of days of menstruation by 9 of 16 women who meet diagnostic criteria for PMDD (unpublished findings).

Laboratory measures

Two studies have used objective measures to quantify daytime sleep characteristics and sleepiness in women with and without PMS [30, 31]. Using a nap protocol, Lamarche and colleagues [31] found no significant differences in sleep architecture during a short mid-afternoon nap between young adult women with severe and minimal premenstrual symptoms. There were no group differences in sleep onset latency: women with severe premenstrual symptoms fell asleep in 6 min on average, and women with minimal symptoms fell asleep in 7 min on average. The short sleep onset latency found for both groups of women suggests that there was a high sleep need during the late-luteal phase regardless of symptom severity, possibly indicating chronic sleep restriction as may be expected in this age group (mean age 26.7 years) [34].

A recent study in our laboratory used the Maintenance of Wakefulness Test (MWT), a measure of "manifest sleepiness", or the effect of sleepiness on outward behavior and abilities [35, 36], to evaluate sleepiness in women with PMS [30]. For the MWT, subjects are instructed to stay awake. This test has been used to discriminate normal subjects from patients with disorders associated with excessive daytime sleepiness, such as narcolepsy and obstructive sleep apnea [36, 37]. Women with PMS and controls were able to maintain wakefulness during the day even under soporific conditions of the MWT in both the symptomatic late-luteal phase and the symptom-free follicular phase [30]. In fact, several women in both groups did not fall asleep during any of the trials. Women with PMS, therefore, are able to maintain wakefulness under soporific conditions even though they *feel* sleepy. Results may have differed if the Multiple Sleep Latency Test (MSLT) had been used. The MSLT is considered a measure of the underlying biologic drive to sleep [35], where subjects are instructed to try to fall asleep. Many patients who fall asleep rapidly when not resisting sleep on the MSLT are able to remain awake if they desire [35]. Using the MSLT in subsequent studies may reveal whether women with PMS have an increased sleep drive in the late-luteal phase, despite their ability to maintain wakefulness under soporific conditions.

As part of the same study, subjects completed the psychomotor vigilance task (PVT), a measure of sustained attention [38] that can be used to measure the effects of sleepiness on the efficiency of brain functioning [36]. The women with PMS performed more poorly on the PVT across the day, with more lapses and slower reaction times, in the late-luteal phase compared with the follicular phase and compared with controls [30]. These performance decrements occurred in the absence of polysomnographic-defined night time sleep disturbances [39], suggesting that some factor other than sleep loss influenced PVT performance in these women [30]. MWT latencies and PVT performance typically change in the same direction during experimental manipulation of sleep loss [40]. However, in the presence of depressed mood, PVT performance and MWT latencies are discordant [41]. These findings suggest that non-sleepiness-related factors may contribute to the poorer performance on the PVT in the late-luteal phase in women with PMS [30]. This psychomotor slowing is modest and unlikely to compromise a woman's ability to execute routine tasks in the premenstrual phase [42].

Summary

Women with PMS as well as some women with minimal premenstrual symptoms may feel sleepier during the day premenstrually and during menstruation compared to other phases of the menstrual cycle, possibly due to sensitivity of the sleep regulatory systems to a changing hormonal environment (decreasing progesterone and estrogen). However, laboratory findings show that women with PMS are able to maintain wakefulness under soporific conditions despite their subjective sleepiness. This apparent lack of objective sleepiness should be confirmed using the MSLT in subsequent studies.

Conclusion

Menstrual-related hypersomnia is a rare and poorly documented disorder. It may represent the severe end of a continuum of hypersomnia experienced by women in association with the hormonal changes of the menstrual cycle. This apparent interaction between female reproductive and sleep regulatory systems should be investigated further. Future case studies of patients with menstrual-related hypersomnia are needed to establish its etiology and to strengthen its standing as a distinct disorder of recurrent hypersomnia.

References

1. **Pocock G**, **Richards C D**. *Human Physiology: The Basis of Medicine.* New York, NY: Oxford University Press, 1999.
2. **Billiard M**, **Guilleminault C**, **Dement W C**. A menstruation-linked periodic hypersomnia. Kleine–Levin syndrome or new clinical entity? *Neurology*, 1975; **25**:436–43.
3. **American Academy of Sleep Medicine**. *International Classification of Sleep Disorders, Revised: Diagnostic and Coding Manual.* Chicago, IL; American Academy of Sleep Medicine, 2001.
4. **American Academy of Sleep Medicine**. *International Classification of Sleep Disorders, Diagnostic and Coding Manual.* (2nd ed.). Westchester, IL: American Academy of Sleep Medicine, 2005.
5. **Arnulf I**, **Zeitzer J M**, **File J**, et al. Kleine Levin syndrome: a systematic review of 186 cases in the literature. *Brain*, 2005; **128**:2763–76.
6. **Guilleminault C**, **Dement W C**. 235 cases of excessive daytime sleepiness. Diagnosis and tentative classification. *J Neurol Sci*, 1977; **31**:13–27.
7. **Andreica B**, **Rauca I**, **Lazar C**, et al. Recurrent hypersomnia – diagnostic difficulties. *Eur Psychiatry*, 2008; **23**:S358.
8. **Sachs C**, **Persson H E**, **Hagenfeldt K**. Menstruation-related periodic hypersomnia: a case study with successful treatment. *Neurology*, 1982; **32**:1376–79.
9. **Bamford C R**. Menstrual-associated sleep disorder: an unusual hypersomniac variant associated with both menstruation and amenorrhea with a possible link to prolactin and metoclopramide. *Sleep*, 1993; **16**: 484–86.
10. **Duffy J P**, **Davison K**. A female case of the Kleine–Levin Syndrome. *Br J Psychiatry*, 1968; **114**:77–84.
11. **Gilbert G J**. Periodic hypersomnia and bulimia. The Kleine–Levin Syndrome. *Neurology*, 1964; **14**:844–50.

12. **Janicki S**, **Franco K**, **Zarko R**. A case report of Kleine–Levin syndrome in an adolescent girl. *Psychosomatics*, 2001; **42**:350–52.

13. **Lhermitte J**. Hypersomnie périodique et menstruation. *Progr Med (Paris)*, 1942; **70**:68–75.

14. **Papy J J**, **Conte-Devolx B**, **Sormani J**, *et al*. [The periodic hypersomnia and megaphagia syndrome in a young female, correlated with menstrual cycle (author's transl)]. *Rev Electroencephalogr Neurophysiol Clin*, 1982; **12**:54–61.

15. **Akerstedt T**, **Gillberg M**. Subjective and objective sleepiness in the active individual. *Int J Neurosci*, 1990; **52**:29–37.

16. **Cajochen C**, **Brunner D P**, **Krauchi K**, *et al*. Power density in theta/alpha frequencies of the waking EEG progressively increases during sustained wakefulness. *Sleep*, 1995; **18**:890–94.

17. **Merryman W**, **Boiman R**, **Barnes L**, *et al*. Progesterone anesthesia in human subjects. *J Clin Endocrinol Metab*, 1954; **14**:1567–69.

18. **Manber R**, **Armitage R**. Sex, steroids, and sleep: a review. *Sleep*, 1999; **22**:540–55.

19. **Lancel M**, **Faulhaber J**, **Holsboer F**, *et al*. Progesterone induces changes in sleep comparable to those of agonistic GABAA receptor modulators. *Am J Physiol*, 1996; **271**:E763–72.

20. **Trachsel L**, **Dijk D J**, **Brunner D P**, *et al*. Effect of zopiclone and midazolam on sleep and EEG spectra in a phase-advanced sleep schedule. *Neuropsychopharmacology*, 1990; **3**:11–18.

21. **Frieboes R M**, **Murck H**, **Stalla G K**, *et al*. Enhanced slow wave sleep in patients with prolactinoma. *J Clin Endocrinol Metab*, 1998; **83**:2706–10.

22. **Frantz A G**. Prolactin. *N Engl J Med*, 1978; **298**: 201–07.

23. **Wise D D**, **Felker A**, **Stahl S M**. Tailoring treatment of depression for women across the reproductive lifecycle: the importance of pregnancy, vasomotor symptoms, and other estrogen-related events in psychopharmacology. *CNS Spectr*, 2008; **13**: 647–62.

24. **Dauvilliers Y**, **Mayer G**, **Lecendreux M**, *et al*. Kleine–Levin syndrome: an autoimmune hypothesis based on clinical and genetic analyses. *Neurology*, 2002; **59**:1739–45.

25. **Driver H S**, **Baker F C**. Menstrual factors in sleep. *Sleep Med Rev*, 1998; **2**:213–29.

26. **Hoddes E**, **Zarcone V**, **Smythe H**, *et al*. Quantification of sleepiness: a new approach. *Psychophysiology*, 1973; **10**:431–36.

27. **Shibui K**, **Uchiyama M**, **Okawa M**, *et al*. Diurnal fluctuation of sleep propensity and hormonal secretion across the menstrual cycle. *Biol Psychiatry*, 2000; **48**:1062–68.

28. **Manber R**, **Bootzin R R**. Sleep and the menstrual cycle. *Health Psychol*, 1997; **16**:209–14.

29. **Mauri M**. Sleep and the reproductive cycle: a review. *Health Care Women Int*, 1990; **11**:409–21.

30. **Baker F C**, **Colrain I M**. Daytime sleepiness, psychomotor performance, waking EEG spectra and evoked potentials in women with severe premenstrual syndrome. *J Sleep Res* 2010; **19**(Suppl 1):214–27.

31. **Lamarche L J**, **Driver H S**, **Wiebe S**, *et al*. Nocturnal sleep, daytime sleepiness, and napping among women with significant emotional/behavioral premenstrual symptoms. *J Sleep Res*, 2007; **16**:262–68.

32. **Theorell-Haglow J**, **Lindberg E**, **Janson C**. What are the important risk factors for daytime sleepiness and fatigue in women? *Sleep*, 2006; **29**:751–57.

33. **American Psychiatric Association**. *Diagnostic and Statistical Manual of Mental Disorders* (4th ed.). Washington, DC: American Psychiatric Press Inc, 1994: 717–18.

34. **Klerman E B**. Clinical aspects of human circadian rhythms. *J Biol Rhythms*, 2005; **20**:375–86.

35. **Mitler M M**, **Carskadon M A**, **Hirshkowitz M**. Evaluating sleepiness. In: Kryger M H, RothT, Dement W C, Eds. *Principles and Practice of Sleep Medicine*. Philadelphia, PA: Elsevier Saunders, 2005: 1417–23.

36. **Shen J**, **Barbera J**, **Shapiro C M**. Distinguishing sleepiness and fatigue: focus on definition and measurement. *Sleep Med Rev*, 2006; **10**:63–76.

37. **Littner M R**, **Kushida C**, **Wise M**, *et al*. Practice parameters for clinical use of the multiple sleep latency test and the maintenance of wakefulness test. *Sleep*, 2005; **28**:113–21.

38. **Dinges D F**, **Powell J W**. Microcomputer analyses of performance on a portable, simple visual RT task during sustained operations. *Behav Res Meth Instr Com*, 1985; **16**:652–55.

39. **Baker F C**, **Kahan T L**, **Trinder J**, *et al*. Sleep quality and the sleep electroencephalogram in women with severe premenstrual syndrome. *Sleep*, 2007; **30**:1283–91.

40. **Dinges D F**, **Arora S**, **Darwish M**, *et al*. Pharmacodynamic effects on alertness of single doses of armodafinil in healthy subjects during a nocturnal period of acute sleep loss. *Curr Med Res Opin*, 2006; **22**:159–67.

41. **Banks S**, **Barnes M**, **Tarquinio N**, et al. Factors associated with maintenance of wakefulness test mean sleep latency in patients with mild to moderate obstructive sleep apnoea and normal subjects. *J Sleep Res*, 2004; **13**:71–78.

42. **Resnick A**, **Perry W**, **Parry B**, et al. Neuropsychological performance across the menstrual cycle in women with and without Premenstrual Dysphoric Disorder. *Psychiatry Res*, 1998; **77**:147–58.

Section 2 Chapter 15

Sleep Disorders and Excessive Sleepiness

Sleepiness due to sleep-related breathing disorders

Jean-Louis Pepin, Sandrine H. Launois, Renaud Tamsier and Patrick Levy

Introduction

Sleep-related breathing disorders in adults include obstructive sleep apnea syndrome (OSA), central sleep apnea (CSA), upper airway resistance syndrome (UARS) and sleep hypoventilation syndrome [1]. This review will mainly focus on sleepiness related to OSA which represents the most common situation in clinical practice and research. Obstructive sleep apnea is due to recurrent episodes of pharyngeal collapse during sleep. These events cause microarousals and nocturnal oxygen desaturation thought to be responsible for sleep fragmentation and, consequently, for excessive daytime sleepiness.

Excessive daytime sleepiness (EDS) is one of the most frequent symptoms experienced by OSA patients, but is not invariably present in these patients. First, this chapter will address the prevalence of sleepiness in OSA and the potential confusion with fatigue, depression and attentional deficits. We will examine the relationship between subjective complaints and objective measurements of sleepiness in OSA patients. The pathophysiology of sleepiness in OSA is specific but actually more complex than the simple link initially proposed with hypoxemia and sleep fragmentation. Potential underlying mechanisms might also include sleep structure disturbances, activation of the hypothalamic–pituitary–adrenal (HPA) axis, inflammation and cytokine production, brain lesions, and the key role of comorbid conditions. In terms of major consequences, sleepiness affects driving abilities through decreased alertness and/or attention deficit. Undiagnosed or untreated OSA patients are indeed at risk for motor vehicle accidents and evaluation of fitness to drive in a patient with OSA is a challenge. Another important hot topic is that sleepiness in OSA is not only a disability in itself, but also a predictor for associated cardiovascular and metabolic comorbidities. We will examine treatment options for EDS caused by OSA, represented mainly by continuous positive airway pressure (CPAP) application, but also to lesser extent by oral appliance treatment. Finally, the specific situation of residual sleepiness in CPAP compliers will be presented in terms of prevalence, pathophysiology, and treatment modalities.

Clinical characteristics of sleepiness in obstructive sleep apnea

In a report of the American Academy of Sleep Medicine dedicated to syndrome definitions, "excessive daytime sleepiness that is not better explained by other factors" is one of the major criteria for the diagnosis of obstructive sleep apnea syndrome (Criterion A [1]). In the same consensus report, severity of OSA is described as having two main components: severity of sleepiness, and the number of overnight abnormal respiratory events. *Mild* severity is defined as sleepiness or involuntary sleep episodes occurring during activities that require little attention such as watching television, reading, or traveling in a vehicle as a passenger. Sleepiness is rated *moderate* when reported during activities that require some attention. Examples include attending concerts, meetings, etc. Sleepiness is considered *severe* when involuntary sleep episodes occur during activities that require active attention (i.e. while eating, during conversation, walking, or driving). In clinical practice, the severity of sleepiness is assessed by the Epworth Sleepiness Scale (ESS) [2].

Despite being a chief symptom of OSA, excessive daytime sleepiness is not universally present in patients. In the Sleep Heart Health Study community-based cohort ($N = 6440$), only 46% of participants

---

Sleepiness: Causes, Consequences and Treatment, ed. Michael J. Thorpy and Michel Billiard. Published by Cambridge University Press. © Cambridge University Press 2011.

with moderate to severe sleep-disordered breathing (apnea–hypopnea index (AHI) ≥15/h) reported sleepiness as defined by an ESS score >10 or a report of at least frequently feeling tired or sleepy [3]. In a recently published large clinical cohort of OSA subjects (*n* = 2882) recruited from five major teaching hospitals in Spain, EDS as defined by an ESS >10 was present only in 1649/2882 (57%) of subjects [4]. A likely explanation for the significant proportion of OSA patients that do not subjectively complain of impaired alertness is that patients can express their complaint with different terms, in particular, "fatigue", "tiredness", or "lack of energy" [5]. In 190 consecutive OSAS patients referred for diagnostic polysomnography, Chervin found that the proportion of patients who preferred the term "sleepiness" to describe their primary problem was only about 22%, while about 40% preferred "lack of energy", 18% preferred "fatigue", and 20% preferred "tiredness" [5]. Additionally, women report feeling sleepy as often as men do, but women are less likely to have an ESS score >10, yet are more likely to report feeling unrested than men [6]. Thus, men and women probably report or express symptoms for OSA differently and ESS may be a more sensitive measure of subjective sleepiness in men than in women [6]. Complaints of subjective sleepiness are also dependent upon the context in which the diagnosis is made. Subjects diagnosed with OSAS after systematic screening of "at-risk" populations have less-subjective symptoms of sleepiness than patients who attend a sleep disorder specialized clinic. These patients suffer from another chronic disease, such as morbid obesity or diabetes, affecting their quality of life and they tend to underestimate their associated sleep problems and daytime sleepiness. Similar observations have been reported in heart failure [7], chronically paced patients [8], or in type 2 diabetic subjects [9].

In clinical practice, sleepiness is in most cases evaluated by the ESS. However, to help assess the impact of OSA on daytime alertness, objective tests can be administered in the sleep laboratory. In OSA patients, studies have yielded somewhat contradictory results, but a poor correlation generally exists between subjective and objective test measures (for review, see [10]). The Multiple Sleep Latency Test (MSLT) measures the propensity to fall asleep in soporific conditions. In a large series of 247 OSA patients, Chervin *et al*. did not find any relationship between ESS and MSLT (Figure 15.1A) [5, 11]. Of note, sleepy, male apneic patients with significant nocturnal desaturations can exhibit two or more sleep onset REM episodes on the MSLT. The Maintenance of Wakefulness Test (MWT) measures the capacity to stay awake in soporific conditions [12]. Again, in OSA, MWT values do not clearly delineate moderate from severe patients (Figure 15.1B) [13]. The Oxford Sleepiness Resistance (OSLER) test represents a simple alternative to the Maintenance of Wakefulness Test [14–16]. The OSLER test is a behavioral test during which the subject, while seated in a dark, quiet room, is instructed to remain awake and press a button each time a dim light flashes. The light-emitting diode flashes regularly for 1 s every 3 s. The subject is instructed to remain awake in this soporific situation for a maximum testing time of 40 min. When the subject fails to respond for 21 s (i.e. seven consecutive illuminations), the test is ended and it is assumed that the patient has fallen asleep. Thus, the OSLER test reproduces many of the MWT characteristics, with the advantage of being a simpler and less expensive tool, which does not require the presence of a trained technician. The results of the OSLER test and MWT correlate well in OSA patients and the OSLER test's capacity to distinguish between control subjects and OSAS patients is demonstrated [14]. In addition to the measurement of sleep latencies, the test is able to identify the probability of microsleep episodes onset. When microsleep is defined as the occurrence of a period of at least 3 s where theta rhythm replaces alpha rhythm, the sensitivity to identify these microsleep episodes by three consecutive errors during the OSlER test is approximately 90% [15]. Thus, in OSA patients, this test measures not only sleep latency but also abnormal fluctuations of alertness level due to attentional deficit.

As stated above, there is poor correlation between the level of alertness reported by patients and the level of alertness objectively quantified using objective testing. However, beyond sleepiness, attentional deficits are likely to contribute in part to daytime functioning impairment and complaints in OSA patients. In OSA, these deficits can be assessed by a variety of neurocognitive tests [17] evaluating sustained or divided attention. When attention performance is measured using the Continuous Performance Test (CPT), assessing sustained and selective attention, and a driving simulator, assessing divided attention, in combination with the evaluation of subjective sleepiness by ESS and of objective behavioral maintenance of wakefulness by the OSLER test, 95% of OSA patients demonstrate alertness and/or attentional impairment [18]

Figure 15.1 Subjective and objective measurements of sleepiness in OSA. (A) Epworth sleepiness scale score is plotted against the mean sleep latency test for 247 patients (modified from [11]). No significant relationship was found between subjective and objective assessment of sleepiness. (B) Mean MWT sleep latencies for moderate and severe OSA groups. Differences between groups did not reach statistical significance (modified from [13]). (C) ESS: Epworth Sleepiness Scale; Beck: Beck depression inventory; OSLER: Oxford sleep resistance test; CPT: continuous performance test; DS: driving simulator; X: abnormal test results. When a combination of three attentional tests is performed in addition to evaluation of subjective sleepiness and depression, 95% of patients had alertness and/or attentional impairment. Even OSA patients with normal subjective sleepiness almost systematically exhibit abnormalities in attentional tasks (modified from [18]).

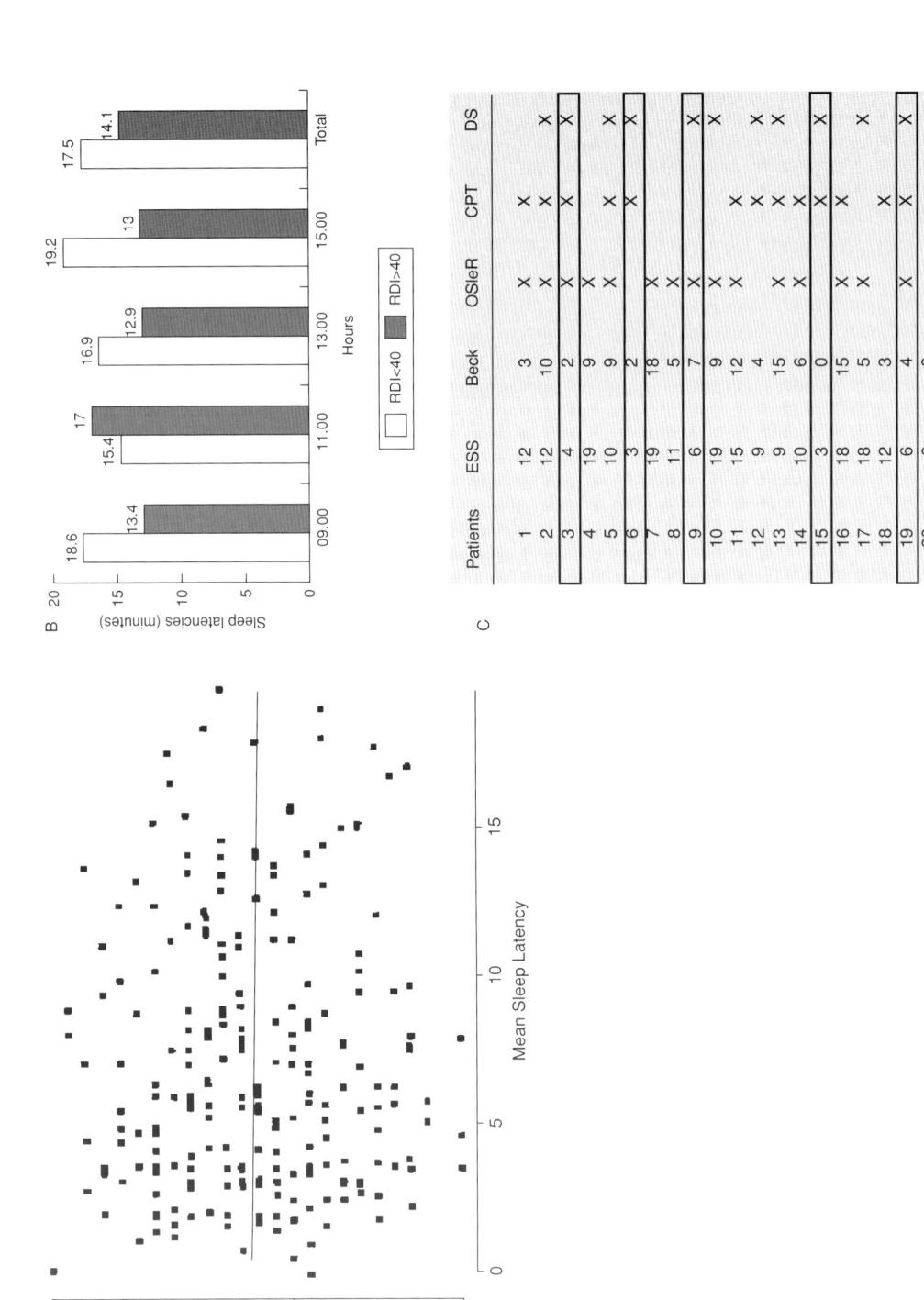

(Figure 15.1C). This means that impairment patterns vary between patients and that even OSA patients with no subjective sleepiness exhibit abnormalities in attention task performance. Such different impairment profiles strengthen the hypothesis that attentional capacity and alertness could be differentially altered and reinforce the need for extended testing in OSA patients, particularly in those without significant EDS. This is a key issue for treatment management, as adherence to CPAP seems difficult in the absence of subjective sleepiness. In this situation, applying a sensitive battery of alertness and attentional tests could improve the identification of patients who could benefit from and respond to CPAP treatment. However, whether these subjects perceive a subjective benefit from CPAP treatment or not remains to be established.

In summary, using one isolated subjective or objective test could lead to not recognizing some patients with impaired alertness and/or attentional deficits. Specific tools should be used to adequately detect deficits in alertness and attention capacity. Whether the different test battery patterns are associated with specific risks of accidents or respond differently to treatment should be studied further.

Pathophysiology of excessive daytime sleepiness in obstructive sleep apnea

Sleep fragmentation and other sleep structure disturbances are classically considered the main causes of daytime sleepiness in OSA patients.

Arousals and excessive daytime sleepiness

In OSA, sleep fragmentation by respiratory event-induced microarousals is overall related to EDS [19]. However, the exact contribution of sleep fragmentation to EDS is still under debate, because of the poor correlation between the number of microarousals per hour of sleep and EDS assessed subjectively or objectively (Figure 15.2A). A hypothesis for this weak relationship is that cortical arousals as defined by the American Sleep Disorders Association (ASDA) are not sensitive enough to detect sleep fragmentation. Sforza et al. have demonstrated evidence for a hierarchy of arousal responses, ranging from autonomic changes to bursts of delta activity on EEG and finally to intrusion of alpha activity into sleep [20]. Therefore, a given stimulus may or may not produce a visible cortical arousal. It is possible that, in certain circumstances, only the first level of the hierarchical arousal response is identifiable, i.e. bursts of autonomic activity. Thus, detection of microarousals by using only autonomic markers such as blood pressure (BP) rises, heart rate variations, or transient dips in pulse transit time (PTT) could provide a more accurate evaluation of sleep fragmentation. However, in OSA, various autonomic markers or arousals and EDS are apparently not better correlated than cortical arousals and EDS [21, 22]. Additional evidence for the limited impact of sleep fragmentation in OSA-related EDS is that suppression of sleep disruption by CPAP only partially explains the changes in EDS after treatment [22].

Sleep architecture and excessive daytime sleepiness

In OSA, daytime sleepiness has also been attributed to poor nocturnal sleep quality. In apneic patients, a positive correlation has been shown between slow-wave activity (SWA) during the first sleep cycle and sleep latencies on MSLT [23]. This suggests that daytime sleepiness in OSA patients may be partly the result of a lack of SWA during the first part of the night (Figure 15.2B). In contrast, two recent studies suggest that sleep architecture and quality is not worse in those OSA subjects exhibiting EDS than in OSA patients who do not [4, 24]. A total of 1649 patients with EDS (mean ± SD ESS = 15 ± 3) and 1233 without EDS (ESS = 7 ± 3) have been studied by Roure et al. [4]. OSA patients with EDS slept longer and more efficiently that patients without EDS [4]. Mediano et al. found that sleepy OSA patients, as defined by an ESS >10 and a mean latency on MSLT <5 min, exhibited shorter night sleep latency and greater sleep efficiency than those without EDS [24]. However, sleep-stage distribution and arousal index did not differ between groups. These findings suggest that sleep organization does not predominantly account for the presence of EDS in apneic patients.

Hypoxemia and excessive daytime sleepiness

Intermittent hypoxemia during sleep could induce neural cell injury and apoptosis through the activation of inflammatory and oxidative pathways. Hypoxia-induced injury occurring specifically in the wakefulness-promoting regions within the CNS

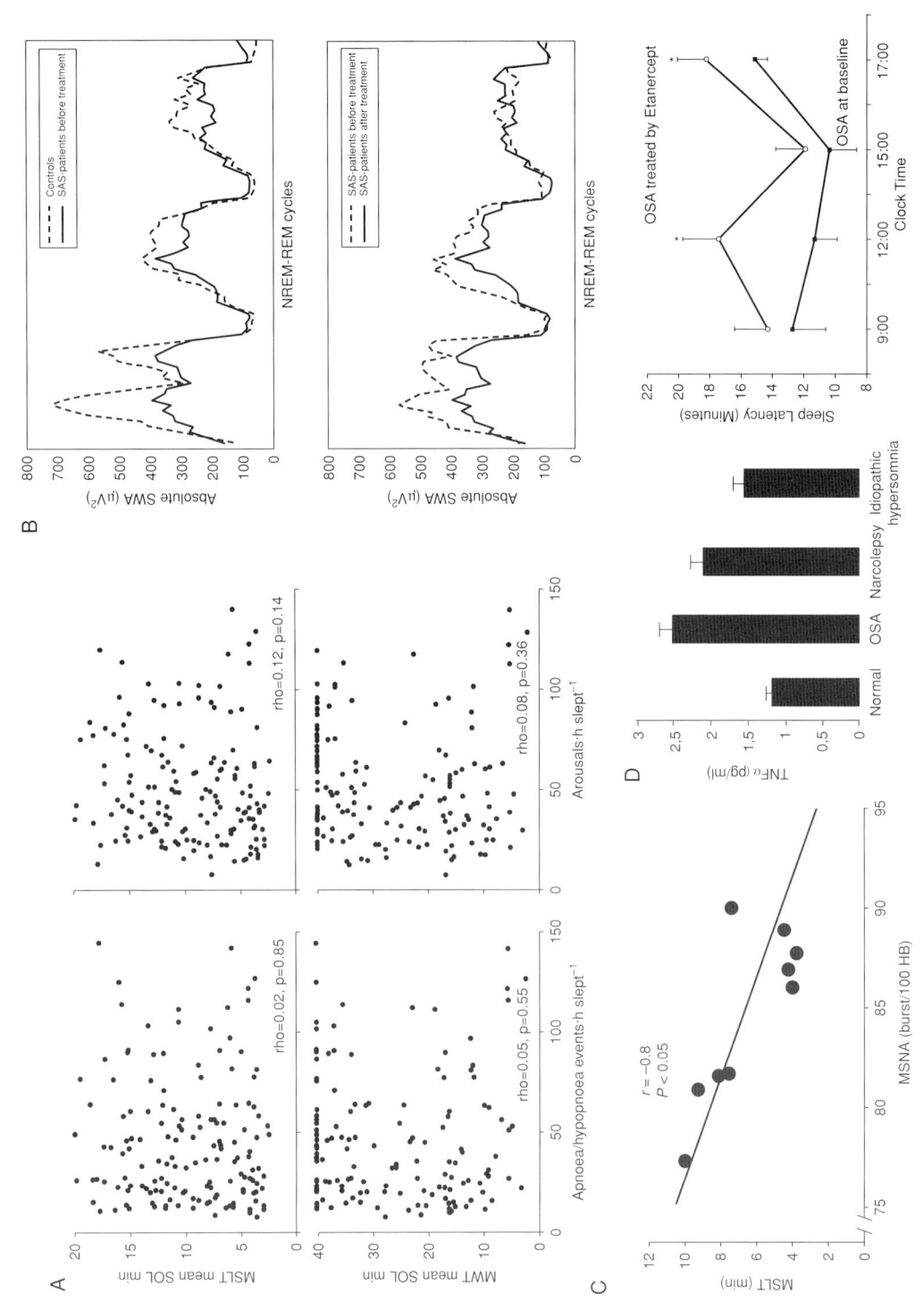

Figure 15.2 Underlying mechanisms for sleepiness in OSA. (A) There is a lack of relationship between objective measures of sleepiness and AHI and sleep fragmentation (modified from [70]). (B) Slow-wave activity (SWA) across three NREM–REM cycles for 10 control subjects and 10 SAS patients before treatment (*top*) and for 10 SAS patients before and after treatment (*bottom*). Note the reduced amount of SWA in OSA compared to controls during the first sleep cycle (Modified from [23]). (C) Linear correlation between muscle sympathetic nerve activity (MSNA) (bursts per 100 heart beats)) and daytime sleep latency on the Multiple sleep latency test (modified from [72]). (D) Increased levels of inflammatory cytokines in different sleep disorders and marked decrease in sleepiness in patients with sleep apnea by etanercept (increase in mean sleep latencies on MSLT, a tumor necrosis factor antagonist (modified from [29]).

could be associated with the occurrence of sleepiness. Indeed, several studies have shown an association between daytime sleepiness and the minimum and mean oxygen saturation, and the number of oxygen desaturation index [24]. In addition, Haba-Rubio *et al.* showed that OSA patients with sleep respiratory disturbances limited to REM sleep (mean AHI for the whole night = 9.7/h) were as sleepy as classic OSA patients exhibiting a threefold greater AHI. The authors suggested that hypoxemia during REM sleep may affect daytime alertness as much as an overall disruption of sleep continuity. Indeed, hypercapnic OSA patients (those with obesity hypoventilation syndrome) with profound REM desaturations due to REM sleep hypoventilation have greater EDS as measured objectively by the OSLER test [25]. The amount of nocturnal hypoxemia is the main determinant of sympathetic system overactivity, a major determinant of OSA cardiovascular consequences. In selected OSA patients without confounding factors (i.e. diabetes mellitus, hypercholesterolemia and brain lesions), daytime sleepiness and sympathetic activity showed a positive correlation (Figure 15.2C). The mechanism underlying this association is unclear, but arterial baroreceptors may be involved as baroreceptor activation decreases arousal and facilitates sleep [26], and possibly sleepiness.

Comorbid conditions

The different mechanisms underlying EDS are complex and not at all limited to sleep deprivation or sleep fragmentation. There is evidence that chronic inflammatory status leading to increased secretion of inflammatory cytokines is associated with sleepiness [27, 28]. This is true not only for sleep apnea but also in narcolepsy or idiopathic hypersomnia. Obesity per se, which is frequently encountered in apneic patients, is a cause of inflammation and increased levels of cytokines and can contribute to daytime hypersomnia [29]. In support for this mechanism, a marked decrease in daytime sleepiness in OSA patients was demonstrated after the administration of etanercept, a tumor necrosis factor-alpha (TNFα) antagonist, which led to decreased levels of TNFα and interleukin-6 (Figure 15.2D) [30]. Based on these studies, Vgontzas and colleagues have hypothesized that the interaction of the HPA axis and pro-inflammatory cytokines determines the level of sleep/arousal within the 24-h cycle. One subtype of obese patients might present with emotional distress, poor sleep, fatigue, HPA axis "hyperactivity," and hypercytokinemia while the other subtype would be associated with no distress, better sleep but more sleepiness, HPA axis "normo or hypoactivity," and hypercytokinemia (see Figure 15.3). This model is particularly interesting as it includes depression, the main determinant for sleepiness in the general population and a contributing factor in OSA [31]. Another strength of this model is to allow understanding of conflicting results on the link between sleep architecture and sleepiness in OSA patients [4, 24].

Other comorbid conditions, including respiratory disease (such as chronic obstructive pulmonary disease or COPD), sleep restriction, insomnia, and nocturnal leg complaints, are important risk factors for sleepiness in individuals with moderate to severe sleep-disordered breathing [3]. In a large series of 1106 subjects referred to a Sleep Disorders Clinic for symptoms consistent with sleep apnea, Basta *et al.* found that not only the severity of OSA but also lack of regular exercise (only in men) and depression were significant predictors of EDS [32].

In summary, Table 15.1 illustrates the obvious discrepancies between studies regarding underlying mechanisms that could account for EDS associated with OSA. Figure 15.3 attempts to summarize and put together the mechanisms involved in OSA-related sleepiness. Obviously, there are many determinants of sleepiness and their respective importance can vary in a given patient. OSA treatment eliminates respiratory events, hence can suppress intermittent hypoxia and, at least partially, improve sleep architecture and sleep fragmentation. However, CPAP has a more limited effectiveness on comorbidities and on inflammation associated with obesity [33]. As a consequence, management of depression, enrolment in physical exercise and weight loss programs should be part of a thorough management of sleepiness in patients with sleep apnea.

Impairment of driving ability: one of the major consequences of sleepiness in OSA

Sleepiness, regardless of its cause, affects driving ability through increased reaction time, inattentiveness or microsleep episodes [34]. As OSA is characterized by impaired daytime alertness and cognitive dysfunction,

2. Sleep Disorders and Excessive Sleepiness

Table 15.1 Determinants of sleepiness in OSA patients: contradictory results from four key studies

	Mediano et al. [24] (n = 40) EDS +	EDS −	Roure et al. [4] (n = 2882) EDS +	EDS −	Kapur et al. [3] (n = 1115) EDS +	EDS −	Basta et al. [32] (men n = 486) EDS + (severe EDS)	EDS − (no EDS)
AHI, events/h	62 ± 18	60 ± 20	36 ± 27	33 ± 25*	32	29*	44 ± 33	38 ± 31
Mean SaO$_2$ (%)	87 ± 6	90 ± 5*	92 ± 5	92 ± 4	93 (during NREM)	93 (during NREM)	NA	NA
Minimum SaO$_2$ (%)	69 ± 12	79 ± 8*	78 ± 12	79 ± 11*	79 (during REM)	80 (during REM)	78 ± 10	81 ± 8*
Total sleep time TST (min)	401 ± 41	379 ± 63	338 ± 67	325 ± 65*	342	342	NA	NA
REM (% of TST)	13 ± 6	14 ± 8	5 ± 4	5 ± 4	18	19	9 ± 9	10 ± 8
SWS (% of TST)	6 ± 8	8 ± 5	11 ± 13	8 ± 10*	15	15	2 ± 4	2 ± 6
Microarousals index (nb/h)	65 ± 20	60 ± 24	37 ± 31	33 ± 23*	28	27	NA	NA
Sleep efficiency (%)	90 ± 7	82 ± 13*	79 ± 22	72 ± 31*	80	79	NA	NA

* Significant differences between EDS− and EDS+, $p < 0.05$. NA: Not available.

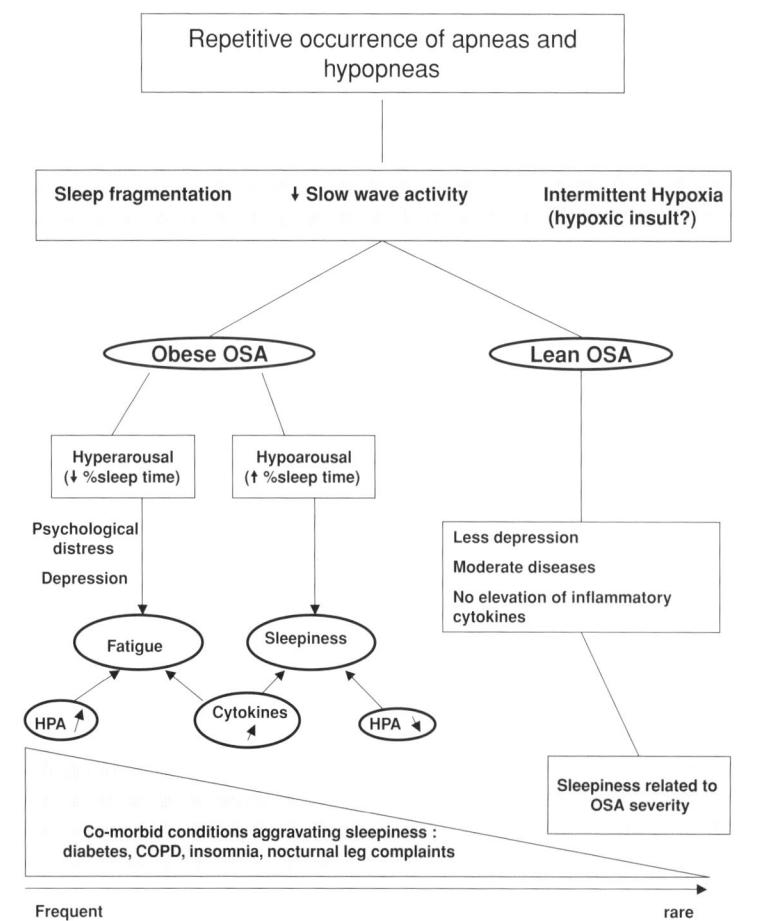

Figure 15.3 Summary of underlying mechanisms explaining sleepiness in OSA.

it is not surprising that undiagnosed or untreated OSA patients are at risk for a variety of accidents and, in particular, motor vehicle accidents (MVA) (see [35] for review).

Specific regulations have been implemented in most countries to evaluate fitness to drive in patients with sleep disorders and/or EDS, sometimes suggesting or imposing tests used to evaluate patients, and outlining the respective responsibility of patients and physicians. While such regulations usually apply only to occupational drivers, evaluation should not be limited to these drivers but should also be performed in any OSA patient who drives. Yet, at present, there is no international consensus on how fitness to drive should be evaluated or whether all OSA patients, regardless of their symptoms, driving history or occupation, should be evaluated.

For obvious reasons, self-reports of driving impairment, automobile accidents or near-accidents may be unreliable [36, 37]. However, these reports are highly correlated with the risk of MVA [36–39] and with decreased performances on a driving simulator [40]. Thus, clinicians evaluating their patient's fitness to drive should systematically assess subjective impairment at the wheel.

Although the AHI or the microarousal index may not accurately predict daytime alertness impairment or the risk of traffic accidents [41], the occurrence of traffic accidents appears to increase with the severity of OSA in most reports (see [35] for review). In addition, a recent Canadian study showed that the seriousness of MVA was linked to the severity of OSA (based on AHI) [42]. Interestingly, in the same study, the body mass index (BMI), independently of OSA, AHI or the ESS score, correlated with the risk of MVA [42]. Some have even advocated the use of BMI measurement as a screening parameter for impaired driving abilities in commercial drivers, as obese drivers were found to be sleepier than non-obese drivers (based on MSLT) and none reported subjective sleepiness [43].

Subjective sleepiness, assessed by the ESS, has been correlated with automobile accidents in some studies [36–39, 44] but not in others [42]. Furthermore, it can be minimized or underestimated by patients and correlates poorly with objective sleepiness [45], or attentiveness [41, 46] in OSA patients.

Objective daytime testing is therefore often required, particularly when an expert opinion is requested by the employer or the national licensing authorities with regards to a patient's fitness to drive.

Real driving condition testing is theoretically possible in OSA patients, following procedures applied to other situations causing sleepiness [47], and is likely to be more relevant to on-road driving risk than in-laboratory testing [48]. However, such tests are currently impractical outside of research protocols. Multiple sleep latency and maintenance of wakefulness tests are considered the gold standards for the objective evaluation of sleepiness and alertness [12]. Rather than the MSLT which measures a variable (the ability to fall asleep) that may not be relevant to driving fitness [40], electrophysiological monitoring of the ability to maintain wakefulness has been advocated as the best means to evaluate fitness to safely perform potentially dangerous tasks in sleepy patients [12]. For the general population, a latency greater than the normal mean minus 2 standard deviations is considered normal. For a 40-min MWT, a latency greater than 19 min is thus "normal" [12]. MWT latency correlates with traffic accident history and driving simulator performances [40, 49] in sleep apnea and control subjects. Yet, one could easily argue that a mean sleep latency of 25 min on a MWT in a truck or bus driver is worrisome. This has led some authors to classify subjects as "sleepy" (latency < 20 min), "alert" (latency 21–34 min) or "fully alert" (latency > 34 min). Performance on a double task driving simulator was significantly linked to these MWT categories, which may be more relevant to driving evaluation than a "normal" or "abnormal" latency [49]. Although MWT can be advocated as a means to test patients whose occupation puts them (and others) at risk, such electrophysiological testing is time-consuming, expensive and can only be performed in sleep laboratories. Thus, MWT may not be a realistic option in a broad clinical setting. The OSLER test [14] correlates well with standard MWT [15, 16]. However, the test validity for routine evaluation of OSA patient alertness as it relates to driving ability has yet to be established. In addition to quantitative measurements of sleepiness or, conversely, of the ability to remain awake, evaluation of attention processes and reaction time also assesses the ability of a patient to perform the complex cognitive task of driving. Numerous tests are available and have been used in OSA patients. Although sophisticated and realistic tools exist, most driving simulators do, in fact, assess reaction time and/or sustained or divided attention performance, rather than on-road driving abilities per se (see [50] for review). Performances fact that RES has a significant impact patient daily life. Using the clinical global impression of severity (CGI-S), patients with RES complain of being moderately ill (60%) or even markedly ill (20%) [67]. In the French multicentric study [66], RES significantly impacted on daily life as these patients had significantly more fatigue, unrefreshing sleep and a greater impairment in energy and emotional quality-of-life domain scores of the Nottingham Health Profile (NHP).

Regarding the underlying mechanisms of RES, it has been proposed that, in a subgroup of subjects, OSA per se may promote irreversible anoxic brain damage affecting the prefrontal cortex [68]. This hypoxic damage may underlie persistent sleepiness and cognitive dysfunction despite treatment. It remains unclear why one individual OSA patient may or may not develop this kind of lesion. The fact that OSA patients with RES were younger and sleepier at the time of diagnosis, with the same range of respiratory event severity compared with those without RES, suggests that patients with RES may represent a subgroup with particular (genetically determined?) brain susceptibility to hypoxic exposure.

Randomized controlled trials using stimulants in RES patients have demonstrated a significant improvement both in terms of symptoms [67] and quality of life [69]. In particular, the activity level subscale of the functional outcomes of the sleep questionnaire, which corresponds to the energy domain of the NHP, has been shown to be significantly improved by stimulants. Stimulants improve subjective and objective alertness without reduction in CPAP compliance [70]. After careful exclusion of all possible causes of sleepiness, it may be justified to initiate treatment with stimulant agents in patients with RES. Some stimulant agents have indeed been approved, at least in some countries, for this indication.

General conclusion

Excessive daytime sleepiness is one of the most frequent symptoms experienced by OSA patients but is not invariably present in these patients. The pathophysiology of sleepiness in OSA is specific, complex and still remains under debate. Hypoxemia, changes in sleep structure and sleep fragmentation are involved, but activity of the hypothalamic–pituitary–adrenal (HPA) axis, inflammation and cytokine production, brain lesions and other comorbid conditions also contribute to EDS. Sleepiness affects driving abilities through hypoalertness and/or attention deficit, increasing the risk for motor vehicle accidents in OSA patients. Evaluation of fitness to drive in a patient with OSA remains a challenge. Importantly, sleepiness in obstructive sleep apnea syndrome is a predictor for associated cardiovascular and metabolic comorbidities. CPAP treatment restores normal alertness except in some patients with residual excessive sleepiness. In this situation sleepiness may justify treatment with stimulants.

References

1. **American Academy of Sleep Medicine Task Force**. Sleep-related breathing disorders in adults: recommendations for syndrome definition and measurement techniques in clinical research. The Report of an American Academy of Sleep Medicine Task Force. *Sleep*, 1999; **22**:667–89.
2. **Johns M W**. A new method for measuring daytime sleepiness: the Epworth sleepiness scale. *Sleep*, 1991; **14**:540–45.
3. **Kapur V K, Baldwin C M, Resnick H E**, *et al*. Sleepiness in patients with moderate to severe sleep-disordered breathing. *Sleep*, 2005; **28**:472–77.
4. **Roure N, Gomez S, Mediano O**, *et al*. Daytime sleepiness and polysomnography in obstructive sleep apnea patients. *Sleep Med*, 2008; **9**:727–31.
5. **Chervin R D**. Sleepiness, fatigue, tiredness, and lack of energy in obstructive sleep apnea. *Chest*, 2000; **118**:372–79.
6. **Baldwin C M, Kapur V K, Holberg C J**, *et al*. Associations between gender and measures of daytime somnolence in the Sleep Heart Health Study. *Sleep*, 2004; **27**:305–11.
7. **Arzt M, Young T, Finn L**, *et al*. Sleepiness and sleep in patients with both systolic heart failure and obstructive sleep apnea. *Arch Intern Med*, 2006; **166**:1716–22.
8. **Garrigue S, Pepin J L, Defaye P**, *et al*. High prevalence of sleep apnea syndrome in patients with long-term pacing: the European Multicenter Polysomnographic Study. *Circulation*, 2007; **115**:1703–09.
9. **Foster G D, Sanders M H, Millman R**, *et al*. Obstructive sleep apnea among obese patients with type 2 diabetes. *Diabetes Care*, 2009; **32**:1017–19.
10. **Fong S Y, Ho C K, Wing Y K**. Comparing MSLT and ESS in the measurement of excessive daytime sleepiness in obstructive sleep apnoea syndrome. *J Psychosom Res*, 2005; **58**:55–60.
11. **Chervin R D, Aldrich M S**. The Epworth Sleepiness Scale may not reflect objective measures of sleepiness or sleep apnea. *Neurology*, 1999; **52**:125–31.

12. **Littner M R**, **Kushida C**, **Wise M**, et al. Practice parameters for clinical use of the multiple sleep latency test and the maintenance of wakefulness test. *Sleep*, 2005; **28**:113–21.

13. **Sauter C**, **Asenbaum S**, **Popovic R**, et al. Excessive daytime sleepiness in patients suffering from different levels of obstructive sleep apnoea syndrome. *J Sleep Res*, 2000; **9**:293–301.

14. **Bennett L S**, **Stradling J R**, **Davies R J**. A behavioural test to assess daytime sleepiness in obstructive sleep apnoea. *J Sleep Res*, 1997; **6**:142–45.

15. **Priest B**, **Brichard C**, **Aubert G**, et al. Microsleep during a simplified maintenance of wakefulness test. A validation study of the OSLER test. *Am J Respir Crit Care Med*, 2001; **163**:1619–25.

16. **Krieger A C**, **Ayappa I**, **Norman R G**, et al. Comparison of the maintenance of wakefulness test (MWT) to a modified behavioral test (OSLER) in the evaluation of daytime sleepiness. *J Sleep Res*, 2004; **13**:407–11.

17. **Beebe D W**, **Groesz L**, **Wells C**, et al. The neuropsychological effects of obstructive sleep apnea: a meta-analysis of norm-referenced and case-controlled data. *Sleep*, 2003; **26**:298–307.

18. **Mazza S**, **Pepin J-L**, **Naegele B**, et al. Most obstructive sleep apnoea patients exhibit vigilance and attention deficits on an extended battery of tests. *Eur Respir J*, 2005; **25**:75–80.

19. **Bennett L S**, **Langford B A**, **Stradling J R**, et al. Sleep fragmentation indices as predictors of daytime sleepiness and nCPAP response in obstructive sleep apnea. *Am J Respir Crit Care Med*, 1998; **158**:778–86.

20. **Sforza E**, **Nicolas A**, **Lavigne G**, et al. EEG and cardiac activation during periodic leg movements in sleep: support for a hierarchy of arousal responses. *Neurology*, 1999; **52**:786–91.

21. **Levy P**, **Pepin J L**. Sleep fragmentation: clinical usefulness of autonomic markers. *Sleep Med*, 2003; 4:489–91.

22. **Bennett L S**, **Barbour C**, **Langford B**, et al. Health status in obstructive sleep apnea: relationship with sleep fragmentation and daytime sleepiness, and effects of continuous positive airway pressure treatment. *Am J Respir Crit Care Med*, 1999; **159**:1884–90.

23. **Heinzer R**, **Gaudreau H**, **Decary A**, et al. Slow-wave activity in sleep apnea patients before and after continuous positive airway pressure treatment: contribution to daytime sleepiness. *Chest*, 2001; **119**:1807–13.

24. **Mediano O**, **Barcelo A**, **de la Pena M**, et al. Daytime sleepiness and polysomnographic variables in sleep apnoea patients. *Eur Respir J*, 2007; **30**:110–13.

25. **Chouri-Pontarollo N**, **Borel J C**, **Tamisier R**, et al. Impaired objective daytime vigilance in obesity–hypoventilation syndrome: impact of noninvasive ventilation. *Chest*, 2007; **131**:148–55.

26. **Rau H**, **Elbert T**. Psychophysiology of arterial baroreceptors and the etiology of hypertension. *Biol Psychol*, 2001; **57**:179–201.

27. **Vgontzas A N**. Does obesity play a major role in the pathogenesis of sleep apnoea and its associated manifestations via inflammation, visceral adiposity, and insulin resistance? *Arch Physiol Biochem*, 2008; **114**:211–23.

28. **Vgontzas A N**, **Bixler E O**, **Chrousos G P**, et al. Obesity and sleep disturbances: meaningful sub-typing of obesity. *Arch Physiol Biochem*, 2008; **114**:224–36.

29. **Vgontzas A N**, **Bixler E O**, **Chrousos G P**. Sleep apnea is a manifestation of the metabolic syndrome. *Sleep Med Rev*, 2005; **9**:211–24.

30. **Vgontzas A N**, **Zoumakis E**, **Bixler E O**, et al. Adverse effects of modest sleep restriction on sleepiness, performance, and inflammatory cytokines. *J Clin Endocrinol Metab*, 2004; **89**:2119–26.

31. **Bixler E O**, **Vgontzas A N**, **Lin H M**, et al. Excessive daytime sleepiness in a general population sample: the role of sleep apnea, age, obesity, diabetes, and depression. *J Clin Endocrinol Metab*, 2005; **90**:4510–15.

32. **Basta M**, **Lin H M**, **Pejovic S**, et al. Lack of regular exercise, depression, and degree of apnea are predictors of excessive daytime sleepiness in patients with sleep apnea: sex differences. *J Clin Sleep Med*, 2008; **4**:19–25.

33. **Levy P**, **Bonsignore M R**, **Eckel J**. Sleep, sleep-disordered breathing and metabolic consequences. *Eur Respir J*, 2009; **34**:243–60.

34. **MacLean A W**, **Davies D R**, **Thiele K**. The hazards and prevention of driving while sleepy. *Sleep Med Rev*, 2003; **7**:507–21.

35. **Ellen R L**, **Marshall S C**, **Palayew M**, et al. Systematic review of motor vehicle crash risk in persons with sleep apnea. *J Clin Sleep Med*, 2006; **2**:193–200.

36. **Masa J F**, **Rubio M**, **Findley L J**. Habitually sleepy drivers have a high frequency of automobile crashes associated with respiratory disorders during sleep. *Am J Respir Crit Care Med*, 2000; **162**:1407–12.

37. **Lloberes P**, **Levy G**, **Descals C**, et al. Self-reported sleepiness while driving as a risk factor for traffic accidents in patients with obstructive sleep apnoea syndrome and in non-apnoeic snorers. *Respir Med*, 2000; **94**:971–76.

38. **Powell N B**, **Schechtman K B**, **Riley R W**, et al. Sleepy driver near-misses may predict accident risks. *Sleep*, 2007; **30**:331–42.

39. **Perez-Chada D**, **Videla A J**, **O'Flaherty M E**, et al. Sleep habits and accident risk among truck drivers: a cross-sectional study in Argentina. *Sleep*, 2005; **28**:1103–08.

40. **Pizza F**, **Contardi S**, **Mondini S**, et al. Daytime sleepiness and driving performance in patients with obstructive sleep apnea: comparison of the MSLT, the MWT, and a simulated driving task. *Sleep*, 2009; **32**:382–91.

41. **Turkington P M**, **Sircar M**, **Allgar V**, et al. Relationship between obstructive sleep apnoea, driving simulator performance, and risk of road traffic accidents. *Thorax*, 2001; **56**:800–05.

42. **Mulgrew A T**, **Nasvadi G**, **Butt A**, et al. Risk and severity of motor vehicle crashes in patients with obstructive sleep apnoea/hypopnoea. *Thorax*, 2008; **63**:536–41.

43. **Dagan Y**, **Doljansky J T**, **Green A**, et al. Body Mass Index (BMI) as a first-line screening criterion for detection of excessive daytime sleepiness among professional drivers. *Traffic Inj Prev*, 2006; **7**:44–48.

44. **Tippin J**, **Sparks J**, **Rizzo M**. Visual vigilance in drivers with obstructive sleep apnea. *J Psychosom Res*, 2009; **67**:143–51.

45. **Cluydts R**, **De Valck E**, **Verstraeten E**, et al. Daytime sleepiness and its evaluation. *Sleep Med Rev*, 2002; **6**:83–96.

46. **Mazza S**, **Pepin J L**, **Naegele B**, et al. Driving ability in sleep apnoea patients before and after CPAP treatment: evaluation on a road safety platform. *Eur Respir J*, 2006; **28**:1020–28.

47. **Philip P**, **Taillard J**, **Klein E**, et al. Effect of fatigue on performance measured by a driving simulator in automobile drivers. *J Psychosom Res*, 2003; **55**:197–200.

48. **Philip P**, **Sagaspe P**, **Taillard J**, et al. Fatigue, sleepiness, and performance in simulated versus real driving conditions. *Sleep*, 2005; **28**:1511–16.

49. **Sagaspe P**, **Taillard J**, **Chaumet G**, et al. Maintenance of wakefulness test as a predictor of driving performance in patients with untreated obstructive sleep apnea. *Sleep*, 2007; **30**:327–30.

50. **George C F**. Driving simulators in clinical practice. *Sleep Med Rev*, 2003; **7**:311–20.

51. **Philip P**, **Akerstedt T**. Transport and industrial safety, how are they affected by sleepiness and sleep restriction? *Sleep Med Rev*, 2006; **10**:347–56.

52. **Vakulin A**, **Baulk S D**, **Catcheside P G**, et al. Effects of alcohol and sleep restriction on simulated driving performance in untreated patients with obstructive sleep apnea. *Ann Intern Med*, 2009; **151**:447–55.

53. **Kapur V K**, **Resnick H E**, **Gottlieb D J**. Sleep disordered breathing and hypertension: does self-reported sleepiness modify the association? *Sleep*, 2008; **31**:1127–32.

54. **Choi J B**, **Nelesen R**, **Loredo J S**, et al. Sleepiness in obstructive sleep apnea: a harbinger of impaired cardiac function? *Sleep*, 2006; **29**:1531–36.

55. **Barcelo A**, **Barbe F**, **de la Pena M**, et al. Insulin resistance and daytime sleepiness in patients with sleep apnoea. *Thorax*, 2008; **63**:946–50.

56. **Ronksley P E**, **Hemmelgarn B R**, **Heitman S J**, et al. Obstructive sleep apnoea is associated with diabetes in sleepy subjects. *Thorax*, 2009; **64**:834–39.

57. **Empana J P**, **Dauvilliers Y**, **Dartigues J F**, et al. Excessive daytime sleepiness is an independent risk indicator for cardiovascular mortality in community-dwelling elderly: the three city study. *Stroke*, 2009; **40**:1219–24.

58. **Montserrat J M**, **Garcia-Rio F**, **Barbe F**. Diagnostic and therapeutic approach to nonsleepy apnea. *Am J Respir Crit Care Med*, 2007; **176**:6–9.

59. **Robinson G V**, **Langford B A**, **Smith D M**, et al. Predictors of blood pressure fall with continuous positive airway pressure (CPAP) treatment of obstructive sleep apnoea (OSA). *Thorax*, 2008; **63**:855–59.

60. **Robinson G V**, **Smith D M**, **Langford B A**, et al. Continuous positive airway pressure does not reduce blood pressure in nonsleepy hypertensive OSA patients. *Eur Respir J*, 2006; **27**:1229–35.

61. **Duran-Cantolla J**, **Aizpuru F**, **Martinez-Null C**, et al. Obstructive sleep apnea/hypopnea and systemic hypertension. *Sleep Med Rev*, 2009; **13**:323–31.

62. **Barbé F**, **Duran-Cantolla J**, **Capote F**, et al. Long-term effect of continuous positive airway pressure in hypertensive with sleep apnea. *AJRCCM*, 2010; **181**:718–26.

63. **McDaid C**, **Duree K H**, **Griffin S C**, et al. A systematic review of continuous positive airway pressure for obstructive sleep apnoea–hypopnoea syndrome. *Sleep Med Rev*, 2009; **13**:427–36.

64. **Santamaria J**, **Iranzo A**, **Ma Montserrat J**, et al. Persistent sleepiness in CPAP treated obstructive sleep apnea patients: evaluation and treatment. *Sleep Med Rev*, 2007; **11**:195–207.

65. **Guilleminault C**, **Philip P**. Tiredness and somnolence despite initial treatment of obstructive sleep apnea syndrome (what to do when an OSAS patient stays hypersomnolent despite treatment). *Sleep*, 1996; **19**(9 Suppl):S117–22.

66. **Pepin J L**, **Viot-Blanc V**, **Escourrou P**, et al. Prevalence of residual excessive sleepiness in CPAP-treated sleep apnoea patients: the French multicentre study. *Eur Respir J*, 2009; **33**:1062–67.

67. **Pack A I**, **Black J E**, **Schwartz J R**, et al. Modafinil as adjunct therapy for daytime sleepiness in obstructive sleep apnea. *Am J Respir Crit Care Med*, 2001; **164**:1675–81.

68. **Tonon C**, **Vetrugno R**, **Lodi R**, et al. Proton magnetic resonance spectroscopy study of brain metabolism in obstructive sleep apnoea syndrome before and after continuous positive airway pressure treatment. *Sleep*, 2007; **30**:305–11.

69. **Dinges D F**, **Weaver T E**. Effects of modafinil on sustained attention performance and quality of life in OSA patients with residual sleepiness while being treated with nCPAP. *Sleep Med*, 2003; **4**:393–402.

70. **Black J E**, **Hirshkowitz M**. Modafinil for treatment of residual excessive sleepiness in nasal continuous positive airway pressure-treated obstructive sleep apnea/hypopnea syndrome. *Sleep*, 2005; **28**:464–71.

71. **Kingshott R N**, **Engleman H M**, **Deary I J**, et al. Does arousal frequency predict daytime function? *Eur Respir J*, 1998; **12**:1264–70.

72. **Donadio V**, **Liguori R**, **Vetrugno R**, et al. Daytime sympathetic hyperactivity in OSAS is related to excessive daytime sleepiness. *J Sleep Res*, 2007; **16**:327–32.

Sleep Disorders and Excessive Sleepiness

Chapter 16: Daytime sleepiness in insomnia patients

Yinghui Low and Andrew D. Krystal

Introduction

Insomnia patients, by definition, have disturbed or non-restorative sleep, and sleep less on average than the general population in terms of both self-reported and objective polysomnographic measures [1–4]. As a result, it would be expected that insomnia patients suffer from at least some degree of sleep deprivation, and should thus have more daytime sleepiness than healthy controls. In this review we evaluate whether insomnia patients are, in fact, sleepier than healthy controls without insomnia.

Daytime sleepiness in insomnia patients vs. healthy controls

Self-report data

A series of studies have been carried out comparing insomnia patients and healthy controls without sleep complaints on measures of daytime sleepiness. All 3 studies in the elderly and 2 in college students detected self-reported sleepiness, whereas sleepiness was found in just 4 out of 10 studies of middle-aged adults with primary insomnia [4–19]. Nearly all of these studies were carried out with primary insomnia patients; however, two in middle-aged adults, one in older adults, and one in college-aged individuals included subjects with insomnia occurring comorbidly with other conditions. The measures used to assess sleepiness included the Stanford Sleepiness Scale [10, 19–21], the Epworth Sleepiness Scale (ESS) [9], and the vigor subscale of the Profile of Mood States [10–13, 15].

In addition, primary insomnia patients were found to have greater fatigue than good sleepers in four of six studies [6–13]. These findings may be relevant to the question of daytime sleepiness in insomnia patients, as it is not clear that fatigue and subjective sleepiness can be validly distinguished from each other. The most common fatigue scale used in these studies was the Fatigue Severity Scale (FSS).

Objective data

In stark contrast, no evidence of excessive daytime sleepiness (EDS) was found in all 10 studies employing the Multiple Sleep Latency Test (MSLT), a physiologic test of daytime sleepiness consisting of four nap opportunities ($N = 512$) [4, 8, 9, 19, 20, 22–25]. In fact, several studies found that insomnia patients were less sleepy than normal controls [9, 21, 22, 25]. This appears to be true for both primary insomnia and insomnia occurring comorbidly with other conditions, as half of these studies compared controls with primary insomnia patients and half with patients with comorbid insomnia [4, 10, 11, 14, 20–24, 26]. Thus, there is no evidence that insomnia patients manifest findings suggestive of daytime sleepiness with objective testing. If anything, they appear to be less sleepy than healthy controls. The absence of decreased sleep latency in the daytime, however, may reflect a general difficulty initiating sleep.

Effect of insomnia therapy on daytime sleepiness in insomnia patients

In order to further assess whether insomnia patients suffer from sleepiness, we assessed the extent to which treatments for insomnia improved some measure related to daytime sleepiness. Only 10 treatment studies reported an outcome measure relevant to daytime sleepiness (see Table 16.1). All of these were subjective measures of insomnia. In 9 out of 10 there was significant improvement in at least one such measure. This included four studies of the treatment of insomnia occurring comorbidly with other conditions [27–30].

Sleepiness: Causes, Consequences and Treatment, ed. Michael J. Thorpy and Michel Billiard. Published by Cambridge University Press. © Cambridge University Press 2011.

16. Daytime sleepiness in insomnia patients

Table 16.1 Summary of randomized, placebo-controlled studies that report daytime sleepiness-related outcomes in patients with primary insomnia

Reference	Sample size	Treatment (duration in weeks)	Outcome
Behavioral therapy studies			
Rybarczyk et al., 2005 [27]	46; age > 55 with medical disorders*	Classroom therapy: stimulus control, sleep restriction, cognitive restructuring, relaxation training, sleep hygiene education (8)	Active treatment was significantly better than the control in number of naps per week
	46; age > 55 with medical disorders*	Control therapy: classroom stress management and wellness training (8)	
Combined behavioral and pharmacotherapy studies			
Jacobs et al., 2004 [39]	14 Primary insomnia; Age 25–64	Stimulus control, sleep restriction, cognitive therapy, and relaxation training (6)	There were no differences between the groups in the effects of treatment on the fatigue and vigor scales of the Profile of Mood States (POMS) scale**
	13 Primary insomnia; Age 25–64	Zolpidem 10 mg nightly (4), then zolpidem 5 mg nightly (1), then zolpidem 5 mg every other night (1)	
	13 Primary insomnia; Age 25–64	The combination of the above 2 therapies (6)	
	14 Primary insomnia; Age 25–64	Placebo pill (6)	
Pharmacotherapy studies			
Krystal et al., 2008 [35]	669 Primary insomnia; Age 18–64	Intermittent (3–7 nights/week) zolpidem-MR 12.5 mg (24)	Likert ratings of morning sleepiness significantly better with zolpidem-MR than placebo; Epworth Sleepiness Scale improved with zolpidem-MR vs. placebo over double-blind treatment period.
	349 Primary insomnia; Age 18–64	Placebo (24)	
Krystal et al., 2003 [31]	593 Primary insomnia; Age 21–69	Eszopiclone 3 mg/night (24)	Eszopiclone better than placebo on Likert ratings of "daytime alertness", throughout 6 months
	195 Primary insomnia; Age 21–69	Placebo (24)	
McCall et al., 2006 [32]	136 Primary insomnia; Age 64–86	Eszopiclone 2mg/night (2)	Eszopiclone is significant vs. placebo for: 1. Reduction of morning sleepiness ratings (trend) 2. Number and cumulative duration (trend) of naps among those who napped 3. Vitality subscale of the SF-36. No difference in Likert ratings of "alertness".
	128 Primary insomnia; Age 64–86	Placebo (2)	
Scharf et al., 2005 [33]	79 Primary insomnia; Age 65–85	Eszopiclone 2 mg/night (2)	Eszopiclone is significant vs. placebo for: 1. Ratings of morning sleepiness, "daytime alertness". 2. Fewer naps and shorter nap duration in those who napped.
	80 Primary insomnia; Age 65–85	Placebo (2)	
Fava et al., 2006 [28]	275 Insomnia + MDD; Age 21–64	Fluoxetine 20–40 mg + eszopiclone 3 mg (8)	Eszopiclone is significant vs. placebo for ratings of "daytime alertness"
	270 Insomnia + MDD; Age 21–64	Fluoxetine 20–40 mg + placebo (8)	

(cont.)

Table 16.1 (cont.)

Reference	Sample size	Treatment (duration in weeks)	Outcome
Soares et al., 2006 [29]	201 Insomnia + menopausal symptoms; Age 40–60 209 Insomnia + menopausal symptoms; Age 40–60	Eszopiclone 3 mg (4) Placebo (4)	Eszopiclone is significant vs. placebo for ratings of "daytime alertness"
Pollack et al., 2008 [30]	301 Insomnia + GAD; Age 18–64 294 Insomnia + GAD; Age 18–64	Escitalopram 10 mg + eszopiclone 3 mg (8) Escitalopram 10 mg + placebo (8)	Eszopiclone is significant vs. placebo for ratings of "daytime alertness"
Walsh et al., 2007 [34]	548 Primary insomnia; Age 21–64 280 Primary insomnia; Age 21–64	Eszopiclone 3 mg/night (24) Placebo (24)	Eszopiclone better than placebo on the Epworth Sleepiness Scale, the Fatigue Severity Scale and the vitality subscale of the SF-36
Walsh et al., 2009 [38]	44 Primary insomnia; Age 65–86 53 Primary insomnia; Age 65–86 52 Primary insomnia; Age 65–86	Placebo (1) EVT201 1.5mg (1) EVT201 2.5mg (1)	EVT201 at 1.5 mg or 2.5 mg is significant vs. placebo for: 1. Longer mean MSLT latency on Day 8 (2 min) 2. No difference in POMS, PVT or RAVLT*** between groups

* Insomnia comorbid with either: osteoarthritis, coronary artery disease, or pulmonary disease.
** POMS, Profile of Mood States; SF-36, short form-36; MDD, Major Depressive Disorder; SSRI, Selective Serotonin Reuptake Inhibitor (in this study only paroxetine, fluoxetine, and sertraline).
*** PVT, psychomotor vigilance test.
RAVLT, Rey Auditory Verbal Learning Test.

Efficacy was found with eszopiclone (seven studies) [28–34], multicomponent cognitive–behavioral therapy (one study) [27], and intermittent dosing with zolpidem-MR (one study) [35]. It would be unreasonable to conclude that therapies which did not have a significant therapeutic effect on daytime sleepiness (see Table 16.1) lacked efficacy on this domain of function, as these studies were not powered to detect non-sleep effects, included relatively fewer subjects, and may not have included patients with sleepiness at baseline [26]. Further, no conclusions should be drawn based on whether studies included measures of daytime sleepiness, because we have no way to determine how often studies employed sleepiness measures but failed to report the findings when no significant improvements in these measures were found with treatment.

Behavioral therapy studies

A study of group multicomponent cognitive–behavioral therapy (stimulus control, sleep restriction, cognitive restructuring, relaxation training, and sleep hygiene education) employed stress management and wellness education as a control therapy, and was carried out in 92 older patients (age > 55) with insomnia occurring comorbidly with either osteoarthritis, coronary artery disease, or pulmonary disease [27]. The multicomponent cognitive–behavioral therapy had a significant advantage over the control therapy in decreasing number of naps per week.

Pharmacotherapy studies

In a 6-month placebo-controlled study of nightly dosing with 3 mg of eszopiclone (the (S)-isomer of zopiclone), efficacy in all measures of sleep [sleep onset latency (SOL), wake time after sleep onset (WASO), awakenings, total sleep time (TST), and quality] at each time point over the 6 months without tolerance was accompanied by significant improvement vs. placebo in self-ratings (0–10 scale) of "daytime alertness" [31]. These effects were sustained during an additional 6 months of open-label eszopiclone treatment which followed the 6-month placebo-controlled phase [36]. These findings were replicated in a second 6-month, randomized, double-blind study ($n = 828$) of eszopiclone 3 mg in adults [34]. However, that study included additional measures related to daytime sleepiness including the ESS, Fatigue Severity Scale (FSS) and the vitality subscale of the SF-36. All of these additional measures were significantly improved in eszopiclone-treated patients vs. placebo throughout the six-month placebo-controlled phase of the study.

In two 2-week studies in elderly patients, eszopiclone 2 mg improved polysomnographic (PSG) and self-reported SOL, WASO, TST, awakenings, and quality vs. placebo and also lowered self-reported morning sleepiness, and decreased the number and duration of naps [32, 33]. In one of the studies, eszopiclone led to greater "daytime alertness" [33]. In the other study, the eszopiclone group had significantly greater improvement than placebo in the vitality subscales of the SF-36 [32].

A 24-week study of 3–7 nights per week "as needed" dosing of zolpidem-MR 12.5 mg reported significant efficacy vs. placebo in ratings of ability to fall and stay asleep as well as global ratings of "morning sleepiness" [37, 38]. In addition, significantly less sleepiness as measured with the ESS was noted in zolpidem-MR-treated subjects compared with placebo over the double-blind treatment period [38].

One study examined the effects of including an insomnia therapy as part of the initial antidepressant regimen in 545 patients with insomnia comorbid with depression [28]. Subjects receiving eszopiclone 3 mg along with fluoxetine 20–40 mg had significantly greater improvement than placebo in sleep measures, non-sleep depression symptoms (measured with the Hamilton Depression Rating Scale), and self-rated "daytime alertness".

A similar study was carried out in patients with insomnia comorbid with generalized anxiety disorder which compared treatment with escitalopram plus eszopiclone 3 mg vs. escitalopram plus placebo [39]. In this study, those receiving escitalopram experienced statistically significantly greater improvement in sleep variables and non-sleep anxiety symptoms (measured with the Hamilton Anxiety Rating Scale) as well as self-rated "daytime alertness".

Greater self-rated daytime alertness was also found in a placebo-controlled trial of eszopiclone 3 mg in women in menopausal-associated insomnia [40]. This effect occurred in conjunction with significant effects on sleep and on sleep disturbance due to hot flushes.

Only one placebo-controlled trial of insomnia patients was carried out which included an objective measure of daytime sleepiness. This study was carried out in elderly patients and found that one week of treatment with an agent which modulates GABA receptor activity at the benzodiazepine binding site resulted in a significant increase in daytime sleep latency by MSLT (2 min, $p<0.03$) [41].

Combined behavioral and pharmacotherapy studies

In a 6-week study, 63 adults with sleep-onset insomnia were randomized to 4 groups, receiving either: cognitive–behavioral therapy (CBT), zolpidem in tapered doses, both CBT and zolpidem, or placebo with no CBT [42]. Sleep parameters were improved in all treatment groups compared to the controls; however, among the groups there was no difference in the pre- to post-treatment changes of fatigue or vigor scale (from the Profile of Mood States scale) results. The authors surmise that this could be a floor effect, since subjects only had moderate pathological levels of fatigue and vigor before treatment.

Discussion

Is insomnia associated with daytime sleepiness?

The current literature suggests that insomnia is frequently associated with greater self-reported daytime sleepiness than is seen in healthy individuals without sleep complaints. However, this is a consistent finding only in two subgroups of insomnia patients: the elderly, and college-aged, although relatively few studies have been carried out in these insomnia subgroups. In adults greater than college age and less than 65 years of age, significantly greater sleepiness compared with controls is inconsistently found, being reported in 4 out of 10 studies. Most of these studies were carried out with primary insomnia patients, so it remains unclear if daytime sleepiness is more commonly associated with comorbid insomnia.

On the other hand, studies measuring objective daytime sleepiness with the multiple sleep latency tests have consistently shown that both primary and comorbid insomnia patients do not have a greater daytime sleep tendency than healthy controls without sleep complaints. In several studies, insomnia patients appeared to be less sleepy than the general population. Thus, we must conclude that insomnia patients are *not* sleepier during the day than controls; however, some subgroups of insomnia patients clearly experience sleepiness during the day.

One explanation that has been proposed that might explain these findings is that insomnia patients have both some degree of daytime sleepiness that they can perceive, and an opposing hyperactivation which counteracts the sleepiness and prevents them from falling asleep when they try to during the day [43].

Insomnia as a 24-h state of hyperarousal

The inconsistent subjective daytime sleepiness, and the objective evidence of equal or less sleepiness in insomnia patients despite the sleep disturbance that characterizes this condition, is consistent with a series of physiologic observations suggesting the hypothesis that insomnia is a generalized state of 24-h hyperarousal [43]. Current evidence for heightened physiological arousal includes increased body temperatures, basal and cerebral metabolic rates, and increased peripheral cortisol and catecholamine levels compared with normal controls [44]. The origin of this hyperarousal remains unestablished. However, a number of hypotheses have been proposed, including genetic factors, an interaction of genetic factors and stress, and cognitive–behavioral responses to stress or sleep disturbance [35, 43, 45, 46]. Further work will be needed to determine whether the indices of hyperarousal observed in insomnia patients are related to the lack of objective sleepiness in insomnia patients and/or the lack of subjective sleepiness in many insomnia patients aged 18–65.

Differences in daytime sleepiness among insomnia subgroups

The reasons why subjective daytime sleepiness seems to be more consistently reported in college-age and older adult insomnia patients are unclear. There may be aspects of insomnia that are present in these groups that are not present or are present less often in insomnia patients aged 18–65.

One possible factor that might explain why reports of daytime sleepiness are relatively common in college-age insomnia patients is the tendency for there to be a delay in the circadian rhythm in this age group. The daytime sleepiness reported by college-aged insomnia patients could be a consequence of their tendency to stay up late and have sleep onset insomnia and the need to wake up for activities scheduled in the morning [45]. Further work will be needed to determine if this circadian tendency might explain the self-reported daytime sleepiness among college-age insomnia patients.

As with college-aged insomnia patients, the reasons why insomnia patients over the age of 65 tend to more consistently report daytime sleepiness than younger adult insomnia patients have not been established. One possibility that cannot be ruled out is that in the elderly, insomnia may be more often associated with comorbid conditions such as pain and acute or chronic diseases [46]. These comorbid conditions might cause sleep disturbance that is more like sleep deprivation than is typical of primary insomnia otherwise and might, therefore, be associated with more daytime sleepiness. While there is no doubt that medical and psychiatric comorbidities are common in older adults, it remains to be determined whether such comorbidities are associated with daytime sleepiness complaints in this population, as few studies comparing patients with comorbid insomnia and controls have been carried out.

Effect of insomnia therapy on daytime sleepiness in insomnia patients

Relatively few placebo-controlled trials of insomnia therapies (a total of 11) included outcome measures related to daytime sleepiness. However, among those 11, significant effects vs. placebo were noted in 10 studies. This included four studies of patients with insomnia occurring with comorbid conditions. Nearly all of the studies carried out assessed sleepiness with Likert ratings of morning sleepiness or daytime alertness. However, three studies noted a decrease in napping and two studies observed significant treatment effects using the Epworth Sleepiness Scale. These studies establish that it is possible for treatment to improve this domain of insomnia, and they provide some indication that subjective daytime sleepiness is a part of the insomnia syndrome at least to some degree.

Given that all of these studies were carried out in adults aged 18–65, it would appear that treatment studies may be more sensitive than comparisons with healthy non-complaining controls as a means of detecting self-reported daytime sleepiness in insomnia patients. Further studies will be needed to determine if this is, in fact, the case. One confounding factor is that the measures used in the treatment studies were not the same ones used in the studies comparing insomnia patients and control populations. Another factor that must be considered is that some of the treatment studies included substantially larger numbers of subjects than some of the comparisons of insomnia and control subjects. As a result, many of the treatment studies had power to detect much smaller effects on daytime sleepiness measures than the comparisons of insomnia patients and controls.

None the less, the findings from treatment studies provide some evidence that there is some degree of self-reported daytime sleepiness in insomnia patients that can be improved with treatment. Only one treatment study has been carried out with an objective measure of insomnia, and this demonstrated a significant effect on the MSLT with therapy. Further studies of the treatment of insomnia using objective outcome measures of daytime sleepiness are clearly warranted.

Summary

Despite the fact that insomnia is characterized by sleep disturbance, studies comparing insomnia patients and healthy controls without sleep complaints suggest that daytime sleepiness is inconsistently reported by insomnia patients. These studies also suggest that daytime sleepiness seems to be a more consistent complaint of college-aged insomnia patients and those over age 65.

More work is needed to determine why subgroups of insomnia patients may be more likely to experience daytime sleepiness and to determine why there is a mismatch between findings when using self-reported and objective measures of daytime sleepiness. Some have hypothesized that this mismatch reflects a hyperarousal state in insomnia that prevents the daytime sleepiness that they experience from becoming manifest in objective daytime sleepiness. There is no direct evidence that this is the case; however, exploring the source of this mismatch will be a fruitful area for future research.

Lastly, the findings of treatment studies provide preliminary evidence that insomnia patients have some degree of daytime sleepiness that can be improved with treatment. These studies provide an additional indication that insomnia patients experience subjective daytime sleepiness and speak to the need for more treatment studies employing objective measures of daytime sleepiness. These studies also suggest the importance of assessing self-reported daytime sleepiness in insomnia treatment studies and when judging the outcome of insomnia therapy in clinical practice.

Acknowledgments

Dr. Krystal would like to disclose research grant and/or consulting support from the following for grants/research support: NIH, Sanofi-Aventis, Cephalon, GlaxoSmithKline, Merck, Neurocrine, Pfizer, Sepracor, Somaxon, Takeda, Transcept, Respironics, Neurogen, Evotec, Astellas, Abbott, Actelion, Arena, Axiom, AstraZeneca, BMS, Eli Lilly, Jazz, Johnson and Johnson, Novartis, Organon, Ortho-McNeil-Janssen, Roche, Kingsdown Inc.

References

1. **Hauri P J**, **Wisbey J**. Wrist actigraphy in insomnia. *Sleep*, 1992; **15**:293–301.
2. **Brezinova V**, **Oswald I**, **Loudon J**. Two types of insomnia: too much waking or not enough sleep. *Br J Psychiatry*, 1975; **126**:439–45.
3. **Zorick F J**, **Roth T**, **Hartze K M**, *et al*. Evaluation and diagnosis of persistent insomnia. *Am J Psychiatry*, 1981; **138**:769–73.
4. **Mendelson W B**, **Garnett D**, **Gillin J C**, *et al*. The experience of insomnia and daytime and nighttime functioning. *Psychiatry Res*, 1984; **12**:235–50.
5. **Liu X**, **Uchiyama M**, **Kim K**, *et al*. Sleep loss and daytime sleepiness in the general adult population of Japan. *Psychiatry Res*, 2000; **93**:1–11.
6. **Fichten C S**, **Creti L**, **Amsel R**, *et al*. Poor sleepers who do not complain of insomnia: myths and realities about psychological and lifestyle characteristics of older good and poor sleepers. *J Behav Med*, 1995; **18**:189–223.
7. **Means M K**, **Lichstein K L**, **Epperson M T**, *et al*. Relaxation therapy for insomnia: nighttime and day time effects. *Behav Res Ther*, 2000; **38**: 665–78.
8. **Seidel W F**, **Ball S**, **Cohen S**, *et al*. Daytime alertness in relation to mood, performance, and nocturnal sleep in chronic insomniacs and noncomplaining sleepers. *Sleep*, 1984; **7**:230–38.
9. **Bonnet M H**, **Arand D L**. 24-Hour metabolic rate in insomniacs and matched normal sleepers. *Sleep*, 1995; **18**:581–88.
10. **Krupp L B**, **LaRocca N G**, **Muir-Nash J**, *et al*. The fatigue severity scale. Application to patients with

multiple sclerosis and systemic lupus erythematosus. *Arch Neurol*, 1989; **46**:1121–23.

11. **Hauri P**, **Fisher J**. Persistent psychophysiologic (learned) insomnia. *Sleep*, 1986; **9**:38–53.

12. **Lichstein K L**, **Means M K**, **Noe S L**, *et al*. Fatigue and sleep disorders. *Behav Res Ther*, 1997; **35**:733–40.

13. **McNair D M**, **Lorr M**, **Droppleman L F**. *Manual for the Profile of Mood States*. San Diego, CA: Educational and Industrial Testing Service, 1971.

14. **Nugent A M**, **Gleadhill I**, **McCrum E**, *et al*. Sleep complaints and risk factors for excessive daytime sleepiness in adult males in Northern Ireland. *J Sleep Res*, 2001; **10**:69–74.

15. **Hauri P J**. Cognitive deficits in insomnia patients. *Acta Neurol Belg*, 1997; **97**:113–17.

16. **Lichstein K L**, **Johnson R S**, **Sen Gupta S**, *et al*. Are insomniacs sleepy during the day? A pupillometric assessment. *Behav Res Ther*, 1992; **30**:283–92.

17. **Riedel B W**, **Lichstein K L**, **Dwyer W O**. Sleep compression and sleep education for older insomniacs: self-help versus therapist guidance. *Psychol Aging*, 1995; **10**:54–63.

18. **Schneider-Helmert D**. Twenty-four-hour sleep–wake function and personality patterns in chronic insomniacs and healthy controls. *Sleep*, 1987; **10**:452–62.

19. **Lichstein K L**, **Wilson N M**, **Noe S L**, *et al*. Daytime sleepiness in insomnia: behavioral, biological and subjective indices. *Sleep*, 1994; **17**:693–702.

20. **Edinger J D**, **Fins A I**, **Sullivan R J**, Jr, *et al*. Do our methods lead to insomniacs' madness? Daytime testing after laboratory and home-based polysomnographic studies. *Sleep*, 1997; **20**:1127–34.

21. **Stepanski E**, **Zorick F**, **Roehrs T**, *et al*. Daytime alertness in patients with chronic insomnia compared with asymptomatic control subjects. *Sleep*, 1988; **11**:54–60.

22. **Edinger J D**, **Glenn D M**, **Bastian L A**, *et al*. Daytime testing after laboratory or home-based polysomnography: comparisons of middle-aged insomnia sufferers and normal sleepers. *J Sleep Res*, 2003; **12**:43–52.

23. **Pedrosi B**, **Rosenthal L**, **Fortier J**, *et al*. Daytime function and benzodiazepine effects in insomniacs compared to normals. *Sleep Res*, 1995; **24**:48.

24. **Stepanski E**, **Lamphere J**, **Badia P**, *et al*. Sleep fragmentation and daytime sleepiness. *Sleep*, 1984; **7**:18–26.

25. **Edinger J D**, **Means M K**, **Carney C E**, *et al*. Psychomotor performance deficits and their relation to prior nights' sleep among individuals with primary insomnia. *Sleep*, 2008; **31**:599–607.

26. **Krystal A R J**, **Caron J**. Efficacy of eszopiclone in the treatment of sleep maintenance insomnia: a subset analysis by baseline wake after sleep onset (WASO). *Sleep*, 2004; **27**:57.

27. **Rybarczyk B**, **Stepanski E**, **Fogg L**, *et al*. A placebo-controlled test of cognitive–behavioral therapy for comorbid insomnia in older adults. *J Consult Clin Psychol*, 2005; **73**:1164–74.

28. **Fava M**, **McCall W V**, **Krystal A**, *et al*. Eszopiclone co-administered with fluoxetine in patients with insomnia coexisting with major depressive disorder. *Biol Psychiatry*, 2006; **59**:1052–60.

29. **Soares C**, **Joffe H**, **Rubens R**, *et al*. Eszopiclone in patients with insomnia during perimenopause and early postmenopause: a randomized controlled trial. *Obstet Gynecol*, 2006; **108**:1402–10.

30. **Pollack M**, **Kinrys G**, **Krystal A**, *et al*. Eszopiclone co-administered with escitalopram in patients with insomnia and comorbid generalized anxiety disorder. *Arch Gen Psychiatry*, 2008; **65**:551–62.

31. **Krystal A D**, **Walsh J K**, **Laska E**, *et al*. Sustained efficacy of eszopiclone over 6 months of nightly treatment: results of a randomized, double-blind, placebo-controlled study in adults with chronic insomnia. *Sleep*, 2003; **26**:793–99.

32. **McCall W V**, **Erman M**, **Krystal A D**, *et al*. A polysomnography study of eszopiclone in elderly patients with insomnia. *Curr Med Res Opin*, 2006; **22**:1633–42.

33. **Scharf M**, **Erman M**, **Rosenberg R**, *et al*. A 2-week efficacy and safety study of eszopiclone in elderly patients with primary insomnia. *Sleep*, 2005; **28**:720–27.

34. **Walsh J K**, **Krystal A D**, **Amato D A**, *et al*. Nightly treatment of primary insomnia with eszopiclone for six months: effect on sleep, quality of life, and work limitations. *Sleep*, 2007; **30**:959–68.

35. **Krystal A D**, **Erman M**, **Zammit G K**, *et al*. Long-term efficacy and safety of zolpidem extended-release 12.5 mg, administered 3 to 7 nights per week for 24 weeks, in patients with chronic primary insomnia: a 6-month, randomized, double-blind, placebo-controlled, parallel-group, multicenter study. *Sleep*, 2008; **31**:79–90.

36. **Roth T**, **Walsh J K**, **Krystal A**, *et al*. An evaluation of the efficacy and safety of eszopiclone over 12 months in patients with chronic primary insomnia. *Sleep Med*, 2005; **6**:487–95.

37. **Krystal A D**, **P M**, **McCall W V**, **Zammitt G**, *et al*. Three-month non-nightly use of zolpidem for the treatment of primary insomnia. *Sleep*, 2002; 25 (Suppl): A68.

38. **Walsh J K**, **Salkeld L**, **Knowles L J**, *et al*. Treatment of elderly primary insomnia patients with EVT 201 improves sleep initiation, sleep maintenance, and daytime sleepiness. *Sleep Med* 2010; **11**:7–8.

39. **Jacobs G D**, **Pace-Schott E F**, **Stickgold R**, *et al*. Cognitive behavior therapy and pharmacotherapy for insomnia: a randomized controlled trial and direct comparison. *Arch Intern Med*, 2004; **164**:1888–96.

40. **Riemann D**, **Spiegelhalder K**, **Feige B**, *et al*. The hyperarousal model of insomnia: a review of the concept and its evidence. *Sleep Med Rev.* 2010; **14**:19–31.

41. **Shekleton J A**, **Rogers N L**, **Rajaratnam S M**. Searching for the daytime impairments of primary insomnia. *Sleep Med Rev* 2010; **14**:47–60.

42. **Brummett B**, **Krystal A D**, **Siegler I C**, *et al*. Associations of a regulatory polymorphism of monoamine oxidase-A gene promoter (MAOA-uVNTR) with symptoms of depression and sleep quality. *Psychosomatic Med*, 2007; **69**:396–401.

43. **Drake C**, **Richardson G**, **Roehrs T**, *et al*. Vulnerability to stress-related sleep disturbance and hyperarousal. *Sleep*, 2004; **27**:285–91.

44. **Brummett B**, **Krystal A D**, **Ashley-Koch A**, *et al*. Sleep quality varies as a function of 5-HTTLPR genotype and stress. *Psychosom Med*, 2007; **69**:285–91.

45. **Calamaro C J**, **Mason T B**, **Ratcliffe S J**. Adolescents living the 24/7 lifestyle: effects of caffeine and technology on sleep duration and daytime functioning. *Pediatrics*, 2009, **123**;e1005–10.

46. **Fetveit A**. Late-life insomnia: a review. *Geriatr Gerontol Int*, 2009; **9**:220–34.

Section 2 Chapter 17

Sleep Disorders and Excessive Sleepiness

Sleepiness in advanced and delayed sleep phase disorders

Scott S. Campbell and Patricia J. Murphy

Introduction

Excessive sleepiness is often considered one of the defining characteristics of the class of sleep disorders referred to as "circadian rhythm sleep disorders", and is noted as a chief complaint of individuals who are eventually diagnosed with such a disorder. Such sleepiness is the consequence of a misalignment between the endogenous circadian clock and schedules imposed by society. This desynchronization between internal and external clocks can affect alertness levels in two ways. First, because the circadian clock governs the timing of sleep and alertness, a misalignment between the clock and societal schedules can result in the "sleepy" portion of the circadian cycle occurring at times typically associated with active wakefulness.

Second, a misalignment between the endogenous pacemaker and external demands can result in truncated sleep periods, leading to insufficient sleep durations and the accumulation of chronic sleep debt which, in turn, results in increased sleepiness during one's waking hours. Additionally, there is growing evidence that circadian desynchronization may not be the sole determinant of sleepiness in circadian rhythm sleep disorders. Independent of the circadian timing system, the homeostatic regulation of sleep, sleepiness, and alertness may be disrupted in these patients, as well. One consequence would be fragmented, disturbed, and non-restorative sleep, which would result in sleepiness during the daytime hours.

Perhaps surprisingly, very few systematically collected data are available in the literature, examining either subjective (e.g. visual analogue scales) or objective (e.g. multiple sleep latency tests (MSLTs)) sleepiness in those with circadian rhythm sleep disorders. The aim of this chapter is to characterize this often problematic, and sometimes debilitating, symptom in two of the most common circadian rhythm sleep disorders – Advanced and Delayed Sleep Phase Disorder (ASPD and DSPD). We will explore the likely causes of the sleepiness associated with the disorders and then briefly discuss approaches to managing sleepiness in the disorders. We begin, however, with a brief introduction to circadian rhythm sleep disorders in general, and to ASPD and DSPD in particular.

Circadian rhythm sleep disorders

Since the first studies of humans in time-free environments, it has been recognized that the timing of major nighttime sleep is governed in large part by the endogenous circadian pacemaker [1, 2]. The dependence of sleep on the biological clock is reflected in the characteristic temporal relationship between sleep propensity and the circadian rhythm of body core temperature. When subjects are studied in environments free of time cues, the onset of major sleep episodes tends to occur in close proximity to the trough of body temperature [3, 4].

Under the entrained conditions of normal daily life, this relationship is altered somewhat, such that major nocturnal sleep is typically initiated five to six hours prior to the temperature minimum and is terminated shortly after the minimum. For most people, this corresponds roughly to sleep onset times of between 11pm and midnight, and wake-up times of between about 6am and 8am. Undoubtedly, because the vast majority of humans exhibit similar timing in sleep–wake behavior, societal demands have evolved to accommodate such biological timetables.

For a small percentage of the population, however, there is a misalignment between the endogenous clock that governs the timing of sleep and the sleep–wake

---

Sleepiness: Causes, Consequences and Treatment, ed. Michael J. Thorpy and Michel Billiard. Published by Cambridge University Press. © Cambridge University Press 2011.

schedule that is desired, or which is regarded as the societal norm. These individuals are said to have circadian rhythm sleep disorders [5, 6]. This class of sleep disorders can be grouped further into two general categories – extrinsic and intrinsic types. Although the current International Classification for Sleep Disorders no longer formally distinguishes between the two, the differentiation is, nevertheless, useful for descriptive purposes. Extrinsic types are those in which the development of the disorder is brought on by an alteration in the environment relative to sleep timing: for example, jet lag, or shift work sleep disorder. Intrinsic types, on the other hand, occur as a result of the endogenous clock being altered relative to the (social) environment. The two most common disorders in this latter category are Delayed and Advanced Sleep Phase Disorders.

Delayed Sleep Phase Disorder (DSPD)

DSPD is probably the most common of the intrinsic circadian sleep disorders, or at least the most commonly diagnosed. Estimates of its prevalence average 0.15% of the population, or approximately 3 in 2000 persons [7, 8]. Based on an early survey, it was estimated that approximately 7% of people diagnosed with disorders of initiating and maintaining sleep meet criteria for DSPD [9]. The average DSPD patient has been reported to be younger than the average non-selected sample of insomniac patients, and many report having experienced the disorder since childhood [7–11].

Of note is that the "adolescent form" of sleep delay, which is associated with a biological shift in circadian rhythms at puberty, occurs in approximately 9% of adolescents [10]. However, this change in sleep timing often remits in young adulthood [12–15], and thus is likely a phenomenon distinct from DSPD. In support of this notion is that apparently only about 1% of adolescents with a sleep delay meet diagnostic criteria for DSPD [13]. In a sample of 14 adult cases studied in depth by Ito and co-workers [16], the mean age of onset was 20.9 years: on average, another 6 years passed before patients sought treatment for the disorder. As would be expected, DSPD patients typically score as "owls", or extreme evening types on morningness–eveningness scales [17–19].

Although the disorder was formally proposed as a clinical entity in 1981 [9], its existence has been known for over a century [20, 21]. Prior to the recognition of DSPD as a discrete disorder, sufferers were typically diagnosed with "sleep onset insomnia" since their major complaint was often an inability to fall asleep at conventional bedtimes. Even today, one criterion for differential diagnosis of DSPD is that the case "does not meet criteria for any other sleep disorder causing inability to initiate sleep or excessive sleepiness." Although the disorder apparently is not gender-specific in adulthood (for example, in the sample studied by Weitzman et al. [9] there were 15 men and 15 women, and in a group of DSPD patients studied by Regestein and Monk [20], there were 19 men and 14 women), there is some evidence for a predominance among males in younger samples.

Clinical depression is exhibited by approximately half those with DSPD [6, 13, 15, 22]. This percentage is similar to those with other forms of insomnia. A recent review also found that bipolar depression is only rarely observed in those with DSPD [18]. However, personality disorders are diagnosed more frequently in those with DSPD compared with other sleep disorder populations, including ASPD [12, 15].

However, unlike individuals who suffer from non-24-h sleep–wake syndrome (see below), case reports of DSPD sufferers reveal that while the disorder is certainly inconvenient and disruptive, it is often less debilitating than other sleep disorders. In many cases, individuals with DSPD are able to schedule their work, school and social lives to accommodate the disorder [see, for example, 9]. Nevertheless, there is at least one instance reported in the literature in which such accommodation was impossible. In this case, criminal proceedings were undertaken against a US Marine Corps lance corporal with DSPD because he could not comply with the schedule of military duty ("failure to go") [23].

In DSPD, the major sleep episode is delayed relative to the desired clock time, resulting in symptoms of sleep-onset insomnia and/or difficulty in awakening at the desired time [5, 6]. DSPD patients typically report an inability to fall asleep before about 2am, and may experience difficulties with sleep onset until as late as 6am.

The criteria employed to diagnose the disorder indicate that when not required to maintain a usual schedule (i.e. awaken early for work or school) but rather are permitted to sleep when they desire, DSPD patients exhibit uninterrupted sleep of normal composition, duration and quality. Yet, the few published reports of polysomnographically recorded sleep in DSPD do not support such a characterization. For example, in their initial description of the disorder, Weitzman and co-workers reported polysomnographic sleep measures in six individuals diagnosed with DSPD. With sleep times scheduled to correspond to subjects' preferred sleep times (average bedtime: 0404h), the investigators reported an average sleep efficiency of only 80% and an average sleep onset latency of 41 min [9].

Thorpy *et al.* [11] reported similar results for 9 adolescent DSPD patients (mean sleep latency: 51.9 min; mean sleep efficiency: 83.9%) and Watanabe and co-workers [24] observed significantly longer sleep onset latencies, more wakefulness after sleep onset and reduced sleep efficiency, and altered distribution of slow-wave sleep (SWS), in 11 DSPD patients sleeping at their habitual (i.e. self-selected) sleep times, when compared to age-matched controls. Similarly, in a case study of DSPD in temporal isolation, we observed longer sleep latency, poorer sleep efficiency, and altered distribution of SWS within sleep episodes initiated and terminated at the discretion of the subject when compared to normal subjects studied under identical conditions [25].

Advanced Sleep Phase Disorder (ASPD)

In ASPD, an individual's circadian sleep tendency is advanced relative to the (societally) desired clock time. This results in symptoms of compelling evening sleepiness, an early sleep onset, and a terminal awakening that is earlier than desired [5, 6]. The disorder is considered to be far less common than DSPD. Indeed, Weitzman *et al.* wrote in 1981 that "there is no clear evidence as yet that there is an advanced sleep phase syndrome" [9, p. 403], and as recently as 1986, its very designation as a pathologic syndrome was still uncertain [26]. Although it is still included in the current ICSD as a type of circadian rhythm sleep disorder, it is considered extremely rare. For example, an epidemiological survey of 10,000 Norwegian adults failed to detect a single case of ASPD [7]. More recently, a handful of families with pedigrees of ASPD have been identified [27, 28].

The fact that the disorder went unrecognized for so long is not entirely surprising. The very symptoms that define ASPD – "early to bed and early to rise" – have, for generations, constituted a philosophy to live by, rather than a disorder to treat. Simply, ASPD may be more easily accommodated by societal norms, and therefore, less likely to be a source of disturbance or complaint.

In contrast to DSPD, which is often characterized by onset in childhood or adolescence (see above), advanced sleep phase syndrome is most frequently reported by middle-aged and older subjects. The late age of onset of ASPS may account, in part, for the presumed rarity of the disorder. Since its very designation as a circadian rhythm sleep disorder stipulates that ASPD is the expression of an altered circadian system, the changes in sleep associated with aging would not have met criteria for diagnosis as ASPD until they were linked to age-related changes in the circadian system.

Although Weitzman *et al.* speculated in 1981 that many older individuals may have advanced sleep phase syndrome [9], such an association was not clearly elucidated until quite recently [29–32]. As such, the large proportion of older individuals who exhibit sleep patterns consistent with ASPD would have been excluded from such a diagnosis.

The earliest case described as ASPD leaves questions concerning the actual nature of the disorder reported [33]. Under entrained conditions, this patient reported habitual bedtimes and rising times of around 2100 h and 0600 h, respectively. Particularly with regard to wake-up time, this is not drastically different from that reported by many normal sleepers with job commitments. A second case report was characterized by features that more closely conform to current criteria for diagnosis of ASPD [34]. The 62-year-old male patient had difficulty maintaining wakefulness in the afternoon and early evening, reporting a usual bedtime of around 1830 h. He would sleep soundly until around 0300 h, when he would awaken alert and refreshed. Although circadian measures (e.g. round-the-clock body core temperature) were not obtained to confirm a phase advance of the biological timing system, and although the case was complicated by the presence of sleep apnea, the authors reported resolution of the problem following chronotherapy (see below).

As mentioned, a number of investigators have recently reported age-related changes in the circadian timing system that may be associated with the sleep patterns often observed in older subjects. The most consistently reported circadian change is a phase advance in various circadian rhythms, including body core temperature [29–32, 35] and melatonin [36–38]. Earlier and more variable bedtimes and rising times, and difficulty maintaining sleep in the second half of the night are the most prominent features of age-related sleep disturbance. This combination of a phase advanced circadian system and an apparent shift in sleep tendency to an earlier clock time may be interpreted to suggest that many middle-aged and older individuals suffer from ASPD.

Sleepiness in DSPD and ASPD – contributing factors

Circadian misalignment

As may be expected in a disorder characterized by the misalignment between the endogenous circadian timing system and societal norms, individuals with ASPD and DSPD often experience reduced levels of alertness at times generally not associated with sleepiness. In the case of DSPD, excessive sleepiness may be experienced for several hours after awakening from a night's sleep, a period typically associated with the highest alertness levels of the day. By the same token, ASPD sufferers often report difficulty maintaining alertness in the early evening which, in normal individuals, includes an approximately 2-h interval often referred to as the "forbidden zone" or "maintenance of wakefulness zone" for sleep [39, 40], based on the finding that it is virtually impossible for healthy adults to initiate sleep at that phase of the circadian cycle. Indeed, a report on three kindreds with ASPD confirmed that these individuals tended to initiate sleep during this time when allowed to sleep at their chosen times [27].

Truncated sleep duration

While there is little doubt that a primary factor underlying such intervals of sleepiness is the circadian timing system itself, there is also little question that the disturbed sleep experienced by DSPD and ASPD sufferers, when trying to conform to societal norms, contributes to their difficulties in maintaining alertness. Difficulties initiating sleep in DSPD and the inability to maintain sleep in ASPD both lead to truncated sleep times [13, 14, 18, 20, 24, 41, 42]. If such shortened sleep episodes continue over a period of days or weeks, the resulting chronic sleep restriction would likely exacerbate the level of sleepiness resulting strictly from circadian misalignment.

"Disordered" sleep

If disturbed nighttime sleep is a contributing factor to the excessive daytime sleepiness reported by many DSPD and ASPD sufferers, one might expect these patients to exhibit difficulty maintaining alertness at times not anchored to a limited portion of the circadian cycle. Such sleepiness would be akin to that observed in disorders such as sleep apnea, in which fragmented nighttime sleep with frequent arousals results in non-restorative sleep and problematic daytime sleepiness.

To our knowledge, however, this issue has rarely been addressed. With regard to whether nighttime sleep in DSPD or ASPD is disturbed, even when it occurs at self-selected times, the evidence is inconsistent. As mentioned, the few reports based on polysomnographic recordings have indicated that sleep is in fact disturbed in DSPD compared to controls [18, 24, 42, 43]. However, a recent study utilizing actigraphy records from a large sample of DSPD and control subjects found no differences in sleep duration or sleep efficiency between groups [44].

Whether daytime sleepiness throughout the waking hours is observed in DSPD or ASPD patients has not yet been adequately characterized. Indeed, we were able to find only two studies in which either subjective or objective assessments of sleepiness, such as visual analogue scales or sleep latency tests, have been obtained periodically throughout the day in individuals with DSPD or ASPD. Studying a group of adolescents with DSPD, Thorpy and co-workers [11] reported that although 82% of their subjects complained of tiredness throughout the day, MSLT sleep latencies were actually longer than those reported for a group of normal adolescents [45], suggesting that the DSPD subjects were, on average, less sleepy. Jones and co-workers [27] carried out MSLTs in 6 individuals with ASPD and 6 normal controls. While it seems that the tests were conducted primarily to rule out narcolepsy and other disorders of excessive daytime sleepiness, the authors found no differences in average latencies between the two groups.

In addition to these two studies, Kripke and co-workers [18] employed actigraphy to examine sleep patterns in a large group of DSPD subjects, including the occurrence of naps. They found that "the DSPD data included daytime sleep and 'naps'" and that many subjects "appeared to nap at all times of day". In contrast, a representative sample from the community "had little sleep out of bed." While this clearly suggests that DSPD subjects may have had higher levels of sleepiness than normals, the authors provide no further details regarding the naps.

In contrast to these findings, the only published case of DSPD studied in temporal isolation [25], we saw little indication that the subject experienced difficulty maintain alertness during his subjective daytime. That is, under conditions in which he was permitted sleep whenever inclined to do so throughout the 14-day protocol (including specific instructions to nap if so inclined), the subject showed no such inclination. This, despite the fact that he continued to exhibit significantly disturbed sleep relative to age-matched norms. Since that report, we have collected data on several additional individuals with DSPD under the same conditions (unpublished) and their PSG records support the virtual absence of napping in this group.

A recent model of human sleep propensity throughout the daytime hours may be relevant to the issue of sleepiness in circadian rhythm sleep disorders. In a simplified variant of the two-process model of sleep regulation, Bes and colleagues found that the well-characterized increase in sleep propensity in the afternoon hours could be accurately modeled by multiplying sleep drive (Process S) by a modified circadian process derived from REM sleep propensity (Process R) [46]. Their model fit experimental data showing the circadian propensity for nighttime sleep, as well as the afternoon nap phase, and evening "forbidden zone."

Germane to the current topic, model simulations in which the timing of the major nocturnal sleep period was altered indicated that the nap phase would be attenuated, or disappear altogether, when the nighttime sleep period was delayed. In contrast, the model suggests, the propensity for daytime sleep would be increased when the nighttime sleep period is advanced. The authors provided evidence for the validity of their model by describing experimental evidence in morning and evening types that matched the model's predictions. However, whether daytime sleep propensity is exacerbated in ASPD, or attenuated in DSPD, remains to be tested systematically.

Treatment of sleepiness in DSPD and ASPD

There are two general approaches to treating sleepiness in DSPD and ASPD. The one that has received the majority of attention seeks to correct the misalignment between the internal clock and societal demands by using various means to reset the circadian timing system. In so doing, it is assumed that portions of the circadian cycle associated with reduced alertness will be more appropriately placed within the 24-h day. An alternative approach does not address the underlying causes of the reduced alertness, but rather uses various techniques to mask periods of unwanted sleepiness. The following section briefly summarizes these two intervention techniques.

Chronotherapy

In this behavioral approach to realigning the endogenous timing system to the 24-h day, bedtimes and rising times are systematically delayed over a period of days until the desired bedtime is achieved. The first such chronotherapy intervention was accomplished by delaying bedtimes for 3 h each night for several consecutive nights [21]. Incremental delays, rather than advances, were selected to take advantage of the fact that most humans exhibit endogenous periods of slightly longer than 24 h, and therefore have a natural tendency to delay. Moreover, a delay in bedtime necessarily increased prior wakefulness, thereby enhancing the likelihood of relatively rapid sleep onset at the new bedtime.

Once achieved, strict adherence to the new sleep–wake schedule is critical to maintaining a positive outcome. Based on subjective reports and sleep logs, Czeisler and co-workers reported "significant and lasting resolution" in all five cases of DSPD studied [21]. Other investigators have reported less success than this original study (see for example [14, 47]), and it should be pointed out, as well, that resolution of the delayed circadian phase in the Czeisler et al. study did not result in improved sleep. In fact, sleep efficiencies did not change following chronotherapy when compared to pre-treatment levels, remaining well below 90% on average.

However, the lack of improvement in sleep quality may not be the most serious problem with chronotherapy. The initial process of realigning the sleep–wake schedule with conventional clock time is demanding, and subsequent compliance is critical. Indeed, the authors hypothesized that a delay in scheduled bedtime for even a single night (e.g. a weekend social engagement) could result in a relapse of symptoms, thus requiring re-implementation of the round-the-clock delaying routine. Few people are willing, or able, to maintain prolonged, strict sleep–wake schedules necessary to make this treatment work.

It is this aspect of the intervention that prohibited Thorpy and co-workers from attempting the chronotherapy routine in their sample of adolescent DSPD patients [11]. Additionally, there is some evidence that the treatment itself may lead to the development of a more debilitating form of circadian rhythm sleep disorder in some patients. Oren and Wehr [48] cite three cases in which the development of Non-24-hour Sleep/Wake Disorder appeared to be the direct consequence of treating DSPD with chronotherapy.

Light treatment

The demonstration in the mid 1980s that timed bright light exposure could be used to effectively reset the human endogenous pacemaker opened the possibility that this procedure may be beneficial in the treatment of DSPD. Rosenthal *et al.* [49] found that a combination of morning bright light exposure (2500 lux for 2 h between 6 and 9am) and afternoon/evening light avoidance phase advanced DSPS patients' temperature minima by an average of 1.45 h. The phase advance was associated with enhanced morning alertness, as measured by sleep latency tests, and by subjective reports of consistently earlier bedtimes. It should be noted that in this study a more liberal set of criteria for the diagnosis of DSPD was employed. For example, individuals who reported usual sleep times as early as 1am and an inability to be alert in the morning between 7am and 9am were included. A substantially greater phase advance would likely be required to alleviate symptoms in more severe cases of DSPD.

Several investigators have reported results that may be relevant to treating sleepiness in ASPD. We compared the effects of evening bright light exposure (~4000 lux for 2 h) with a dim red light control condition (<50 lux for 2 h), in older subjects with sleep maintenance insomnia and significant phase advances of the circadian system [30]. Following 12 consecutive days of treatment, subjects in the bright light condition exhibited a significant increase in sleep efficiency (baseline: 77.5%; post-treatment: 90.1%), the result of an average 1-h decline in wakefulness within the night. In contrast, those receiving dim light exposure showed no significant change in sleep efficiency, wakefulness within sleep, or any other sleep parameter measured.

Similar findings were reported by Lack and Schumacher [50] using exposure to evening bright light in a group of early morning awakening insomniacs. In that study, subjects were exposed to either 4 h of evening bright light (2500 lux), or dim red light (200 lux), for two consecutive days (2000–2400 h on the first night, 2100–0100 h on the second). Bright light produced improvements in sleep, as measured by wrist actigraphy and subjective assessment. Self-reported sleep duration increased significantly, whereas, actigraph movement time in the first 6 h of sleep declined significantly following treatment. The dim light group showed no such changes in sleep measures. The same results were obtained in a subsequent study of nine subjects with early morning awakening insomnia [37]. Following two consecutive days of bright light exposure (2500 lux from 2000 h to 2400 h), actigraphically measured total sleep time increased by an average of 1.2 h.

In all three studies described above, improvement in sleep was accompanied by significant delays in the circadian course of body core temperature. We observed an average phase delay of 3.1 h following treatment. Lack and Schumacher observed phase delays in the temperature minimum of 3–4 h, and Lack and Wright [37] reported an average delay of 1.85 h. Although we found no significant change in the average ability of subjects to maintain wakefulness throughout the day (using the Repeated Test of Sustained Wakefulness), it should be pointed out that these older subjects were not excessively sleepy at baseline. We should also emphasize that all subjects were able to maintain wakefulness for the entire 20-min test administered at 1800 h. It is still conceivable, therefore, that the improved nighttime sleep quality, and the circadian clock resetting, may be beneficial to ASPD patients complaining of early evening sleepiness.

In addition to its phase-shifting properties, exposure to bright light has also been shown to directly enhance alertness in healthy subjects and in some patient samples. (For a brief review of this topic, see [49].) For example, a group of pathologically sleepy subjects (as a result of obstructive sleep apnea) exhibited significantly reduced sleep tendency on sleep latency tests that were immediately preceded by 2 h of bright light exposure. In a subset of subjects, the effect carried over to a subsequent latency test before which no bright light was administered. Similarly, in a group of healthy subjects working a simulated night shift during which they were exposed to 1000 lux ambient light, we observed improvements in both alertness and cognitive performance when compared to a dim light condition. Although we know of no study that has examined the effects of enhanced ambient light specifically

10. **Carskadon M A**, **Vieira C**, **Acebo C**. Association between puberty and delayed phase preference. *Sleep*, 1993; **16**:258–62.

11. **Thorpy M J**, **Korman E**, **Spielman A J**, et al. Delayed sleep phase syndrome in adolescents. *J Adolesc Health Care*, 1988; **9**:22–27.

12. **Dagan Y.** Circadian rhythm sleep disorders (CRSD). *Sleep Med Rev*, 2002; **6**:45–54.

13. **Ohayon M M**, **Roberts R E**, **Zulley J**, et al. Prevalence and patterns of problematic sleep among older adolescents. *J Am Acad Child Adolesc Psychiatry*, 2000; **39**:1549–56.

14. **Sack R L**, **Auckley D**, **Auger R R**, et al. Circadian rhythm sleep disorders: part II, advanced sleep phase disorder, delayed sleep phase disorder, free-running disorder, and irregular sleep–wake rhythm. An American Academy of Sleep Medicine review. *Sleep*, 2007; **30**:1484–501.

15. **Shirayama M**, **Shirayama Y**, **Iida H**, et al. The psychological aspects of patients with delayed sleep phase syndrome (DSPS). *Sleep Med*, 2003; **4**:427–33.

16. **Ito A**, **Ando K**, **Hayakawa T**, et al. Long-term course of adult patients with delayed sleep phase syndrome. *Jap J Psychiatry Neurol*, 1993; **47**:563–67.

17. **Horne J A**, **Ostberg O**. A self-assessment questionnaire to determine morningness–eveningness in human circadian rhythms. *Int J Chronobiol*, 1976; **4**:97–110.

18. **Kripke D F**, **Rex K M**, **Ancoli-Israel S**, et al. Delayed sleep phase cases and controls. *J Circadian Rhythms*, 2008; **6**:6.

19. **Mundey K**, **Benloucif S**, **Harsanyi K**, et al. Phase-dependent treatment of delayed sleep phase syndrome with melatonin. *Sleep*, 2005; **28**:1271–78.

20. **Regestein Q R**, **Monk T H**. Delayed sleep phase syndrome: a review of its clinical aspects. *Am J Psychiatry*, 1995; **152**:602–08.

21. **Czeisler C A**, **Richardson G S**, **Coleman R M**, et al. Chronotherapy: resetting the circadian clocks of patients with delayed sleep phase insomnia. *Sleep*, 1981; **4**:1–21.

22. **Yamadera W**, **Sasaki M**, **Itoh H**, et al. Clinical features of circadian rhythm sleep disorders in outpatients. *Psychiatry Clin Neurosci*, 1998; **52**:311–16.

23. **de Beck T W**. Delayed sleep phase syndrome – criminal offense in the military? *Military Med*, 1990; **155**:1–14.

24. **Watanabe T**, **Kajimura N**, **Kato M**, et al. Sleep and circadian rhythm disturbances in patients with delayed sleep phase syndrome. *Sleep*, 2003; **26**:657–61.

25. **Campbell S S**, **Murphy P J**. Delayed sleep phase disorder in temporal isolation. *Sleep*, 2007; **30**:1225–28.

26. Diagnostic classification of sleep and arousal disorder, 1st edition prepared by the Sleep Disorders Classification Committee, H P Roffwarg, Chairman. *Sleep*, 1979; **2**: 1–130.

27. **Jones C R**, **Campbell S S**, **Zone S E**, et al. Familial advanced sleep-phase syndrome: a short-period circadian rhythm variant in humans. *Nat Med*, 1999; **5**:1062–65.

28. **Satoh K**, **Mishima K**, **Inoue Y**, et al. Two pedigrees of familial advanced sleep phase syndrome in Japan. *Sleep*, 2003; **26**:416–17.

29. **Campbell S S**, **Gillin J C**, **Kripke D F**, et al. Gender differences in the circadian temperature rhythms of healthy elderly subjects: relationships to sleep quality. *Sleep*, 1989; **12**:529–36.

30. **Campbell S S**, **Dawson D**, **Anderson M W**. Alleviation of sleep maintenance insomnia with timed exposure to bright light. *J Am Geriatr Soc*, 1993; **41**:829–36.

31. **Czeisler C A**, **Dumont M**, **Duffy J F**, et al. Association of sleep–wake habits in older people with changes in output of circadian pacemaker. *Lancet*, 1992; **340**:933–36.

32. **Moe K E**, **Prinz P N**, **Vitiello M V**, et al. Healthy elderly women and men have different entrained circadian temperature rhythms. *J Am Geriatr Soc*, 1991; **39**:383–87.

33. **Kamei R**, **Hughes L**, **Miles L**, et al. Advanced sleep phase syndrome studied in a time isolation facility. *Chronobiologia*, 1979; **6**:115.

34. **Moldofsky H**, **Musisi S**, **Phillipson E A**. Treatment of a case of advanced sleep phase syndrome by phase advance chronotherapy. *Sleep*, 1986; **9**:61–65.

35. **Monk T H**, **Buysse D J**, **Reynolds C F**, et al. Circadian temperature rhythms of older people. *Exp Gerontol*, 1995; **30**:455–74.

36. **Lack L C**, **Mercer J D**, **Wright H**. Circadian rhythms of early morning awakening insomniacs. *J Sleep Res*, 1996; **5**:211–19.

37. **Lack L**, **Wright H**. The effect of evening bright light in delaying the circadian rhythms and lengthening the sleep of early morning awakening insomniacs. *Sleep*, 1993; **16**:436–43.

38. **Monk T H**. Aging human circadian rhythms: conventional wisdom may not always be right. *J Biol Rhythms*, 2005; **20**:366–74.

39. **Lavie P**. Ultrashort sleep–waking schedule. III. 'Gates' and 'forbidden zones' for sleep. *Electroencephalogr Clin Neurophysiol*, 1986; **63**:414–25.

40. **Strogatz S H**, **Kronauer R E**, **Czeisler C A**. Circadian regulation dominates homeostatic control of sleep length and prior wake length in humans. *Sleep*, 1986; **9**:353–64.

41. **Uchiyama M**, **Okawa M**, **Shibui K**, *et al*. Poor recovery sleep after sleep deprivation in delayed sleep phase syndrome. *Psychiatry Clin Neurosci*, 1999; **53**:195–97.

42. **Uchiyama M**, **Okawa M**, **Shibui K**, *et al*. Altered phase relation between sleep timing and core body temperature rhythm in delayed sleep phase syndrome and non-24-hour sleep–wake syndrome in humans. *Neurosci Lett*, 2000; **294**:101–04.

43. **Okawa M**, **Uchiyama M**. Circadian rhythm sleep disorders: characteristics and entrainment pathology in delayed sleep phase and non-24-h sleep–wake syndrome. *Sleep Med Rev*, 2007; **11**:485–96.

44. **Chang A**, **Reid K J**, **Gourineni R**, *et al*. Sleep timing and circadian phase in delayed sleep phase syndrome. *J Biol Rhythms*, 2009; **24**:313–21.

45. **Carskadon M A**, **Dement W C**. Multiple sleep latency tests during the constant routine. *Sleep*, 1992; **15**:396–99.

46. **Bes F**, **Jobert M**, **Schulz H**. Modeling napping, post-lunch dip, and other variations in human sleep propensity. *Sleep*, 2009; **32**:392–98.

47. **Morgenthaler T I**, **Lee-Chiong T**, **Alessi C**, *et al*. Practice parameters for the clinical evaluation and treatment of circadian rhythm sleep disorders. An American Academy of Sleep Medicine report. *Sleep*, 2007; **30**:1445–59.

48. **Oren D A**, **Wehr T A**. Hypernyctohemeral syndrome after chronotherapy for delayed sleep phase syndrome. *N Engl J Med*, 1992; **327**:1762.

49. **Rosenthal N E**, **Joseph-Vanderpool J R**, **Levendosky A A**, *et al*. Phase-shifting effects of bright morning light as treatment for delayed sleep phase syndrome. *Sleep*, 1990; **13**:354–61.

50. **Lack L**, **Schumacher K**. Evening light treatment of early morning insomnia. *Sleep Res*, 1993; **22**:225.

51. **Campbell S S**, **Dijk D J**, **Boulos Z**, *et al*. Light treatment for sleep disorders: consensus report. III. Alerting and activating effects. *J Biol Rhythms*, 1995; **10**:129–32.

52. **Dahlitz M**, **Alvarez B**, **Vignau J**, *et al*. Delayed sleep phase syndrome response to melatonin. *Lancet*, 1991; **337**:1121–24.

53. **Oldani A**, **Ferini-Strambi L**, **Zucconi M**, *et al*. Melatonin and delayed sleep phase syndrome: ambulatory polygraphic evaluation. *Neuroreport*, 1994; **6**:132–34.

54. **Kayumov L**, **Brown G**, **Jindal R**, *et al*. A randomized, double-blind, placebo-controlled crossover study of the effect of exogenous melatonin on delayed sleep phase syndrome. *Psychosom Med*, 2001; **63**:40–48.

55. **Zee P**, **Wang-Weigand S**, **Ogrinc F**, **Roth T**. The use of ramelteon to advance sleep timing and melatonin phase in delayed sleep phase disorder. *Sleep*, 2009; **32**(Abstract supplement):A47–48.

56. **Rajaratnam S M**, **Polymeropoulos M H**, **Fisher D M**, *et al*. Melatonin agonist tasimelteon (VEC-162) for transient insomnia after sleep-time shift: two randomised controlled multicentre trials. *Lancet*, 2009; **373**:482–91.

57. **Okawa M**, **Mishima K**, **Nanami T**, *et al*. Vitamin B12 treatment for sleep–wake rhythm disorders. *Sleep*, 1990; **13**:15–23.

58. **Uchiyama M**, **Okawa M**, **Shibui K**, *et al*. Poor compensatory function for sleep loss as a pathogenic factor in patients with delayed sleep phase syndrome. *Sleep*, 2000; **23**:553–58.

Section 2 Chapter 18

Sleep Disorders and Excessive Sleepiness

Shift work disorder and sleepiness

Torbjörn Åkerstedt

Shift work disrupts circadian and homeostatic sleep regulation and is probably the most common cause of sleepiness in society. We will organize the present topic according to the particular sleepiness indicators – mainly survey self-descriptions, physiological measures, and dense sampling of subjective momentary ratings of sleepiness. We will also discuss more integrated issues, such as the severity of sleepiness, sleepiness-related accidents, the regulation of sleepiness in shift work, and shift work disorder. It should be mentioned that the concept of "fatigue" is often used interchangeably with "sleepiness". They are not exactly the same, however, and the differential definition of the two is constantly debated [1, 2]. Here we see sleepiness as "a drive to fall asleep" [3], measurable as a subjective perception or as physiological and behavioral changes. There is no consensus on fatigue, however, but here we see fatigue as a reduced inclination for activity, due to excessive extension in time or intensity of that activity.

Shift work

The concept of shift work describes an arrangement of work hours through which the daily duration of production/service extends to cover 16 or 24 h, usually by dividing the time into two or three 8-h "shifts" (with some variation). Normally, the first step of extending production beyond a day shift is to introduce a morning and evening shift (6am to 2pm and 2pm to 10pm, respectively). When necessary, also a night shift may be used to cover the remaining 8 h.

In Europe, workers often alternate between shifts and work the same shift 2–4 times in succession and then switch to a new shift. In North America, permanent shifts are more common. In transport, health care and the service sector, the shifts may be more variable in placement and duration (roster work), but the principle remains – one alternates between different shifts. Even the permanent night worker alternates – between a night shift and a day life during his/her days off.

Usually, the night shift is the most problematic one, causing disturbed circadian rhythms, disturbed sleep, and excessive sleepiness [4], and several medical disorders deriving from these disturbances [5]. However, early morning hours also present problems and will be brought up here, as will some aspects of non-work shift-like activity, such as driving at night for other reasons than work.

Survey studies of sleepiness

The first documentation of perceived sleepiness or fatigue among shift workers was obtained in survey studies [6–9]. Most shift workers were shown to experience sleepiness (or sometimes fatigue) in connection with, mainly, night shift work, whereas day work is associated with no, or marginal, sleepiness.

A more palpable variety of sleepiness is reports of involuntary sleep in shift workers [10]. Between 10 and 20% report falling asleep during night work and shift work is usually one of the strongest predictors of falling asleep at work. Disturbed sleep is usually one of the other high-ranking predictors in survey studies.

The popular Epworth Sleepiness Scale has not been used very frequently in relation to shift work, but one recent study showed values of 9.2 in night workers, and 8.6 in rotating shift workers, and 8.0 in day workers [11].

Physiological sleepiness

The reports of involuntary sleep at work should be observable in the studies of physiological sleepiness indicators during work. As discussed elsewhere

---

Sleepiness: Causes, Consequences and Treatment, ed. Michael J. Thorpy and Michel Billiard. Published by Cambridge University Press. © Cambridge University Press 2011.

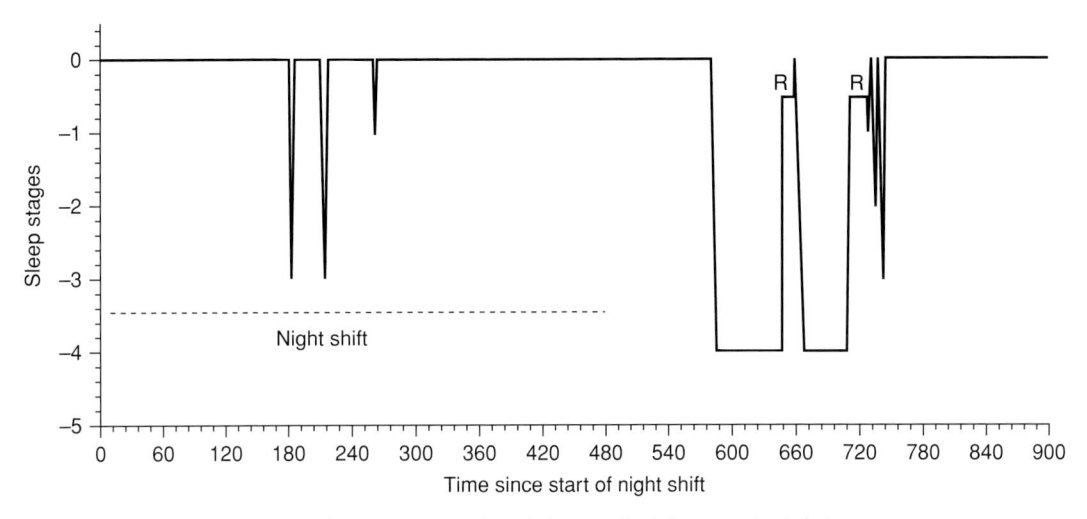

Figure 18.1 Hypnogram for one shift worker across 24 h, including a night shift, post-night shift sleep.

in this volume, sleepiness appears physiologically as increased levels of EEG alpha (8–12 Hz) and theta (4–8 Hz) activity, and as slow eye movements [12], or long eye closure durations [13]. Especially the 5–9 Hz band seems to reflect sleepiness [14]. These changes are also related to performance impairment [15].

In one of the first EEG studies of night workers at work (train drivers) we found that a quarter showed pronounced increases in alpha (8–12 Hz) and theta (4–8 Hz) activity, as well as slow eye movements (SEM), towards the early morning, but these were absent during day driving [16]. The correlations with ratings of sleepiness were quite high ($r = .74$). In some instances obvious performance lapses, such as driving against a red light, occurred during bursts of SEMs and of alpha/theta activity. The pattern is very similar in truck drivers during long-haul (8–10 h) night drives [17, 18], and similar results have been demonstrated for aircrew during long-haul flights [19].

In process operators there was found not only sleepiness-related increases in alpha and theta activity, but also fully fledged sleep during the night shift (but not during other shifts) [20, 21]. Such incidents of actual sleep occurred in approximately a quarter of the subjects (Figure 18.1). Usually, they occurred during the second half of the night shift and never in connection with any other shift. Importantly, sleep on the job was not condoned by the company, nor was there any official awareness that sleep would or could occur during work hours. Interestingly, the subjects were unaware of having slept, but were aware of sleepiness. In hospital interns on call there was observed "attentional failures" (defined as sleep intrusions in the EEG), particularly during early morning work [22]. This was reduced when continuous on-call duty across days was broken up to permit relatively normal amounts of sleep each day.

Increased alpha and theta activity have also been demonstrated in truck drivers driving a truck simulator at night [23], or in power station operators during a night shift [24], or in shift workers driving a simulator after a regular night shift [25]. In the latter, eye blink durations were also used and showed a strong increase after night work. The electrooculogram (EOG) was also strongly affected in a simulator study that studied driving at different times of day [26]. In that study, not only blink durations increased, but blink amplitude decreased with night driving. All studies also showed large increases in subjective sleepiness and the driving simulator studies showed impaired performance in the form of increased variation in lateral position.

In general, one gets the impression that laboratory/simulator studies show clearer results than field studies. The reason may be that real work situations contain much more stimulation than the laboratory. It is also possible that many individuals start counteracting sleepiness when sleepiness symptoms start to appear. This probably prevents sleepiness from appearing in many physiological indicators, since EEG and EOG signs of sleepiness only occur at higher levels of sleepiness, when the individual is "fighting sleep" and has reached a maximum level of sleepiness [12].

With respect to the Multiple Sleep Latency Test (MSLT), which is the standard clinical polysomnographic measure of sleepiness, only data from post-night shift bedtimes exist in field studies [27]. Essentially they indicate short (<5 min) latencies, attesting to excessive sleepiness according to clinical criteria [28]. The reason for the lack of field studies with this method is probably the difficulty of getting workers off from work to perform the 20-min MSLT several times during a night shift, finding a suitably quiet place to make the measurements, and getting workers to wear electrodes (for fast hook-up to the polysomnograph) while working. However, there have been a large number of "simulated" night shift studies showing short latencies; for example, Czeisler et al. [29], who studied individuals suffering from shift work (sleep) disorder and found a mean MSLT of 2 min during the night shift. Even if a controlled and soporific laboratory situation may enhance sleepiness, the observed values were very low, indicating considerable sleepiness.

Clearly, night work involves bouts of physiological sleepiness in many, but not all, shift workers. While sleep during work should not occur in any occupational group, it is difficult to judge how serious night shift sleepiness is – except for a few isolated cases, the sleep intrusions have not been explicitly linked to a particular accident risk or performance impairment.

Momentary subjective sleepiness

EEG measures give some indication of the pattern of sleepiness in relation to shift work, that is, incidents of sleep intrusions are frequently seen during the second half of a night shift. However, high-frequency (every 2 h, for example) subjective ratings give more detailed information about sleepiness patterns and permit data collection across long time periods, across many shifts and days off. The overall impression is moderate to high sleepiness during the night shift and no sleepiness at all during the day shifts [30].

In order to be able to compare different studies and look for common patterns, we have brought together some of our own studies of work hours. This has the advantage of the same rating scale being used in many different situations, the Karolinska Sleepiness Scale (KSS) [12]. The KSS ranges from 1 to 9, with 1 = very alert, 3 = rather alert, 5 = neither alert nor sleepy, 7 = sleepy but no difficulty remaining awake, 9 = very sleepy (fighting sleep, an effort to remain awake). Phys-

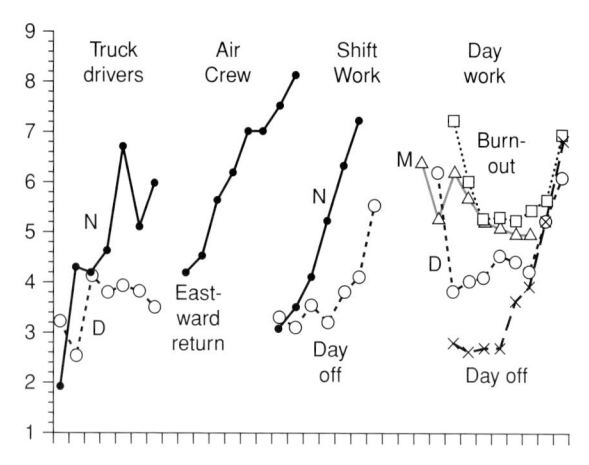

Figure 18.2 Subjective sleepiness in truck drivers during a night and a day shift;, in air crew during a westward flight from Stockholm to Los Angeles, starting at 9am and ending at 9pm Central European Time (CET) or 11 am West Coast Time (WCT); at two points = 2 and 4 h after landing (11pm and 01am CET); in shift workers on a night shift 10pm to 6am and on a day shift from 2pm to 10pm (first two points represent 2 and 4h before start of shift); in patients with burnout; Morning shift (M) workers working 6am to 2pm, in day workers (D – 8am to 5pm) during the working week and during a day off (Sunday).

iological intrusions of sleep in the EEG or EOG usually start at level 7 and dominate the recording at level 9. Its validity is discussed below.

Day and shift work

Normal day work is associated with a characteristic pattern of sleepiness. The most obvious observation in this type of study is the high level of sleepiness in the morning, low levels during the afternoon, and return to relatively high levels of sleepiness in the evening. Figure 18.2 (rightmost) describes this pattern in a group of healthy normals and a group high on burnout [31]. The former show levels of 3–4 on the KSS. During the weekend this level drops even further, to below 3, while the burnout subjects remain at relatively high working week levels. The same part of the figure also includes sleepiness levels for a morning shift [32]. The values are very similar to those in the burnout group, between 5 and 6. The morning shift effect usually seems to be similar to mid night shift levels (see below) but seems, on the other hand, to be present throughout the entire shift [30]. The morning shift sleepiness leads to an early afternoon nap in about a third of the workers [33, 34].

The leftmost part of the figure shows ratings of truck drivers while driving during the day and

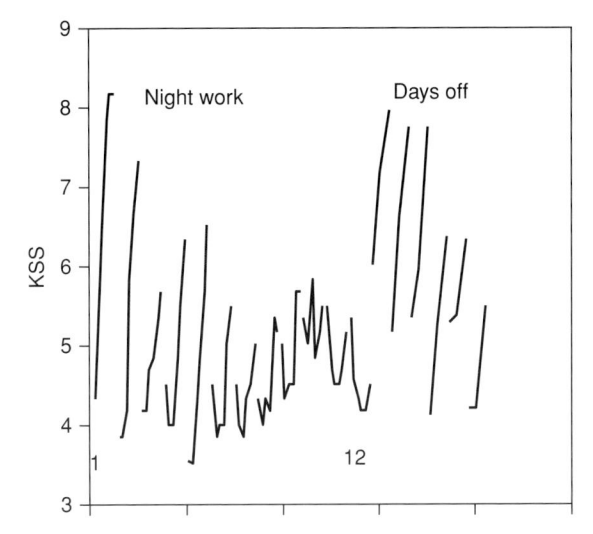

Figure 18.3 Subjective sleepiness across 12 days of 12-h night shifts on a North Sea oil platform and during the subsequent 7 days off (ashore).

during the night [17]. Note the decrease of sleepiness in the early morning of the night drive, which for the most part is due to the legally required break. The next section of the figure describes the sleepiness of aircrew during a return flight from Los Angeles to Stockholm, after a two-day layover [30]. This essentially corresponds to biological night work since the flight takes place during the window of circadian low. Very high levels of sleepiness are reached. The next section shows the night shift and day off for the first shift in a rapidly rotating shift system [35]. High levels are reached (>7) towards the end of the night shift, while levels during the day off are quite low (3–4).

Adjustment under special conditions

Figure 18.3 concerns adjustment to night work under rather special circumstances. Adjustment to night shifts normally does not occur because shifts alternate and because of the exposure to daylight when returning home from the night shift. The latter counteracts the expected delay of the circadian clock [36]. However, when light is not interfering, as happens on North Sea oil production platforms, adjustment does occur since work is carried out indoors and the light cycle is adjusted to the work/sleep pattern [37]. In the figure the sleepiness pattern during the fortnight of night work changes day by day and the steep night shift (12 shifts) was reversed by day 4–5. Return to day-life on days off required a new adjustment period with initial high sleepiness and a reversal by day 4–5.

A comment on the relevance of subjective ratings

The effects of shift work on subjective sleepiness are profound, but an important question is the relation to function and safety. Such a relation is found in most studies [26, 38–40]. The relationship seems distinctly curvilinear, such that physiological intrusions of sleep and impaired performance start to appear at level 7 of the KSS and become very frequent at level 9 [12]. However, it has been suggested that the relation may be rather moderate [41–43]. In particular, performance impairment during accumulation of partial sleep loss seems to increase more rapidly than subjective sleepiness.

It seems quite likely, however, that a subjective rating is very context-dependent (as are performance measures), that is, it may need to be measured under the same conditions as the performance test. This is usually characterized by total control of the context, high work load, and often a great deal of boredom. Subjective ratings under such conditions become much higher [44, 45] and closely reflect the performance changes. Yang et al. have suggested that a self-rating of sleepiness after a minute of sitting quietly with closed eyes may solve the discrepancy problem [46].

Performance and accidents at work

If sleepiness is as pronounced as suggested in connection with night work, there should be a link with performance errors and accidents. Considerable amounts of results support this assumption, but it should be emphasized that almost none of the relevant studies demonstrate a link between *explicit* sleepiness and risk. Rather, sleepiness is inferred from the setting of the accident – mainly night shifts or night activity in general. In the present section we extend the discussion to include not only what happens during work hours, but also to non-work activities during the night, particularly driving. Below we have divided the material into industry/health care and road transport, since particularly the latter has been the target for much research recently, with a special focus on developing drowsiness warning devices.

Industry and health care

With respect to errors or impaired performance in shift work, a classic study is that of Bjerner et al. [47], who showed that errors in meter readings over a period of 20 years in a gas works had a pronounced peak on the night shift. There was also a secondary peak during the afternoon. Similarly, Brown [48] demonstrated that telephone operators connected calls considerably slower at night. Wojtczak-Jaroszowa found that the speed of spinning threads in a textile mill went down during the night [49]. Dorrian et al. [50] demonstrated that the fatigue of train drivers on a particular work schedule was related to the fuel costs because of uneconomical ways of using speed and braking. From conventional industrial operations most studies show a night shift dominance [51–53], but not all.

One of the most convincing field studies of work hours and safety thus far may be that of Landrigan et al. [22]. They studied interns on call and showed that reduction of total work hours from 80 to 60 h/week, together with a maximal shift duration of 16 h (instead of 24–36 h), produced a 50% reduction in serious errors. Also sleepiness was reduced and the number of "attention failures" (similar to "micro-sleeps") as indicated by EEG/EOG was greatly reduced during night work [54]. The hours of sleep per day (across a week) increased from 6.6 to 7.4 h. It was concluded that the protection of sleep and the reduction of total hours was responsible for the effects. Interestingly, the number of hours worked per week correlated ($r = 0.57$) with mean sleep duration per week. Fifty-five hours of work per week seemed to be compatible with 56 h of sleep per week (mean of 8 h/day). At 70 h of work per week mean sleep duration was 7 h/day. Other research has demonstrated that fatigue/sleepiness starts to accumulate below that level [55]. In another study, the effect of prior night work did not affect complications after procedures, unless prior sleep had been less than 6 h [56].

Another carefully designed study from car manufacturing seems to indicate a moderate increase (30–50%) in accident risk on the night shift [57]. Åkerstedt et al. [58] showed that fatal occupational accidents were higher in shift workers in a prospective study of shift workers (controlling for physical work load, stress, and other factors). Among nurses, maintaining a diary for sleep, sleepiness and errors, it was found that days with a "struggle to stay awake" (which may be seen as an indicator of sleepiness) coincided with days with errors at work [59]. Basner et al. [60] further demonstrated that airport security personnel showed sizeable impairment during night work in ability to detect dangerous objects in the scanning procedure.

It is also believed that the (nighttime) nuclear plant meltdown at Chernobyl was due to human error related to work scheduling [61]. Similar observations have been made for the Three Mile Island reactor accident and the near-miss incidents at the David Beese reactor in Ohio and at the Rancho Seco reactor in California. The (US) National Transportation Safety board (NTSB) also found that the *Exxon Valdez* accident in 1989 was due to fatigue, caused by reduced sleep and extended work hours [62]. These are all anecdotal, however. The extent of fatal, fatigue-related accidents is considered to lie around 30% [63] in the air-traffic sector and somewhat lower in the maritime sector.

Road transport

Road transport is the area where the link between safety and night work sleepiness is most pronounced. Harris [64], Hamelin [65] and others [66] convincingly demonstrated that single vehicle truck accidents have by far the greatest probability of occurring at night (early morning). In particular, night workers are at risk [67, 68]. Furthermore, the NTSB found that 30–40% of all US truck accidents are fatigue-related (and grossly underestimated in conventional reports). The latter investigation was extended to search for the immediate causes of fatigue-induced accidents [69]. It was found that the most important factor was the amount of sleep obtained during the proceeding 24 h and split-sleep patterns, whereas the length of time driven seemed to play a minor role.

Interestingly, the accident risk is increased in the early morning (when sleepiness is assumed to be maximal) for all types of driving accidents, except for those due to overtaking [70]. The risk at that time is increased 5.5-times for all types of accidents, and by 10 for accidents leading to death. The most pronounced effect, however, is for single-vehicle accidents, which are particularly linked to falling asleep incidents. Young age increases risk several times and male gender doubles the risk [71].

In a rather unique case-control study, Connor et al. [72] interviewed individuals who had been involved in a car accident and found that retrospective sleepiness ratings from before a crash showed high Odds Ratio for higher sleepiness: OR = 8.2 compared to drivers who had been interviewed without having been involved in a crash. Also, night driving and short prior sleep increased the accident risk. This may be the first, and almost the only, study that has linked a sleepiness measure to actual accidents. Crummy *et al.* [73] carried out a somewhat similar study. They interviewed 112 injured drivers and found that 50% had at least one sleep-related risk factor; 20% had two or more. Being a shift worker, driving at night, reporting high sleepiness (KSS > 5) were related to sleep-related accidents.

Another approach has been to carry out field studies with long-term video recording of the driver and the traffic situation and fatigue/sleepiness (estimated through video scoring). The results suggest that inattention, frequently caused by sleepiness, to be the most prevalent cause of near accidents [74, 75]. Philip *et al.* equipped cars with lane trackers and conducted driving experiments on French motorways. A reduction to 2 h of sleep caused a considerable increase in "illegitimate" line crossings and in subjective sleepiness [76], presumably related to accident risk.

The link between sleepiness and risk/performance has also been studied extensively in simulator studies and both subjective sleepiness as well as increased alpha or theta activity or long eye blink durations is associated with unintentional line crossings [40, 77]. As discussed above, the relation is almost exponential, that is, incidents/accidents seem to occur only at the highest level of sleepiness, that of "fighting sleep", level 9 on the KSS scale. In a systematic driving simulator study of sleepiness and "hitting" a rumble strip, a clear relation between "hits" and subjective sleepiness, lateral variability of the vehicle, and EEG/EOG indications of sleepiness was found [78]. The hits occurred on the average at 8.1 units of the KSS.

The strength of sleepiness

Above, it was concluded that EEG and EOG measures show that incursions of sleep during work/activity and accidents occur during particularly night work, when sleepiness is at its peak. Comparisons with alcohol effects indicate that late night sleepiness causes behavioral impairment similar to that of 0.05–0.08% blood alcohol levels [79, 80]. This suggests that sleepiness is a powerful force. On the other hand, there seems to exist a notion of sleepiness being easily handled by "pulling oneself together" with a little effort. This leads to the thoughts of the possibility of establishing critical levels of sleepiness at which the effect becomes imperative. The search for levels may probably start with subjective sleepiness, since there are relatively few studies of physiological indicators and these have quite different approaches.

Apparently, individuals are aware of their sleepy state since subjective ratings of sleepiness are increased before a real road accident [72], and before driving off the road in a driving simulator [40, 81]. This suggests that the afflicted person either fails to realize that his/her state is dangerous or that sleepiness, while perceived as high, still seems possible to handle but that there is an attempt to "turn off" consciousness by the brain without a final warning, somewhat like the state instability characterizing states of sleep loss [82, 83]. The instability occurs at relatively high levels of sleep loss (24 h awake), and involves short, relatively frequent reductions of prefrontal cortex metabolism, combined with high levels that seem related to efforts to fight sleepiness.

Another glimpse of the imperative nature of sleepiness comes from a driving simulator study of the effects of rumble strips [78]. It was found that hitting a rumble strip in the morning after being awake during the night was associated with strong pre-hit increases in EEG alpha/theta activity, eye closure duration, lateral variability of the vehicle and high sleepiness levels (KSS = 8.1 on the 9-step scale) (Figure 18.4). Thus, sleepiness was undoubtedly present. However, the high level was maintained during at least 5 min before hitting the rumble strip, and no further increase was seen immediately before the hit. This suggests a combination of high perceived and physiological and behavioral sleepiness, combined with state instability.

Another observation in the study by Anund *et al.* [78] was that the hit immediately reduced EOG, EEG and driving variability to intermediate levels of sleepiness and the vehicle was brought back to the proper lane by the driver. The increased alertness was reversed in 2–4 min and a new hit occurred some minutes later. This was repeated seven more times on average. Apparently, the alerting effects of a hit were extremely temporary and irresistible sleepiness returned very rapidly, despite major efforts to remain awake.

In another study with 100 video-equipped cars [75], there were large numbers of incidents associated with sleepiness, as judged by video recording of

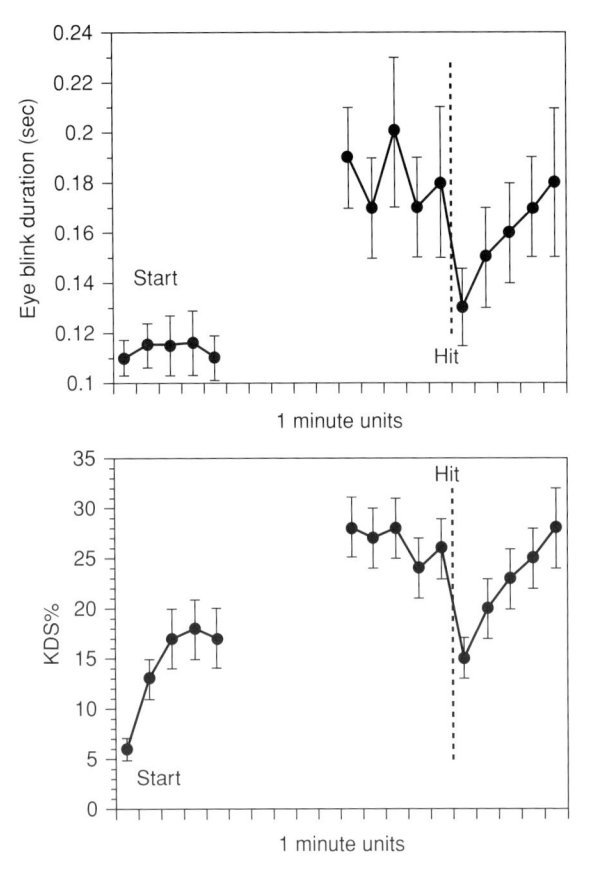

Figure 18.4 Eye blink duration and sleep intrusions (alpha/theta activity or slow eye movements) while driving for 1 h in a driving simulator after sleep loss. First 5 min of the drive and 5 min before and after the first incidence of hitting a rumble strip ("Hit"). KDS = karolinska drowsiness score.

the driver's face. However, the analysis was not detailed and did not contain subjective sleepiness or physiology.

Severe and non-acceptable sleepiness levels

The severity discussion raises the question of whether there is a quantitative level of sleepiness that might be dangerous or "unacceptable" considering a putative right of individuals to lead their lives at reasonable levels of alertness. With the present availability of physiological data there does not seem to be any possibility of merging studies to construct "norms". However, there are a number of studies with subjective measures available that might be used.

We noted above that the KSS level 3–4 characterized subjective sleepiness during day work [31]. The weekend, with more sleep, showed even lower levels, below 3. Similar levels are seen in shift workers during their days off [30, 35]. Shift workers in connection with night work usually vary from 4 early during the night shift, to reach around 7 towards the end [30, 35]. During morning work, levels around 5–6 are usually seen [30].

The values above may be compared with those in individuals with a very negative attitude to shift work [35]. That group reached a maximum of 7.2 on the night shift, 5.2 on the afternoon shift and 5.9 on the morning shift, while they fell below 4 during days off. The corresponding values for those with a positive attitude was 5.7, 3.9, 4.8 and <4, respectively. Similarly, Czeisler et al. [29] showed that workers diagnosed with shift work disorder (SWD) had a mean KSS value of 7 out of 9 on the night shift. The latter are averages (no end-of-shift values were given), which probably means that the maximum may have been close to 9, that is, very high.

One might also compare the shift work values with the daytime values 5–6 that characterize subjects high on burnout [31] and patients with a burnout diagnosis at slightly higher levels [84].

The overview of sleepiness levels suggests that shift workers spend much of their waking time well above the levels of day workers. Most of this time may not be spent at levels extreme enough to constitute safety hazards, but the common levels of 5–6 appear to constitute a reduced quality of living, particularly if these levels dominate the working week, such as is the case with individuals with low tolerance for shift work. Based on the group mean data from different studies of shift workers it seems that two-hourly ratings of sleepiness may result in 3 out of 8 ratings above 5. During days with morning shifts, most ratings (7) may exceed 5. In connection with evening shifts there may occur 2 such ratings (during the last part of the shift), while days off may involve 1 such rating. A well-adjusted shift worker with two shifts of each type and two days off would then accumulate 26 above-5 ratings out of 48 possible ratings. Shift workers with a low tolerance appear to show 5, 8, 4 and 1 such ratings, that is 36/48, while burnout subjects may show 48/48 such ratings. A tentative level for good adjustment to shift work would then be <50% two-hourly ratings at levels >5. Risk levels for low tolerance would center around 70%. At present, the suggested levels are rough estimates and merely an indication of direction, but it should be possible to make a systematic approach trying to evaluate more detailed issues, while accounting for age, gender, type of task, etc. It remains to be seen if such levels are related to exits from shift work or increased sickness absence.

Causes of sleepiness in shift work and a model

Possible causes

In the introduction the main regulatory factors of alertness (and sleep) were briefly mentioned – circadian phase, time awake and prior sleep duration. These are discussed in greater detail elsewhere in this volume. Briefly, however, the main interfering factor for the shift worker is the displacement of work to the "window of circadian low", when metabolism is slow and sleepiness/fatigue is induced [85, 86]. The number of hours spent awake will have similar effects on the different types of sleepiness [86, 87].

After the night shift, the subsequent sleep is interfered with by the rising circadian phase. The latter effect was observed early by Foret and Lantin [27] in the first polysomnographic study of night work and sleep. They found an almost linear decrease in sleep duration from a bedtime at midnight to noon. If bedtime is further delayed, sleep duration starts to increase again and reaches a maximum around 1900h (with 36 h of time awake) [88]. Previous polysomnographic studies suggest sleep durations around 5.5–6 h [27]. This is also the outcome of a meta-analysis of questionnaire studies [89].

The shortening is due to the fact that sleep is terminated after only 4–6 h without the individual being able to return to sleep. The sleep loss is primarily taken out of stage 2 sleep ("basic" sleep) and stage REM sleep (dream sleep). Stages 3 and 4 ("deep" sleep) do not seem to be affected. Furthermore, the time taken to fall asleep (sleep latency) is usually shorter. Also, night sleep before a morning shift is reduced, but the termination is through artificial means and the awakening usually difficult and unpleasant [90].

However, 6 h or slightly below this amount should not cause much of an impairment of alertness. Several laboratory studies have found that this amount of sleep curtailment may affect sleepiness only marginally [43], at least acutely. Over time it may have effects, since 7 h appear to be necessary for long-term maintenance of alertness [55, 91]. In a recent study of sleepiness in a driving simulator, it was shown that subjective sleepiness increased as a function of sleep restriction (to 4 h),

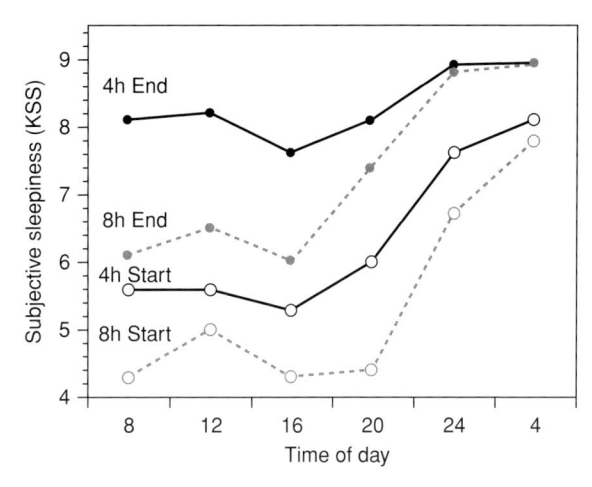

Figure 18.5 Subjective sleepiness during six 1-h drives at different times of day in a driving simulator, preceded by 8 or 4 h of sleep. Ratings are given for the start and the end of the drive.

time on task (start to end of drive) and a combination of time awake and time of day, reaching maximum possible sleepiness around 4 in the morning [26] (Figure 18.5). Lateral variability and slow eye closure durations showed similar effects and interactions with sleep loss (no main effect). Notably, the sleep restriction effect tends to disappear towards the end of the drive and during the window of circadian low. This was interpreted as a ceiling effect; one cannot be subjectively more sleepy than "fighting sleep".

Fragmentation of sleep, i.e. frequent awakenings, leads to effects similar to those of sleep reduction [92]. However, the rate of awakenings needs to exceed 5/h in order to cause significant effects on sleepiness. However, the PSG studies of shift workers' sleep do not seem to indicate sleep fragmentation and questionnaire data do not indicate any difference in sleep quality between shift workers and day workers [93]. The polysomnographic studies of sleep after the night shift do not indicate any fragmentation or reduced sleep efficiency.

Time on task is another important factor, but has not been investigated extensively. Classical studies of performance show the so-called "vigilance decrement", i.e. a gradual impairment of performance with time on task [94]. It is present in all types of performance, such as, for example, reaction time [95] or driving a simulator [96]. Subjective ratings or EEG/EOG variables are less common, but EEG or EOG indicators of sleepiness show a rather steep increase with time on task in the typical boring vigilance test situation [25, 26, 96]. Real

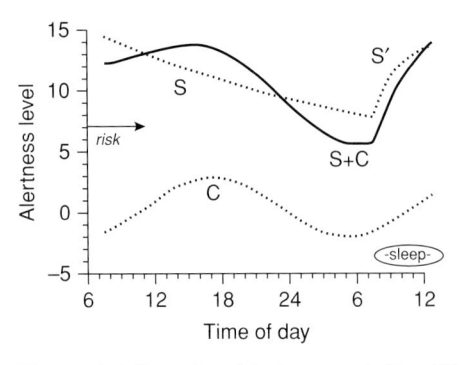

Figure 18.6 Illustration of the homeostatic (S and S′) and circadian (C) influences on sleepiness, as well as the sum of the two factors. The arrow indicates where sleep EEG and EOG intrusions usually start.

driving has been studied only once (with control for prior sleep, prior time awake and time of day) and it was demonstrated that unintended line crossings during night driving increased with time of driving (8, 4, 2 h), as did subjective ratings of sleepiness [97]. However, it is not clear if the effect is present during day driving. Philip *et al.* found no such effect, but permitted two-hourly breaks, which may have prevented time-on-task effects [98].

Modeling sleepiness

The regulatory factors of sleepiness and sleep have been brought together to form mathematical models for alertness or performance prediction for use as tools for evaluating work or sleep–wake schedules that deviate from traditional daytime orientation. The first (two-process) model mainly addressed the question of sleep regulation and, by inference, the need for sleep or fatigue/sleepiness [99]. Its main components were factors representing homeostatic effects of time awake and amount of prior sleep and a circadian component representing the effect of the biological clock on metabolism and performance (see Figure 18.6). The homeostatic factors are usually seen as having an exponential relation to sleepiness (for example, a steep initial fall of alertness after awakening, with a gradual flattening out towards an asymptote of very low alertness after 24 h of time awake). The circadian component is usually represented as a sinusoid function with a 24-h period. For a review of present models, see Mallis *et al.* [100].

The first model to focus explicitly on sleepiness was inspired by the model of Borbély *et al.* and also included sleep inertia. It was called The Three Process Model of Alertness (TPM) [101], and was subsequently expanded to include prediction of sleep duration and sleep latency [102, 103], and validated against EEG parameters and laboratory performance tests [104, 105]. Several other models predict sleepiness or fatigue and most include laboratory performance validations [106–108] and the predictive accuracy is rather similar [109]. The TPM (or SWP – sleep–wake predictor) was recently validated against road accident data (interviews with victims on prior sleep/wake pattern) [110]. The results show a 10-fold increase from very low to very high predicted alertness, or a hazard ratio of 1.72 per unit of the 9 unit output scale (controlling for alcohol involvement). An important finding was that moderate amounts of alcohol potentiated the circadian/homeostatic effect several thousand times.

Folkard and Akerstedt [111] have developed a model for identifying the risk factors in shift work scheduling using published data. The results show that, apart from the night shift, accident risk rises with the number of consecutive shifts (particularly night shifts), the duration of the shift and the absence of breaks. Sleep loss may play a role for the effect of number of successive shifts since one may assume that each night shift contributes to an accumulation of sleep loss [112]. However, the duration of the shift and the effect of time between breaks are more likely to be fatigue effects. But this is, of course, speculation.

Special cases

Even if the main problem in shift work is the night shift, and perhaps also the morning shift, there are other issues that may be of importance. One such concern attempts to show that clockwise shift changes should be less negative for performance than counterclockwise ones, but the results are not encouraging [113–115].

There has also been a continuous discussion of whether permanent shifts are better than rotating ones. While some have argued that permanent night work may have benefits in terms of circadian adjustment to shift work, there is little support for this argument [116]. Interestingly, day sleep does not seem to improve much across a series of night shifts [117, 118]. It appears, however, that night workers' sleep is slightly better (longer) than rotating workers on the night shift [119, 120]. The same lack of adjustment is reported in subjective sleep reports [121]. The assumed explanation for non-adjustment is the conflict with the external light–dark cycle [121]. Strict control over exposure to light and darkness can facilitate complete or partial circadian adaptation to permanent night work schedules [36, 122, 123].

Rapid shift rotation is reported to be associated with reduced total sleep duration compared to slower rotations (e.g. at least 3 weeks per shift schedule [89]). Rapid counterclockwise rotations appear to especially disrupt sleep immediately prior to the night shift [124]. These effects are thought to be less severe for workers experiencing a clockwise rotation because of the natural tendency of the circadian clock to delay to a later hour [125]. However, in another study, changing the shift schedule from three days on each of the three shifts to one with a fast-forward rotation morning-evening-night (M-E-N), that is "rapid rotation", caused a reduction of sleepiness during work hours [126]. Presumably the reason is that the new schedule gives a possibility for speedy recovery immediately after the morning and night shifts. The question of speed of rotation needs more experimental work.

Also, monotonous work causes sleepiness in terms of EEG/EOG changes, as well as in subjective ratings [127]. The effect was similar to that of a 50% sleep reduction. Presumably the driving simulator studies discussed above reflect corresponding effects of monotony.

Overtime work may exacerbate the effects of night work on sleepiness. In a field study of shift workers, Son et al. [128] showed strong effects of night shifts and overtime work on high levels of subjective sleepiness (KSS>7). A similar finding was made by Dahlgren et al. during a week of experimental overtime work [129]. Also, monotonous work increases sleepiness [127]. One could also conceive of longer shifts, since they would leave more days free for recuperation. This is probably not applicable to all occupations because of too high a work load, but in many studies shifts up to 12 h have been shown not to affect performance negatively [130], and they seem to be very attractive to the employees. Findings from other studies, however, of shifts 10 h and greater indicate increased sleepiness [128] and risk of accidents [131, 132].

The total duration of night work is another issue. Dumont et al. [133] found that the amount of sleep–wake and related disturbances in present day workers were related to their previous experience of night work. Guilleminault et al. [134] found an overrepresentation of former shift workers with different clinical sleep–wake disturbances appearing at a sleep clinic.

We have also shown that in pairs of twins discordant on night work exposure, the exposed twin reports somewhat deteriorated sleep quality and health after retirement [135].

Individual differences, a disorder and countermeasures/treatment

Clinicians and researchers find large differences between individuals in their tolerance to shift work, to the extent that those most afflicted need treatment. Below is discussed individual differences, the diagnosis Shift Work Disorder, and possible ways of counteracting or treating intolerance to shift work.

Individual differences

For a long time researchers have tried to identify individual differences that relate to the ability to handle work schedules that involve the night. In most cases, however, factors such as age, gender, personality, circadian type and others have failed to account for shift work tolerance [136], although increasing age seems to have a negative impact on the ability to sleep during the daytime. However, with particular reference to sleepiness, young individuals are more prone to falling asleep at work [137]. They also are overrepresented in late night road accidents (controlling for exposure) [71], and show higher levels of sleepiness in driving simulator studies [138]. These observations are in line with the observations of close to pathological sleepiness levels in teenagers [139] and with the ability to sleep much longer than older individuals when given unlimited time in bed [140]. The data clearly point to a loss of sleepiness with increasing age.

Using another approach, Axelsson et al. [35] selected a group (50% women) of paper mill workers with a very positive and negative attitude to their work hours, respectively, and followed them through a shift cycle with actigraphy, sleepiness ratings (KSS), and questionnaires. The main multivariate predictor of intolerance became sleepiness/fatigue, with family/work conflict as the second predictor. The low tolerance group rated consistently higher during all three shifts, but sleep duration did not differ. Age, gender, personality, diurnal type, etc., did not contribute. Those with low tolerance accounted for 8% of all employees (550). The results suggest that the main problem of shift workers is fatigue/sleepiness.

The reason for the low tolerance is unknown, but one possibility is a greater need for sleep or low quality of daytime sleep. Another possibility is a suboptimal relation between sleep and the circadian acrophase. Neither hypothesis has been tested formally. However, Koller *et al.* [141] noted that night nurses with problems exhibited an unshifted melatonin rhythm with a peak during the night shift. A similar observation was made by Burch *et al.* [142], who showed that a low work/sleep melatonin ratio in permanent night workers was associated with fatigue and accident risk, i.e. too much melatonin was circulating during the night shift. The question of low tolerance to shift work clearly needs research efforts.

Shift work disorder

The recognition of individuals with a low tolerance to shift work led to the diagnosis "Shift work sleep disorder" (SWSD), defined by the *Diagnostic and Statistical Manual of Mental Disorders* (DSM IV) [143] as "report of difficulty falling asleep, staying asleep, or non-restorative sleep for at least one month"; and it must be associated with "a work period that occurs during the habitual sleep phase". The *International Classification of Sleep Disorders* (ICSD) [144] bases the diagnosis of shift work disorder (SWD – "sleep" has been dropped) on four criteria: (1) complaint of insomnia or excessive sleepiness temporally associated with a recurring work schedule that overlaps the usual time for sleep; (2) symptoms must be associated with the shift work schedule over the course of at least one month; (3) circadian and sleep-time misalignment as demonstrated by sleep log or actigraphical monitoring for 7 days or more; and finally (4) sleep disturbance is not explainable by another sleep disorder, a medical or neurological disorder, mental disorder, medication use or substance use disorder. An important point is that in the change from SWSD to SWD, the focus has changed somewhat from "sleep" to insufficient restitution from sleep. To a large extent, this means that fatigue and sleepiness have come into focus.

The prevalence of SWD is not clear, since there is a lack of operational definition of the criteria [145]. However, one estimate arrives at 10% of the shift workers with night work, using the criteria (sleep difficulties or sleepiness sometimes or often at a severity level of 6 on a 1–10 scale [11]). In another study, mentioned above, a figure of 8% in a sample of rotating shift workers was found when using "a very negative or rather negative attitude to the present work hours" as a criterion [35].

Czeisler *et al.* [29] did not estimate the prevalence but used ICSD1 criteria as well as MSLT values of <6 min during a simulated night shift, as well as a sleep efficiency of <87.5% during day sleep (8 h time in bed) after a night shift. The resulting group showed a mean MSLT during the night shift of 2 min, a sleepiness rating of 7 on the Karolinska Sleepiness Scale [12] and sleep duration of 6 h. MSLT and sleepiness ratings are clearly at levels indicating excessive sleepiness, whereas the sleep duration seems very similar to most other studies. Waage *et al.* [146] made an estimate of 23.3% SWD in a sample of shift workers on North Sea oil platforms alternating between 12 night and day shifts. The authors used a question on whether the workers had substantially more difficulties sleeping or being alert during periods of night work than they had during day work or days off. While these studies give some information on individuals that may suffer from SWD, they do not seem to have ruled out underlying primary insomnia (seen during non-shift work periods), and there still has been no attempt to set clear operational and quantitative criteria.

Countermeasures

As brought up above, the main problem for shift workers is the misalignment of the sleep–wake pattern and the circadian system. Countermeasures, or treatments, focus on this misalignment. The most obvious countermeasure is to eliminate the misalignment through leaving employment that requires night work. This, however, may not always be socially or economically feasible.

As discussed above, there has also been a number of attempts at schedule design for better shift work. This includes rapid (1–2 shifts of the same type in sequence), rather than slow, rotation [116]. Even if sleep will be somewhat shorter after the night shift, there is no partial adjustment of the biological clock and recovery after the night shift occurs immediately. Clockwise rotation (morning–evening–night shift sequence) is another way of ameliorating negative effects, if one uses a counterclockwise shift system [114]. Both approaches should, however, be considered experimental, and scientific support is rather limited.

Permanent night work may be an alternative. This permits more of a permanent, but modest, circadian phase delay that may make sleepiness less pronounced. If the night shift, in addition, ends early, at 5am instead of 6am, sleep may be extended by almost an hour.

An important possibility may be self-selected work hours. Such systems usually involve a computerized selection system that makes sure that all temporal needs of production are covered and may permit rewards for selecting unpopular shifts [147]. In general, influence over work hours is an important factor in coping with shift work [148].

About a third of shift workers add an afternoon nap as a boost before the next night shift [149]. The duration of the nap is a function of the amount of prior (main) sleep. There are rather few field studies of the effects of this type of napping, but the effects on night shift alertness seem positive [150–153]. The Schweitzer *et al.* study also combined caffeine with a nap and found improved alertness on the night shift [150]. Most other studies have been carried out under simulated conditions and, while showing impressive results, may not be representative for what happens in real work situations. There may sometimes arise worries about possible negative effects of splitting sleep into two or more segments. However, there is no evidence for this. Mollicone *et al.* [154] studied different kinds of split sleep schedules and found no performance differences between them, or between them and solid sleep episodes. Only the total amount of sleep per 24 h was important for maintaining performance.

Another approach is light exposure during the early half of the night shift [155]. Alertness is enhanced due to the direct effects of light and to the delay of the circadian phase [112]. A number of other studies exist, the bulk of which are laboratory simulations of night shift work. Again, there is a need for real-life studies. Still, results from a 10-day laboratory experiment suggest an interesting countermeasure [156]. It used morning sleep (with light treatment during the first 4 h of work) or evening sleep (with light treatment during the last hours of the shift) after simulated night work. The result was a reduction of attention lapses during the last night shift for the evening sleep group. This suggests that stabilizing the day orientation of the circadian rhythm, together with decreased homeostatic sleep pressure before the night shift, improves alertness during the night shift. This may be one way of ameliorating night shift sleepiness (and SWD).

Treatment

Unsystematic reports indicate that hypnotics are relatively frequently used by shift workers. However, alertness-enhancing drugs, such as modafinil, is another possibility, and SWD is one of the indications for treatment. In one clinical trial, treatment with 200 mg of modafinil reduced extreme sleepiness in patients with shift-work sleep disorder and resulted in a small but significant improvement in performance and subjective alertness, as compared with placebo [29]. However, the residual sleepiness that was observed in the treated patients underscores the need for the development of interventions that are even more effective. In a subsequent study, armodafinil, with more than double the half-time of modafinil, significantly improved wakefulness during scheduled night work, raising mean nighttime sleep latency above the level considered to indicate severe sleepiness during the daytime [157]. Armodafinil also significantly improved measures of overall clinical condition, long-term memory, and attention.

The hormone melatonin is a chronobiotic and an inducer of sleepiness [158, 159]. Theoretically, it should be possible to use it in relation to shift work, but it should then be applied after the night shift, immediately before daytime sleep. This does not seem to work well, however [159]. Also theoretically, evening melatonin might be useful for getting to sleep before an early morning shift. There are no data to support this, however.

Conclusions

Shift work that includes night shifts causes high levels of sleepiness that may constitute a major safety risk, particularly in transport work, but also in health care and industry. The reason is a misalignment between the night-oriented work/rest pattern and the day-oriented circadian system. The impact of sleepiness is very powerful and lapses of consciousness may occur at high levels of sleepiness without any additional warning. Particularly vulnerable subjects, around 8–10% are at a special risk and may be diagnosed with "Shift Work Disorder". This is a group which also suffers from increased sleepiness during other shifts and spends much of its waking hours at pathological sleepiness levels. Countermeasures/treatment include naps, improved sleep schedules, light treatment, alertness-enhancing drugs, rapid shift rotation, and clockwise shift rotation.

References

1. **Horne J**. The semantics of sleepiness. *Sleep*, 2003; **26**:763; author reply 4.

2. **Dement W C**, **Hall J**, **Walsh J K**. Tiredness versus sleepiness: semantics or a target for public education? *Sleep*, 2003; **26**:485–86.

3. **Dement W C**, **Carskadon M A**. Current perspectives on daytime sleepiness: the issues. *Sleep*, 1982; **5**:56–66.

4. **Åkerstedt T**. Shift work and disturbed sleep/wakefulness. *Occup Med*, 2003; **53**:89–94.

5. **Knutsson A**. Health disorders of shift workers. *Occup Med*, 2003; **53**:103–08.

6. **Andersen JE**. *Three-Shift Work*. Copenhagen: Socialforskningsinstituttet, 1970.

7. **Verhaegen P**, **Maasen A**, **Meers A**. Health problems in shift workers. In: Johnson L C, Tepas D J, Colquhoun W P, Colligan M J, Eds. *Biological Rhythms and Shift Work*. New York, NY: Spectrum, 1981: 271–82.

8. **Paley M J**, **Tepas D I**. Fatigue and the shiftworker: firefighters working on a rotating shift schedule. *Hum Factors*, 1994; **36**:269–84.

9. **Thiis-Evensen E**. Shift work and health. Proceedings of the XII International Congress of Occupational Health (Helsinki). Helsinki, 1957: 97–105.

10. **Prokop O**, **Prokop L**. Ermüdung und Einschlafen am Steuer. *Zentralblatt für Verkehrsmedizin, Verkehrspsychologie und angrenzende Gebiete* 1955; **1**:19–30.

11. **Drake C L**, **Roehrs T**, **Richardson G**, *et al.* Shift work sleep disorder: prevalence and consequences beyond that of symptomatic day workers. *Sleep*, 2004; **27**:1453–62.

12. **Åkerstedt T**, **Gillberg M**. Subjective and objective sleepiness in the active individual. *Int J Neurosci*, 1990; **52**:29–37.

13. **Wierwille W W**, **Ellsworth L A**. Evaluation of driver drowsiness by trained raters. *Accid Analys Prevent*, 1994; **26**:571–81.

14. **Cajochen C**, **Khalsa S B S**, **Wyatt J K**, *et al.* EEG and ocular correlates of circadian melatonin phase and human performance decrements during sleep loss. *Am J Physiol*, 1999; **277**:R640–9.

15. **Dinges D F**, **Mallis M M**. Managing fatigue by drowsiness detection: can technological promises be realized? In: Hartley L, Ed. *Managing Fatigue in Transportation*. Oxford: Elsevier Science, 1998.

16. **Torsvall L**, **Åkerstedt T**. Sleepiness on the job: continuously measured EEG changes in train drivers. *Electroencephalogr Clin Neurophysiol*, 1987; **66**: 502–11.

17. **Kecklund G**, **Åkerstedt T**. Sleepiness in long distance truck driving: an ambulatory EEG study of night driving. *Ergonomics*, 1993; **36**:1007–17.

18. **Mitler M M**, **Miller J C**, **Lipsitz J J**, *et al.* The sleep of long-haul truck drivers. *N Engl J Med*, 1997; **337**:755–61.

19. **Rosekind M R**, **Graeber R C**, **Dinges D F**, *et al.* Crew factors in flight operations IX: effects of planned cockpit rest on crew performance and alertness in longhaul operations. Technical Memorandum. Moffett Field, CA.: NASA Technical Memorandum, September 1994. Report No.: A-94134.

20. **Torsvall L**, **Åkerstedt T**, **Gillander K**, *et al.* Sleep on the night shift: 24-hour EEG monitoring of spontaneous sleep/wake behavior. *Psychophysiology*, 1989; **26**:352–58.

21. **Åkerstedt T**, **Kecklund G**, **Knutsson A**. Spectral analysis of sleep electroencephalography in rotating three-shift work. *Scand J Work Environ Health* 1991; **17**:330–36.

22. **Landrigan C P**, **Rothschild J M**, **Cronin J W**, *et al.* Effect of reducing interns' work hours on serious medical errors in intensive care units. *N Engl J Med*, 2004; **351**:1838–48.

23. **Gillberg M**, **Kecklund G**, **Åkerstedt T**. Sleepiness and performance of professional drivers in a truck simulator – comparisons between day and night driving. *J Sleep Res*, 1996; **5**:12–15.

24. **Gillberg M**, **Kecklund G**, **Göransson B**, *et al.* Operator performance and signs of sleepiness during day and night work in a simulated thermal power plant. *Int J Ind Erg*, 2003; **31**:101–09.

25. **Åkerstedt T**, **Peters T**, **Anund A**, *et al.* Impaired alertness and performance while driving home from the night shift – a driving simulator study. *J Sleep Res*, 2005; **14**:17–20.

26. **Åkerstedt T**, **Ingre M**, **Kecklund G**, *et al.* Reaction of sleepiness indicators to partial sleep deprivation, time of day and time on task in a driving simulator – the DROWSI project. *J Sleep Res* 2010; **19**:298–309.

27. **Foret J**, **Lantin G**. The sleep of train drivers: an example of the effects of irregular work schedules on sleep. In: Colquhoun W P, Ed. *Aspects of Human Efficiency Diurnal Rhythm and Loss of Sleep*. London: The English Universities Press Ltd, 1972: 273–81.

28. **Roehrs T**, **Roth T**. Multiple sleep latency test: technical aspects and normal values. *J Clin Neurophysiol*, 1992; **9**:63–67.

29. **Czeisler C A**, **Walsh J K**, **Roth T**, *et al.* Modafinil for excessive sleepiness associated with shift-work sleep disorder. *N Engl J Med*, 2005; **353**:476–86.

30. **Lowden A**, **Kecklund G**, **Axelsson J**, *et al*. Change from an 8-hour shift to a 12-hour shift, attitudes, sleep, sleepiness and performance. *Scand J Work Environ Health*, 1998; **24**(suppl 3):69–75.

31. **Söderström M**, **Ekstedt M**, **Åkerstedt T**, *et al*. Sleep and sleepiness in young individuals with high burnout scores. *Sleep*, 2004; **17**:1369–77.

32. **Gillberg M**. Permanent 12-hour day and night shifts: subjective alertness and sleep quality. *Scand J Work Environ Health*, 1998, **24**(suppl 3):76–81.

33. **Knauth P**, **Rutenfranz J**. Duration of sleep related to the type of shift work. In: Reinberg A, Vieux N, Andlauer P, Eds. *Night and Shift Work: Biological and Social Aspects*. Oxford: Pergamon Press, 1981.

34. **Tepas D I**. Shiftworker sleep strategies. *J Hum Ergol*, 1982; **11**:325–36.

35. **Axelsson J**, **Åkerstedt T**, **Kecklund G**, *et al*. Tolerance to shift work – how does it relate to sleep and wakefullness? *Int Arch Occup Environ Health*, 2004; **77**:121–29.

36. **Smith M R**, **Eastman C I**. Night shift performance is improved by a compromise circadian phase position: study 3. Circadian phase after 7 night shifts with an intervening weekend off. *Sleep*, 2008; **31**:1639–45.

37. **Bjorvatn B**, **Stangenes K**, **Oyane N**, *et al*. Subjective and objective measures of adaptation and readaptation to night work on an oil rig in the North Sea. *Sleep*, 2006; **29**:821–29.

38. **Gillberg M**, **Kecklund G**, **Åkerstedt T**. Relations between performance and subjective ratings of sleepiness during a night awake. *Sleep*, 1994; **17**:236–41.

39. **Dorrian J**, **Lamond N**, **Dawson D**. The ability to self-monitor performance when fatigued. *J Sleep Res*, 2000; **9**:137–44.

40. **Ingre M**, **Akerstedt T**, **Peters B**, *et al*. Subjective sleepiness and accident risk avoiding the ecological fallacy. *J Sleep Res*, 2006; **15**:142–48.

41. **Rogers N L**, **Dinges D F**. Subjective surrogates of performance during night work. *Sleep*, 2003; **26**:790–91.

42. **Dinges D F**. The nature of sleepiness: causes, contexts, and consequences. In: Stunkard A, Baum A, Eds. *Perspectives in Behavioral Medicine: Eating, Sleeping, and Sex*. Hillsdale, NJ: Lawrence Erlbaum, 1989: 147–79.

43. **Van Dongen H P A**, **Dinges D F**. Sleep debt and cumulative excess wakefulness. *Sleep*, 2003; **26**:249.

44. **Horne J**, **Burley C V**. We know when we are sleepy : subjective versus objective measurements of moderate sleepiness in healthy adults. *Biol Psychol*, 2010; **83**:266–68.

45. **Akerstedt T**, **Kecklund G**, **Axelsson J**. Effects of context on sleepiness self-ratings during repeated partial sleep deprivation. *Chronobiol Int*, 2008; **25**:271–78.

46. **Yang C-M**, **Lin F-W**, **Spielman A J**. A standard procedure enhances the correlation between subjective and objective measures of sleepiness. *Sleep*, 2004; **27**:329–32.

47. **Bjerner B**, **Holm Å**, **Swensson Å**. Diurnal variation of mental perfomance. A study of three-shift workers. *Br J Ind Med*, 1955; **12**:103–10.

48. **Brown R C**. The day and night performance of teleprinter switchboard operators. *J Occup Psychol*, 1949; **23**:121–26.

49. **Wojtczak-Jaroszowa J**, **Pawlowska-Skyga K**. Night and shift work I: Circadian variations in work. *Med Pr*, 1967; **18**:1–10.

50. **Dorrian J**, **Hussey F**, **Dawson D**. Train driving efficiency and safety: examining the cost of fatigue. *J Sleep Res*, 2007; **16**:1–11.

51. **Andlauer P**. The effect of shift working on the workers' health. European Productivity Agency, TU Information Bulletin, **29**, 1960.

52. **Quaas M**, **Tunsch R**. Problems of disablement and accident frequency in shift and night work. *Studia Laboris et Salutis*, 1972; **4**:52–65.

53. **Smith P**. A study of weekly and rapidly rotating shift workers. *Int Arch Occup Environ Health*, 1979; **43**:211–20.

54. **Lockley S W**, **Cronin J W**, **Evans E E**, *et al*. Effect of reducing interns' weekly work hours on sleep and attentional failures. *N Engl J Med*, 2004; **351**:1829–37.

55. **Van Dongen H P**, **Maislin G**, **Mullington J M**, *et al*. The cumulative cost of additional wakefulness: dose–response effects on neurobehavioral functions and sleep physiology from chronic sleep restriction and total sleep deprivation. *Sleep*, 2003; **26**:117–26.

56. **Rothschild J M**, **Keohane C A**, **Rogers S**, *et al*. Risks of complications by attending physicians after performing nighttime procedures. *JAMA*, 2009; **302**:1565–72.

57. **Smith L**, **Folkard S**, **Poole C J M**. Increased injuries on night shift. *Lancet*, 1994; **344**:1137–39.

58. **Åkerstedt T**, **Fredlund P**, **Gillberg M**, *et al*. A prospective study of fatal occupational accidents – relationship to sleeping difficulties and occupational factors. *J Sleep Res*, 2002; **11**:69–71.

59. **Dorrian J**, **Tolley C**, **Lamond N**, *et al*. Sleep and errors in a group of Australian hospital nurses at work and during the commute. *Appl Ergon*, 2008; **39**:605–13.

60. **Basner M**, **Rubinstein J**, **Fomberstein K M**, *et al*. Effects of night work, sleep loss and time on task on

119. **Kripke D F, Cook B, Lewis O F.** Sleep of night workers: EEG recordings. *Psychophysiology*, 1971; 7:377–84.

120. **Bryden G, Holdstock T L.** Effects of night duty on sleep patterns of nurses. *Psychophysiology*, 1973; 10:36–42.

121. **Åkerstedt T.** Adjustment of physiological circadian rhythms and the sleep–wake cycle to shift work. In: Monk T H, Folkard S, Eds. *Hours of Work*. Chichester: John Wiley, 1985: 185–98.

122. **Uchiyama S, Kurasawa T, Sekizawa T,** et al. Job strain and risk of cardiovascular events in treated hypertensive Japanese workers: hypertension follow-up group study. *J Occup Health*, 2005; 47:102–11.

123. **Horowitz T S, Cade B E, Wolfe J M,** et al. Efficacy of bright light and sleep/darkness scheduling in alleviating circadian maladaptation to night work. *Am J Physiol Endocrinol Metab*, 2001; 281:E384–91.

124. **Signal T L, Gander P H.** Rapid counterclockwise shift rotation in air traffic control: effects on sleep and night work. *Aviat Space Environ Med*, 2007; 78:878–85.

125. **Czeisler C A, Duffy J F, Shanahan T L,** et al. Stability, precision, and near-24-hour period of the human circadian pacemaker. *Science*, 1999; 284:2177–81.

126. **Viitasalo K, Kuosma E, Laitinen J,** et al. Effects of shift rotation and the flexibility of a shift system on daytime alertness and cardiovascular risk factors. *Scand J Work Environ Health*, 2008; 34:198–205.

127. **Sallinen M, Harma M, Akila R,** et al. The effects of sleep debt and monotonous work on sleepiness and performance during a 12-h dayshift. *J Sleep Res*, 2004; 13:285–94.

128. **Son M, Kong J O, Koh S B,** et al. Effects of long working hours and the night shift on severe sleepiness among workers with 12-hour shift systems for 5 to 7 consecutive days in the automobile factories of Korea. *J Sleep Res*, 2008; 17:385–94.

129. **Dahlgren A, Kecklund G, Akerstedt T.** Overtime work and its effects on sleep, sleepiness, cortisol and blood pressure in an experimental field study. *Scand J Work Environ Health*, 2006; 32:318–27.

130. **Lowden A, Åkerstedt T.** Sleep and wake patterns in aircrew on a 2-day layover on westward long distance flights. *Aviat Space Environ Med*, 1998; 69:596–602.

131. **Scott L D, Hwang W T, Rogers A E,** et al. The relationship between nurse work schedules, sleep duration, and drowsy driving. *Sleep*, 2007; 30:1801–07.

132. **Barger L K, Cade B E, Ayas N T,** et al. Extended work shifts and the risk of motor vehicle crashes among interns. *N Engl J Med*, 2005; 352:125–34.

133. **Dumont M, Montplaisir J, Infante-Rivard C.** Insomnia symptoms in nurses with former permanent nightwork experience. In: Koella W P, Obal F, Schulz H, Visser P, Eds. *Sleep '86*. Stuttgart: Gustav Fischer Verlag, 1988: 405–06.

134. **Guilleminault C, Czeisler S, Coleman R,** et al. Circadian rhythm disturbances and sleep disorders in shift workers (EEG Supl no. 36). In: Buser P A, Cobb W A, Okuma T, Eds. *Kyoto Symposia*. Amsterdam: Elsevier, 1982: 709–14.

135. **Ingre M, Åkerstedt T.** Effect of accumulated night work during the working lifetime, on subjective health and sleep in monozygotic twins. *J Sleep Res*, 2004; 13:45–48.

136. **Harma M.** Workhours in relation to work stress, recovery and health. *Scand J Work Environ Health*, 2006; 32:502–14.

137. **Åkerstedt T, Knutsson A, Westerholm P,** et al. Work organization and unintentional sleep: results from the WOLF study. *Occup Environ Med*, 2002; 59:595–600.

138. **Anund A, Kecklund G, Peters B,** et al. Driver impairment at night and its relation to physiological sleepiness. *Scand J Work Environ Health*, 2008; 34:142–50.

139. **Gibson E S, Powles A C, Thabane L,** et al. "Sleepiness" is serious in adolescence: two surveys of 3235 Canadian students. *BMC Publ Health*, 2006; 6:116.

140. **Klerman E B, Dijk D J.** Age-related reduction in the maximal capacity for sleep – implications for insomnia. *Curr Biol*, 2008; 18:1118–23.

141. **Koller M, Härmä M, Laitinen J T,** et al. Different patterns of light exposure in relation to melatonin and cortisol rhythms and sleep of night workers. *J Pineal Res*, 1994; 16:127–35.

142. **Burch J B, Yost M G, Johnson W,** et al. Melatonin, sleep, and shift work adaptation. *J Occup Environ Med*, 2005; 47:893–901.

143. **APA.** *Diagnostic and Statistical Manual of Mental Disorders* (4th Ed.). Washington, DC: American Psychiatric Association, 2000.

144. **AASM.** *International Classification of Sleep Disorders – Diagnostic and Coding Manual*. AASM, 2001.

145. **Sack R L, Auckley D, Auger R R,** et al. Circadian rhythm sleep disorders: part I, basic principles, shift work and jet lag disorders. An American Academy of Sleep Medicine review. *Sleep*, 2007; 30:1460–83.

146. **Waage S, Moen B E, Pallesen S,** et al. Shift work disorder among oil rig workers in the North Sea. *Sleep*, 2009; 32:558–65.

147. **Lowden A, Åkerstedt T.** Self-selected work hours – work satisfaction, health and social life. In: Knauth

S H P, Folkard G C S, Eds. *Shiftwork in the 21st Century*. Frankfurt am Main: Peter Lang GmbH, 2000: 345–50.

148. **Costa G, Sartori S, Åkerstedt T**. Influence of flexibility and variability of working hours on health and well-being. *Chronobiol Int*, 2006; **23**:1125–37.

149. **Åkerstedt T, Torsvall L, Gillberg M**. Shift work and napping. In: Dinges D F, Broughton R, Eds. *Sleep and Alertness: Chronobiological, Behavioral, and Medical Aspects of Napping*. New York, NY: Raven Press, 1989: 205–20.

150. **Schweitzer P K, Randazzo A C, Stone K**, et al. Laboratory and field studies of naps and caffeine as practical countermeasures for sleep–wake problems associated with night work. *Sleep*, 2006; **29**:39–50.

151. **Garbarino S, Mascialino B, Penco M S**, et al. Professional shift-work drivers who adopt prophylactic naps can reduce the risk of car accidents during night work. *Sleep*, 2004; **27**:1295–302.

152. **Purnell M T, Feyer A-M, Herbison G P**. The impact of a nap opportunity during the night shift on the performance and alertness of 12-h shift workers. *J Sleep Res*, 2002; **11**:219–27.

153. **Signal T L, Gander P H, Anderson H**, et al. Scheduled napping as a countermeasure to sleepiness in air traffic controllers. *J Sleep Res*, 2009; **18**:11–19.

154. **Mollicone D J, Van Dongen H P, Rogers N L**, et al. Response surface mapping of neurobehavioral performance: testing the feasibility of split sleep schedules for space operations. *Acta Astronautica*, 2008; **63**:833–40.

155. **Boivin D B, James F O**. Light treatment and circadian adaptation to shift work. *Ind Health*, 2005; **43**:34–48.

156. **Santhi N, Aeschbach D, Horowitz T S**, et al. The impact of sleep timing and bright light exposure on attentional impairment during night work. *J Biol Rhythms*, 2008; **23**:341–52.

157. **Czeisler C A, Walsh J K, Wesnes K A**, et al. Armodafinil for treatment of excessive sleepiness associated with shift work disorder: a randomized controlled study. *Mayo Clin Proc*, 2009; **84**:958–72.

158. **Skene D J**. Optimization of light and melatonin to phase-shift human circadian rhythms. *J Neuroendocrinol*, 2003; **15**:438–41.

159. **Smith M R, Lee C, Crowley S J**, et al. Morning melatonin has limited benefit as a soporific for daytime sleep after night work. *Chronobiol Int*, 2005; **22**:873–88.

Section 2 Sleep Disorders and Excessive Sleepiness

Chapter 19

Sleepiness in healthcare workers

Brian Abaluck and Christopher P. Landrigan

Insufficient sleep among healthcare providers is a primary contributor to medical error [1]; the sixth leading cause of death in America [1]. Current Accreditation Council for Graduate Medical Education (the professional body responsible for monitoring residents' training in general, and work hours in particular) regulations [2] permit residents to work up to 80–88 h per week on average, in shifts as long as 30 h, and actual work hours often exceed even these limits. The hours of nurses and attending physicians are not regulated at a national level in the USA and can sometimes equal or exceed those of residents. Numerous studies have demonstrated impaired performance associated with these work hours [3].

In this chapter, we will briefly review the manner in which sleep deprivation and circadian misalignment lead to impaired performance among healthcare providers. We will then review the data directly assessing the effects of long work hours and sleep deprivation on patient and provider safety, and we will discuss how the healthcare system, hospitals, and individual providers can begin to address this issue.

Sleep and circadian determinants of physician-in-training performance

Several sleep and circadian factors affect the performance of physicians-in-training as well as other healthcare providers [4]. First, healthcare professionals must work through their circadian nadirs, during which performance degrades. In addition, long shifts lead to acute sleep deprivation and chronic sleep restriction, which – irrespective of circadian misalignment – can lead to poor performance and an increased risk of error. Third, sporadic, brief sleep periods in the hospital lead to recurrent episodes of sleep inertia, or impairment present immediately following awakening from sleep.

Circadian misalignment

The suprachiasmatic nucleus (SCN), located within the hypothalamus, drives a 24-h oscillation of alertness and sleepiness [5]. In most individuals, alertness reaches its nadir, and sleepiness peaks, between 2 and 6am, shortly before habitual wake time. Such reduced alertness may impair any work performed at night and may contribute to higher rates of accidents among night shift workers [6]. The circadian system does not adapt to large rapid changes in work schedules, leading to persistent mismatch of drive and state, mimicking jet lag. A state of jet lag may persist in many healthcare workers whose shifts vary day to day and week to week.

Acute and chronic sleep deprivation

American residents routinely work shifts lasting from 24 to 30 h [7]. In most institutions, there is no scheduled nap or break period. Sleep may therefore occur, if at all, in sporadic and variable patterns. Sleep deprivation dramatically impacts performance; after 16–18 h of wakefulness, alertness and performance decline rapidly [8]. The combination of prolonged wakefulness and wakefulness during the circadian nadir lead to synergistic impairment greater than the sum of the impairment associated with each [9]. A 2005 meta-analysis suggests that sleep loss impairs performance in both physicians and non-physicians [10]. In both physicians and others, acute sleep loss impairs vigilance, memory, verbal intelligence, reaction time, and numerous other cognitive functions. In physicians in particular, sleep loss has been found to disproportionately impair performance on clinical tasks, as

Sleepiness: Causes, Consequences and Treatment, ed. Michael J. Thorpy and Michel Billiard. Published by Cambridge University Press. © Cambridge University Press 2011.

compared with performance on tests of vigilance, memory, or verbal intelligence, although there is considerable variance in the performance of these tasks.

In addition to acute sleep restriction, residents suffer chronic sleep restriction. Chronic partial sleep deprivation induces cognitive deficits that do not recover immediately. Young adults sleep 8.5 h per night, on average, when given the opportunity [11]. Residents working extended shifts report averages 2 h lower [1, 12]. In one study of non-residents, subjects restricted to 6 or 4 h of time in bed over 14 days suffered frequent lapses in psychomotor vigilance (PVT), which persisted even after 2 days of 8 h in bed of recovery sleep [13]. In another study, subjects restricted to 3, 5, and 7 h of time in bed for 7 consecutive nights demonstrated dose-dependent declines in vigilance [14]. Subjects restricted to 5 and 7 h nightly did not demonstrate complete recovery of baseline vigilance after 3 days of 8-h recovery sleep periods. This contrasts with the pattern of recovery after total sleep deprivation, where vigilance has been found to normalize in one to two nights of unlimited sleep time [15]. Furthermore, lag in performance rebound appears to be longer following chronic partial sleep deprivation than following a single night of complete sleep loss [16]. Few data exist directly assessing the effects of chronic sleep restriction over weeks to months in interns or residents. However, the amount of recovery sleep interns and residents can obtain is frequently limited by their persistent heavy work schedules. In addition, post-call recovery sleep often occurs during the day, likely leading to a reduction in its quality and duration. Thus, it is likely that chronic sleep restriction contributes meaningfully to cognitive impairment and error among interns and residents, even though there are limited data on this issue to date.

It is worth noting that in laboratory experiments, while performance declines over weeks of sleep restriction, self-assessment of fatigue plateaus [13], such that individuals tend to believe they are tolerating chronic sleep loss better than objective measures indicate is in fact the case. Generally, self-assessment alone guides healthcare professionals. Interns, experiencing progressive chronic sleep deprivation over the course of a busy month in a hospital setting, will continue to make important decisions, even as their self-assessment of impairment becomes progressively less accurate. Such discrepancy between self-assessed fatigue and performance in healthcare workers may contribute to error.

Sleep inertia

Given their chronic sleep restriction, residents generally attempt to sleep when possible during overnight shifts. These naps are often ended by beeping pagers. Each page may represent a variety of requests. A nurse may require an order to be entered into a computer or (still more commonly) handwritten in a chart. He or she may inform a resident that a patient is "crashing" and requires emergent care. Another physician may ask a resident to see one of his or her patients in consultation, or to admit a patient from the emergency room. Unfortunately, during the first 15–30 min after sleeping, impairment (as measured by PVT performance) may exceed that suffered after 24 h of sleep deprivation [17]. Alertness remains submaximal for several hours [17]. Thus, in the current American system, residents frequently make crucial decisions while in their most impaired states.

Healthcare provider sleep restriction harms physicians and patients

Resident-physicians, work hours, and safety

Despite the accumulation of evidence that acute and chronic sleep restriction impairs performance; that sleep inertia impairs performance on awakening; and that circadian misalignment impairs performance at night, debate has persisted regarding the impact of long work hours on healthcare workers and their patients. Opponents of work hour changes make several arguments. Many note that a system involving shorter shifts requires more handoffs, which are a potential source of error. Some educators have expressed concerns that decreasing work hours would lead to poorer training. In addition, some critics have simply suggested that medical errors due to resident sleep deprivation are not a concern, as safety nets in hospitals catch errors made by sleep-deprived trainees before they harm patients. In the context of conflicting concerns, researchers over the past decade have sought to quantify the effects of extended shifts upon providers and patients, and the effects of work hour reduction on patient safety.

In April 2002, The Harvard Work Hours, Health, and Safety Group emailed all students graduating from US medical schools who were matched by the National Resident Matching Program into US residencies [18]. A web-based baseline survey regarding work hours, extended shifts, motor vehicle crashes, near-miss incidents (near-miss motor vehicle crashes in which property damage or bodily harm was narrowly avoided), serious errors, adverse patient events, and percutaneous injuries was completed by 2737 first-year residents, or interns. At least one follow-up web-based survey was completed by 2554 interns. Investigators gathered 17 003 total monthly reports from interns. Participants were 53% female, 79% medical (non-surgical) specialties, and 85% US medical school graduates. Interns worked an average of 3.9 ± 3.4 extended-duration (24 h) shifts averaging 32.0 ± .7 h per month. They reported 6.5 ± 4.5 days off per month. Interns reported a mean of 70.7 ± 26.0 weekly in-hospital hours and reported sleeping 3.2 ± 4.2 of these hours. In 7% of the cohort, 3–4 weeks of sleep diaries were obtained. These diaries correlated strongly with sleep reports obtained via a monthly web-based survey form ($r = .94, p < .0001$).

Extended-duration work shifts were associated with an increased likelihood of motor vehicle crashes [19]. Interns reported 320 crashes, 40% occurring during the commute from work. The odds ratio of reporting a crash following an extended-duration shift compared to a non-extended shift was 2.3 (95% CI 1.6–3.3). Furthermore, every extended work shift increased the likelihood of a motor vehicle crash by 9.1% (95% CI 3.4–14.7%) and increased the risk of a crash during the commute from work by 16.2% (95% CI 7.8–24.7). In months requiring five or more extended shifts, compared to months requiring no extended shifts, the odds ratio of falling asleep while driving was 2.39 (95% CI 7.8–24.7), and of falling asleep while stopped in traffic was 3.69 (95% CI 3.6–3.77). Confirmatory police reports, insurance claims, repair records, vehicle photographs, medical records, or detailed descriptions substantiating reported crashes were obtained in 82% of crashes.

Extended-duration work shifts also increased the likelihood of fatigue-related, self-reported medical errors [13]. Intra-individual rates of error during months where interns worked no extended shifts, one to four extended shifts, and five or more extended shifts were compared. Reported fatigue-related errors more than tripled (OR 3.5, 95% CI 3.3–3.7) in months with one to four extended shifts and increased sevenfold (OR 7.5, 95% CI 7.2–7.8) in months with five or more extended shifts; reported fatigue-related adverse events, respectively, increased almost ninefold (OR 8.7, OR 3.4–22) and sevenfold (OR 7.0, 4.3–11).

Extended shifts also increased the risk of percutaneous injury [14]. In addition, the risk of percutaneous injury was found to be increased during nighttime hours. Interns reported 500 injuries, noting that fatigue and attentional lapse, both of which may result from sleep restriction, were the most common reasons for occupational exposures [20]. Exposure frequencies were doubled at night (OR 2.04, 95% CI 1.98–2.11) compared with days, and increased significantly during daytime hours after extended shifts (OR 1.61, 95% CI 1.45–1.78), as compared with days that did not follow extended shifts.

Nurses, work hours, and safety

Nurses have also been found to make more errors and suffer an increased risk of occupational injury when working extended shifts. Trinkoff and colleagues surveyed 2273 nurses between 2002 and 2004 [21]. Of respondents, 16.3% reported a needlestick injury. The likelihood of experiencing a needlestick injury correlated with hours worked per day, weekends worked per month, night shifts, and working 13 or more hours per day. Regarding medical error, Rogers et al. surveyed 393 randomly selected members of the American Nursing Association about their work hours and errors in 5317 shifts. Thirty-nine percent of shifts exceeded 12.5 h, and shifts of >12.5 h were associated with a tripling of risk of error (OR = 3.29, $P = .001$) [22]. Another study involved 502 randomly selected nurses from the American Association of Critical Care Nursing who reported 6017 shifts [23]. 67% of shifts exceeded 12 h. Shifts >12.5 h were associated with a doubling of error (OR = 1.94, $p = .03$).

Attending physicians, work hours, and safety

In contrast to the growing literature regarding residents and nurses, few data have been accrued regarding the effects of attending physicians' extended shifts on patient safety. Once American physicians finish training, there are no regulations to limit their work hours. To begin assessing the relationship between attending sleep deprivation and complication rates, Rothschild et al. recently conducted a retrospective study of the risk of complications of procedures performed following attendings' overnight shifts [24]. Complication rates of surgeons and obstetricians post-call were compared with complication rates on matched procedures when surgeons and obstetricians were not post-call. Overall, being on call was not associated with a change in complication rates. However, following call nights when surgeons/obstetricians had <6 h of sleep opportunity, as defined by the window between the last procedure of call and the first procedure post-call, complication rates increased significantly (OR 1.72, 95% CI 1.02–2.89, 3.4 vs. 6.2%), suggesting that senior physicians may also perform poorly when sleep deprived.

A randomized trial of reducing intern work hours

The above studies identifying associations between extended shifts and poor outcomes share two primary limitations. First, all data were self-reported. As such, they may suffer from recall or other biases. For example, it is possible that interns or nurses may believe that they err more frequently during extended shifts and thus may be more likely to note perceived errors during these shifts. Second, these studies, which are intra-individually controlled but not randomized, cannot establish causation. While errors may be more frequent during extended shifts, the intensity and nature of work may also vary during such shifts, making determination of causation complex. During extended shifts, for example, interns may be more likely to be admitting patients or performing procedures, an activity potentially more conducive to making an error or experiencing an occupational injury than seeing established inpatients. (This limitation does not hold in assessing driving risk, however, as the nature of driving is unlikely to significantly vary following extended vs. non-extended shifts.)

To address the questions of correlation vs. causation and the issue of recall bias, the Intern Sleep and Patient Safety Study randomized interns to traditional and intervention schedules and used an established two-tiered error collection methodology to determine if a reduction in work hours led to a reduction in overall and intern-specific rates of serious medical errors. Randomization allows inference of causation over correlation, and the use of a two-tiered system for determining error, where reviewers at the second level were blinded as to whether an event being rated was collected on the traditional or intervention schedule, reduces the risk of reporting bias. We present the Intern Sleep and Patient Safety Study below [2].

AHRQ and NIOSH funded researchers in the Harvard Division of Sleep Medicine to assess the impact of work hour reconfiguration upon internal medicine interns rotating through the medical intensive care unit and the cardiac care unit at a tertiary care teaching hospital. Consenting interns were randomized either to a control group, where they worked the unit schedule of 24–30 h call every third day – the "traditional" schedule – or to an experimental group working the "intervention" schedule. On the intervention schedule, interns were scheduled to work no more than 16 h consecutively and no more than 63 h in a week (see Figure 19.1 for illustration of schedule). Even distribution of rotations throughout the year minimized learning and seasonal effects.

Interns were monitored extensively. They compiled daily work logs. Third-party study staff documented work hours on most shifts (75%), and correlation between diary-reported and observed work hours was high ($r = .98$). Interns also compiled sleep logs. At least 3 days per week, interns underwent ambulatory electroencephalographic monitoring. Reported and EEG sleep were likewise highly correlated ($r = .94$). Primary outcomes included attentional failure and error. Attentional failure was defined as the presence of slow rolling eye movements upon electrooculography (part of electroencephalographic monitoring), which are indicative of sleep pressure and the transition from wake to sleep. Non-blinded researchers initially assessed slow rolling eye movements, and blinded observers confirmed their findings. Regarding error, trained physician observers constantly observed interns, and trained critical care nurses reviewed medical records, collected solicited and voluntary reports of errors from unit staff, and gathered data from the hospital's error-reporting systems. These non-blinded observers collected information on any errors, regardless of who was involved or why, and all error reports were assessed in a second stage by blinded evaluators.

On the traditional schedule, 17 of 20 interns worked more than 80 h (mean 85 h). On the intervention schedule, all interns worked fewer than 80 h per week (mean of 65.4 h). Interns on the traditional schedule averaged 45.9 h of sleep per week, while interns on the intervention schedule averaged 51.7 h of sleep.

Outcome measures demonstrated substantial changes. Interns on the intervention schedule suffered half the rate of attentional failures at night as those on the traditional schedule ($p = .02$). On the

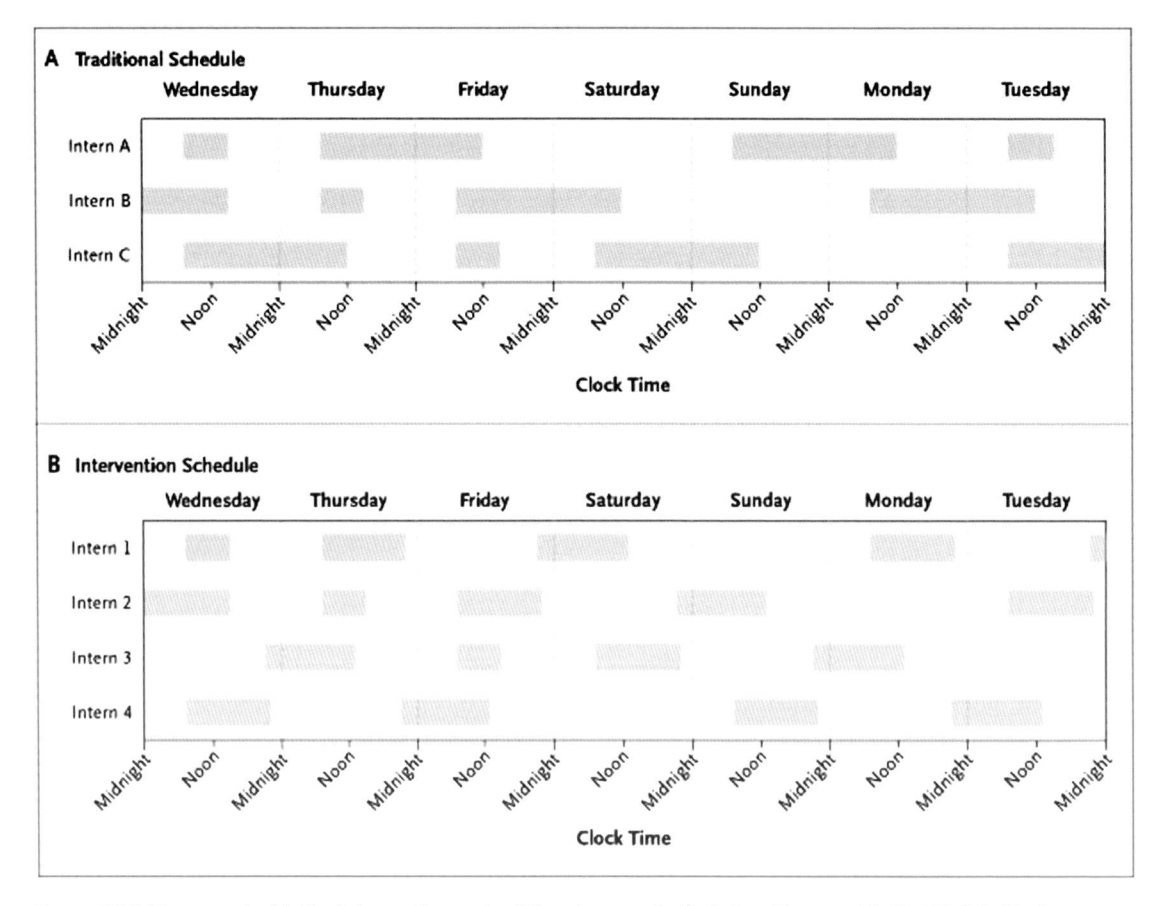

Figure 19.1 Hours worked in the intervention vs. traditional groups in the Intern Sleep and Patient Safety Study.
Dark bars represent shifts worked in traditional (top) vs. intervention (bottom) schedule in the Intern Sleep and Patient Safety Study.

intervention schedule, interns made far fewer errors than they made on the traditional schedule, despite some reported problems with handoffs. Interns on the intervention schedule made 100 serious errors per 1000 patient days, compared with 136 per 1000 patient days on the traditional schedule (36% more, $P < .001$). Diagnostic errors occurred with particularly elevated frequency on the traditional schedule, occurring more than 5 times as often ($p < .001$). Overall rates of errors (those involving interns and all other staff) were similarly much higher on the traditional schedule, but this difference was driven entirely by the difference in intern error rates; errors committed by non-intern providers (whose schedules were not changed as part of this intervention) did not change significantly on the intervention schedule. The Intern Sleep and Patient Safety study demonstrated that elimination of traditional, extended shifts improved the safety of care delivery.

Provider sleep deprivation and mood

In addition to its effect on patient and provider safety, repeated sleep deprivation among healthcare providers can lead to mood disturbances. A cohort of interns at a major academic center experienced depression, anger, and fatigue that worsened across the first five months of internship and then stabilized. A subsequent intern cohort demonstrated development of depression and burnout [25]. Among interns in this cohort who were not chronically sleep-deprived or depressed at the onset of internship, chronic sleep deprivation (report of <42 h of sleep over the prior 7 nights) moderated the development of depression during internship.

Sleep restriction and resident learning

As learning is central to medical residency, any factor impairing resident learning is of concern. Many physicians who oppose work hour reforms have expressed concern that their disciplines require greater than 80 h per week over many (3–10) years for trainees to attain competence. While there are some data demonstrating that increased experience (both at an individual and hospital level) correlates with better outcomes, there are also data that lack of sleep precludes learning. Over the last decade, an expanding body of literature has established a clear link between sleep and learning [26]. Sleep may play a key role in diverting neural networks, otherwise involved in conscious processing, to memory consolidation and enhancement [27].

Medical students and residents must learn facts and principles (forms of declarative memory) and intuition and procedures (forms of no declarative memory) over the course of their training. Sleep appears to benefit all classes of memory; in no class of memory has sleep been shown to have no benefit [28]. Not only does sleep allow for the solidification of memory against competing stimuli, but sleep potentiates learning of visual and procedural tasks; researchers have demonstrated that performance on procedural and visual tasks, following initial training, improves after several hours of non-training, but only if the non-training period involves sleep [28]. Thus, without sleep, learning suffers. These data suggest that the current system of overnight call and extended work hours may impair resident learning. Data in residents showing that overnight call hinders learning, however, are currently lacking.

Current US regulations do not adequately address healthcare provider sleep restriction

The Accreditation Council for Graduate Medical Educations (ACGME) implemented work hour regulations in July 2003 [2]. The ACGME mandated that all physicians-in-training must:

(1) work no more than 80 h per week (or in some cases 88 h), averaged over 4 weeks;
(2) have at least one day in seven off, averaged over 4 weeks;
(3) work no more than 30 consecutive hours, including time for patient care transitions, didactic learning, and continuing care for existing patients; no new patients may be admitted after 24 h of continuous duty;
(4) have a 10-h period free of work between all daily duty periods and after an extended shift; and
(5) work extended overnight shifts (24+ h) no more often than one night in three, averaged over 4 weeks.

Such regulations, if violated, can potentially lead to probation and, if unresolved, to loss of program accreditation to train residents. Unfortunately, even with perfect adherence to the above limits, residents would still be working hours which, evidence suggests, lead to an increased risk of occupational injury and medical error. Furthermore, several studies, including a nationwide cohort study, have found that interns frequently exceed work hour limits in the majority (62%) of in-hospital months [7].

In light of the perpetuation of traditional 24–30-h shifts under current regulations, as well as the frequent violations of even these limits, it is not surprising that patient outcomes have not been shown to change substantially in most populations following implementation of the ACGME regulations. A Medicare analysis – the largest study conducted to date – showed no differential improvement in either medical or surgical outcomes in teaching hospitals after implementation of the new work hour rules [29]. A VA study showed some improvement in outcomes for medical but not surgical patients [30]. Another large study in community hospitals likewise showed some improvement in medical but not surgical patients [31].

While there are reasons to believe that the current ACGME regulations for residents are inadequate to effectively address fatigue-related errors, they are the only national regulations in place in the USA regarding healthcare providers' work hours. There are no nationwide work hour limits for either attending physicians or for nurses in the United States.

In contrast to the professionally enforced American regulations for residents, European regulations limit the work hours of all healthcare professionals by law, although enforcement varies from country to country. The European Working Time Directive limits all healthcare workers to 48 h per week [32]. European Courts consider sleep time in the hospital to contribute to work hours [33]. In New Zealand, an agreement between the resident union and the government limits residents to 72 h per week (with a formal agreement to work toward 60 h per week) in shifts no longer than 16 h.

Several recent expert panels have recommended major changes in US resident and nurse work hours

In 2004, the Sleep Research Society convened a Presidential Task Force to review literature on work hours, sleep restriction, and safety and to develop work hour regulations for residents. In 2006, the Task Force recommended the following [34].

(1) Weekly work hours of physicians-in-training should be limited to an optimal maximum of 60 h of work per week, and a fixed maximum limit of 80 h of work in any week.
(2) Consecutive work should be limited to an optimal limit of 12 h of consecutive work, with a maximum limit of 18 consecutive hours of work in any setting, including time for the transition of patient care information.
(3) Physicians-in-training should have 16 h free of all duties following a shift of ≥18 consecutive hours, and at least 10 h free of all duties after work shifts of shorter than 18 consecutive hours.
(4) Physicians-in-training should have at least 36 consecutive hours free of work including two consecutive nocturnal periods once every seven days, and a 60-h consecutive period free of work once every four weeks.
(5) Physicians-in-training who are assigned to patient care responsibilities in an emergency department or other high-intensity setting where the probability and/or potential consequence of a medical error is high should work no more than 12 continuous hours in that setting.
(6) Physicians-in-training should not be scheduled to work an 18-h shift more often than every third night.

The National Sleep Foundation and Sleep Research society have endorsed these guidelines.

In late 2008, the Institute of Medicine (IOM) convened a Task Force to assess residents' duty hour limits [34]. The IOM recommended several revisions to the 2003 ACGME regulations.

(1) Limit work hours to either: (a) 30 h, with a mandatory 5-h period of protected time for sleep at night, or (b) 16 h without protected time for sleep.
(2) Residents should have 10 h after a day shift, 12 h after a night shift, and 14 h after any extended duty shift.
(3) Residents should work no more than four consecutive night shifts, with each 3- or 4-night series followed by at least 48 h off work.
(4) Residents should have at least 5 days, including at least one 48-h period, off per month.
(5) All moonlighting counts against the 80-h workweek.

In a separate report, the Institute of Medicine also recommended work hour limits for nurses [35]. Based upon the evidence regarding nurses' sleep deprivation and safety, the Institute of Medicine has suggested that nurses' shifts be limited to 12 consecutive hours. Although work hour limits for nurses do exist in some hospitals and systems (e.g. the Veterans Affairs (VA) healthcare system), the USA does not currently regulate nurse work hours across all hospitals.

Concerns about reducing provider work hours

Cost

Some academic physicians argue that the costs of reducing resident work hours would be prohibitive. A recent cost–benefit analysis estimated that the institution of 2008 IOM recommendations would cost academic medical centers $1.6 billion [36]. However, if error decreased by 11.3%, the authors estimate that the intervention would be cost-neutral for society. The only randomized evidence regarding elimination of 30-h shifts, and substitution with 16-h shifts, suggests that errors could in fact decrease by more than double this amount with widespread implementation of a 16-h shift limit.

Handoffs

Another potential objection to work hour reform is that shorter shifts may increase error by increasing transitions of care, or handoffs. An AHRQ survey in 2008 found that 51% of 160 176 hospital staff agreed that "important patient care information is lost during shift changes" [37]. Retrospective studies of emergency room patients, of hospitalized surgery patients, and of outpatients found that handoffs contributed to 24, 28, and 20% of errors, respectively [38–40]. Shorter shifts magnify the importance of transitions of care by increasing their frequency and, in many cases, by increasing the likelihood that the provider responsible for any given patient at any given time is not the provider who admitted the patient to the hospital. However, in the Intern Sleep and Patient Safety Study, those interns on the intervention schedule committed significantly fewer errors than those on the traditional schedule, despite performing more handoffs. While managing handoffs is an important patient safety goal, this study demonstrates that increased handoffs do not necessarily lead to more errors. In implementing systems with reduced hours, however, attention should be paid to optimizing the handoff. Each handoff should be complete and standardized. Ongoing research is evaluating the roles of rounding tools and technology to improve handoffs. In parallel, the Agency for Healthcare Research and Quality has recommended that communication among professionals in high-risk, information-rich fields entail standardized communication strategies, such as "SBAR" (Situation Background Assessment Recommendation).

Education

While sleep deprivation can impair learning, as discussed above, critics of work hour reduction have raised concerns that reduced hours in the hospital could lead to fewer educational opportunities. In fact, in several studies conducted to date evaluating the effects on education of eliminating or reducing 24-h work shifts in the USA, obstetrical and surgical case volume has generally been preserved, and standardized exam scores have remained stable or improved [41–44]. That said, preservation or improvement of educational opportunities with work hour reduction typically requires substantial reorganization of curricula, which is an important challenge in implementing care systems with reduced resident work hours, as discussed below.

We suggest additional evidence-based principles of work hour reform

Schedule designs should incorporate knowledge of circadian physiology. Work hour limitations are necessary but not sufficient to reduce fatigue-related impairment. For example, the European Working Time Directive limits workers to 48 h per week. Switching rapidly from a week of day work into a week where a resident works six consecutive 8-h night shifts meets such a requirement, but is likely not the best schedule for patient safety, as the rapid transition from day to night results in circadian misalignment, and as recurrent nights lead to progressive chronic sleep restriction (due to most night workers' difficulties sleeping during the day, at an adverse circadian phase).

While such an example represents an extreme case, predicting the effectiveness of any novel schedule is difficult. In part, this difficulty in prediction results from the dearth of research regarding non-traditional physician schedules. However, testing of diverse schedules, and publication of outcomes of physician alertness and patient safety associated with these schedules, would provide significant benefit to those redesigning schedules in their own institutions. While the Intern Sleep and Patient Safety Study showed a clear reduction of error committed by those working an intervention schedule, this schedule was only one of many possible schedules that might reduce work hours; it remains unknown which one or ones may be best in various circumstances. Ideally, future testing of a variety of strategies, in single- or multi-center studies, would allow local leaders to select the most appropriate of many from a suite of options.

Implementation of any novel schedule should include regular hour reporting of its participants and mechanisms for modifying attempted schedules as needed; often, unpredicted problems arise with new schedules that must be addressed expeditiously.

We suggest the following guidelines, based upon our own experience and the literature, to inform schedule design [45].

(1) Minimize consecutive nights on duty. Sleep between consecutive night shifts is poor and leads to chronic sleep deprivation.
(2) Allow a day off after a night on duty to allow for recovery from acute sleep restriction.
(3) Minimize duration of night shifts to minimize sleep while on shift to minimize sleep inertia.
(4) Allow extended recovery after extended day shifts.
(5) If rotating between multiple shifts (e.g. day, afternoon, night), rotate in the delay direction (early shift, afternoon shift, night shift) rather than in the advance direction (night shift, morning shift, afternoon shift).
(6) Provide sleep education to healthcare professionals. Such education should include the following:

a. education regarding the importance of napping before each night shift to interrupt built-up sleep pressure from the day;
   b. education about the importance of maximizing sleep between non-extended shifts to minimize chronic sleep restriction. Most healthy young individuals attain peak cognitive function only by sleeping 8–9 h per night;
   c. training in strategic caffeine use. Caffeine is most effective taken in small, frequent doses. Caffeine may impair one's ability to evaluate one's own sleepiness and lead to negative behavioral side-effects at high doses. In addition, it is important to modulate its use as a sleep opportunity approaches so that sleep is not impaired by the caffeine.

(7) Plan adequate recovery sleep following long shifts when designing schedules.
(8) Design planned naps on duty where possible and necessary, ideally followed by 15 min of coverage by another provider, in order to minimize sleep inertia.
(9) Screen providers for sleep disorders, which may increase the risk of fatigue-related errors.

Challenges

The above principles provide guidance in how to implement pragmatic circadian-based schedules that minimize the risk of fatigue-related errors, but the actual implementation of such schedules is invariably challenging. Each institution faces its own set of barriers and constraints in establishing safer work schedules. These may include concerns about provider workforce, continuity of care, and medical education. Plans must be in place to adequately staff units with implementation of shorter work hours, handoffs of care must be optimized, and residents' curricula reorganized to ensure high-quality education in a new system.

In addition, an up-front investment of resources is generally necessary to implement successful work hour reforms. While reduction of work hours could potentially be cost-neutral for society (given the potential to reduce costly adverse events, as discussed above) there is a cost to hiring the providers needed to implement the change. Often, when work hour reductions are mandated, hospital departments or residency programs are expected inappropriately to bear the cost of this change on a limited budget, and find themselves in the difficult position of trying to get the same amount of work done with the same funds and same number of providers, each of whom is present for fewer hours per week. As savings due to improved care do not generally accrue to hospital departments and programs, they cannot reap the financial benefits of an improved, more efficient system. Such a misalignment of incentives can impede improvement. Overcoming this barrier requires high-level policy changes, where the costs of reorganizing care in an evidence-based, improved manner are shared between departments, hospital administration, and most importantly healthcare system payers, who are the beneficiaries in most systems of more efficient care.

Conclusion

Sleepiness continues to play a central and largely avoidable role in healthcare. Lab- and field-based studies show us that extended resident shifts impair cognition and likely impair learning. Such impairment translates into error, poor patient care, and resident harm. Reduction of provider work hours is a powerful means of addressing the high rate of avoidable error and injury in hospitals, but making this change requires substantial changes in scheduling, an up-front investment of resources and effort to establish a new infrastructure, and changes in healthcare professionals' approach to work hours, safety, teamwork, and professionalism.

References

1. **Institute of Medicine**. *To Err is Human: Building A Safer Health System*. Retrieved 15 September 2009 from: http://www.iom.edu/Reports/1999/ To-Err-is-Human-Building-A-Safer-Health-System.aspx
2. **ACGME**. *Common Program Requirements – Duty Hour Requirements. Retrieved* 15 September 2009 from http://www.acgme.org/acWebsite/dutyHours/dh_ComProgrRequirmentsDutyHours0707.pdf
3. **Arnedt J T, Owens J, Crouch M**, *et al*. Neurobehavioral performance of residents after heavy night call vs after alcohol ingestion. *JAMA*, 2005; **294**:1025–33.
4. **Lockley S W, Barger L K, Ayas N T**, *et al*. Effects of health care provider work hours and sleep deprivation on safety and performance. *Jt Comm J Qual Patient Saf*, 2007; **33**:7–18.

5. **Jewett M E, Kronauer R E**. Interactive mathematical models of subjective alertness and cognitive throughput in humans. *J Biol Rhythms*, 1999; **14**:588–97.

6. **Folkard S, Lombardi D A**. Modeling the impact of the components of long work hours on injuries and "accidents". *Am J Ind Med*, 2006; **49**: 953–63.

7. **Landrigan C P, Barger L K, Cade B E**, *et al*. Interns' compliance with accreditation council for graduate medical education work-hour limits. *JAMA*, 2006; **296**:1063–70.

8. **Jewett M E, Kronauer R E**. Interactive mathematical models of subjective alertness and cognitive throughput in humans. *J Biol Rhythms*, 1999; **14**:588–97.

9. **Dijk D J, Lockley S W**. Integration of human sleep–wake regulation and circadian rhythmicity. *J Appl Physiol*, 2002; **92**:852–62.

10. **Philibert I**. Sleep loss and performance in residents and nonphysicians: a meta-analytic examination. *Sleep*, 2005; **28**:1392–402.

11. **Rajaratnam S M, Middleton B, Stone B M**, *et al*. Melatonin advances the circadian timing of EEG sleep and directly facilitates sleep without altering its duration in extended sleep opportunities in humans. *J Physiol*, 2004; **561**:339–51.

12. **Barger L K, Cade B E, Ayas N T**, *et al*. Extended work shifts and the risk of motor vehicle crashes among interns. *N Engl J Med*, 2005; **352**:125–34.

13. **Van Dongen H P, Maislin G, Mullington J M**, *et al*. The cumulative cost of additional wakefulness: dose–response effects on neurobehavioral functions and sleep physiology from chronic sleep restriction and total sleep deprivation. *Sleep*, 2003; **26**:117–26.

14. **Belenky G, Wesensten N J, Thorne D R**, *et al*. Patterns of performance degradation and restoration during sleep restriction and subsequent recovery: a sleep dose–response study. *J Sleep Res*, 2003; **12**:1–12.

15. **Jay S M, Lamond N, Ferguson S**, *et al*. The characteristics of recovery sleep when recovery opportunity is restricted. *Sleep*, 2007; **30**:353–60.

16. **Van Dongen H P, Dinges D F**. Sleep, circadian rhythms, and psychomotor vigilance. *Clin Sports Med*, 2005; **24**:237–49, vii–viii.

17. **Jewett M E, Wyatt J K, Ritz-De C A**, *et al*. Time course of sleep inertia dissipation in human performance and alertness. *J Sleep Res*, 1999; **8**:1–8.

18. **Barger L K, Cade B E, Ayas N T**, *et al*. Extended work shifts and the risk of motor vehicle crashes among interns. *N Engl J Med*, 2005; **352**:125–34.

19. **Barger L K, Ayas N T, Cade B E**, *et al*. Impact of extended-duration shifts on medical errors, adverse events, and attentional failures. *PLoS Med*, 2006; 3:e487.

20. **Ayas N T, Barger L K, Cade B E**, *et al*. Extended work duration and the risk of self-reported percutaneous injuries in interns. *JAMA*, 2006; **296**:1055–62.

21. **Trinkoff A M, Le R, Geiger-Brown J**, *et al*. Work schedule, needle use, and needlestick injuries among registered nurses. *Infect Control Hosp Epidemiol*, 2007; **28**:156–64.

22. **Rogers A E, Hwang W T, Scott L D**, *et al*. The working hours of hospital staff nurses and patient safety. *Health Aff (Millwood)*, 2004; **23**:202–12.

23. **Scott L D, Rogers A E, Hwang W T**, *et al*. Effects of critical care nurses' work hours on vigilance and patients' safety. *Am J Crit Care*, 2006; **15**:30–37.

24. **Rothschild J M, Keohane C A, Rogers S**, *et al*. Risks of complications by attending physicians after performing nighttime procedures. *JAMA*, 2009; **302**:1565–72.

25. **Rosen I M, Gimotty P A, Shea J A**, *et al*. Evolution of sleep quantity, sleep deprivation, mood disturbances, empathy, and burnout among interns. *Acad Med*, 2006; **81**:82–85.

26. **Stickgold R, Walker M P**. Sleep and memory: the ongoing debate. *Sleep*, 2005; **28**:1225–27.

27. **Diekelmann S, Wilhelm I, Born J**. The whats and whens of sleep-dependent memory consolidation. *Sleep Med Rev*, 2009; **13**:309–21.

28. **Stickgold R**. How do I remember? Let me count the ways. *Sleep Med Rev*, 2009; **13**:305–08.

29. **Volpp K G, Rosen A K, Rosenbaum P R**, *et al*. Mortality among hospitalized Medicare beneficiaries in the first 2 years following ACGME resident duty hour reform. *JAMA*, 2007; **298**:975–83.

30. **Volpp K G, Rosen A K, Rosenbaum P R**, *et al*. Mortality among patients in VA hospitals in the first 2 years following ACGME resident duty hour reform. *JAMA*, 2007; **298**:984–92.

31. **Shetty K D, Bhattacharya J**. Changes in hospital mortality associated with residency work-hour regulations. *Ann Intern Med*, 2007; **147**:73–80.

32. **British Medical Association**. *The Final Countdown to the European Working Time Directive – a Guide for Junior Doctors*. Retrieved 15 September 2009 from http://www.bma.org.uk/images/FinalCountdown_tcm41-158037.pdf.

33. **Mayor S, Burgermeister J, Kosner K**, *et al*. Over the limit? *BMJ*, 2004; **329**:310.

34. **Czeisler C A**. The Gordon Wilson Lecture. Work hours, sleep and patient safety in residency training. *Trans Am Clin Climatol Assoc*, 2006; **117**:159–88.

35. **Institute of Medicine**. *Keeping Patients Safe: Transforming the Work Environment of Nurses.* Retrieved 15 September 2009 from http://www.iom.edu/Reports/2003/Keeping-Patients-Safe-Transforming-the-Work-Environment-of-Nurses.aspx.

36. **Nuckols T K**, **Bhattacharya J**, **Wolman D M**, *et al.* Cost implications of reduced work hours and workloads for resident physicians. *N Engl J Med*, 2009; **360**:2202–15.

37. **AHRQ**. *Hospital Survey on Patient Safety Culture: 2008 Comparative Database Report. 2008 March.* Retrieved 15 September 2009 from: http://www.ahrq.gov/qual/patientsafetyculture/.

38. **Kachalia A**, **Gandhi T K**, **Puopolo A L**, *et al.* Missed and delayed diagnoses in the emergency department: a study of closed malpractice claims from 4 liability insurers. *Ann Emerg Med*, 2007; **49**:196–205.

39. **Greenberg C C**, **Regenbogen S E**, **Studdert D M**, *et al.* Patterns of communication breakdowns resulting in injury to surgical patients. *J Am Coll Surg*, 2007; **204**:533–40.

40. **Gandhi T K**, **Kachalia A**, **Thomas E J**, *et al.* Missed and delayed diagnoses in the ambulatory setting: a study of closed malpractice claims. *Ann Intern Med*, 2006; **145**:488–96.

41. **McElearney S T**, **Saalwachter A R**, **Hedrick T L**, *et al.* Effect of the 80-hour work week on cases performed by general surgery residents. *Am Surg*, 2005; **71**:552–55.

42. **Barden C B**, **Specht M C**, **McCarter M D**, *et al.* Effects of limited work hours on surgical training. *J Am Coll Surg*, 2002; **195**:531–38.

43. **de Virgilio C**, **Yaghoubian A**, **Lewis R J**, *et al.* The 80-hour resident workweek does not adversely affect patient outcomes or resident education. *Curr Surg*, 2006; **63**:435–39.

44. **Kelly A**, **Marks F**, **Westhoff C**, *et al.* The effect of the New York State restrictions on resident work hours. *Obstet Gynecol*, 1991; **78**:468–73.

45. **Landrigan C P**, **Czeisler C A**, **Barger L K**, *et al.* Effective implementation of work-hour limits and systemic improvements. *Jt Comm J Qual Patient Saf*, 2007; **33**:19–29.

Section 2 Chapter 20

Sleep Disorders and Excessive Sleepiness

Sleepiness in the military: operational implications and research imperatives

Thomas J. Balkin

Fatigue, exertion, and privation constitute in war a special principle of destruction, not essentially belonging to contest, but more or less inseparably bound up with it, and certainly one which especially belongs to strategy.
von Clausewitz, On War (1873) [1].

Military strategy has always been about creating battlefield advantages and exploiting those advantages. The most obvious advantages are those within the physical realm, including superior weaponry or firepower, superior manpower, and occupation of easily defended terrain. Clearly, in conventional warfare, any force possessing such advantages constitutes a formidable foe.

Historically, however, such advantages have rarely proven insurmountable. Military history is rife with examples of battles won by forces which, although physically inferior, gained the upper hand by outwitting the enemy – often by coupling tactics involving deception (i.e. causing the enemy to deploy its resources inappropriately) with the "element of surprise." Among the best-known modern examples of such battles was the allied invasion of Normandy in World War II, which was preceded by extensive efforts to mislead the German forces regarding the likely location and timing of the invasion [2].

Although the capacity for strategic thinking is clearly important in the planning and preparation stages, it becomes more critical during actual engagement with the enemy, when plans need to be altered in real time to reflect battlefield exigencies. In fact, battles are generally won not because of the brilliance of the initial plan, but because of the brilliance of individuals who, while engaged in the battle, have both the mental wherewithal to recognize a battlefield opportunity when it appears and the initiative to seize and capitalize on that opportunity. Indeed, Field Marshall Helmuth Carl Bernard von Moltke's famous observation that "No battle plan ever survives contact with the enemy" [3] can be considered an acknowledgment of the criticality of mental acuity [manifested as situational (battlefield) awareness, problem-solving ability, and creativity] during the heat of battle.

Given that relatively greater mental acuity constitutes a military advantage, it is reasonable to postulate that military strategists throughout the ages might have specifically endeavored to optimize the cognitive readiness of their own troops while endeavoring to diminish the cognitive readiness of the enemy. Indeed, the observation by Pericles (~432 BC) that "I am more afraid of our own mistakes than of our enemy's designs" [4] suggests that the importance of mental perspicacity on the battlefield has long been appreciated.

An obvious way to reduce the enemy's mental acuity would be to ensure that they were deprived of adequate sleep. Of course, sleep deprivation has been the object of scientific investigation for only the past 114 years (i.e. Patrick and Gilbert are credited with the first scientific study of sleep deprivation in 1896 [5]) and an explicit understanding of the effects of sleep loss on militarily relevant higher-order cognitive capabilities such as planning, problem-solving, and creativity [6] has emerged only over the past few decades. Nevertheless, it is likely that early military strategists had at least an implicit understanding of the mental readiness-related advantages that can be conferred by depriving an enemy of rest – if not sleep, per se. And although Sun Tzu's (~476–221 BC) advice in *The Art of War* that "If he [the enemy] is taking his ease, give him no rest" [7] does not suggest that the enemy should be deprived of sleep per se, it is nevertheless clear that the sustained harassment that Sun Tzu counsels would inevitably involve the sort of

Sleepiness: Causes, Consequences and Treatment, ed. Michael J. Thorpy and Michel Billiard. Published by Cambridge University Press. © Cambridge University Press 2011.

nighttime operations that preclude adequate sleep for the enemy.

Nighttime operations

Most ancient battles were conducted (or at least initiated) in daylight. For conventional warfare, this was a logical necessity since (a) generals needed to be able to see the battlefield to make informed real-time decisions about deployment of resources, (b) much of the real-time communication on the battlefield was via flags ("battle standards") – so coordinated actions were dependent upon the visibility of these flags (although horns were also used for communication, they were less useful for specifying the positions of the various divisions within an army), and (c) soldiers were thought to be heartened and reassured by the sight of their commanders on the battlefield – and to have their resolve steeled by the fact that their commanders could also see them (i.e. should they be tempted to turn and flee).

Given the necessity of daylight for optimal effectiveness of large ancient armies, it is not surprising that nighttime raids have traditionally been favored by smaller forces – especially by guerrillas who prefer to take advantage of darkness (and perhaps their enemy's "sleep inertia") to harass stronger enemies at night [8]. However, nighttime attacks have not been conducted solely by guerrillas – nor solely for the purpose of harassment. Early military doctrine/conventional wisdom had it that armies who felt themselves to be at a relative disadvantage in terms of military strength *should* attack under the cloak of darkness, when the stronger army's ability to communicate was greatly diminished – thus fostering confusion and panic and neutralizing the physical advantages of that stronger force by diminishing its ability to effectively marshal its superior resources to its own defense.

The Battle of Gaugamela

The challenge for any ancient military strategist who wanted to deprive his enemy of sleep would have been figuring out how to do so without exacting a comparable toll on his own troops. In the annals of ancient military history, there is probably no better example of a strategy that achieved such an outcome than that employed by Alexander the Great at the Battle of Gaugamela:

It was the year 331 BC, Alexander was 25 years old, and he was in the midst of his campaign to conquer the known world. He and his army of approximately 47 000 troops had invaded Persia, winning several skirmishes, and a significant battle at Issus. Darius III was the king of Persia and the leader of its army, and after his initial losses to Alexander he mustered a force that was conservatively estimated to be 100 000 troops (a significant advantage in terms of manpower, although it is likely that many of these troops were poorly trained compared to Alexander's professional troops). Darius also held significant advantages in terms of his numbers of scythed chariots and cavalry – and he reportedly had 15 war elephants, which were at that time considered to be especially terrifying and effective weapons.

In order to take maximum advantage of his superiority in the number of chariots, it was important for Darius to meet Alexander's army on a flat battleground, where these vehicles would have optimal maneuverability. Accordingly, he positioned his army to meet Alexander's on the plains of Guagamela – and there are even some reports that he prepared this chosen battle site by removing vegetation and smoothing out mounds so as to further facilitate maneuverability.

When Alexander arrived at Guagamela, he was advised by at least one of his generals to attack Darius' larger force at night – consistent with what would have been the "conventional military wisdom" of the time. Since this was also what the Persians expected, Darius ordered his army to stand ready (in full armor, with horses yoked to chariots, etc.) all night, to repel the expected nighttime attack. However, Alexander decided to wait until morning to launch his attack (and he even allegedly "overslept" on the morning of the attack) – which meant that he and his army were relatively rested and refreshed, whereas Darius and his army were relatively sleep-deprived by the time the battle started.

Needless to say, Alexander defeated Darius III at Guagamela (in fact, he almost managed to kill him), and although Darius managed to escape with his life, this loss ultimately resulted in the collapse of the Persian Empire about a year later. (For those interested, a detailed description of the Battle of Guagamela can be found in [9].)

Of course, it is impossible to know what Alexander was thinking when he decided to delay his attack at Guagamela until morning – whether this was a deliberate attempt to deprive the enemy forces of sleep and thus reduce their military effectiveness, or merely a "happy accident" with that fortuitous outcome.

Likewise, it is impossible to know whether, or to what extent, Darius' army might have fared any better had they obtained sleep on the prior night. However, as perhaps the greatest military strategist in history, it would be difficult to conceive of the possibility that Alexander made this decision without (a) anticipating that Darius would keep his army at the ready all night long while (b) the Macedonian army slept (or at least rested), and that (c) this would confer military advantage to his Macedonian army on the following day. Otherwise, Alexander surely would have attacked at night.

Sleepiness and the Cold War

Although the extent to which Alexander purposely endeavored to deprive the Persian army of sleep at Gaugamela can never be known for certain, it is likely that sleep- and sleepiness-related considerations have figured prominently (albeit, sometimes implicitly) in military strategy and tactics across the ages. And while it is beyond the scope of this chapter to review and describe all past battles in which sleep loss/sleepiness were likely to have played a role, it is useful to illustrate the manner in which sleep/sleepiness has remained a militarily relevant factor in modern times. This is best illustrated by the presumed military strategy of the former USSR/Warsaw Pact nations during the Cold War:

From the period of 1945 to 1991, considerable tensions over the political, economic, and military configuration of the post-WWII world were manifested as mutual distrust and competition between the west (the US and other NATO nations) and the east (the USSR and other Eastern Bloc/Warsaw Pact nations). In part, these tensions were both reflected by, and fueled by, an arms race in which both sides sought military advantage in what, if it degenerated to that point, would be a war fought for dominion over all of Europe (and in effect, domination of the rest of the modern world).

During this period, the Soviet Union built the largest (in terms of number of troops) military in the world, investing heavily in the development and stockpiling of both conventional and nuclear weapons. However, it was generally considered that the technological superiority of western weapons effectively offset the Soviets' numerical advantage, at least in the early years of the Cold War. During the latter years, the technological gap between eastern and western weapons systems narrowed, increasingly tipping the scales in favor of the Warsaw Pact.

The presumed Soviet plan for a conventional invasion of Western Europe was simple – and heavily predicated on what was known about sleepiness, fatigue, and performance: Essentially, the Soviets would mass their troops in Eastern Europe, and invade the West in two "waves." The purpose of the first of these waves was not so much to "win" its battles with the NATO forces as to continuously "engage" those forces for 2–3 consecutive days, at which point it was expected that troops on both sides of the conflict would be rendered "militarily ineffective" [10] by virtue of sleep deprivation and fatigue. At that point, the second wave of the invasion (consisting of well-rested, well-slept troops) would be sent into Western Europe, where they would encounter little effective resistance (since the NATO forces would not have any "fresh" troops remaining to meet this second wave).

No such invasion ever occurred because (a) the West deployed short-range nuclear weapons in Europe as a deterrence to invasion, and (b) efforts at that time by the Soviet Union to get the United States to forswear a "first strike" with nuclear weapons (i.e. to promise not to be the first to launch nuclear missiles in a conflict with the USSR) were rebuffed. (Clearly, the use of nuclear weapons could have shortened the time course of a war in Europe to such an extent that "sleep loss-induced deficits in military effectiveness" would not have been a factor). Interestingly, it can therefore be argued that the ultimate utility of deploying nuclear weapons in Europe during the Cold War was that it neutralized the considerable Soviet advantage in troop alertness that would have assured them of victory in a conventional war against NATO forces!

Military sleep research

Of course, the attention of military sleep researchers has always been (and thankfully, is likely to always remain) focused more within the realms of neurophysiology and psychology than on issues related to military strategy and global politics. Specifically, military sleep researchers have mostly been dedicated to performing studies with an ultimate aim of sustaining the "military effectiveness" (ability to perform those tasks required to successfully achieve mission objectives) of sleepy soldiers. Accordingly, the military sleep researcher's mission has generally included efforts to (a) determine the nature of sleep loss-induced performance deficits [11]; (b) quantify the relationship between sleepiness and performance [12]; and to

(c) devise and test interventions to sustain performance in sleepy soldiers [13]. Over the past 25+ years, the ultimate goal of these lines of research has been to develop a comprehensive sleep/performance management system.

The Walter Reed Sleep/Performance Management System: an overview

Today, conventional (non-nuclear) warfare remains the "norm" for military conflicts around the world. Most conflicts involving US troops are continuous, 24-h per day, high OPTEMPO (operational tempo) endeavors that result in night work, disturbed or restricted sleep, and (occasionally) rapid deployment across multiple time zones. Because the soldiers' mental readiness for combat is primarily a function of the adequacy (duration and quality) of recent sleep, efforts by military sleep research laboratories have traditionally been focused on development of tools and strategies for monitoring, preventing and/or reversing the decrementing effects of sleep loss and fatigue on operationally relevant cognitive performance capabilities, and transitioning the results of such studies into a fieldable, easy-to-use tool for commanders and military medical personnel. The culmination of this effort, spearheaded by the Walter Reed Army Institute of Research (WRAIR), is a comprehensive sleep/performance management system (SPMS) with three components.

1. The "Sleep Watch Actigraph" is a wrist-worn (wear-and-forget) digital signal-processing device that was developed at WRAIR. This device measures and records wrist movement data, and transduces these data into valid records of objectively determined sleep/wake state (with a resolution of 1 min) for up to 6 weeks before a battery change or data download is required.
2. The Sleep, Activity, Fatigue and Task Effectiveness (SAFTE) model [14] is a mathematical algorithm being developed to predict cognitive readiness based on two factors that mediate cognitive performance: (a) sleep/wake history and (b) time of day. With sleep/wake data provided by the Sleep Watch Actigraph and with the operational implications of these data made clear by the model, informed decisions regarding optimal application (timing and dosage) of pharmacological countermeasures are possible.

Also, it is likely that the model will be used interactively before and during military missions to optimize and update sleep/wake and work schedules. Future developments of the model will supersede current sleep/performance prediction models by (a) predicting the rate of recovery from sleep loss (current models only predict rate of decline during sleep loss), (b) specifying sources of individual variability in resilience during sleep loss (current models are based on group mean data), and (c) predicting the efficacy of fatigue countermeasures (e.g. caffeine, modafinil, etc.). These improvements to the model, in addition to studies aimed at validating the model in the operational environment, currently constitute the major aims of the research program.

3. Pharmacological countermeasures (e.g. caffeine, modafinil, D-amphetamine, etc.) are investigated to determine their relative efficacy for restoring alertness, for their safety (side-effect) profiles, and for their effects on various aspects of militarily relevant cognitive performance (vigilance, problem-solving, situation awareness, etc.). Similarly, sleep-inducing/enhancing medications (zolpidem, melatonin, etc.) have been studied to determine potential usefulness as sleep aids in the operational environment (to enhance sleep following travel across time zones, following night work, under non-sleep-conducive environmental conditions, etc.) [e.g. 15]. Again, in addition to measures of safety and efficacy, military researchers focus on the militarily relevant performance effects of these compounds – reflecting the ultimate aim of the SPMS to sustain the military effectiveness of the soldiers in the field.

The chronically sleep-restricted soldier

Although planned military operations occasionally require personnel to stay awake (and militarily effective) for up to 72 h, such missions are more the exception than the rule. In part, this is because it has long been recognized that the military effectiveness of soldiers is, on average, neutralized after 24–48 h of continuous wakefulness [10] – and commanders who plan such missions are increasingly aware of the risks that they incur. Far more common, and perhaps nearly ubiquitous in modern military operations, is chronic sleep restriction – in which soldiers habitually obtain some sleep each day, albeit not enough to maintain optimal (or perhaps even nominal) levels of alertness and cognitive performance. Findings from the recent Mental Health Assessment Team (MHAT) V survey of military personnel in Operation Enduring Freedom (OEF) and Operation Iraqi Freedom (OIF) revealed that soldiers report an average of 5.6 h of sleep per night [16] – significantly less than the 7–8 h of nightly sleep that is typically recommended. And there can be little doubt that this chronic sleep loss is currently taking a toll, as revealed by analyses showing: (a) as self-reported hours of nightly sleep decline, the likelihood of self-reported "accidents or mistakes that affected the mission" increase, and (b) as self-reported hours of nightly sleep decline, likelihood of self-reported "abuse of a noncombatant" increases. In fact, for those soldiers reporting 5–6 h of sleep per night, 6–8% reported making errors or having accidents that impacted their missions, and approximately 5–7% reported engaging in activities that they considered to be "abuse of a noncombatant" (i.e. an Iraqi or Afghani civilian) (unpublished findings based on MHAT-V data, not included in the final report [16], but currently being prepared for publication).

Sleep restriction studies

It is striking that most of what is currently known about the effects of sleep loss comes from total sleep deprivation (TSD) studies. This is, at least in part, because scientists (including military scientists) studying sleep loss effects have typically made the implicit and parsimonious assumption that the effects of TSD and partial sleep deprivation (i.e. PSD or sleep restriction) differ only in terms of the rapidity and extent to which they produce sleepiness and its attendant deficits in alertness and neurocognitive performance. Such studies have produced a wealth of data over the years. In fact, over the past 10 years, studies conducted at WRAIR alone have revealed that total sleep deprivation produces deficits in capabilities ranging from simple reaction time [17] to problem-solving [18], moral reasoning [19], humor appreciation [20], risk-taking behavior [21], decision-making [22], and ability to differentiate odors [23].

Because the qualitative equivalence of TSD and chronic sleep restriction effects have been assumed but never demonstrated empirically, and because chronic sleep restriction (CSR) is far more prevalent in the operational environment than TSD, military sleep researchers have recently begun to focus more specifically on the effects of chronic sleep restriction.

Early studies on the effects of sleep restriction were generally conducted for the express purpose of determining whether, and to what extent, adaptation to long-term (weeks/months) partial sleep loss might develop. Results from such studies did actually suggest the possibility of adaptation. After an initial decline, performance and subjective alertness tended to improve over ensuing weeks and months of continued sleep restriction [24]. However, in those early studies, the subjects did not actually sleep in the laboratory every night, so it was not possible to objectively verify that the assigned restricted sleep schedules were faithfully maintained for the duration of the study.

More recent studies have failed to reveal evidence of adaptation. In one such study by Belenky et al. [25] at the Walter Reed Army Institute of Research, daytime alertness and performance changes were determined and quantified during chronic sleep restriction vs. sleep augmentation. Sixty-six normal volunteers spent either 3 h ($n = 18$), 5 h ($n = 16$), 7 h ($n = 16$), or 9 h ($n = 16$) daily time in bed (TIB) for 7 days (restriction/augmentation) followed by 3 days with 8 h daily TIB (recovery). In the 3-h TIB group, speed (mean and fastest 10% of responses) on the Psychomotor Vigilance Task (PVT) declined, and PVT lapses (reaction times greater than 500 ms) increased across the 7 days of sleep restriction. In the 7- and 5-h TIB groups, speed initially declined, then stabilized at a relatively (compared to baseline) reduced level. In the 9-h group, speed and lapses remained at baseline levels. All subjects then underwent 3 nights of recovery with 8 h time in bed (TIB) per night. No evidence of physiological or behavioral adaptation to sleep restriction was found. To the contrary, it was revealed that PVT performance declined in a sleep dose-dependent manner, and either leveled off at a reduced level or continued to decline across the entire sleep restriction period (see Figure 20.1). Among the most interesting, and least expected, findings from this study was the evidence of "carry-over" effects of sleep restriction into the "recovery sleep" phase. PVT performance in the 3- and 5-h TIB groups declined, and remained below baseline, for the entire 3-day recovery sleep phase – although it was estimated that full recovery of performance (to pre-restriction baseline levels) following a comparable level of TSD would normally occur following 1–2 nights of recovery sleep. Also, it was found that self-ratings of sleepiness, which had also increased

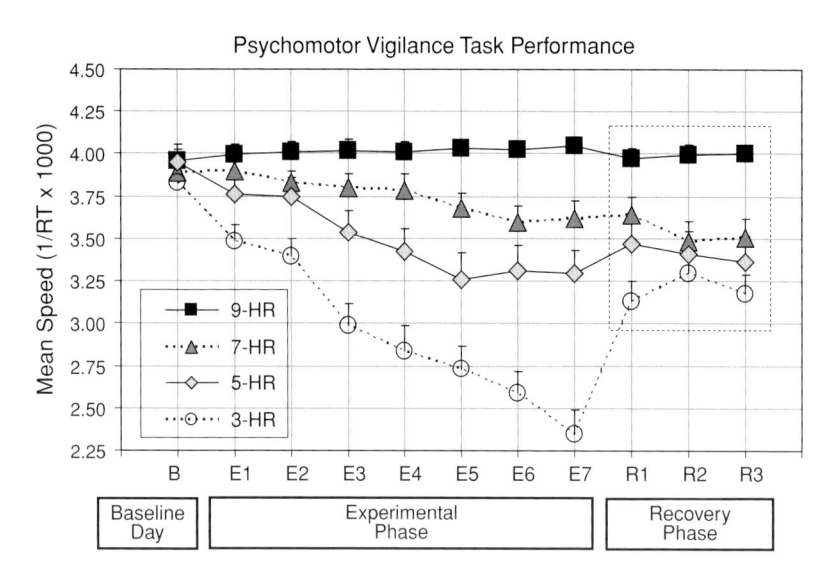

Figure 20.1 PVT performance across 1 baseline day (B), seven days (E1–E7), of 3, 5, 7, or 9 h TIB per night, and three days of recovery sleep (R1– R3, with 8 h TIB per night). Dashed box highlights performance during the recovery sleep period. RT = Reaction Time. Adapted from Belenky et al. [25] with permission.

in a dose-dependent manner across the sleep restriction phase in the 3-h TIB group, rebounded to baseline levels after a single night of recovery sleep. This suggested that although there was no evidence of physiological adaptation to restricted sleep (i.e. reflected by an improved ability to perform on the PVT across days), some subjective habituation to the restricted sleep regime had occurred.

Of course, for logistical reasons, laboratory studies of sleep restriction have been of relatively short duration – including only 7–14 consecutive nights of restricted sleep. Therefore, it remains possible that sleep restriction periods of longer duration (i.e. months) would reveal evidence of adaptation. However, this seems unlikely, since (a) prior studies in patients with sleep disorders such as sleep apnea have revealed no evidence of behavioral or physiological adaptation to chronic sleep disruption [26], and (b) there is evidence that short (but otherwise normal) sleepers tend to carry a relatively increased chronic sleep debt – a debt that can only be "paid off" with sleep. For example, in an elegant study by Klerman and Dijk [27], it was found that subjects who habitually obtain relatively less sleep at home fall asleep faster on the multiple sleep latency test, and obtain more recovery sleep when afforded the opportunity to do so over several days/nights in a "sleep extension" paradigm, than those who habitually obtain relatively more sleep.

So why did PVT performance of subjects in the 3-h TIB group fail to recover fully during the 3-night recovery sleep phase? There were three possibilities: (a) the 3-h TIB group accrued a greater level of sleep debt than anticipated across the 7 nights of sleep restriction; and/or (b) the amount of recovery sleep afforded by three 8-h TIB recovery nights was inadequate (i.e. faster recovery would have been evident with a more extended opportunity for nightly sleep during the recovery period – e.g. 10 h TIB per night); and/or (c) the sleep restriction period had resulted in a change to the physiological "set point" for sleep maintenance processes (i.e. the physiological threshold at which awakening from sleep occurs had been lowered) without changing the absolute amount of sleep needed to attain and maintain a normal (i.e. pre-study baseline) level of neurocognitive performance.

Next, in order to partially replicate findings from the Belenky et al. study [25] and to determine how long it would take for PVT performance to fully recover following 7 nights of sleep restricted to 3 h TIB, a second sleep restriction study (SR-2) was conducted [28]. In that study, PVT performance of a 3-h TIB group was again measured across 7 days and nights of sleep restriction, but the recovery sleep phase was extended from three nights with 8 h TIB (i.e. as in SR-1) to seven nights with 8 h TIB. This was done in the hope of capturing the point at which full recovery occurs (or, to at least capture enough data points to draw a line and predict when recovery should be complete based on its slope). Another difference between SR-1 and SR-2 was that in SR-2 subjects were required to extend their nightly TIB at home to 10 h (verified with wrist actigraphy) for one week prior to reporting to the laboratory. This was an effort to ensure that all subjects began the study with a similar (i.e. minimal) level of chronic sleep

Figure 20.2 A comparison of PVT performance across two sleep restriction (SR) studies. In SR-1, the subjects maintained their normal sleep/wake schedule for the week prior to the study (E1–E7). In SR-2, sleep was extended to 10 h TIB for the week prior to the study (E1–E7). Sleep was restricted to 3 h TIB during the 7-day restriction period (R1–R7) in both studies. Dashed box indicates daytime performance during the recovery sleep periods (8 h TIB per night). BL = baseline, RT = Reaction Time.

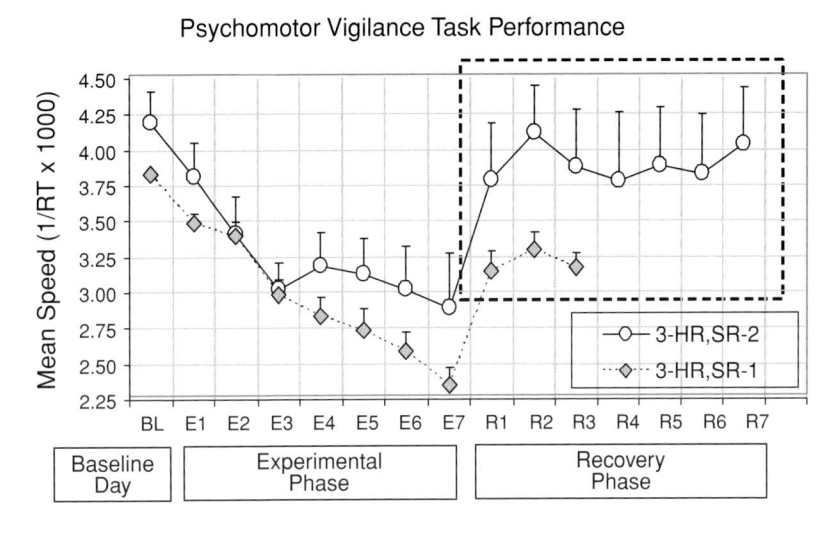

debt, and to thereby help ensure minimal variability in PVT performance and other measures of sleepiness on the baseline day.

However, much to the initial chagrin of the researchers, the most interesting finding from SR-1 was not replicated in SR-2. As shown in Figure 20.2, recovery of PVT performance was nearly complete after only one night of recovery sleep.

Methodologically, the only differences between the 3-h TIB condition in the two studies was that (a) the number of recovery sleep nights was increased for SR-2, and (b) subjects were asked to extend their nightly TIB for 1 week prior to initiation of sleep restriction in SR-2. (Subjects in SR-1 were merely asked to maintain their normal sleep schedules before reporting to the laboratory.) Since it was unlikely that increasing the number of post-restriction recovery sleep nights from three to seven could retroactively facilitate recuperation on the first recovery night, the only reasonable hypothesis to explain the disparity between the two sets of findings was that prior sleep extension had somehow facilitated post-restriction recovery. To test this hypothesis, a third sleep restriction study (SR-3) was conducted in which half of the subjects were randomly assigned to the "sleep extension" condition (1 week with 10 h TIB per night) and half were assigned the "Habitual Sleep" group (in which they maintained their typical nightly sleep schedule of approximately 7 h of sleep per night) [29]. Then both groups underwent 7 nights of sleep restriction with 3 h TIB, followed by 5 nights of recovery sleep with 8 h TIB. As predicted (and consistent with the implications from the first two studies), recovery from sleep restriction was relatively enhanced in the Extended Sleep group, with greater recovery of PVT performance over the first nights of recovery sleep. Also, performance remained relatively elevated over the last several days of sleep restriction (see Figure 20.3). This suggested that sleep extension had effectively "banked" the extra sleep (or, alternatively, used that extra sleep to "pay down a chronic sleep debt") – with the beneficial effects of that increased sleep manifested as both (a) improved performance during the last days of the sleep restriction period, and (b) enhanced recovery from sleep restriction – even though one week of sleep restriction separated the sleep extension phase from the recovery sleep phase of the study. These results suggest that sleep is "banked", and that soldiers in the field should therefore take every opportunity to sleep – not only during missions but prior to missions – because every hour of sleep obtained can mean relatively enhanced performance extending at least one week into the future.

The physiological basis of TSD vs. CSR differences: a hypothesis

Although the physiological processes underlying the long-term effects of "nightly sleep duration" are not yet known, one possibility is suggested by the still-unfolding "adenosine story," as described by Strecker et al. [30]: Adenosine (AD) and adenosine receptor agonists promote sleep. During acute sleep loss, extracellular adenosine accumulates in the brain (especially the basal forebrain, BF) of both animals [31] and humans [32]. During subsequent sleep, AD levels

Psychomotor Vigilance Task Performance

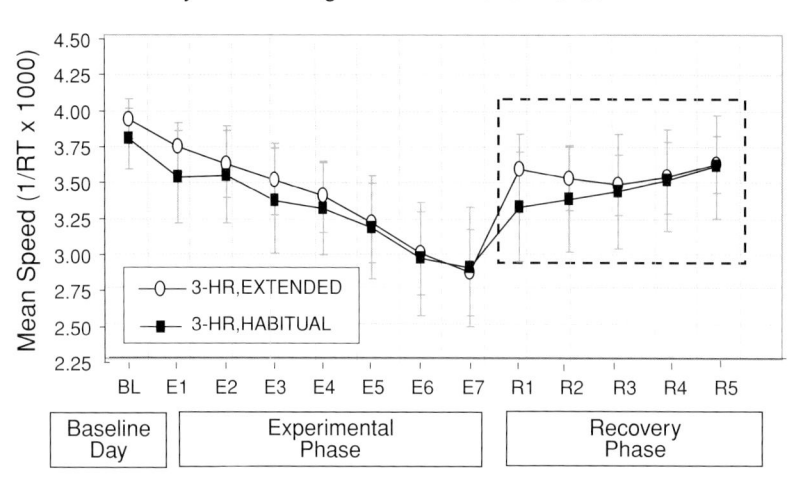

Figure 20.3 A comparison of PVT performance across two sleep restriction (SR) conditions: In the "3-HR, Habitual" condition, subjects maintained their normal sleep/wake schedule (~7 h of sleep per night) for the week prior to the study (E1–E7), followed by 7 nights of sleep restriction with 3 h TIB, then 5 nights (R1–R5) of recovery sleep with 8 h TIB. The "3-HR, Extended" condition was identical, except that TIB was 10 h per night for the week prior to the baseline day. BL = baseline, RT = Reaction Time. Adapted from Rupp et al. [29] with permission.

decline, thereby facilitating post-sleep wakefulness via disinhibition of cholinergic BF neurons [33].

Like acute sleep deprivation, sleep fragmentation procedures also initially result in increased extracellular AD in BF. However, with continued, longer-term (5 days) exposure to sleep fragmentation procedures, AD levels in rats' BF wane [31], suggesting a fatigued capacity for production and/or release of extracellular AD in the BF. This reduction in extracellular AD is accompanied by a concomitant upregulation of AD_{A1} receptors [33], and it has been hypothesized that this upregulation may be the mechanism by which heightened adenosinergic tone/homeostatic pressure is maintained [30]. In other words, instead of a direct reflection of extracellular AD in the BF, the sleep homeostat may be a synergistic function reflecting the relative balance between the level of extracellular AD in the BF and the density of AD_{A1} receptors in that region.

If this hypothesis is correct, then it suggests a mechanism that may explain the observation that recovery from multiple days of sleep restriction is slower than recovery from acute, total sleep deprivation [25]: with acute sleep deprivation there is an initial increase in extracellular AD levels. However, because TSD studies are typically of relatively limited duration, recovery sleep is initiated well before extracellular AD levels begin to wane in the BF, and well before upregulation of AD_{A1} receptors is precipitated. Therefore, the "normal" balance between AD_{A1} receptors and exogenous AD in the BF – as well as homeostatic pressure to sleep – is quickly restored by recovery sleep.

However, with extended sleep restriction, an initially increased level of extracellular AD in the BF eventually wanes despite continued sleep loss (as it does across multiple days of sleep fragmentation in animals). Over days of sleep restriction, waning extracellular AD levels are offset by upregulation of AD_{A1} receptors – a process that serves to maintain homeostatic pressure to sleep. Following sleep restriction, adequate (recovery) sleep restores the normal, baseline capacity to produce/release AD in the BF more quickly than AD_{A1} receptors in that region can be downregulated, resulting in an "imbalance" that effectively amplifies suppression of cholinergic BF neurons. This imbalance is manifested as depressed alertness and performance until such time as downregulation of AD_{A1} receptors (to levels typical of normal sleep and alertness) occurs. Until then, the relative imbalance in the levels of extracellular AD and density of AD_{A1} receptors could manifest as the sort of "failure to recover" following multiple days of sleep restriction that was reported by Belenky et al. [25].

New and future military sleep research efforts

Sleep and mild traumatic brain injury (mTBI)

Mild traumatic brain injury (mTBI), has been called the "signature injury of the Iraq War", with estimates of the number of soldiers who have experienced mTBI (i.e. concussions) ranging as high as 20% of deployed forces [34]. Of these, up to 80% may experience post-concussion syndrome (PCS) [35] – a cluster of symptoms that can persist for several months after the mTBI event. For this reason, military sleep researchers have begun to turn their attention and efforts toward the study of sleep and mTBI.

Previous research indicates that "sleep disturbance" is among the most common, and most persistent, symptoms of mTBI and PCS. However, little is known about (a) the role of habitual sleep duration/status in determining sensitivity/resilience to mTBI events (i.e. mediating the severity of the functional brain changes that characterize mTBI), (b) the extent to which severity of sleep disturbance generally reflects severity of (i.e. serves as a physiological marker of) mTBI, or (c) the role (if any) that sleep plays in facilitating recovery from mTBI. Given findings that sleep mediates brain plasticity and various aspects of learning and memory [36], it is reasonable to hypothesize that sleep also facilitates the learning processes that are integral to TBI rehabilitation – and perhaps even aspects of physiological recovery. Eventually, delineation of the relationships between sleep and mTBI might (a) provide a strategy for prevention/mitigation of mTBI injuries, (b) provide a sleep-related physiological marker of mTBI (i.e. to aid in its diagnosis), and (c) suggest a treatment strategy (i.e. sleep enhancement to speed recovery).

Sleep and post-traumatic stress disorder (PTSD)

Combat veterans have high rates of PTSD, a disorder characterized by sleep disturbance. In fact, sleep disturbance is reported by 87% PTSD patients [37]. Approximately 44% of combat veterans with PTSD report difficulty initiating nighttime sleep compared to 6% of combat veterans without PTSD; and 91% of combat veterans with PTSD report difficulty maintaining nighttime sleep, compared to 63% of combat veterans without PTSD [38]. Furthermore, sleep complaints following exposure to traumatic events are predictive of a subsequent diagnosis of PTSD [39], suggesting the possibility that sleep disturbances may not only reflect PTSD, they may actually mediate the relationship between traumatic experiences and symptomatology.

Whether, or the extent to which, sleep plays a role in psychological resilience and PTSD is unknown. However, the recent finding that sleep loss leads to deactivation of the prefrontal cortex, which in turn leads to disinhibition of the amygdala and hyper-responsiveness to emotional stimuli [40], suggests a potential mediating role for sleep in the development of PTSD and other psychological disorders. Based on such findings, it is reasonable to hypothesize that "good sleepers" may be impacted less by traumatic events (as reflected by amygdalar activation) than "poor sleepers" – and this difference may reflect differences in susceptibility to PTSD. Knowledge gained from further study of the relationships between sleep and PTSD may ultimately be translated into strategies by the military to (a) improve resilience to the stressors that precipitate PTSD and other anxiety disorders (i.e. by improving sleep in the operational environment), and (b) facilitate recovery from PTSD and related disorders, by improving sleep during recovery and rehabilitation.

References

1. **von Clausewitz C**. *On War*. [The complete translation by Colonel JJ Graham]. London, 1873. http://www.clausewitz.com/readings/OnWar1873/TOC.htm
2. **Breuer W B**. *Hoodwinking Hitler: The Normandy Deception*. Westport, CT: Praeger Publishers, 1993.
3. **Hughes D J**. (ed.). *Moltke on the Art of War: Selected Writings*. New York, NY: Presidio Press, 1993.
4. **Luce T J**. *The Greek Historians*. London: Routledge, 1997.
5. **Patrick G T W, Gilbert J A**. On the effects of loss of sleep. *Psychol Rev*, 1896; **3**:469–83.
6. **Goel N, Rao H, Durmer J S, Dinges D F**. Neurocognitive consequences of sleep deprivation. *Semin Neurol*, 2009; **29**:320–39.
7. **Sun Tzu**. *The Art of War*. Mineola, NY: Dover Publications Inc., 2002.
8. **Asprey R B**. *War in the Shadows: The Guerrilla in History*. Lincoln, NE: iUniverse Inc., 2002.
9. **Arrian F, De Selincourt A, Hamilton J R**. *The Campaigns of Alexander*. London: Penguin Books, 1971.
10. **Haslam D**. The military performance of soldiers in continuous operations: Exercise Early Call I and II. In: Johnson L, Tepas D, Colquhoun W, Colligan M, Eds. *Advances in Sleep Research*, vol 7. New York, NY: Spectrum, 1981: 435–58.
11. **Balkin T J, Rupp T, Picchioni D, Wesensten N J**. Sleep loss and sleepiness: current issues. *Chest*, 2008; **134**:653–60.
12. **Rajaraman S, Gribok A V, Wesensten N J**, *et al*. An improved methodology for individualized

performance prediction of sleep-deprived individuals with the two-process model. *Sleep*, 2009; **32**:1377–92.

13. **Wesensten N J, Killgore W D, Balkin T J.** Performance and alertness effects of caffeine, dextroamphetamine, and modafinil during sleep deprivation. *J Sleep Res*, 2005; **14**:255–66.

14. **Hursh S R, Redmond D P, Johnson M L**, *et al.* Fatigue models for applied research in warfighting. *Aviat Space Environ Med*, 2004; **75**:A44–53.

15. **Wesensten N J, Balkin T J, Belenky G L.** Effects of daytime administration of zolpidem and triazolam on performance. *Aviat Space Environ Med*, 1996; **67**:115–20.

16. **Mental Health Advisory Team (MHAT) V Report.** 14 February 2008. http://www.armymedicine.army.mil/reports/mhat/mhat_v/mhat-v.cfm

17. **Lim J, Dinges D F.** Sleep deprivation and vigilant attention. *Ann N Y Acad Sci*, 2008; **1129**:305–22.

18. **Killgore W D, Kahn-Greene E T, Lipizzi E L**, *et al.* Sleep deprivation reduces perceived emotional intelligence and constructive thinking skills. *Sleep Med*, 2008; **9**:517–26.

19. **Killgore W D, Killgore D B, Day L M**, *et al.* The effects of 53 hours of sleep deprivation on moral judgment. *Sleep*, 2007; **30**:345–52.

20. **Killgore W D, McBride S A, Killgore D B**, *et al.* The effects of caffeine, dextroamphetamine, and modafinil on humor appreciation during sleep deprivation. *Sleep*, 2006; **29**:841–47.

21. **Killgore W D, Grugle N L, Killgore D B**, *et al.* Restoration of risk-propensity during sleep deprivation: caffeine, dextroamphetamine, and modafinil. *Aviat Space Environ Med*, 2008; **79**:867–74.

22. **Killgore W D, Balkin T J, Wesensten N J.** Impaired decision making following 49 h of sleep deprivation. *J Sleep Res*, 2006; **15**:7–13.

23. **Killgore W D, McBride S A.** Odor identification accuracy declines following 24 h of sleep deprivation. *J Sleep Res*, 2006; **15**:111–16.

24. **Webb W B, Agnew H W.** The effects of a chronic limitation of sleep length. *Psychophysics*, 1974; **11**:256–74.

25. **Belenky G, Wesensten N J, Thorne D R**, *et al.* Patterns of performance degradation and restoration during sleep restriction and subsequent recovery: a sleep dose–response study. *J Sleep Res*, 2003; **12**:1–12.

26. **Bedard M A, Montplaisir J, Malo J**, *et al.* Persistent neuropsychological deficits and vigilance impairment in sleep apnea syndrome after treatment with continuous positive airways pressure (CPAP). *J Clin Exp Neuropsychol*, 1993; **15**:330–41.

27. **Klerman E B, Dijk D J.** Interindividual variation in sleep duration and its association with sleep debt in young adults. *Sleep*, 2005; **28**:1253–59.

28. **Wesensten N J, Reichardt R, Balkin T J.** Chronic sleep restriction and resatiation. I. Recovery of psychomotor vigilance performance. *Sleep*, 2005; **28**:A136 (abstract).

29. **Rupp T L, Wesensten N J, Bliese P D, Balkin T J.** Banking sleep: realization of benefits during subsequent sleep restriction and recovery. *Sleep*, 2009; **32**:311–21.

30. **Strecker R E, Basheer R, McKenna J T, McCarley R W.** Another chapter in the adenosine story. *Sleep*, 2006; **29**:426–28.

31. **McKenna J T, Tartar J L, Ward C P**, *et al.* Sleep fragmentation elevates behavioral, electrographic and neurochemical measures of sleepiness. *Neuroscience*, 2007; **146**:1462–73.

32. **Zeitzer J M, Morales-Villagran A, Maidment N T**, *et al.* Extracellular adenosine in the human brain during sleep and sleep deprivation: an in vivo microdialysis study. *Sleep*, 2006; **29**:455–56.

33. **Porkka-Heiskanen T, Strecker R E, Thakkar M**, *et al.* Adenosine: a mediator of the sleep-inducing effects of prolonged wakefulness. *Science*, 1997; **276**:1265–68.

34. **Hoge C W, McGurk D, Thomas J L**, *et al.* Mild traumatic brain injury in U.S. soldiers returning from Iraq. *N Engl J Med*, 2008; **358**:453–63.

35. **Hall R C, Hall R C, Chapman M J.** Definition, diagnosis, and forensic implications of postconcussional syndrome. *Psychosomatics*, 2005; **46**:195–202.

36. **Vassalli A, Dijk D J** Sleep function: current questions and new approaches. *Eur J Neurosci*, 2009; **29**:1830–41.

37. **Kilpatrick D G, Resnick H S, Freedy J R**, *et al.* Posttraumatic stress disorder field trial: evaluation of the PTSD construct – criteria A through E. In: Widiger T A, Frances A J, Pincus H A, *et al.*, Eds. *DSM-IV Sourcebook*. Washington, DC: American Psychiatric Press, 1994: 803–46.

38. **Neylan T C, Marmar C R, Metzler T J**, *et al.* Sleep disturbances in the Vietnam generation: findings from a nationally representative sample of male Vietnam veterans. *Am J Psychiatry*, 1998; **155**:929–33.

39. **Koren D, Arnon I, Lavie P**, *et al.* Sleep complaints as early predictors of posttraumatic stress disorder: a 1-year prospective study of injured survivors of motor vehicle accidents. *Am J Psychiatry*, 2002; **159**:855–57.

40. **Yoo S S, Gujar N, Hu, P.** The human emotional brain without sleep – a prefrontal amygdala disconnect. *Curr Biol*, 2007; **17**:R877–78.

Section 2 Chapter 21

Sleep Disorders and Excessive Sleepiness

Time-zone transitions and sleepiness

Jim Waterhouse

In memory of Professor Thomas Reilly

Long journeys are associated with "travel fatigue" and, if they cross multiple time zones, "jet lag" also. Both conditions are associated with increased sleepiness, which, in the current article, will be treated as a subjective assessment that is synonymous with "fatigue" and lack of "alertness". However, the causes of the two conditions differ [1–3].

Travel fatigue and jet lag

The symptoms of travel fatigue (Table 21.1) include a general weariness, and travellers often nap during the journey. This nap reflects boredom as much as sleep deprivation, although sleep loss might be present if the journey necessitated rising earlier than normal, or if the previous night's sleep had been poor due to apprehension about the journey. Dehydration and sitting in cramped conditions are contributory factors.

Advice to combat travel fatigue

Making full preparations for the journey – arriving in good time and having made arrangements at the final destination, for example – minimizes the disruption and possible problems [4]. Dehydration can be combated by water and fruit juice, but coffee, tea and alcohol, which can accentuate fluid loss by diaphoresis or diuresis, should be avoided. Performing stretching exercises or taking a brief stroll, if possible, will reduce the risks of cramp and deep vein thrombosis; wearing support stockings that prevent pooling of the blood might help [5].

After reaching the destination, rehydration, a brief nap and a shower are recommended. Nocturnal sleep should present no problems since local times at destination and place of departure coincide. The symptoms of travel fatigue will have dissipated substantially by the next day.

Jet lag

Jet lag (Table 21.1) occurs only if more than two time zones have been traversed rapidly, the symptoms increasing with the number of time zones crossed [1–3]. The symptom causing most inconvenience is poor nocturnal sleep. After eastward flights, sleep onset tends to be delayed (by local time), with difficulty in waking in the morning; after westward flights, the traveller feels tired in the late afternoon and evening and tends to wake early. Travel in either direction is accompanied by fractionated nocturnal sleep. These deteriorations in sleep are associated with increased daytime sleepiness which, in turn, contributes to increased irritability, negative effects upon mood, motivation and the ability to concentrate, and poorer cognitive and physical performance.

Jet lag is always associated with sleepiness and fatigue, but the perceived importance of other symptoms depends upon the time of assessment. Thus, jet lag is correlated, in the morning, with poor sleep the night before; during the daytime, with decreased abilities to concentrate and to maintain motivation; and, in the evening, with not feeling ready for sleep [6].

Jet lag is due to desynchrony between individuals' new environment (whose timing alters in accord with the new time zone) and their "body clock" (which is slow to adjust from the old time zone). The symptoms regress as the normal synchrony between the body clock and the new environment is re-established. The cause of jet lag is fundamentally different from that of travel fatigue, therefore (Table 21.1).

Sleepiness: Causes, Consequences and Treatment, ed. Michael J. Thorpy and Michel Billiard. Published by Cambridge University Press. © Cambridge University Press 2011.

Table 21.1 Travel fatigue and jet lag

A. Travel fatigue
Symptoms:
General fatigue (due to boredom)
Increased incidence of headaches

Causes:
Disruption of sleep and normal routine
Hassles associated with the journey
Dehydration

Advice:
Before the journey: Arrange documentation, inoculations, etc. Make arrangements for arrival at the final destination
During the journey: Drink plenty of water or fruit juice – avoid alcohol, tea, coffee
On reaching the destination: Relax and rehydrate (not alcohol, tea or coffee). Take a brief nap, if needed, but not too near normal bedtime

B. Jet lag
Symptoms:
Poor sleep in the new time zone
Negative subjective changes when awake – increases in sleepiness and irritability, decreases in motivation and the ability to concentrate
Poorer objective measures of physical and cognitive performance during the daytime
Gastrointestinal disturbances, decreased interest in food

Causes:
Slow adjustment of the body clock to the new time zone – the clock-driven endogenous component of a circadian rhythm is out of synchrony with the new environment.
Increased internal drive for sleep (sleepiness) following any sleep loss

C. Differences between travel fatigue and jet lag
Origin and symptoms:
Travel fatigue is associated with any long journey; jet lag needs more than two time zones to be crossed rapidly
Travel fatigue affects a narrower range of variables (compare parts A and B of this Table)

Time-course of recovery:
Travel fatigue is almost completely finished by the next day, the traveller having been able to have a good night's sleep; jet lag lasts considerably longer (particularly disturbed sleep), with inter-individual differences in problems experienced

Main cause:
Travel fatigue is due to the disruption of the normal daily routine and the hassles associated with travel; jet lag is due to a temporary loss of the normal synchrony between the traveller's body clock and environment

In order to understand the implications of this loss of synchrony and ways of re-establishing the normal synchrony, some basic concepts in chronobiology need to be understood.

Circadian rhythms

A key physiological concept is "homeostasis" – maintaining a variable within narrow limits in spite of tendencies of the individual's environment and activities to produce change. For example, thermoregulatory reflexes keep core body temperature within the range 35–40 °C, whether the subject is active or asleep, and even though environmental temperatures vary over a far wider range. However, when repeated measurements are made over the course of 24 h in subjects who are active in the daytime and sleeping at night, temperature and other variables show daily rhythms that are in synchrony with the individual's sleep–wake cycle. The rhythms tend to fall into two groups: (a) those that peak during the daytime and are associated with the active phase of the individual (core temperature, cognitive and physical performance, alertness and adrenaline, for example); and (b) those that peak during nocturnal sleep and are associated with fasting and recuperation (for example, growth hormone, cortisol and pineal melatonin, which is secreted only in darkness) [7, 8].

Endogenous and exogenous components of a rhythm

It might be supposed that such rhythms result from the sleep–activity cycle: during the daytime, individuals are physically and mentally active, and eat and

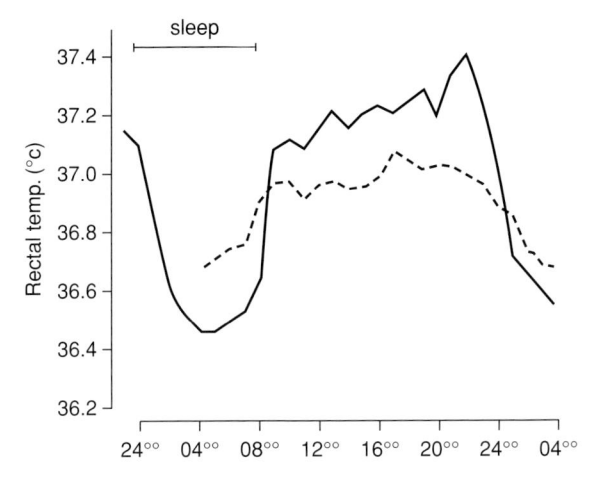

Figure 21.1 Mean circadian changes in core (rectal) temperature measured hourly in 8 subjects: living normally and sleeping from 24:00 to 08:00 h (solid line); woken at 04:00 h and spending the next 24 h on a "constant routine" (dashed line). (Taken with permission from [8].)

drink in a stimulating environment; at night, they sleep in the quiet. This explanation is only partially correct, as can be demonstrated by a "Constant Routine" [8]. In this protocol, the subject is required for a period of at least 24 h: to remain awake, sedentary (or lying down) and relaxed in an environment of constant temperature, humidity, and lighting; to engage in restful activities, generally reading or listening to music; and to take identical and regularly spaced meals. With this protocol, it is observed (Figure 21.1) that the rhythm of core temperature does not disappear, even though its amplitude decreases. Therefore, three deductions can be made.

(i) The remaining temperature rhythm must arise internally. It is described as the "endogenous" component of the original rhythm and is attributed to a "body clock".
(ii) An effect of the individual's environment and lifestyle does exist (the two rhythms differ); this difference is termed the "exogenous" component of the original rhythm.
(iii) In subjects living conventionally, these two components are in phase, both raising core temperature in the daytime and lowering it at night. That is, exogenous and endogenous components of a rhythm are normally synchronized.

Differences exist in causes of the exogenous component and the relative importance of exogenous and endogenous components [7, 8]. For core temperature, blood pressure and airway caliber, for example, the exogenous component consists of rises due to physical and mental activity and falls when lying down and sleeping, whereas the melatonin rhythm is affected far more by bright light, which suppresses its secretion. Several hormones are modified by food ingestion, and antidiuretic hormone by fluid intake and posture. Rhythms of heart rate, blood pressure, water excretion by the kidneys and sleep-mediated growth hormone secretion have larger exogenous than endogenous components whereas the rhythms of excretion of potassium in the urine and, particularly in sedentary subjects studied indoors, of plasma melatonin and cortisol have smaller exogenous than endogenous components. Core temperature in sedentary individuals has exogenous and endogenous components of similar magnitude (compare the amplitudes of the curves in Figure 21.1).

The body clock

The site of the body clock and its circadian nature

The suprachiasmatic nuclei (SCN), paired groups of cells in the base of the hypothalamus, are the site of the body clock in mammals [9, 10]. One of the strongest pieces of evidence (from a large body of data) is that only these cells show a daily rhythmicity in activity when cultured in vitro in constant conditions. There is a large degree of evolutionary conservation between species with regard to clock mechanisms, their molecular biochemistry and genetics. In brief, nuclear "clock genes" are transcribed into "clock mRNAs" which are then translated into "clock proteins" in the cytoplasm. These proteins are responsible for the rhythmic processes (neural activity, transmitter production, etc.) seen in SCN cells. Some of these proteins form complexes that move back into the nucleus and inhibit the transcription of the clock genes. The decline in clock-protein production that results means that the clock genes are not inhibited and so reactivate, a new cycle beginning. In humans, the whole cycle takes just over 24 h, a result confirmed by studies of rhythmic changes in individuals living in time-free conditions (in caves or laboratories isolated from time cues, for example). For this reason, these rhythms are called circadian (Latin: "about a day").

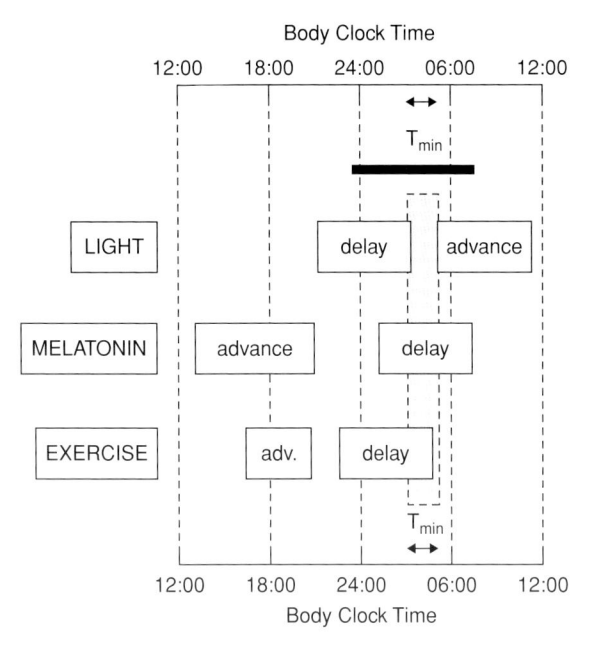

Figure 21.2 Simplified phase-response curves to light, melatonin and exercise; times are shown when the stimulus causes a phase advance (adv.) or phase delay of the body clock. T_{min} (gray box and double arrow) indicates normal range of times for the core temperature minimum. Bar indicates normal time of sleep. (Based on [3].)

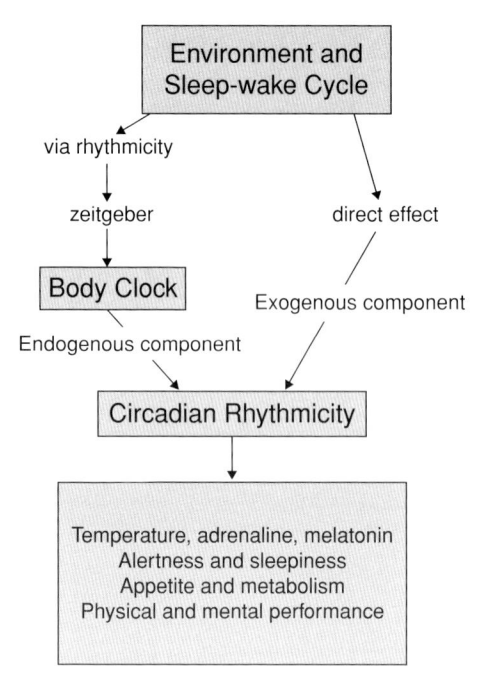

Figure 21.3 The endogenous (driven by the body clock) and exogenous (driven by the environment) components of a circadian rhythm, together with the role as a zeitgeber of environmental rhythms and the sleep–wake cycle. Some of the variables affected by the circadian system are also shown.

Adjustment of the body clock

To synchronize with the environment, such a circadian clock and the rhythms it produces need to be adjusted to a 24-h day. This is achieved by zeitgebers (German: "time-givers") – rhythms resulting, directly or indirectly, from the environment. In humans, the most important zeitgebers are the light–dark cycle [11] and the regular release into the blood stream of melatonin during the hours of darkness [12]. Rhythms in eating and physical, cognitive and social activities might have a weak role also.

Zeitgebers adjust the body clock by advancing or delaying it according to the stage of the circadian cycle, a relationship which is called a phase-response curve (PRC). Bright light (as found outdoors) advances the body clock when present in the 6 h immediately after the trough of the body temperature rhythm (the trough normally being mid-sleep, see Figure 21.1) and delays it when present in the 6 h before this trough. Weaker light (as found indoors) produces smaller phase shifts, an effect that is important for those who have little exposure to the natural alternation of daylight and darkness [13]. A pathway from the retina directly transmits light information to the SCN.

Simplified PRCs for light, melatonin and exercise are shown in Figure 21.2.

Zeitgebers normally act in harmony to adjust circadian rhythms. For example, in the evening declining light and the onset of melatonin secretion advances the body clock (via the melatonin PRC) and the lack of light means that the clock is not delayed (via the light PRC); in the morning, bright light advances the body clock and suppresses melatonin release, so preventing the clock delay that melatonin would produce at this time (see Figure 21.2).

Roles of the body clock

The body clock transmits its rhythmic output to regions of the brain controlling temperature regulation, hormone release, feeding and sleep. As a result, the physiology, biochemistry and behavior of the whole body become rhythmic, with a phase determined by the SCN (Figure 21.3). The whole body is geared towards a daytime "active" mode and a nocturnal "recovery and restitution" mode. These endogenous components of the circadian rhythms are normally synchronized to the environment and lifestyle, the exogenous components; in the evening, individuals relax in a quiet environment and, in the morning, activity increases in a more dynamic environment.

Sleep, wake and sleepiness

The circadian rhythms of sleep, sleepiness and cognitive and physical performance are of most concern to the traveller across time zones. The ease of getting to sleep (sleep propensity), of staying asleep and waking up are influenced by external (how conducive to sleep is the environment) and internal (body clock and time-since-waking) influences. Laboratory studies can optimize the environment, maximizing the possibility of falling asleep. Sleep can then be predicted by a model [14] which postulates two factors: (1) a "sleep homeostat", which monitors the increasing need for restitutive sleep as time awake increases (although its detailed mechanism is unknown); and (2) a circadian factor which is phased opposite to the circadian rhythm of core temperature. Sleep onset is easiest when core temperature is at its trough or falling rapidly and the skin of the distal limbs is warm due to cutaneous vasodilatation [15, 16]. The fall in core temperature is promoted by clock-mediated changes to thermal reflexes (decreasing the "set-point") and melatonin-induced vasodilatation [17, 18]. (This effect of melatonin has given rise to the concept that it acts as a "natural hypnotic" or soporific.) Conversely, sleep is most difficult when the temperature is at its peak or rising rapidly. Spontaneous waking from sleep is more likely when core temperature is high or rising and less likely if core temperature is low or falling.

Accepting that core temperature is normally minimum around 05:00 h (see Figure 21.1), then the conventional times of attempting sleep – between about 23:00 (core temperature falling most quickly) and 08:00 h (rising most quickly) – are synchronized closely to the circadian rhythm of core temperature [19]. Consolidated and extended sleep is more difficult at other times. In the daytime, core temperature is too high and "sleep pressure" (due to the sleep homeostat) is likely to be small (the problems after eastward flights); by contrast, if an individual stays up until 04:00 h, then the increased sleep pressure and low core temperature will facilitate the onset of sleep, but the rising core temperature will terminate it prematurely (the problem after westward flights).

Sleepiness can be considered the subjective correlate of sleep propensity. In practice, alertness, the opposite of sleepiness, has been modelled in a manner closely analogous to that of sleep propensity (see [20], for example). Alertness is predicted from increasing time awake (which decreases alertness and increases sleepiness) and a circadian factor (alertness being parallel to core temperature and sleepiness being phased opposite and parallel to sleep propensity). The models predict that sleep propensity, alertness and sleepiness will be abnormal if the sleep–wake cycle is disrupted and/or the normal synchrony between the body clock and the environment is lost.

Mood and cognitive and physical performance

The rhythms of mood (including the ability to concentrate and general motivation) and most types of physical and cognitive performance are in phase with core temperature, a causal link often being postulated [21, 22]. Mood and cognitive performance are also affected negatively by time awake and sleep loss, with mood and complex cognitive tasks showing a greater deterioration. This deterioration is often referred to as "fatigue", but it is a centrally induced process and distinct from muscular fatigue. However, physical performance is not immune to the effects of time awake because, whilst there is little effect upon muscle strength, cognitive components (decision-making, the processing of sensory information and motivation, for example) will deteriorate [22].

Summary of the interactions between circadian rhythms and time awake

The normal position

Measured circadian rhythms are combined effects from a body clock (endogenous component) and the environment (exogenous component) that are normally in synchrony. Increasing time awake increases mental fatigue, sleep propensity and sleepiness, and decreases alertness and general performance. In the first part of the waking day, the effects of time awake are small and the rising phase of the circadian rhythms (temperature, adrenaline, for example) enables performance to improve. In the afternoon, the effects of increasing time awake are combated by peak values of the circadian rhythm and an active environment. During the evening, the falling phase of circadian rhythms, increasing time awake and the tendency to relax in a quiet environment all lead to declines in alertness,

Table 21.2 Changes due to the body clock with time of day in sleep, sleepiness and cognitive performance. Results for home time and immediately after flights to the west or east across eight time zones.

	24:00–08:00 h	Local time of day 08:00–16:00 h	16:00–24:00 h
Home time zone:			
Sleep and sleepiness	Easy to remain asleep	Low sleepiness	Sleepiness increases
Cognitive performance	–	Improves to high values	Deteriorates
Immediately after 8 time zones to west:			
Sleep	Easy onset, premature waking	Sleepiness increases	High sleepiness
Cognitive performance	–	Deteriorates	Poor
Immediately after 8 time zones to east:			
Sleep	Low sleepiness, delayed sleep	Sleepiness high	Low sleepiness
Cognitive performance	–	Poor	Improves to high values

Note: Sleepiness and the ease of sleep will increase, and cognitive performance will decrease, with increasing time spent awake, particularly following partial sleep loss.

cognitive performance and physical performance, coupled with rises in sleep propensity and sleepiness. Such changes accord well with our being diurnal.

Problems associated with alterations to the sleep–wake cycle

The body clock is robust; transient changes in routine (waking in the middle of the night or taking a nap in the daytime, for example) do not change its phase. Such robustness normally has ecological advantage, but causes problems whenever individuals' sleep–wake cycles are changed – travelling to a new time zone, for example [1–3, 23]. Environmental time cues change whereas the body clock is slow to adjust to the new time zone, and so normal synchrony between endogenous and exogenous components of a circadian rhythm is lost.

Several problems will arise due to such desynchrony. Sleep propensity and sleepiness will continue to peak around the trough of the endogenous core temperature rhythm, but this will now be around 12:00 h local time in Beijing (8 time zones to the east of the UK) and 20:00 h in Los Angeles (8 time zones to the west). Sleep propensity and sleepiness in the new night (midnight–08:00 h) will be less than normal and poorer sleep will be obtained because this time in Beijing will correspond to 16:00–24:00 h and, in Los Angeles, to 08:00–16:00 h by *body time*. After eastward flights, sleep onset will be delayed (core temperature still too high) and waking up the next day will be more difficult (around the temperature trough); after westward flights, getting to sleep will not be difficult (temperature only just on its rising phase) but premature waking will occur (continuing rise in core temperature). After flights in either direction, sleep will be inadequate and this will lead to sleepiness and associated negative effects the next day. In these regards, the effects of jet lag differ from those of travel fatigue (where a good night's sleep is possible). The negative effects of partial sleep deprivation upon cognitive and physical performance will be additional to those due to the inappropriate timing of the endogenous circadian components of these variables.

There will also be effects due to the sleep homeostat: after an eastward flight, local sleep times are advanced, decreasing sleep propensity and sleepiness; after a westward flight, the delay of local sleep times increases time awake, this partially offsetting sleep difficulties due to the body clock.

Table 21.2 summarizes some of the problems associated with jet lag.

Advice on dealing with jet lag

Jet lag exists while the body clock remains unadjusted to the new time zone, and the numerous symptoms comprising jet lag attest to the multitude of circadian rhythms influenced by this clock (Figure 21.3). Adjustment of the body clock requires inputs from appropriate time zeitgebers in the new time zone. Symptoms of jet lag regress at different rates, loss of enjoyment of food disappearing before aspects of sleep and cognitive performance, for example [6, 24]. This difference reflects the relative importance of the endogenous and exogenous components of a rhythm. If the endogenous component is weak (enjoyment of food) then negative effects from a partially adjusted body clock (after a couple of days in the new time zone) will be unimportant; if the endogenous component is stronger, then effects persist until full adjustment of the body clock.

General principles regarding methods for dealing with jet lag

For sojourns of only a few days, adjustment of the body clock is not possible and "body time" will remain on "home time" (time in the zone just left). Travellers are advised to arrange appointments to coincide with daytime, and to avoid times that coincide with night, on home time. Thus, after eastward flights, the new afternoon is preferable and the new morning is to be avoided (coincident with morning and night, respectively, on home time); after westward flights, the new morning is preferable and the late afternoon and evening are to be avoided.

For sojourns lasting more than a few days, adjustment of the body clock is advised [1–3, 23]. Even following the advice below, adjustment takes about one day per time zone crossed after eastward flights and slightly less after westward transitions. Arriving in the new time zone well before an important event is advised, therefore.

Flights to the west (delaying the body clock required) are generally associated with less jet lag because: (1) it is easier to get to sleep the first night, the sleep homeostat increasing sleepiness and sleep propensity in proportion to time awake; (2) the body clock tends to run with a period slightly greater than 24 h, so delaying it is easier; and (3) exposure to the natural light–dark cycle at the destination naturally promotes appropriate adjustment of the body clock (see below).

Adjustment can be achieved pharmacologically (using "chronobiotics" [25], substances that adjust the phase of the body clock) or behaviorally (using zeitgebers [1–3, 23]). Substances can also be used to ameliorate the symptoms of jet lag, even if they do not adjust the body clock, in much the same way that a headache, but not its cause, can be alleviated by a painkiller.

What to do before and during the flight

Small adjustments of the sleep–wake cycle in the days before the flight might be possible – retiring and rising earlier than usual before eastward flights, and later than usual before westward ones [26], so starting the process of phase shifting the body clock. However, changes in excess of 2 h are generally inconvenient and lead to the problems associated with night work.

Travellers are advised to adopt destination time as soon as entering the aircraft and to use this time to determine whether to nap (night on destination time) or to stay awake [27]. When staying awake is recommended, strolling round the cabin or using the in-flight entertainment system is advised. The type and timing of meals should reflect destination time; unfortunately, full meals are often offered soon after take-off and just before landing, but some carriers now allow passengers to choose their mealtimes.

What to do after the flight

Pharmacological approaches to promote alertness and sleep

Drugs to promote alertness and sleep are covered in other articles in this book; only a general account, pertaining to healthy travellers undergoing time-zone transitions, is given here.

Several drugs, often studied in a military context, have been shown to sustain performance during extended periods without sleep [28, 29]. The value of such drugs is contentious because they also reduce the ability to initiate and sustain sleep, extended use can lead to drug dependence, and effects on mood and cognitive performance have not been investigated in detail. Therefore, these drugs are unacceptable for use by civilian aircrew and normal travellers.

By contrast, caffeine is widely used [30], a dose equivalent to about two cups of coffee temporarily improving alertness after sleep loss. Also, it was found that, following a night of total sleep deprivation, caffeine increased sleep latency but more so with a daytime than a nocturnal recovery sleep [31]. It must be remembered that daytime sleep in the new time zone might coincide with "night" by body time. Drinking coffee with breakfast might help waking up but, during the evening, might prevent nocturnal sleep.

Soporific drugs and short-acting hypnotics have been investigated for ameliorating poor nocturnal sleep in the new time zone [32, 33]. Taken before retiring, they promote sleep without sleepiness the next day, but detailed effects upon cognitive and physical performance have not been established; hypnotics with a longer half-life would be unsuitable due to residual effects on alertness and psychomotor performance. Further work is required to ascertain which drugs might benefit the traveller's sleep without compromising performance the following day, but such drugs are generally believed to be unnecessary [34].

Several reviews consider the use of melatonin and its synthetic analogues to treat sleep problems [35–38]. In doses up to about 3 mg, melatonin acts as a natural soporific and produces no effects on performance the following morning. It also reduces "jet lag", although this has often been assessed without details of the time of assessment or reference to a particular symptom. Such results indicate melatonin's value, but the lack of long-term toxicological data, no obligation for undesirable side-effects following use to be recorded (melatonin does not currently have a license), and no guarantee as to the purity of some of the formulations available all lead to the recommendation to take melatonin only under medical supervision. A meta-analysis [36] stated: "There is no evidence that melatonin is effective in treating…sleep disorders accompanying sleep restriction, such as jet lag", but also concluded that melatonin was safe with use up to a period of three months.

The exact role played by melatonin in treating jet lag is unclear; it might be shifting the body clock and/or exerting a soporific effect. For appropriate clock adjustment, the timing of ingestion is critical (Figure 21.2) and this might be inconvenient after certain time-zone transitions (ingestion required at night) or counterproductive after others (required during the daytime) due to the soporific effect that occurs whenever it is taken. In practice, melatonin is taken a few hours before sleep is required, invoking its soporific effect.

It is possible that a variety of drugs (including higher doses of melatonin) might adjust the body clock – act as "chronobiotics" [25] – but far more work on these substances is required.

Use of light and dark to adjust the body clock

The light PRC is the basis of advice promoting adjustment of the body clock. Few field studies have investigated shifts of the body clock produced by timed light exposure, but the following advice is based upon the well-established chronobiological principles that were considered above [1–3, 7, 8, 11, 13, 23].

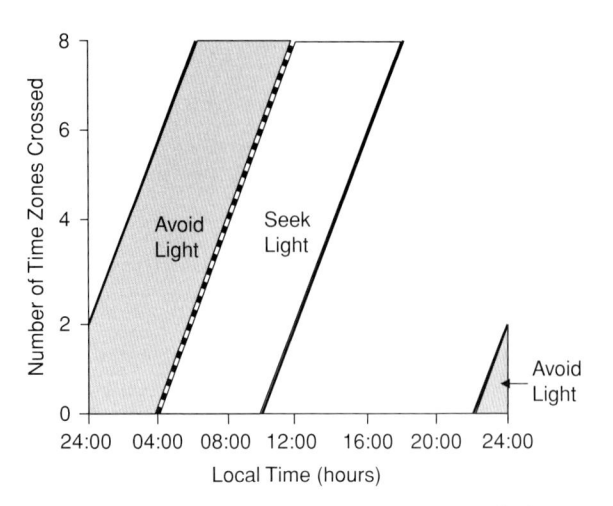

Figure 21.4 Times of light avoidance and exposure on the first day after EASTWARD transitions across up to eight time zones. Dashed line indicates temperature minimum (04:00 h). (Taken with permission from [25].)

Eastward flights across up to eight time zones

After an eastward flight across up to eight time zones, the body clock needs to be advanced. This requires light exposure in the 6 h after the core temperature minimum and light avoidance in the 6 h before it, which would shift the body clock in the wrong direction (Figure 21.2). These "body" times must be converted to the new local time. Figure 21.4 shows this conversion applied to the first day in the new time zone.

To illustrate the use of Figure 21.4, consider an eastward flight over eight time zones. Light has to be avoided between 06:00 and 12:00 h local time (22:00–04:00 h on unadjusted body time) and sought from 12:00 to 18:00 h by local time (04:00–12:00 h body time). (In devising this Figure, the individual's mid-sleep was assumed to be 04:00 h; if mid-sleep differs from this, then all times need to be adjusted accordingly. Thus, if the individual's time of mid-sleep is 03:00 h, then these times become 05:00–11:00 h and 11:00–17:00 h for avoidance and exposure, respectively.) Local times of avoidance and exposure are advanced 1–2 h each day until light avoidance coincides with nocturnal sleep. Morning light after waking should be avoided for the first few days. This can be difficult, particularly when arriving, since many flights are overnight and land in the morning. The only solution is to wear sunglasses that are as dark as possible (not jeopardizing safety) until the dimmer indoor light at the hotel is reached. In general, when light is to be

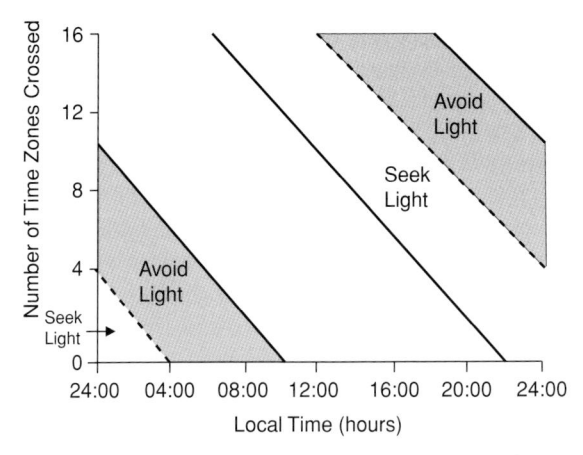

Figure 21.5 Times of light avoidance and exposure on the first day after WESTWARD time-zone transitions and EASTWARD transitions across more than eight time zones. Eastward time-zone transitions in excess of 8 h (X h) are to be treated as westward transitions of [24 − X] h. Dashed line indicates temperature minimum (04:00 h). (Taken with permission from [25].).

avoided, undertaking indoor activities away from windows is recommended.

Eastward flights across more than eight time zones and all westward flights

For eastward flights across more than eight time zones, and for all westward flights, the aim is to delay the body clock. (For example, eastward flights across 10 time zones are to be treated as westward flights across 14 time zones requiring a *delay* of the body clock.) To delay the body clock requires light exposure in the 6 h before the temperature minimum and avoidance in the 6 h afterwards. Once again, body time has to be converted into local time, and this has been done (assuming mid-sleep is at 04:00 h) for the first day after arrival (Figure 21.5). The local times of light avoidance can, if necessary, be delayed 2 h each subsequent day until they coincide with the local night.

The fact that eastward flights crossing more than eight time zones require the body clock to be delayed rather than advanced reflects the fact that the body clock tends to run slow with a natural period slightly in excess of 24 h, large delays being more easily accomplished than large advances. Phase-delaying the body clock has another advantage. After flights to the east across 10 time zones, for example, greatest sleepiness and worst performance are initially at about 14:00 h local time (04:00 h body time); delaying the body clock makes this performance trough progressively later on subsequent days, avoiding times when individuals wish to be most active. If the body clock were advanced, the time of feeling most sleepy and performing worst would be more intrusive, advancing from 14:00 h through the morning.

Conveniently, living in synchrony with the local population and being exposed to the local light–dark cycle after westward flights results in light exposure/avoidance close to the times recommended in Figure 21.5. For example, after a flight across eight time zones, light is initially required at 14:00–20:00 h, and should be avoided between 20:00 and 02:00 h, local time – requirements that accord with the natural light–dark cycle in the new environment. By contrast, after a flight to the east, such "natural" behavior results in light exposure at the wrong time (see Figure 21.4). For example, after a flight across eight time zones, light is required at 12:00–18:00 h, and should be avoided between 06:00 and 12:00 h, local time. The eastward traveller who tries to promote adjustment by "getting out and about" at the first opportunity will cause the body clock to delay (due to morning exposure to light) as well as to advance (afternoon exposure to light), and this will prolong the time taken for body clock adjustment.

Combined approaches

Advice exists on times for melatonin ingestion combined with light exposure and avoidance (for example: [39, 40]), and more elaborate protocols have been reported, including a field study of the combined use of evening melatonin ingestion, light and exercise (training sessions) in athletes [41]. In some cases, there can be doubt as to exactly how subjects were interpreting "jet lag", and distinguishing between promoting adjustment of the body clock and overcoming the symptoms of jet lag is difficult. More studies that address such problems are required before detailed protocols can be recommended.

Accepting that the timing and composition of meals, and exercising at appropriate times, act as zeitgebers, these variables might be used to combat jet lag [42]. However, any effects are small, and the exercise and feeding regimens required would be unacceptable to most travellers. Nevertheless, exercise can be used as an adjunct to light exposure (*activity* outdoors with friends) and light avoidance (meeting friends indoors *to chat*), and meals can underpin the new local time.

Figure 21.6 summarizes advice on dealing with the problems of jet lag.

1. For ANY journey that will take a long time, consider the advice on Travel Fatigue
2. Then consider the following tree:

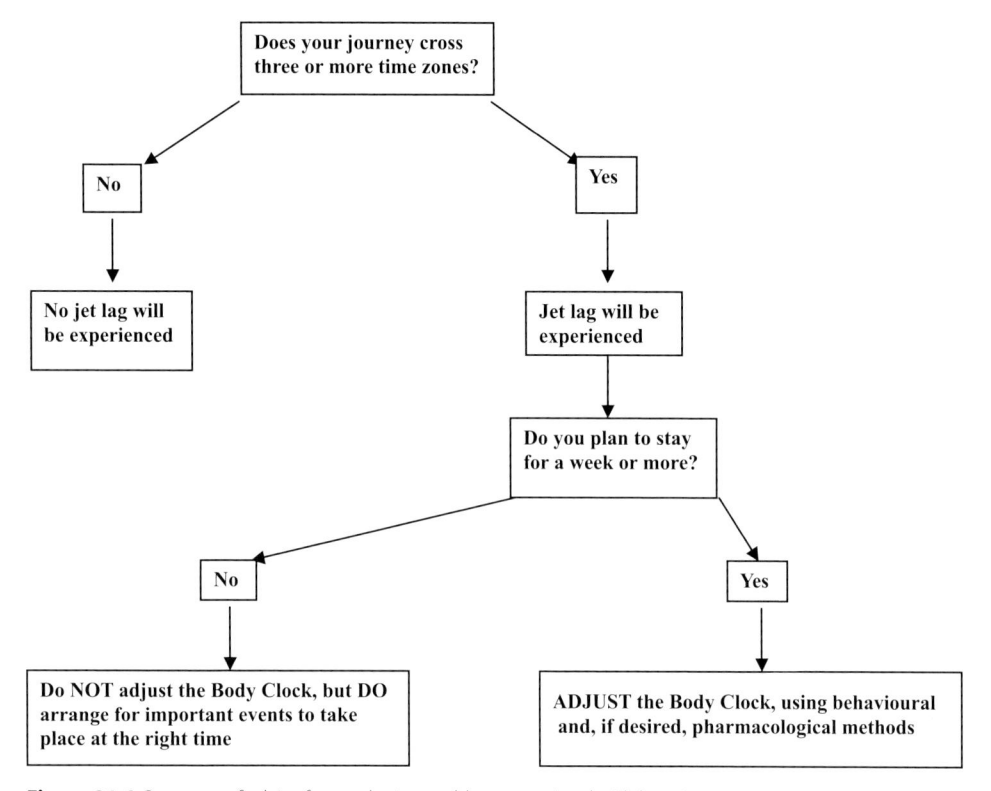

Figure 21.6 Summary of advice for combating problems associated with long journeys.

Differences between individuals

Some individuals suffer more jet lag than others; can they be predicted? Some aircrew undergo frequent long-haul flights across time zones; how do they react to the possibility of continual jet lag?

Personal attributes

It has been argued that jet lag will be less marked in the young rather than the aged, in athletically fit rather than unfit subjects, and in those with rigid rather than flexible sleep habits. Supporting evidence is sparse and ambiguous.

Individuals can also be distinguished with regard to chronotype. "Larks" (morning types) go to sleep and get up early and perform important tasks in the first part of the waking day; "owls" (evening types) are the opposite. The groups differ in the phasing of their temperature and cognitive performance rhythms (larks being 2–4 h earlier), differences being partly due to the body clock [43]. The differences in phase are thought to reflect larks possessing a body clock that runs slightly faster than average, implying less difficulties after eastward flights and more after ones to the west. Owls would be expected to behave in the opposite manner. Such differences have not been found experimentally and, anyway, the majority of the population is an "intermediate" chronotype – neither a lark nor an owl.

Recent work [44, 45] has found that polymorphism exists in one of the human clock genes, *PER3*. Changes in part of this gene are associated with being an "extreme lark" or "extreme owl"; extreme larks also suffer more adverse consequences of sleep deprivation and disruption, implying they might suffer more marked jet lag.

Even so, there is little evidence that personal attributes influence markedly the amount of jet lag experienced; rather, appropriate planning of the trip seems more important. For example, jet lag was less marked in travellers whose flight times minimized the interval between the last nocturnal sleep on "old" time and the first nocturnal sleep by "new" time, a difference that could not be attributed to the amount of in-flight sleep [24].

Aircrew

Investigations of aircrew will indicate if individuals become sensitized to frequent time-zone transitions or if they develop a tolerance and/or "coping mechanisms". However, the position is complex to interpret because necessary safety and commercial considerations severely limit scientific investigation. In addition, a simple time-zone transition followed by rest days is comparatively rare, many long-haul flights occurring during the night (adding problems due to night work) and days in the new time zone often include local, short-haul flights.

Nevertheless, data indicate that aircrew suffer from sleepiness and other symptoms of jet lag [46–48]. When the duty roster requires a return home after only a few days, aircrew sleep at night by "home time" throughout the trip [49]; with longer stays away from home, adjustment of sleep times to the new time zone is attempted after westward flights, but aircrew often retain home time or adjust sleep times only partially after eastward flights [50]. Commercial airlines do not promote the use of melatonin and, with the exception of coffee, other substances to promote sleep or wakefulness are prohibited.

There is no evidence that aircrew are chronobiologically "special", therefore, but they are aware of the problems associated with sleepiness, and often take naps before flights or whenever opportunities arise, in order to prepare for, and recuperate from, work [27]. The symptoms of jet lag do not appear to modify with continual time-zone transitions; instead, they become accepted as a necessary concomitant of the job. Individuals tolerate the adverse effects and adopt personal regimens that minimize them; in this, they resemble those who have worked at night for years and developed "coping mechanisms".

References

1. **Reilly T, Waterhouse J, Edwards B**. Some chronobiological and physiological problems associated with long-distance journeys. *Trav Med Inf Dis*, 2009; **7**:88–101.
2. **Reilly T, Edwards B, Waterhouse J**, et al. Jet lag and air travel: implications for performance. *Clin Sports Med*, 2005; **24**:367–80.
3. **Waterhouse J, Reilly T, Atkinson G**, et al. Jet lag: trends and coping strategies. *Lancet*, 2007; **369**:1117–29.
4. **DeHart R**. Health issues of air travel. *Ann Rev Public Health*, 2003; **24**:133–51.
5. **Philbrick J, Shumate R, Siadaty M**, et al. Air travel and venous thromboembolism: a systematic review. *J Gen Intern Med*, 2007; **22**:107–14.
6. **Waterhouse J, Nevill A, Finnegan J**, et al. Further assessments of the relationship between jet lag and some of its symptoms. *Chronobiol Int*, 2005; **22**: 107–22.
7. **Reilly T, Atkinson G, Waterhouse J**. *Biological Rhythms and Exercise*. Oxford: Oxford University Press, 1997.
8. **Minors D, Waterhouse J**. *Circadian Rhythms and the Human*. Bristol: John Wright, 1981.
9. **Clayton J, Kyriacou C, Reppert S**. Keeping time with the human genome. *Nature*, 2001; **409**:829–31.
10. **Reppert S, Weaver D**. Molecular analysis of mammalian circadian rhythms. *Ann Rev Physiol*, 2001; **63**:647–78.
11. **Khalsa S, Jewett M, Cajochen C**, et al. A phase response curve to single bright light pulses in human subjects. *J Physiol*, 2003; **549**:945–52.
12. **Lewy A, Bauer V, Ahmed S**. The human phase response curve (PRC) to melatonin is about 12 hours out of phase with the PRC to light. *Chronobiol Int*, 1998; **15**:71–83.
13. **Waterhouse J, Minors D, Folkard S**, et al. Light of domestic intensity produces phase shifts of the circadian oscillator in humans. *Neurosci Lett*, 1998; **245**:97–100.
14. **Borbely A, Ackermann P, Trachsel L**, et al. Sleep initiation and initial sleep intensity: interaction of homeostatic and circadian mechanisms. *J Biol Rhythms*, 1989; **4**:149–60.
15. **Åkerstedt T, Gillberg T**. The circadian variation of experimentally displaced sleep. *Sleep*, 1981; **4**: 159–69.
16. **Kräuchi K**. The human sleep–wake cycle reconsidered from a thermoregulatory point of view. *Physiol Behav*, 2007; **90**:236–45.
17. **Murphy P, Campbell S**. Nighttime drop in body temperature: a physiological trigger for sleep onset? *Sleep*, 1997; **20**:505–11.
18. **Shochat T, Luboshitzky R, Lavie P**. Nocturnal melatonin onset is phase locked to the primary sleep gate. *Am J Physiol – Regulat Integrat Comp Physiol*, 1997; **42**:R364–70.
19. **Dijk D-J, Czeisler C**. Contribution of the circadian pacemaker and the sleep homeostat to sleep

propensity, sleep structure, electroencephalographic slow waves, and spindle activity in humans. *J Neurosci*, 1995, **15**:3526–38.

20. **Åkerstedt T**, **Folkard S**. Validation of the S and C components of the three-process model of alertness regulation. *Sleep*, 1995; **18**:1–6.

21. **Waterhouse J**, **Minors D**, **Åkerstedt T**, *et al*. Rhythms of human performance. In Takahashi J, Turek F, Moore R, Eds. *Handbook of Behavioral Neurobiology: Circadian Clocks*. New York, NY: Kluwer Academic/Plenum Publishers, 2001: 571–601.

22. **Reilly T**, **Waterhouse J**. Sports performance: is there evidence that the body clock plays a role? *Eur J Appl Physiol*, 2009; **106**:321–32.

23. **Reilly T**, **Waterhouse J**, **Edwards B**. A review on some of the problems associated with long-distance journeys. *Clin Ter*, 2008; **159**:117–27.

24. **Waterhouse J**, **Edwards B**, **Nevill A**, *et al*. Do subjective symptoms predict our perception of jet lag? *Ergonomics*, 2000; **43**:1514–27.

25. **Dawson D**, **Armstrong S**. Chronobiotics – drugs that shift rhythms. *Pharmacol Ther*, 1996; **69**:15–36.

26. **Eastman C**, **Gazda C**, **Burgess H**. Advancing circadian rhythms before eastward flight: a strategy to prevent or reduce jet lag. *Sleep*, 2005; **28**:33–44.

27. **Nicholson A**. Sleep and intercontinental flights. *Travel Med Infect Dis*, 2006; **4**:336–39.

28. **Caldwell J A**, **Caldwell J L**. Fatigue in military aviation: an overview of US military-approved pharmacological countermeasures. *Aviat Space Environ Med*, 2005; **76**(Suppl 5):C39–51.

29. **Schwartz J**. Pharmacologic management of daytime sleepiness. *J Clin Psychiat*, 2004; **65**(Suppl 16):46–49.

30. **Walsh J**, **Muehlbach M**, **Schweitzer P**. Hypnotics and caffeine as countermeasures for shiftwork-related sleepiness and sleep disturbance. *J Sleep Res*, 1995; **4**(Suppl):80–83.

31. **Carrier J**, **Fernandez-Bolanos M**, **Robillard R**, *et al*. Effects of caffeine are more marked on daytime recovery sleep than on nocturnal sleep. *Neuropsychopharmacology*, 2007; **32**:964–72.

32. **Walsh J**. Pharmacologic management of insomnia. *J Clin Psychiat*, 2004; **65**:41–45.

33. **Richardson G**, **Mitrzyk B**, **Bramley T**. Circadian rhythmicity and the pharmacologic management of insomnia. *Am J Man Care*, 2007; **13**:S125–28.

34. **Lemmer B**. The sleep–wake cycle and sleeping pills. *Physiol Behav*, 2007; **90**:285–93.

35. **Altun A**, **Ugur-Altun B**. Melatonin: therapeutic and clinical utilization. *Int J Clin Pract*, 2007; **61**:835–45.

36. **Buscemi N**, **Vandermeer B**, **Hooton N**, *et al*. Efficacy and safety of exogenous melatonin for secondary sleep disorders and sleep disorders accompanying sleep restriction: meta-analysis. *BMJ*, 2006; **332**:385–88.

37. **Srinivasan V**, **Spence D**, **Pandi-Perumal S**, *et al*. Jet lag: therapeutic use of melatonin and possible application of melatonin analogs. *Travel Med Infect Dis*, 2008; **6**:17–28.

38. **Herxheimer A**, **Petrie K**. Melatonin for the prevention and treatment of jet lag (Cochrane review). In: The Cochrane Library 2002, Issue 4, Oxford update software.

39. **Revell V**, **Burgess H**, **Gazda C**, *et al*. Advancing human circadian rhythms with afternoon melatonin and morning intermittent bright light. *J Clin Endocrinol Metab*, 2006; **91**:54–59.

40. **Parry B**. Jet lag: minimizing its effects with critically timed bright light and melatonin administration. *J Mol Microbiol Biotechnol*, 2002; **4**:463–66.

41. **Cardinali D**, **Bortman G**, **Liotta G**, *et al*. A multifactorial approach employing melatonin to accelerate resynchronization of sleep–wake cycle after a 12 time-zone westerly transmeridian flight in elite soccer athletes. *J Pineal Res*, 2002; **32**:41–46.

42. **Atkinson G**, **Edwards B**, **Reilly T**, *et al*. Exercise as a synchroniser of human circadian rhythms: an update and discussion of the methodological problems. *Eur J Appl Physiol*, 2007; **99**:331–41.

43. **Kramer C**, **Kerkhof G**, **Hofman W**. Age differences in sleep–wake behavior under natural conditions. *Pers Ind Diff*, 1999; **27**:853–60.

44. **Archer S**, **Robilliard D**, **Skene D**, *et al*. A length polymorphism in the circadian clock gene Per3 is linked to delayed sleep phase syndrome and extreme diurnal preference. *Sleep*, 2003; **26**:413–15.

45. **Mongrain V**, **Dumont M**. Increased homeostatic response to behavioral sleep fragmentation in morning types compared to evening types. *Sleep*, 2007; **30**:773–80.

46. **Caldwell J A**, **Caldwell J L**, **Schmidt R**. Alertness management strategies for operational contexts. *Sleep Med Rev*, 2008; **12**:257–73.

47. **Ariznavarreta C**, **Cardinali D**, **Villanua M**, *et al*. Circadian rhythms in airline pilots submitted to long-haul transmeridian flights. *Aviat Space Environ Med*, 2002; **73**:445–55.

48. **Eriksen C, Åkerstedt T**. Aircrew fatigue in trans-atlantic morning and evening flights. *Chronobiol Int*, 2006; **23**:843–58.
49. **Lowden A, Åkerstedt T**. Retaining home-base sleep hours to prevent jet lag in connection with a westward flight across nine time zones. *Chronobiol Int*, 1998; **15**:365–76.
50. **Carvalho-Bos S, Waterhouse J, Edwards B**, *et al*. The use of actimetry to assess changes to the rest–activity cycle. *Chronobiol Int*, 2003, **20**:1039–59.

Section 2 Chapter 22

Sleep Disorders and Excessive Sleepiness

Restless legs syndrome and periodic limb movements and excessive sleepiness

Anil N. Rama, Rajive Zachariah and Clete A. Kushida

History

Restless legs syndrome (RLS) is a common neurological condition characterized by unpleasant sensations in the legs, occurring at rest, especially at bedtime. The paresthesias are accompanied by an irresistible urge to move the limbs, which results in a temporary relief of the symptoms. RLS can be associated with fatigue and excessive daytime sleepiness (EDS), although these are not diagnostic criteria. In most patients with RLS, periodic limb movements of sleep (PLMS) are observed. These are stereotyped, periodic, jerking movements typically consisting of flexion of the ankle, knee, and hip. Periodic limb movements of sleep are sometimes accompanied by a cortical arousal resulting in sleep fragmentation and subsequent excessive daytime sleepiness, although this is controversial. The International Restless Legs Study Group formally defined criteria for restless leg syndrome in 1995, and revised criteria for diagnosis in 2002 [1].

Restless legs syndrome can occur as an idiopathic and often hereditary condition (primary RLS), or in association with a variety of other conditions (secondary RLS). This latter form of RLS is associated with uremia, iron deficiency, polyneuropathy, pregnancy, fibromyalgia, rheumatoid arthritis, Sjogren syndrome, radiculopathy, cobalamin deficiency, folate deficiency, and attention-deficit hyperactivity disorder. Dopamine agonists are now considered the treatment of choice for primary RLS and periodic limb movement disorder (PLMD). This article reviews the clinical features, natural history, laboratory investigations, genetics, pathology, and management of both disorders.

Clinical findings

Restless legs syndrome

The diagnostic criteria for RLS, summarized in Table 22.1, are as follows: (1) an urge to move the legs, usually accompanied or caused by uncomfortable and unpleasant sensations in the legs (sometimes the urge to move is present without the uncomfortable sensations and sometimes the arms or other body parts are involved in addition to the legs); (2) the urge to move or unpleasant sensations begin or worsen during periods of rest or inactivity such as lying or sitting; (3) the urge to move or unpleasant sensations are partially or totally relieved by movement, such as walking or stretching, at least as long as the activity continues; and (4) the urge to move or unpleasant sensations are worse in the evening or night than during the day or only occur in the evening or night (when symptoms are very severe, the worsening at night may not be noticeable but must have been previously present) [2].

Table 22.1 Diagnostic criteria for restless legs syndrome

- The patient reports an urge to move the legs, usually accompanied by unpleasant sensations in the legs.
- The urge to move the legs or unpleasant sensations is worsened during periods of sleep or inactivity.
- The urge to move the legs or unpleasant sensations is relieved by movement.
- The urge to move the legs or unpleasant sensations is worsened during periods of sleep or inactivity
- The condition is not better explained by another current sleep disorder, medical or neurological disorder, mental disorder, medication use, or substance use disorder.

Sleepiness: Causes, Consequences and Treatment, ed. Michael J. Thorpy and Michel Billiard. Published by Cambridge University Press. © Cambridge University Press 2011.

Common descriptions of RLS symptoms include creeping, crawling, tingling, cramping, pulling, pain, electric, tension, itching, stinging, nervousness, growing pains, and burning. The bilateral or unilateral sensory symptoms are usually unpleasant (but not painful) and are described as affecting the depth of the extremity (as opposed to affecting the superficial skin). The majority of the patients describe these symptoms between the ankle and knees, but the entire leg as well as arms and torso could be involved. Volitional movements such as walking, stretching, or shaking their legs attenuates the sensory symptoms in most patients.

RLS is often associated with chronic sleep loss and subsequent EDS, although this is controversial. Large epidemiological surveys have shown that self-reported symptoms of RLS were correlated with sleepiness. A poll given by the National Sleep Foundation found that 9.7% of respondents met the criteria for RLS symptoms (an uncomfortable urge to move the legs occurring at least a few times a week, and which worsens at night) [3]. This subgroup was also more likely to report having fatigue, missing events, being late to work, making errors at work, and driving drowsy than respondents that had not reported RLS symptoms. A larger international study (16 202 adults) corroborated these data using the questionnaire and the Short-Form-36 Health Survey (SF-36), finding that the 2.7% of respondents with medically significant RLS (greater than two occurrences per week, with a complaint of moderate to severe distress) had a quality of life below population norms [4]. Comparative data suggested that RLS sufferers had SF-36 scores similar to those of patients in US populations with other chronic medical conditions, such as type 2 diabetes mellitus and clinical depression. Another survey noted that RLS symptoms were associated with poorer self-reported general health, including depressive and anxiety symptoms, in addition to EDS [5].

Several studies have utilized a variety of ratings scales to correlate sleepiness with RLS in clinical populations. Studies evaluating RLS patients using the Epworth Sleepiness Scale (ESS) and Fatigue Severity Scale (FSS) have demonstrated the daytime impacts of RLS [6]. A review of 26 studies that assessed sleepiness in RLS patients by ESS scores summarily found that untreated subjects with idiopathic RLS have a 20–25% increased risk for daytime sleepiness compared to population norms [7]. Patients with an ESS score >10 were considered sleepy, and the proportion of sleepy RLS patients was estimated at 22%. However, one study of multiple sclerosis patients with RLS that evaluated patients using the Pittsburg Sleep Quality Index (PSQI), Expanded Disability Status Scale (EDSS), FSS, and ESS scores noted that while greater disability, fatigue, and poorer sleep were associated with RLS, EDS (defined as an ESS score >10) was not correlated with RLS [8]. The reduced sleep quality associated with RLS has also been reported to have other secondary outcomes, such as depression and reduced quality of life as measured by Center for Epidemiological Studies – Depression Scale (CES-D), and RLS Quality of Life Instrument (RLS-QLI) [9]. Depression, in particular, may also result in decrements in sleep quality and quantity, with consequent fatigue and/or sleepiness.

Objective measures of sleepiness by sleep latency have not positively associated RLS with sleepiness. One study measuring a number of polysomnographic parameters in 45 RLS patients versus age- and sex-matched controls found that RLS patients exhibited longer sleep onset latencies (according to the 10-min criterion but not to the one-epoch criterion) [10]. A community-based study using polysomnography also reported that sleep latency increased progressively as RLS symptom frequency increased from 5–15 days per month to 16–23 days per month to 6–7 days per week [11]. Still, the study also reported a significant correlation between the sleep arousal index and self-reported sleepiness measured by the ESS.

Periodic limb movement disorder

Periodic limb movement disorder (PLMD) is a disorder characterized by limb movements while asleep that may result in a complaint of insomnia and excessive daytime sleepiness. Periodic limb movements affecting the lower extremities can be described as intermittent extensions of the big toe and dorsiflexion of the ankle with occasional flexion of the knee and hip. The movements are often bilateral, but may predominate in one leg or alternate between legs. Periodic limb movements may affect the upper extremity and manifest as intermittent flexion at the elbow. Periodic limb movements of sleep are predominant in the first half of the night and show a typical pattern of progressive decline through the course of the night.

While RLS is a clinical diagnosis made by the characteristic symptoms of the disorder, the diagnosis of PLMD is made by polysomnography utilizing electromyography (EMG) recordings from the tibialis anterior muscles. Movements are counted if they last

Triazolam (Halcion®) at a dose of 0.25 mg or 0.50 mg is effective in diminishing daytime sleepiness and in improving sleep continuity and duration in patients with PLMS. Interestingly, although the frequency of periodic limb movements were unchanged, the frequency of associated arousals decreased after treatment [78].

Alprazolam (Xanax®) has also been suggested to possibly control the symptoms of RLS [79].

Adrenergic agonists

Clonidine (Catapres®) at a mean dosage of 0.05 mg per day has been shown to reduce the sensory symptoms of RLS but not the number of periodic limb movements of sleep. Therefore, clonidine may be an effective treatment for RLS patients who do not have a large number of periodic limb movements [80].

Antiepileptic drugs

Gabapentin (Neurontin®) improves the sensory and motor symptoms in RLS and also improves sleep architecture and reduces the number of periodic limb movements in sleep [81]. In a head-to-head study of gabapentin versus ropinirole, both drugs were similarly effective in the treatment of RLS and periodic limb movements of sleep [82]. The starting dose of gabapentin was 300 mg at bedtime with a mean dose of 800 mg and range of 300–1200 mg. A gabapentin prodrug, gabapentin enacarbil, that has better absorption and less interpatient variability in plasma concentrations compared to gabapentin, has been shown to significantly improve RLS and PLMS vs. placebo, but is currently not FDA approved.

Carbamazepine (Tegretol®, Tegretol XR®, Carbatrol®, Atretol®, Epitol®) has been shown to be effective in treatment of the sensory discomfort of RLS [83, 84]. However, treatment with carbamazepine does not modify the pattern of nocturnal myoclonus and its relationship to arousal during sleep [85].

Slow-release valproic acid at a dose of 600 mg has also been reported to decrease the subjectively rated intensity of RLS complaints and the duration of its symptoms [86].

Opioids

Oxycodone (Roxicodone®, OxyContin®, Percolone®, OxyIR®, OxyFAST®, Endocodone®, Supeudol®) at an average dose of 15.9 mg subjectively reduces leg sensations and motor restlessness and improves daytime alertness. Furthermore, oxycodone significantly reduces the number of periodic limb movements and arousals during sleep [87]. When naloxone is given parentally to patients treated with opioids for RLS and PLMS, their signs and symptoms of RLS and periodic limb movements reappeared [88]. Long-term effectiveness ranging from 1 to 23 years has been documented in patients taking opioids for the treatment of RLS and periodic limb movements of sleep [89].

Methadone at a dose of 15.5 mg/day is considered an investigational treatment [90]. It should be used cautiously because of its respiratory depressant effect.

N-Methyl-D-aspartate (NMDA) antagonists

Amantadine (Symmetrel®, Endantadine®) started at 100 mg per day and increased to a maximum of 300 mg per day resulted in subjective improvement of RLS in 52% of patients. The mean effective dose was 227 mg per day [91].

Oral ketamine has also been used to treat restless legs syndrome [92].

Other medications

Bupropion (Wellbutrin®) is not associated with antidepressant-induced PLMD and does not significantly worsen RLS. In contrast, treatment with bupropion is associated with a reduction in the objective measures of PLMD [93]. Consequently, bupropion may be appropriate for patients with depression and PLMD.

Folate may ameliorate the symptoms of RLS in patients with acquired folate deficiency and those with familial symptomatology [94].

Selegiline (Eldepryl®, Endantadine®) has been shown to decrease the number of periodic limb movements of sleep. The alerting effect associated with the medication did not have a significant effect on sleep efficiency or sleep-onset latency [95].

Entacapone (Comptan®) is a catechol-*O*-methyltransferase inhibitor that increases the duration of action of carbidopa/levodopa. When given in conjunction with carbidopa/levodopa, it resulted in longer periods of symptomatic relief in a patient with RLS [96].

Tramadol (Ultram®) is a central analgesic that has fewer side-effects and a lower abuse potential than opioids. Tramadol given at a dose range of 50–150 mg per day for 15–24 months resulted in clear amelioration of symptoms in 10 of 12 patients. No major tolerance against treatment effect emerged among those who needed only a single evening dose [97].

Special cases

Kidney transplantation in uremic patients has been reported to successfully treat RLS [98].

An intrathecal pump delivering morphine and bupivacaine resulted in resolution of RLS symptoms in two patients [99].

Conclusions

Restless legs syndrome and periodic limb movement disorder are common neurological entities that may be associated with insomnia and excessive daytime sleepiness. Considerable research has been directed towards elucidating the basic mechanisms and optimizing the management of RLS and PLMD. The goal of future research should be directed towards the application of the fundamental principles learned in the laboratory to the clinical setting.

References

1. **Byrne R**, **Sinha S**, **Chaudhuri K R**. Restless legs syndrome: diagnosis and review of management options. *Neuropsychiatr Dis Treat*, 2006; **2**:155–64.
2. **American Academy of Sleep Medicine**. *International Classification of Sleep Disorders: Diagnostic and Coding Manual* (2nd Ed.). Westchester, IL: AASM, 2005.
3. **Phillips B**, **Hening W**, **Britz P**, et al. Prevalence and correlates of restless legs syndrome: results from the 2005 National Sleep Foundation Poll. *Chest*, 2006; **129**:76–80.
4. **Allen R P**, **Walters A S**, **Montplaisir J**, et al. Restless legs syndrome prevalence and impact: REST general population study. *Arch Intern Med*, 2005; **165**:1286–92.
5. **Winkelman J W**, **Finn L**, **Young T**. Prevalence and correlates of restless legs syndrome symptoms in the Wisconsin Sleep Cohort. *Sleep Med*, 2006; **7**:545–52.
6. **Gerhard R**, **Bosse A**, **Uzun D**, et al. Quality of life in restless legs syndrome. Influence of daytime sleepiness and fatigue. *Med Klin (Munich)*, 2005; **100**:704–09 [in German].
7. **Fulda S**, **Wetter T C**. Is daytime sleepiness a neglected problem in patients with restless legs syndrome? *Mov Disord*, 2007; **22**(Suppl 18):S409–13. Erratum in: *Mov Disord*, 2008; 23:1200–02.
8. **Moreira N C**, **Damasceno R S**, **Medeiros C A**, et al. Restless leg syndrome, sleep quality and fatigue in multiple sclerosis patients. *Braz J Med Biol Res*, 2008; **41**:932–37.
9. **Cuellar N G**, **Strumpf N E**, **Ratcliffe S J**. Symptoms of restless legs syndrome in older adults: outcomes on sleep quality, sleepiness, fatigue, depression, and quality of life. *J Am Geriatr Soc*, 2007; **55**:1387–92.
10. **Hornyak M**, **Feige B**, **Voderholzer U**, et al. Polysomnography findings in patients with restless legs syndrome and in healthy controls: a comparative observational study. *Sleep*, 2007; **30**:861–65.
11. **Winkelman J W**, **Redline S**, **Baldwin C M**, et al. Polysomnographic and health-related quality of life correlates of restless legs syndrome in the Sleep Heart Health Study. *Sleep*, 2009; **32**:772–78.
12. **American Academy of Sleep Medicine**. *The AASM Manual for the Scoring of Sleep and Associated Events: Rules, Terminology, and Technical Specifications*. Westchester, IL: The American Academy of Sleep Medicine, 2008.
13. **Ferri R**, **Gschliesser V**, **Frauscher B**, et al. Periodic leg movements during sleep and periodic limb movement disorder in patients presenting with unexplained insomnia. *Clin Neurophysiol*, 2009; **120**:257–63.
14. **Mendelson W B**. Are periodic leg movements associated with clinical sleep disturbance? *Sleep*, 1996; **19**:219–23.
15. **Mahowald M W**. Con: assessment of periodic leg movements is not an essential component of an overnight sleep study. *Am J Respir Crit Care Med*, 2001; **164**:1340–41; discussion 1341–42.
16. **Chervin R D**. Periodic leg movements and sleepiness in patients evaluated for sleep-disordered breathing. *Am J Respir Crit Care Med*, 2001; **164**:1454–58.
17. **Coleman R M**, **Bliwise D L**, **Sajben N**, et al. Epidemiology of periodic movements during sleep. In Guilleminault C, Lugaresi E, Eds. *Sleep/Wake Disorders. Natural History, Epidemiology and Long Term Evolution*. New York, NY: Raven Press, 1988: 217–29.
18. **Feinsilver S H**. Sleep in the elderly. What is normal? *Clin Geriatr Med*, 2003; **19**:177–88, viii.
19. **Garcia-Borreguero D**, **Egatz R**, **Winkelmann J**. Epidemiology of restless legs syndrome: the current status. *Sleep Med Rev*, 2006; **10**:153–67.
20. **Allen R P**, **Earley C J**. Defining the phenotype of the restless legs syndrome (RLS) using age-of-symptom-onset. *Sleep Med*, 2000; **1**:11–19.
21. **Gamaldo C E**, **Earley C J**. Restless legs syndrome: a clinical update. *Chest*, 2006; **130**:1596–604.

22. **Bayard M**, **Avonda T**, **Wadzinski J**. Restless legs syndrome. *Am Fam Phys*, 2008; **78**:235–40.

23. **Ondo W**, **Tan E K**, **Mansoor J**. Rheumatologic serologies in secondary restless legs syndrome. *Mov Disord*, 2000; **1**:321–23.

24. **Bonati M T**, **Ferini-Strambi L**, **Aridon P**, *et al*. Autosomal dominant restless legs syndrome maps on chromosome 14q. *Brain*, 2003; **126**:1485–92.

25. **Ondo W G**, **Vuong K D**, **Wang Q**. Restless legs syndrome in monozygotic twins: clinical correlates. *Neurology*, 2000; **55**:1404–06.

26. **Kemlink D**, **Plazzi G**, **Vetrugno R**. Suggestive evidence for linkage for restless legs syndrome on chromosome 19p13. *Neurogenetics*, 2008; **9**:75–82.

27. **Stefansson H**, **Rye D B**, **Hicks A**, *et al*. A genetic risk factor for periodic limb movements in sleep. *N Engl J Med*, 2007; **357**:639–47.

28. **Winkelmann J**, **Schadrack J**, **Wetter T C**, *et al*. Opioid and dopamine antagonist drug challenges in untreated restless legs syndrome patients. *Sleep Med*, 2001; **2**:57–61.

29. **Montplaisir J**, **Lorrain D**, **Godbout R**. Restless legs syndrome and periodic leg movements in sleep: the primary role of dopaminergic mechanism. *Eur Neurol*, 1991; **31**:41–43.

30. **Connor J R**, **Wang X S**, **Allen R P**. Altered dopaminergic profile in the putamen and substantia nigra in restless leg syndrome. *Brain*, 2009; **132**:2403–12.

31. **Trenkwalder C**, **Hening W A**, **Walters A S**, *et al*. Circadian rhythm of periodic limb movements and sensory symptoms of restless legs syndrome. *Mov Disord*, 1999; **14**:102–10.

32. **Earley C J**, **Connor J R**, **Beard J L**, *et al*. Abnormalities in CSF concentrations of ferritin and transferring in restless legs syndrome. *Neurology*, 2000; **54**:1698–700.

33. **Allen R P**, **Barker P B**, **Wehrl F**, *et al*. MRI measurement of brain iron in patients with restless legs syndrome. *Neurology*, 2001; **56**:263–65.

34. **Connor J R**, **Boyer P J**, **Menzies S L**, *et al*. Neuropathological examination suggests impaired brain iron acquisition in restless legs syndrome. *Neurology*, 2003; **61**:304–09.

35. **Allen R P**, **Mignot E**, **Ripley B**, *et al*. Increased CSF hypocretin-1 (orexin-A) in restless legs syndrome. *Neurology*, 2002; **59**:639–41.

36. **Kallweit U**, **Siccoli M M**, **Poryazova R**, *et al*. Excessive daytime sleepiness in idiopathic restless legs syndrome: characteristics and evolution under dopaminergic treatment. *Eur Neurol*, 2009; **62**:176–79.

37. **Nicolas A**, **Lespérance P**, **Montplaisir J**. Is excessive daytime sleepiness with periodic leg movements during sleep a specific diagnostic category? *Eur Neurol*, 1998; **40**:22–26.

38. **Gamaldo C**, **Benbrook A R**, **Allen R P**, *et al*. Evaluating daytime alertness in individuals with Restless Legs Syndrome (RLS) compared to sleep restricted controls. *Sleep Med*, 2009; **10**:134–38, 39.

39. **Edinger J D**, **Fins A I**, **Sullivan R J**, *et al*. Comparison of cognitive-behavioral therapy and clonazepam for treating periodic limb movement disorder. *Sleep*, 1996; **19**:442–44.

40. **Paulson G W**. Restless legs syndrome. How to provide symptom relief with drug and nondrug therapies. *Geriatrics*, 2000; **55**:35–38, 43–44, 47–48.

41. **Aldrich M S**, **Shipley J E**. Alcohol use and periodic limb movements of sleep. *Alcohol Clin Exp Res*, 1993; **17**:192–96.

42. **Lutz E G**. Restless legs, anxiety, and caffeinism. *J Clin Psychiatry*, 1978; **39**:693–98.

43. **Dorsey C M**, **Lukas S E**, **Cunningham S L**. Fluoxetine-induced sleep disturbance in depressed patients. *Neuropsychopharmacology*, 1996; **14**:437–42.

44. **Markkula J**, **Lauerma H**. Mianserin and restless legs. *Int Clin Psychopharmacol*, 1997; **12**:53–58.

45. **Hargrave R**, **Beckley D J**. Restless legs syndrome exacerbated by sertraline. *Psychosomatics*, 1998; **39**:177–78.

46. **Paik I H**, **Lee C**, **Choi B M**, *et al*. Mianserin-induced restless legs syndrome. *Br J Psychiatry*, 1989; **155**:415–17.

47. **Agargun M Y**, **Kara H**, **Ozbek H**, *et al*. Restless legs syndrome induced by mirtazapine. *J Clin Psychiatry*, 2002; **63**:1179.

48. **Sanz-Fuentenebro F J**, **Huidobro A**, **Tejadas-Rivas A**. Restless legs syndrome and paroxetine. *Acta Psychiatr Scand*, 1996; **94**:482–84.

49. **Kraus T**, **Schuld A**, **Pollmacher T**. Periodic leg movements in sleep and restless legs syndrome probably caused by olanzapine. *J Clin Psychopharmacol*, 1999; **19**:478–79.

50. **Wetter T C**, **Brunner J**, **Bronisch T**. Restless legs syndrome probably induced by risperidone treatment. *Pharmacopsychiatry*, 2002; **35**:109–11.

51. **Morgan L K**. Letter: Restless legs: precipitated by beta blockers, relieved by orphenadrine. *Med J Aust*, 1975; **2**:753.

52. **Terao T**, **Terao M**, **Yoshimura R**, **Abe K**. Restless legs syndrome induced by lithium. *Biol Psychiatry*, 1991; **30**:1167–70.

53. **Chen J T**, **Garcia P A**, **Alldredge B K**. Zonisamide-induced restless legs syndrome. *Neurology*, 2003; **60**:147.

54. **Alldredge B K**. Zonisamide-induced restless legs syndrome. *Neurology*, 2003; **60**:147.

55. **Ohayon M M**, **Roth T**. Prevalence of restless legs syndrome and periodic limb movement disorder in general population. *J Psychosom Res*, 2002; **53**:547–54.

56. **Lavigne G L**, **Lobbezoo F**, **Rompre P H**, et al. Cigarette smoking as a risk factor or an exacerbating factor for restless legs syndrome and sleep bruxism. *Sleep*, 1997; **20**:290–93.

57. **Silber M H**, **Richardson J W**. Multiple blood donations associated with iron deficiency in patients with restless legs syndrome. *Mayo Clin Proc*, 2003; **78**:52–54.

58. **Barton J C**, **Wooten V D**, **Acton R T**. Hemochromatosis and iron therapy of Restless Legs Syndrome. *Sleep Med*, 2001; **2**:249–51.

59. **Brindani F**, **Vitetta F**, **Gemignani F**. Restless legs syndrome: differential diagnosis and management with pramipexole. *Clin Interv Aging*, 2009; **4**:305–13.

60. **Montplaisir J**, **Denesle R**, **Petit D**. Pramipexole in the treatment of restless legs syndrome: a follow-up study. *Eur J Neurol*, 2000;**7**(Suppl 1):27–31.

61. **Bogan R K**, **Fry J M**, **Schmidt M H**, et al. Ropinirole in the treatment of patients with restless legs syndrome: a US-based randomized, double-blind, placebo-controlled clinical trial. *Mayo Clin Proc*, 2006; **81**:17–27.

62. **Saletu M**, **Anderer P**, **Saletu B**, et al. Sleep laboratory studies in restless legs syndrome patients as compared with normals and acute effects of ropinirole. 2. Findings on periodic leg movements, arousals and respiratory variables. *Neuropsychobiology*, 2000; **41**:190–99.

63. **Estivill E**, **de la Fuente V**. The use of ropinirole as a treatment for restless legs syndrome. *Rev Neurol*. 1999 May 16–31;**28**(10):962–3.

64. **Oertel W H**, **Benes H**, **Garcia-Borreguero D**, et al. Efficacy of rotigotine transdermal system in severe restless legs syndrome: a randomized, double-blind, placebo-controlled, six-week dose-finding trial in Europe. *Sleep Med*, 2008; **9**:228–39.

65. **Wetter T C**, **Stiasny K**, **Winkelmann J**, et al. A randomized controlled study of pergolide in patients with restless legs syndrome. *Neurology*, 1999; **52**:944–50.

66. **Staedt J**, **Hunerjarger H**, **Ruther E**, **Stoppe G**. Pergolide: treatment of choice in Restless Legs Syndrome (RLS) and Nocturnal Myoclonus Syndrome (NMS). Long term follow up on pergolide. Short communication. *J Neural Transm*, 1998; **105**:265–68.

67. **Winkelmann J**, **Wetter TC**, **Stiasny K**, et al. Treatment of restless legs syndrome with pergolide – an open clinical trial. *Mov Disord*, 1998; **13**:566–69.

68. **Trenkwalder C**, **Hening WA**, **Montagna P**, et al. Treatment of restless legs syndrome: an evidence-based review and implications for clinical practice. *Mov Disord*, 2008; **23**:2267–302.

69. **Stiasny K**, **Robbecke J**, **Schuler P**, **Oertel W H**. Treatment of idiopathic restless legs syndrome (RLS) with the D2-agonist cabergoline – an open clinical trial. *Sleep*, 2000; **23**:349–54.

70. **Trenkwalder C**, **Stiasny K**, **Pollmacher T**, et al. L-dopa therapy of uremic and idiopathic restless legs syndrome: a double-blind, crossover trial. *Sleep*, 1995; **18**:681–88.

71. **Saletu M**, **Anderer P**, **Högl B**, et al. Acute double-blind, placebo-controlled sleep laboratory and clinical follow-up studies with a combination treatment of rr-L-dopa and sr-L-dopa in restless legs syndrome. *J Neural Transm*, 2003; **110**:611–26.

72. **Moyer D E**, **Zayas-Bazan J**, **Reese G**. Restless legs syndrome: diagnostic time-savers, Tx tips. *J Fam Pract*, 2009; **58**:415–23.

73. **Högl B**, **García-Borreguero D**, **Kohnen R**. et al. Progressive development of augmentation during long-term treatment with levodopa in restless legs syndrome: results of a prospective multi-center study. *J Neurol*, 2010; **257**:230–37.

74. **Earley C J**, **Allen R P**. Pergolide and carbidopa/levodopa treatment of the restless legs syndrome and periodic leg movements in sleep in a consecutive series of patients. *Sleep*, 1996; **19**:801–10.

75. **Boghen D**, **Lamothe L**, **Elie R**, et al. The treatment of the restless legs syndrome with clonazepam: a prospective controlled study. *Can J Neurol Sci*, 1986; **13**:245–47.

76. **Mitler M M**, **Browman C P**, **Menn S J**, et al. Nocturnal myoclonus: treatment efficacy of clonazepam and temazepam. *Sleep*, 1986; **9**:385–92.

77. **Horiguchi J**, **Inami Y**, **Sasaki A**, et al. Periodic leg movements in sleep with restless legs syndrome: effect of clonazepam treatment. *Jpn J Psychiatry Neurol*, 1992; **46**:727–32.

78. **Doghramji K**, **Browman C P**, **Gaddy J R**, **Walsh J K**. Triazolam diminishes daytime sleepiness and sleep fragmentation in patients with periodic limb movements in sleep. *J Clin Psychopharmacol*, 1991; **11**:284–90.

causation – see Faubel et al. [5] for a discussion of these possibilities).

Sleep quality, insomnia, sleepiness, and behavioral and socio-psychological correlates of sleep duration

Most epidemiological studies investigating sleepiness and the behavioral and psychological characteristics of long sleepers have examined the extremes of sleep duration relative to each other; few have focused specifically on differences between long and midrange sleepers. In this context, epidemiological studies have reported that long sleepers have an increased likelihood of depression, anxiety/worry, medication use, lack of activity, lower socioeconomic status, medical, dietary, heart, breathing, and sleep problems [41]. Long sleepers are also more likely to be under 25 and over 65 [6], although some investigators have found that total sleep time decreases with age in a more or less linear manner [42]. As for sex differences, some studies reported that men sleep longer than women [5, 42, 43], others reported that women sleep more than men [44, 45], while still others reported no sex difference in sleep duration [1].

Although epidemiological studies spanning approximately 50 years have reported negative health and psychological outcomes associated with both short and long sleep lengths, only a few of these studies directly or indirectly addressed nighttime sleep quality and daytime sleepiness in these populations. Some studies reported no difference in sleepiness between long and midrange sleepers [1]. Nevertheless, most indicate more sleep fragmentation and daytime sleepiness among long sleepers relative to midrange sleepers [7, 37, 46], a higher incidence of DIMS and non-refreshing sleep [7], and a higher incidence of feeling "non-energetic" and "tired" or having feelings of "exceptional tiredness" [44]. A recent Japanese study also found that sleepiness was associated with long sleep, but only on weekends/non-working days, and only in one of two different large Japanese companies [47].

In contrast with such large-scale study findings, an elaborately designed laboratory investigation compared small samples of healthy young adults who were long and midrange sleepers [30]. The author reported that long sleepers had lower scores on ratings of depression and anger-hostility and higher scores on ratings of cheerfulness, energy and activation, as measured by an adjective checklist. In addition, longer sleepers functioned with better speed and accuracy on a vigilance task. Although daytime sleepiness was not directly examined in this study, one might speculate that the cheerful, energetic and well-functioning long sleepers were probably not simultaneously experiencing daytime sleepiness or fatigue.

Biological factors associated with long sleep, long sleepers and sleepiness

Physiological basis of sleep duration

It has been hypothesized that individual differences in habitual sleep duration have a physiological basis. Existing empirically supported models of sleep regulation postulate that duration and timing of sleep are regulated by an interaction between a circadian pacemaker, which programs daily cycles in sleep propensity, and a sleep homeostat, which tracks increases in sleep pressure [48–50]. Each component is controlled by a separate brain mechanism; these components may differ between individuals and affect habitual sleep duration.

A third factor, process W, was recently proposed [51] to account for the drop in alertness in the first few hours after awakening. Brain mechanisms have also been described for the wake drive or arousal factor [52]. A four-process model of sleep and wakefulness was proposed a decade later [25]. This model incorporates a sleep drive, which consists of the circadian and homeostatic components of the two-process model, a wake drive, which is composed of chronobiological factors, and environmental factors such as posture, physical activity, and the soporific/alerting nature of a situation.

Circadian aspects and properties of sleep in long sleepers

In an early laboratory investigation of nighttime sleep, Taub [30] showed that healthy young adult habitually long sleepers (9.5–10 h of nocturnal sleep) had higher daytime body temperature, more REM and Stage 2 sleep, and a larger number of awakenings than habitual midrange sleepers (7–8 hours of nocturnal sleep). However, the two groups did not differ on sleep onset latency or wakefulness after sleep onset. He also found that the average daily level of oral temperature was significantly lower in midrange than long sleepers. Results such as these suggest that circadian factors are implicated in habitual long sleep.

A series of important studies conducted more recently by Aeschbach and colleagues [9, 10] investigated circadian factors in carefully selected small samples of habitually long (>9 h) and short (<6 h) sleepers under constant environmental conditions. Aeschbach and colleagues showed that markers of "the biological night" indicate that sleep duration in long sleepers is due to delayed offset in the morning, and not to advanced onset in the evening [10]. For example, the nocturnal interval of high plasma melatonin levels was longer in long than in short sleepers; the interval of low body temperature was longer, as was the nocturnal interval of increasing plasma cortisol levels. They also demonstrated that long sleepers initiate sleep closer to the circadian body temperature peak than short sleepers (i.e. long sleepers have less tolerance to sleep pressure than short sleepers) [9]. Aeschbach and colleagues concluded that differences in the circadian pacemaker's program contribute to habitual sleep length because the pacemaker programs a longer biological night in long sleepers than in those who sleep for shorter periods [10].

Genetic aspects

A large study of monozygotic (MZ) and dizygotic (DZ) same-sex twin pairs showed that total sleep times are more closely related in MZ than in DZ pairs [53]. In their thoughtful review, Taheri and Mignot [54] indicated that EEG studies on smaller samples confirm the discrepancy between MZ and DZ twins, and concluded that genetic factors influence sleep duration through circadian factors.

The studies reviewed above suggest that not only are habitual long sleepers physiologically programmed, but also that long sleep is a heritable characteristic.

Consequences of extended sleep

Since there are few studies that explore directly the characteristics of habitual long sleepers across the lifespan, here we include findings on the physiological and psychological effects of artificially extending nocturnal sleep (i.e. exploring sleep that is experimentally lengthened) and on weekend/non-workday "catch-up" sleep.

Dubbed the "Rip Van Winkle Effect" [55], there is a commonly observed phenomenon when adults sleep longer than usual: they often report persistent feelings of fatigue, lethargy, sleepiness and irritability which can persist several hours after wakening [19]. These feelings of sleepiness and fatigue may then lead to an increased desire to sleep, thereby perpetuating the cycle of longer sleep and more sleepiness.

This phenomenon was studied in a student population [19], where it was found that the experience of "sleeping late" is related to feeling worn out, lethargic, irritable, and "having difficulty getting going." But are these experiences due to extended sleep, per se? Because this study [19] confounded extended sleep with other variables, it is difficult to ascertain whether the findings are due to long sleep time, prior sleep deprivation or circadian factors, such as substantially later than habitual wake times.

It is possible, in experimental settings, to increase sleep duration by 2–3 h through increasing time in bed. In one such study of extended sleep in healthy young adults whose habitual sleep length was 7–8 h, the consequences of extending sleep to between 9 and 11 h were reports of increased daytime sleepiness and worsened mood [18]. In addition, performance deficits were observed, including slowed reaction times, lowered vigilance and increased difficulty with mathematical tasks. Although this study eliminated the confound of prior sleep deprivation, it is still not possible to conclude that extending sleep results in greater sleepiness and poorer daytime outcomes because this study continued to confound total nocturnal sleep time with circadian factors.

In a more conclusive, tightly controlled experimental study of ad lib sleep extension in healthy habitual midrange sleeper (7–8 h per night) young adults, Taub [17] showed that an extension of habitual nocturnal sleep by an average of 2.1 h was associated with more time spent in REM and Stage 2 sleep and that it had adverse effects on daytime fatigue and sleepiness (as well as decrements in performance). These negative results on extended long sleep stand in contrast with Taub's [30] earlier findings on habitual long sleepers (9.5–10 h of nocturnal sleep with no experimentally induced sleep extension) who, despite longer Stage 2 and REM sleep, experienced significantly higher energy and activation than midrange sleepers (7–8 h of nocturnal sleep) on questionnaire measures. Such findings suggest that there are no adverse consequences to long sleep in healthy long sleepers when this is their habitual sleep/wake pattern. The subjective and objective adverse effects were only evident when "oversleeping" took place (i.e. extended sleep). These negative effects of extended sleep held true for both midrange and long sleeper participants [16, 17, 56].

Additional support for the notion that habitual long sleep is different from extended sleep was provided by Ohayon in his large-scale study [57]. This showed that the likelihood of having non-refreshing sleep (a possible proxy for daytime sleepiness) was associated with shorter nocturnal sleep time and with longer extra sleep on weekends/non-workdays. This is similar to the findings reported by Taub and Berger [16, 56], who demonstrated that all deviations from one's habitual sleep/wake pattern (i.e. sleep deprivation, sleep extension and sleep phase shifting relative to one's habitual sleep period), regardless of whether individuals are habitually long or midrange sleepers, negatively affect performance and mood. All result in more fatigue, greater sleepiness and less energy than habitual sleep. Based on their findings, they concluded that these negative effects were primarily due to disruption of an established circadian sleep–wake pattern, and that sleeping fewer, more, or different hours than one typically does are all associated with sleepiness.

Thus, the literature shows that "extended sleep" is not a proxy for habitual long sleep. Even though the two have some similar characteristics (e.g. longer Stage 2 and REM sleep durations in both habitual and extended long sleep than in habitual midrange sleep) [17, 30], Aeschbach et al.'s [10] data on sleep-related physiological characteristics suggest that the circadian pacemaker programs a longer biological night in long sleepers, compared with those who sleep for shorter periods.

Sleepiness in healthy habitually long and midrange sleepers without insomnia

A second look at our own data

In an article entitled, "Long sleepers sleep more and short sleepers sleep less: a comparison of older adults who sleep well" [58], we showed that differences between long and short sleepers reported in the literature on sleep-related, personality and daytime factors disappeared once we excluded individuals with DIMS insomnia from consideration. Since we had not looked at midrange sleepers in this investigation, we reanalyzed the sleepiness and fatigue data for this chapter.

It can be seen in Table 23.1 that we did not find significant differences between older ($n = 54$, mean age = 71) good habitual long (=>8 h nocturnal sleep time) and midrange (7–7.9 h) sleepers on either the Stanford Sleepiness Scale [24] or the single-item fatigue measure administered in our investigation. As a replication, we also reanalyzed data from our study of college students, where we used the same measures [59]. Here, we were surprised to find that midrange and long sleepers differed significantly on sleepiness. What could account for the difference between the college student and older adult samples? Was the difference due to measurement error or power issues? After considerable detective work, we found a much simpler explanation: our older adult data set included only *good* sleepers, while the college student findings were derived from an unselected sample. The discrepancy, we realized to our chagrin, was due to a failure to exclude participants with insomnia! Once this was done, it can be seen in Table 23.1 that the findings on 33 college students (mean age = 20) replicate the "no significant differences" finding obtained on older adults.

But non-significant findings are not very compelling. Therefore, we reanalyzed sleepiness and fatigue data from 30 older (mean age = 63) midrange and long sleeper adults from our current research on individuals diagnosed with sleep apnea (a primary sleep disorder that is associated with fragmented sleep) who had not yet initiated treatment [32]. Here we also used the Stanford Sleepiness Scale [24] as well as some different measures to evaluate fatigue and sleepiness. Nevertheless, as can be seen in Table 23.1, we again found no significant differences after filtering the data to rule out participants with insomnia.

As an additional check on our findings, we correlated Stanford Sleepiness Scale [24] scores with total nocturnal sleep time in all three samples. The results, presented in Table 23.1, again show small and non-significant correlations. In addition, both long and midrange sleepers reported going to bed between 10:45 PM and 11:45 PM; there was no consistent or significant relationship between total sleep time and bed time among the three samples. Although not significant, the difference in sleep times is more readily reflected in arising times, since arising time in all three samples of midrange sleepers was earlier than in the three long sleeper samples. This is consistent with Aeschbach et al.'s [10] findings, and represents a behavioral reflection of the sleep onset and offset data in biological studies of long and short sleepers.

Table 23.1 Comparisons on demographic, daytime, and lifestyle variables of short and long sleepers: means, standard deviations and test results

	Older adults sample (n = 54) [58]				College student sample sample (n = 33) [59]				Sleep apnea sample (n = 30) [32]			
Total sleep time:	Long sleeper ≥ 8 h	Midrange sleeper 7–7.9 h	Test	Sig. p =	Long sleeper ≥ 8 h	Midrange sleeper 7–7.9 h	Test	Sig. p =	Long sleeper ≥ 8 h	Midrange sleeper 7–7.9 h	Test	Sig. p =
Demographic variables												
Sex[3]												
Number of females	16	24	$\chi^2(1, 54) = .58$	0.446	9	7	$\chi^2(1, 33) = .75$	0.387	9	7	$\xi^2(1, 30) = .26$	0.183
Number of males	4	10			7	10			11	3		
Age												
Mean	69.53	71.24	t(50) = −.97	0.338	19.00	20.06	t(31) = −1.25	0.223	63.45	61.10	t(28) = −.56	0.581
SD	5.82	6.35			1.93	2.84			12.15	7.43		
N	20	34			16	17			20	10		
Sleep variables												
Total Nocturnal Sleep Time (TST)												
Mean	8.20	7.15	t(52) = 12.78	0.000	8.52	7.12	t(31) = 9.71	0.000	8.78	7.05	t(28) = −3.33	0.002
SD	0.40	0.23			0.55	0.22			1.62	0.16		
N	20	34			16	17			20	10		
Total Nocturnal Sleep Time Needed												
Mean									8.58	7.70	t(28) = 1.38	0.179
SD									1.96	0.54		
N									20	10		
Usual bed time (PM)												
Mean	23.06	23.21	t(52) = −.68	0.500	23.78	23.66	t(31) = −.65	0.519	22.74	23.23	t(28) = −.96	0.343
SD	0.49	0.80			1.47	0.98			1.31	1.30		
N	20	34			16	17			20	10		
Usual time up (AM)												
Mean	7.84	7.37	t(52) = 2.00	0.051	8.14	7.52	t(31) = 1.32	0.198	8.31	7.73	t(28) = −.79	0.434
SD	0.62	0.93			1.68	0.81			2.13	1.27		
N	20	34			16	17			20	10		

(cont.)

Table 23.1 (cont.)

	Older adults sample (n = 54) [58]				College student sample (n = 33) [59]				Sleep apnea sample (n = 30) [32]			
Total sleep time:	Long sleeper ≥ 8 h	Midrange sleeper 7–7.9 h	Test	Sig. p =	Long sleeper ≥ 8 h	Midrange sleeper 7–7.9 h	Test	Sig. p =	Long sleeper ≥ 8 h	Midrange sleeper 7–7.9 h	Test	Sig. p =

Daytime functioning variables

Stanford Sleepiness Scale[1] (1–7) [24]

Mean	2.00	1.74	t(52) = .69	0.494	2.06	2.56	t(31) = 1.44	0.160	3.50	2.95	t(28) = −.93	0.362
SD	1.75	1.08			0.93	1.03			1.58	1.34		
N	20	34			16	17			20	10		

Sleepy during the day[1] (10 = very sleepy)

Mean									5.10	5.15	t(28) = .05	0.958
SD									2.37	2.56		
N									20	10		

Empirical Sleepiness Scale[1,2] (0–18) [31]

Mean									5.25	5.00	t(28) = −0.15	0.878
SD									4.44	3.56		
N									20	10		

Q Subscale: Sleepy[1,2]

Mean									20.04	19.74	t(28) = −0.53	0.603
SD									1.53	1.41		
N									18	10		

Empirical Fatigue Scale[1,2] (3–18) [31]

Mean					2.19	2.41	t(31) = .44	0.663	10.10	9.50	t(28) = −.37	0.711
SD					1.42	1.50			4.13	4.14		
N					16	17			20	10		

Fatigue attributed to sleep problems (days/wk)[3]

Mean	0.80	0.56	t(52) = .54	0.590								
SD	2.14	1.13										
N	20	34										

Note. TST and the difference between Usual bed time and Usual time up are not equal because all scores are based on estimates by the subjects.

Note. Correlation between TST and SSS for Students r(32) = −.27, p = .143; for Older Adults r(52) = .14, p = .321; for Sleep Apnea Sample r(26) = .29, p = .141.

[1] Higher scores indicate greater sleepiness or fatigue.

[2] The Empirical Sleepiness Scale consists of 6 items from the Epworth Sleepiness Scale. The Empirical Fatigue Scale consists of 6 items 6-point Likert-scaled items [31]. The Q Subscale: sleepy is a composite measure of sleep items [32, 64].

[3] Because Chi-square tests on the proportion of male and female subjects showed no significant differences, data for males and females are combined.

In summary, all of our own results indicate that habitual long and midrange sleepers do not differ on sleepiness or fatigue *provided they do not have diagnosable DIMS insomnia*. This led us to review findings on long sleepers and sleepiness conducted by others in studies where the research was not carried out with a pathology focus.

What others' studies show

Investigations conducted outside the U-shaped pathology lens have also found that long sleepers who do not have insomnia are no sleepier than midrange sleepers. A series of studies on a large sample of college students from Daniel Taylor's lab at the University of North Texas also show that long sleep is not pathological. For example, findings on 951 undergraduates indicate that total nocturnal sleep time, based on 1 week of daily sleep diary, was weakly and *negatively* related to Epworth Sleepiness Scale scores, even when participants with insomnia were not excluded from the sample [60]. In addition, total sleep time was positively related to better sleep quality. These results indicate that the longer participants reported sleeping, the *less* sleepy they felt and the *better* the quality of their sleep. Similarly, sleep diary data from 315 midrange and 269 long sleeper college students who did not experience DIMS insomnia [61] show that long sleepers (= >8 h nocturnal sleep time) experienced significantly *less* sleepiness, *less* fatigue and *better* sleep quality than midrange (7–7.9 h) sleepers (see Table 23.2). In addition, the number of hours of sleep that students indicated needing to function at their best during the day (long sleepers $M = 8.7$ h, midrange $M = 8.5$ h) was closer to being met for long than for midrange sleepers ($M = 8.6$ h, $M = 7.5$ h, respectively). That approximately 8.5 h of sleep per night is most desirable is not restricted to college students. Consistent with this view are findings from a representative sample of the Sleep in America Poll [2, p. 12], which show that 29% of respondents, the largest group, indicated needing between 8 and 9 h of sleep to function at their best during the day.

Other studies on college as well as adult non-clinical populations also failed to show the U-shaped relationship. For example, another study of college students [62] also found *negative* correlations between total sleep time and Stanford Sleepiness Scale [24] as well as Epworth Sleepiness Scale [25] scores. Similarly, in healthy middle-aged to older adults with no sleep complaints, the correlations between total nocturnal sleep times and these two measures of sleepiness were also small and *negative* [63]. In addition, an older study on sleep duration and sleepiness in a community sample of middle-aged adults failed to find significant differences between those who reported long (>8 h) and midrange duration (6–8 h) of nocturnal sleep [1]: this was true of both males and females.

Such findings suggest that if there is, indeed, a relationship between sleepiness and total sleep time in otherwise healthy individuals with no insomnia, that this relationship is small, negative and, if anything, that habitual long sleepers are likely to feel less not more sleepy than midrange sleepers.

Summary

Is long sleep associated with sleepiness? Yes

The literature shows that extended sleep (i.e. occasional long sleep, which has circadian ramifications), even in good sleepers, can be associated with sleepiness. In addition, if comorbidities such as insomnia, negative affectivity, psychological and medical disorders are not ruled out, then self-reported habitual long sleep is frequently related to daytime sleepiness. However, long sleep in these individuals is likely to be associated both with physical and psychological disorders, as well as with disproportionately long bed times, which also appear to be associated with sleepiness. Among these individuals, the hypothesis that it is long bed time, rather than long sleep time, that is related to sleepiness, needs further investigation. There is also the possibility that these daytime sleepiness findings are related not so much to nocturnal sleep but to 24-h sleep time, which incorporates daytime napping.

Because so many of the studies were conducted with a pathology lens, and because the U-shaped distribution is so ingrained in the literature, studies which fail to find the predicted U-shaped relationship are seen as deficient in some way, and limitations sections often provide lengthy explanations for why this relationship was not found. Moreover, non-significant results rarely see print.

Are habitual long sleepers especially sleepy? No

On the other hand, studies conducted without the pathology lens and those where insomnia, a

Table 23.2 Sleepiness, fatigue, and sleep quality in college students without insomnia

	Midrange sleepers (7–7.9 h)		Long sleepers (≥8 h)		Test	
	M	(SD)	M	(SD)	F	p =
Total sleep time (TST) (minutes)	450.71	(17.54)	518.90	(34.62)	939.73	0.001
Ideal amount of sleep desired	507.25	(64.37)	521.43	(64.99)	6.98	0.008
Minimum amount of sleep needed	351.67	(82.86)	370.00	(85.75)	6.88	0.009
Sleep quality[1]	7.20	(1.39)	7.42	(1.32)	3.94	0.048
Epworth Sleepiness Scale (25)[2]	8.80	(3.38)	8.15	(3.62)	4.91	0.027
Multidimensional fatigue Inventory: general fatigue [65][2]	11.63	(3.28)	10.54	(3.20)	16.50	0.001

Note. Based on a significant multivariate analysis of variance. Data were provided by: Taylor and Bramoweth [61].
[1] Sleep Quality is a self-report 1–10 scale with higher scores indicating higher sleep quality.
[2] Higher scores indicate greater sleepiness or fatigue.

comorbidity of most psychiatric conditions, has been removed, typically show either no significant differences between midrange and long sleepers or show that long sleepers are *less* sleepy. These studies also demonstrate that long sleepers get as much sleep as they would like, unlike midrange sleepers, who would like to sleep substantially longer. Moreover, phase delay, phase advance, and extended sleep have a similar impact on habitual long sleepers and on those who habitually sleep less, although it is possible that naturally long sleepers may be especially vulnerable to negative effects of sleep loss.

Conclusions and recommendations

Our review of the many indirect and few direct findings related to sleepiness in long sleepers has led us to believe that sleep length is simply a manifestation of natural variability in sleep need that is normally distributed in the population, in a manner similar to an individual's height, for example. Consistent with this view are conclusions from a recent laboratory study which took into account both variability in sleep need as well as vulnerability to sleep loss [27]. Based on their findings, the authors suggested that the daily mean sleep need is 8.2 h with a huge standard deviation: 2.6 h. Such a finding would appear to eliminate the category of "long sleeper" all together and put sleep length on a continuum. That this is a reasonable way to proceed is suggested by findings of the most recent Sleep in America Poll [2], which provides the following breakdown of total sleep times: 28% of adults report sleeping 8 h or more; 20% report sleeping less than 6 h; 23% 6 to less than 7 h; and 28% 7 to less than 8 h.

Might life circumstances induce more daytime sleepiness in habitual long sleepers than in their midrange sleep counterparts? Possibly. One can predict, for example, from the similar bedtimes of long sleepers and their counterparts who sleep for shorter periods, as well as from data indicating that shorter sleepers appear to tolerate homeostatic pressure better than long sleepers, that long sleepers might experience more daytime sleepiness when they must chronically cope with the 9 to 5 schedules of the working world. But how would the four-process model of sleep, with its addition of environmental and motivational factors, alter such a prediction? These remain outstanding questions for future research in the relatively unexplored field of individual differences in sleepiness and habitual sleep duration across the lifespan.

References

1. **Bliwise D L, King A C, Harris R B**. Habitual sleep durations and health in a 50–65 year old population. *J Clin Epidemiol*, 1994; **47**:35–41.
2. **National Sleep Foundation**. 2009 Sleep in American Poll: Summary of findings. Retrieved 2 November 2009, from http://www.sleepfoundation.org/sites/default/files/2009%20Sleep%20in%20America%20SOF%20EMBARGOED.pdf..

3. **Grandner M A**, **Drummond S P A**. Who are the long sleepers? Towards an understanding of the mortality relationship. *Sleep Med Rev*, 2007; **11**:341–60.

4. **Chen J C**, **Brunner R L**, **Ren H**, *et al*. Sleep duration and risk of ischemic stroke in postmenopausal women. *Stroke*, 2008; **39**:3185–92.

5. **Faubel R**, **Lopez-Garcia E**, **Guallar-Castillon P**, *et al*. Sleep duration and health-related quality of life among older adults: a population-based cohort in Spain. *Sleep*, 2009; **32**:1059–68.

6. **Basner M**, **Fomberstein K M**, **Razavi F M**, *et al*. American time use survey: sleep time and its relationship to waking activities. *Sleep*, 2007; **30**:1085–95.

7. **Grandner M A**, **Kripke D F**. Self-reported sleep complaints with long and short sleep: a nationally representative sample. *Psychosom Med*, 2004; **66**:239–41.

8. **Vincent N**, **Cox B**, **Clara I**. Are personality dimensions associated with sleep length in a large nationally representative sample? *Compr Psychiatry*, 2009; **50**:158–63.

9. **Aeschbach D**, **Postolache T T**, **Sher L**, *et al*. Evidence from the waking electroencephalogram that short sleepers live under higher homeostatic sleep pressure than long sleepers. *Neuroscience*, 2001; **102**:493–502.

10. **Aeschbach D**, **Sher L**, **Postolache T T**, *et al*. A longer biological night in long sleepers than in short sleepers. *J Clin Endocrinol Metab*, 2003; **88**:26–30.

11. **Anderson C**, **Platten C R**, **Horne J A**. Self-reported 'sleep deficit' is unrelated to daytime sleepiness. *Physiol Behav*, 2009; **96**:513–17.

12. **Youngstedt S D**, **Kline C E**, **Zielinski M R**, *et al*. Tolerance of chronic 90-minute time-in-bed restriction in older long sleepers. *Sleep*, 2009; **32**:1467–79.

13. **Goldman S E**, **Stone K L**, **Ancoli-Israel S**, *et al*. Poor sleep is associated with poorer physical performance and greater functional limitations in older women. *Sleep*, 2007; **30**:1317–24.

14. **Creti L**, **Libman E**, **Baltzan M**, *et al*. Impaired sleep in chronic fatigue syndrome: how is it best measured? *J Health Psychol*, 2010; **15**:596–607.

15. **Libman E**, **Creti L**, **Baltzan M**, *et al*. Sleep apnea and psychological functioning in chronic fatigue syndrome. *J Health Psychol*, 2009; **14**:1251–67.

16. **Taub J M**, **Berger R J**. Performance and mood following variations in the length and timing of sleep. *Psychophysiology*, 1973; **10**:559–70.

17. **Taub J M**. Effects of ad lib extended-delayed sleep on sensorimotor performance, memory and sleepiness in the young adult. *Physiol Behav*, 1980; **25**:77–87.

18. **Taub J M**, **Globus G G**, **Phoebus E**, *et al*. Extended sleep and performance. *Nature*, 1971; **233**:142–43.

19. **Globus G G**. A syndrome associated with sleeping late. *Psychosom Med*, 1969; **31**:528–35.

20. **Kaplan K A**, **Harvey A G**. Hypersomnia across mood disorders: a review and synthesis. *Sleep Med Rev*, 2009; **13**:275–85.

21. **Lichstein K L**, **Durrence H H**, **Taylor D J**, *et al*. Quantitative criteria for insomnia. *Behav Res Ther*, 2003; **41**:427–45.

22. **Fichten C**, **Libman E**, **Bailes S**, *et al*. Characteristics of older adults with insomnia. In: Lichstein K L, Morin C M, Eds. *Treatment of Late Life Insomnia*. New York, NY: Sage, 2000: 37–80.

23. **American Psychiatric Association**. *Diagnostic and Statistical Manual of Mental Disorders [Text Revision]* (4th Ed.). Arlington, VA: American Psychiatric Association, 2000.

24. **Hoddes E**, **Zarcone V**, **Smythe H**, *et al*. Quantification of sleepiness – new approach. *Psychophysiology*, 1973; **10**:431–36.

25. **Johns M W**. A new method for measuring daytime sleepiness – the Epworth Sleepiness Scale. *Sleep*, 1991; **14**:540–45.

26. **Akerstedt T**, **Gillberg M**. Subjective and objective sleepiness in the active individual. *Int J Neurosci*, 1990; **52**:29–37.

27. **Van Dongen H P A**, **Rogers N L**, **Dinges D F**. Sleep debt: theoretical and empirical issues. *Sleep Biol Rhythms*, 2003; **1**:5–13.

28. **Cluydts R**, **De Valck E**, **Verstraeten E**, *et al*. Daytime sleepiness and its evaluation. *Sleep Med Rev*, 2002; **6**:83–96.

29. **Saarenpaa-Heikkila O**, **Laippala P**, **Koivikko M**. Subjective daytime sleepiness and its predictors in Finnish adolescents in an interview study. *Acta Paediatr*, 2001; **90**:552–57.

30. **Taub J M**. Behavioral and psychological correlates of a difference in chronic sleep duration. *Biol Psychol*, 1977; **5**:29–45.

31. **Bailes S**, **Libman E**, **Baltzan M**, *et al*. Brief and distinct empirical sleepiness and fatigue scales. *J Psychosom Res*, 2006; **60**:605–13.

32. **Bailes S**, **Libman E**, **Baltzan M**, *et al*. Fatigue: the forgotten symptom of sleep apnea. Available from: sally.bailes@mail.mcgill.ca. 2009.

33. **Hossain J L**, **Ahmad P**, **Reinish L W**, *et al*. Subjective fatigue and subjective sleepiness: two independent

33. consequences of sleep disorders? *J Sleep Res*, 2005; **14**:245–53.

34. **Ohayon M M**. From wakefulness to excessive sleepiness: what we know and still need to know. *Sleep Med Rev*, 2008; **12**:129–41.

35. **Hammond E C**. Some preliminary findings on physical complaints from a prospective-study of 1,064,004 men and women. *Am J Public Health Nations Health*, 1964; **54**:11–23.

36. **Youngstedt S D**, **Kripke D F**. Long sleep and mortality: rationale for sleep restriction. *Sleep Med Rev*, 2004; **8**:159–74.

37. **Kripke D F**, **Garfinkel L**, **Wingard D L**, *et al*. Mortality associated with sleep duration and insomnia. *Arch Gen Psychiatry*, 2002; **59**:131–36.

38. **Tamakoshi A**, **Ohno Y**. Self-reported sleep duration as a predictor of all-cause mortality: results from the JACC Study, Japan. *Sleep*, 2004; **27**:51–54.

39. **Kripke D F**, **Simons R N**, **Garfinkel L**, *et al*. Short and long sleep and sleeping pills. Is increased mortality associated? *Arch Gen Psychiatry*, 1979; **36**:103–16.

40. **Horne J**. Short sleep is a questionable risk factor for obesity and related disorders: statistical versus clinical significance. *Biol Psychol*, 2008; **77**:266–76.

41. **Patel S R**, **Malhotra A**, **Gottlieb D J**, *et al*. Correlates of long sleep duration. *Sleep*, 2006; **29**:881–89.

42. **Ohayon M M**, **Carskadon M A**, **Guilleminault C**, *et al*. Meta-analysis of quantitative sleep parameters from childhood to old age in healthy individuals: developing normative sleep values across the human lifespan. *Sleep*, 2004; **27**:1255–73.

43. **Habte-Gabr E**, **Wallace R B**, **Colsher P L**, *et al*. Sleep patterns in rural elders: demographic, health, and psychobehavioral correlates. *J Clin Epidemiol*, 1991; **44**:5–13.

44. **Kronholm E**, **Harma M**, **Hublin C**, *et al*. Self-reported sleep duration in Finnish general population. *J Sleep Res*, 2006; **15**:276–90.

45. **Natale V**, **Adan A**, **Fabbri M**. Season of birth, gender, and social–cultural effects on sleep timing preferences in humans. *Sleep*, 2009; **32**:423–26.

46. **Kripke C**, **Brunner R**, **Freeman R**, *et al*. Sleep complaints of postmenopausal women. *Clin J Women's Health*, 2001; **1**:8.

47. **Fukasawa K**, **Aikawa H**, **Okazaki I**, *et al*. Perceived sleepiness of non-shift working men in two different types of work organization. *J Occup Health*, 2006; **48**:230–38.

48. **Borbely A A**. A two process model of sleep regulation. *Hum Neurobiol*, 1982; **1**:195–204.

49. **Daan S**, **Beersma D G**, **Borbely A A**. Timing of human sleep: recovery process gated by a circadian pacemaker. *Am J Physiol*, 1984; **246**:R161–83.

50. **Dijk D J**, **Czeisler C A**. Contribution of the circadian pacemaker and the sleep homeostat to sleep propensity, sleep structure, electroencephalographic slow waves, and sleep spindle activity in humans. *J Neurosci*, 1995; **15**:3526–38.

51. **Folkard S**, **Akerstedt T**. Towards a model for the prediction of alertness and/or fatigue on different sleep/wake schedules. In: Oginski A, Polorki J, Rutenfranz J, Eds. *Contemporary Advances in Shift-work Research: Theoretical and Practical Aspects in the Late Eighties*. Krakow: Medical Academy, 1987: 231–40.

52. **Lin J S**. Brain structures and mechanisms involved in the control of cortical activation and wakefulness, with emphasis on the posterior hypothalamus and histaminergic neurons. *Sleep Med Rev*, 2000; **4**:471–503.

53. **Heath A C**, **Kendler K S**, **Eaves L J**, *et al*. Evidence for genetic influences on sleep disturbance and sleep pattern in twins. *Sleep*, 1990; **13**:318–35.

54. **Taheri S**, **Mignot E**. The genetics of sleep disorders. *Lancet Neurol*, 2002; **1**:242–50.

55. **Taub J M**, **Berger R J**. Extended sleep and performance – Rip Van Winkle Effect. *Psychon Sci*, 1969; **16**:204–05.

56. **Taub J M**, **Berger R J**. Altered sleep duration and sleep period time displacements: effects on performance in habitual long sleepers. *Physiol Behav*, 1976; **16**:177–84.

57. **Ohayon M M**. Prevalence and correlates of nonrestorative sleep complaints. *Arch Intern Med*, 2005; **165**:35–41.

58. **Fichten C S**, **Libman E**, **Creti L**, *et al*. Long sleepers sleep more and short sleepers sleep less: a comparison of older adults who sleep well. *Behav Sleep Med*, 2004; **2**:2–23.

59. **Alapin I**, **Fichten C S**, **Libman E**, *et al*. How is good and poor sleep in older adults and college students related to daytime sleepiness, fatigue, and ability to concentrate? *J Psychosom Res*, 2000; **49**:381–90.

60. **Vatthauer K**. Psychological, demographic, academic, and sleep predictors of academic performance in college students. Unpublished thesis: University of North Texas. Available November 2009, from KarlynVatthauer@my.unt.edu; 2009.

61. **Taylor D J**, **Bramoweth A D**. Long sleepers in a sample of college students. Unpublished raw data available from AdamBramoweth@my.unt.edu. 2009.

62. **Pilcher J J, Ginter D R, Sadowsky B**. Sleep quality versus sleep quantity: relationships between sleep and measures of health, well-being and sleepiness in college students. *J Psychosom Res*, 1997; **42**:583–96.

63. **Pilcher J J, Schoeling S E, Prosansky C M**. Self-report sleep habits as predictors of subjective sleepiness. *Behav Med*, 2000; **25**:161–68.

64. **Bailes, S, Baltzan, M, Rizzo, D**, *et al*. The Sleep Symptoms Checklist: useful for screening but not diagnosis. *Sleep*, 2008; **31**(Abstract Supplement), #0514, p. A171.

65. **Smets E M A, Garssen B, Bonke B, De Haes J C**. The Multidimensional Fatigue Inventory (MFI) psychometric qualities of an instrument to assess fatigue. *J Psychosom Res*, 1995, **39**:315–25.

Section 2 Sleep Disorders and Excessive Sleepiness

Chapter 24

Sleepiness in children

Sanjeev V. Kothare and Joseph Kaleyias

Definition

Sleep is defined as a reversible behavioral state of decreased responsiveness and interaction with the environment [1]. Sleepiness is often regarded as the opposite of alertness. Alertness is defined as the inherent ability of the brain to sustain attentive wakefulness with little or no external stimulation. Daytime sleepiness is defined by the International Classification of Sleep Disorders, second edition (ICSD-2) as "the inability to stay awake during the major waking episodes of the day, resulting in unintended lapses into drowsiness or sleep" [2]. Hypersomnia is characterized by recurrent episodes of excessive daytime sleepiness (EDS) or prolonged nighttime sleep that affects the everyday life of the patient [3].

Prevalence

The precise prevalence of EDS in children is unknown. Questionnaire-based estimates suggest that up to 40% of children and adolescents report sleep problems that either restrict or disrupt sleep [4]; 33% of the teenagers report falling asleep during school in another study conducted in the USA [5], whereas daytime sleepiness has been more specifically reported in 17–21% of school-aged children and adolescents [6]. A cross-sectional survey with 9261 school children in Japan demonstrated that 25% reported sleepiness always and 47% often [7]. Clinical surveys have reported EDS as a complaint in up to 68% of normal high-school children [8].

The clinical presentation of EDS in children

Although sleepiness is a problem commonly encountered in adults, children suffering from EDS are frequently not recognized or erroneously labeled as "lazy," inattentive, and/or lacking motivation [9]. The excessively sleepy child can be difficult to detect, although identification is important to correct the underlying cause.

Identification and characterization of excessive sleepiness is one of the most important roles for the sleep clinician. The cornerstone for the prompt recognition of the "sleepy" child is the knowledge of the normal sleep patterns including the total sleep time, which is age dependent [10, 11]. In addition, normal daytime napping habits of infants and children are also important to consider when evaluating suspected EDS. Normal infants nap twice a day for 1–2 h during each nap. This is reduced to 1 nap of 1–2 h between 2 and 5 years of age. Most children do not nap after the age of 5, except infrequently on the weekends [11].

Clues to childhood daytime sleepiness may be (1) sleeping longer hours than children of his/her age, (2) daytime naps beyond normal for age, (3) being sleepy when other children of same age are active and alert, and (4) sleeping more than previously [12].

As a general rule in a school-age child, habitually falling asleep while travelling in a car for less than 30 min or while reading or watching television, or regularly napping on return home from school in the afternoon, should raise suspicion about pathological daytime sleepiness [3].

It is often difficult to separate sleepy tiredness from physical tiredness. It is also important to realize that sleepiness can be caused by coexisting dual pathology, such as depression or chronic fatigue syndrome, with the presence of both sleepy tiredness and physical tiredness.

Causes of sleepiness

Mechanisms of daytime sleepiness have been shown in Figure 24.1. Causes of EDS [3, 9, 11, 13–18] are divided

---

Sleepiness: Causes, Consequences and Treatment, ed. Michael J. Thorpy and Michel Billiard. Published by Cambridge University Press. © Cambridge University Press 2011.

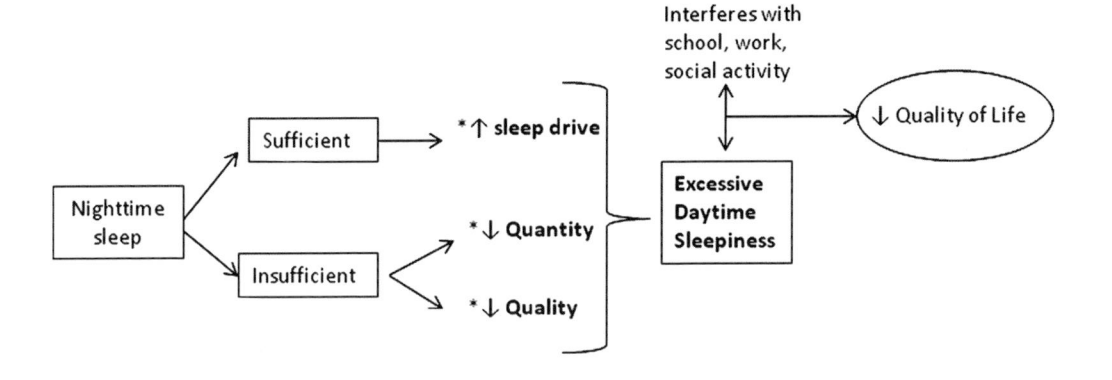

Figure 24.1 Mechanisms for excessive daytime sleepiness.

Factors associated with sleepiness
1. Biologic rhythm (homeostatic-circadian)
2. Environmental
3. Social
4. Psychological
5. Age
6. Sleep disorders [primary/secondary]

into three categories: (1) insufficient nighttime sleep, (2) fragmented nighttime sleep, and (3) an increased need of sleep (Table 24.1).

Sleep deprivation (reduced sleep quantity) is the most common cause of hypersomnolence at all ages, followed by sleep fragmentation (reduced sleep quality). Disorders that increase sleep drive (hypersomnias of central origin) such as idiopathic hypersomnia or narcolepsy are relatively rare causes of EDS.

Assessment of EDS in children

History

A detailed history is crucial in evaluating patients with EDS [12]. The sleep history may be obtained from the patient, parent, guardian, teacher, and/or daycare provider and is crucial in planning appropriate diagnostic procedures in arriving at a specific diagnosis [14]. Important points in the sleep history should include total daily 24-h sleep time, daily sleep patterns (bed-onset and sleep-onset time) on weekdays and weekends and during summer, daytime naps, number of nocturnal awakenings, snoring, witnessed apneas (pauses in breathing), symptoms of Restless Legs Syndrome (dysesthesias in the legs in the late evening at rest relieved by movement), twitching in sleep that might be a reflection of periodic limb movements of sleep (PLMS), and nocturnal symptoms suggestive of gastroesophageal reflux, asthma, or pain. The patient should be asked whether daytime sleep bouts are refreshing and recuperative. Medical conditions and drug or caffeine use can be significant contributors to EDS; if suspected, appropriate evaluation should ensue for these issues as well. Sedentary habits like television watching and excessive snacking that are linked to obesity and obstructive sleep apnea (OSA) should be explored [5, 19]. The long-term use of any sedating medications should also be noted [20]. Patients with migraine, neuromuscular disorders, epilepsy, autism, and attention-deficit hyperactivity disorder can have associated sleep disturbances, including EDS. The sleep history taking can be facilitated by mnemonics like "SIFT" and "BEARS" [12, 21] (Table 24.2).

Physical examination

Obesity, assessed by elevated age-appropriate body mass index, craniofacial anomalies (micrognathia, midfacial hypoplasia), tonsillar hypertrophy, enlarged tongue base, "adenoid face," deviated nasal septum, swollen inferior turbinates, high arched palate, and mouth breathing may be associated with OSA. Dark pigmentation on the neck (linea nigricans) may be an indicator of insulin resistance that is seen in the obese population and patients with epilepsy on antiepileptic drugs such as valproate.

2. Sleep Disorders and Excessive Sleepiness

Table 24.1 Causes of excessive daytime sleepiness in children [3, 9, 11, 13–18]

Insufficient sleep	Fragmented sleep	Increased need of sleep [hypersomnias of central origin]

Insomnia
1. Adjustment insomnia
2. Psychophysiological insomnia
3. Paradoxical insomnia
4. Idiopathic insomnia
5. Behavioral insomnia of childhood
    Sleep-onset association
    Limit-setting association
    Combined type
6. Inadequate sleep hygiene
7. Insomnia due to alcohol, medications, drugs
8. Insomnia due to mental/medical disorder
    (ADHD, PDD, Depression, Bipolar)
Circadian rhythm sleep disorders
1. Delayed sleep phase syndrome
2. Non-24-h sleep–wake schedule
3. Sleep entrainment difficulties
    Blindness
    Developmental delay
    Mental retardation
	Behavioral disorders
	Sleep-onset association disorder
	Respiratory-related disorders
	Obstructive sleep apnea syndrome
	Upper airway respiratory syndrome
	Hypoventilation
	Central sleep apnea
	Movement disorders
	Periodic limb movement disorder
	Restless legs syndrome
	Bruxism
	Head banging/body rocking
	Parasomnias
	Night terrors
	Sleep talking
	Sleep walking
	Confusional arousals
	Medical causes
	Asthma, eczema, cystic fibrosis, gastroesophageal reflux, epilepsy
	Environmental causes
	Noise/light, co-sleeping
		Temporary hypersomnolence
		1. Behaviorally induced insufficient sleep syndrome
		2. Hypersomnia due to medical condition
		    Neurologic disorders (head trauma, increased intracranial pressure)
		    Medical disorders (infection, metabolic)
		3. Hypersomnia due to drug or substance
		4. Non-organic hypersomnia
		    (not due to substance abuse or known physiological condition)
		5. Organic hypersomnia
		    [physiological (organic) Hypersomnia, unspecified]
		    Recurrent hypersomnolence
		    Depression
		    Kleine–Levin syndrome
		    Menstrual-associated
		Persistent hypersomnolence
		1. Narcolepsy with cataplexy
		2. Narcolepsy without cataplexy
		3. Narcolepsy due to medical conditions
		    • *Inherited disorders* (Prader Willi syndrome, Niemann–Pick C, Myotonic dystrophy type I)
		    • *Hypothalamic lesions* (craniopharyngioma, astrocytoma, vascular, infection, traumatic, degenerative)
		    • *Head trauma*
		4. Narcolepsy unspecified
		5. Idiopathic hypersomnia with long sleep time
		6. Idiopathic hypersomnia without long sleep time

Linea nigricans, reflecting insulin resistance, has been found to be a risk factor to obstructive sleep apnea syndrome (OSAS) [22].

Measures of sleepiness

The evaluation of patients who show EDS relies on subjective measures (meticulously obtained history, sleep logs, and sleep-quality questionnaires) and supplemented by objective measures (appropriate sleep diagnostic tests) (Table 24.3).

Subjective measures of EDS

Subjective measures of EDS consist of sleep logs (diary), use of validated scales for quantifying sleepiness, and assessing sleep habits via sleep questionnaires.

1. Sleep logs

Sleep logs give an estimate of the number, duration, and timing of daily episodes of nocturnal sleep, daytime naps, and wake periods. These can be used to evaluate sleep–wake habits over weeks to months, including weekdays and weekends [23]. Eating times can also be indicated. These are further validated using actigraphy [24] (see later). They are frequently used before the Multiple Sleep Latency Test (MSLT), and may reveal evidence of chronically insufficient sleep with the prerequisite that they are accurately completed [25].

2. Clinical sleep scales

Three clinical sleep scales have been used to assess sleepiness: (1) Stanford Sleepiness Scale (SSS) [26], (2) Epworth Sleepiness Scale (ESS) [27], and (3) Pediatric Daytime Sleepiness Scale (PDSS) [28]. SSS and ESS

Table 24.2 Pediatric sleep history for evaluation of EDS [12, 21]

Pediatric sleep history
- SLEEP HISTORY
- total daily 24-h sleep time
- daily sleep patterns (bed-onset and sleep-onset time)
- daytime naps (refreshing or not)
- number of nocturnal awakenings
- snoring, witnessed apneas (pauses in breathing),
- dysesthesias in the legs in the late evening at rest, relieved by movement (symptoms of Restless Legs Syndrome)
- twitching in sleep (a reflection of periodic limb movements of sleep)
- weekdays and weekends

	SIFT		BEARS
Situation	When does the child feel sleep/tired?	Bedtime problems	Does the child have any problems falling asleep at bedtime?
Impairment	To what extent does sleepiness interfere with daily life?	EDS	Does the child feel sleepy a lot during the day? In school? In the car?
Frequency	How often does the child feel sleepy?	Awakenings during the night	Does he/she wake up a lot at night?
Tools	Use tools like ESS to determine presence/degree of EDS	Regularity and duration of sleep	What time does the child usually go to bed on school nights? At weekends? How much sleep does he/she usually get?
		Sleep-disordered breathing	Parent: does your child snore loudly at night? Patient: has anyone ever told you that you snore loudly at night?

EDS, excessive daytime sleepiness; ESS, Epworth Sleepiness Scale.

Table 24.3 Subjective and objective measures of hypersomnias [12]

Subjective measures	Objective measures
Sleep history	**Actigraphy**
Sleep logs	Nocturnal polysomnography
Clinical sleep scales	Multiple sleep latency test
• Stanford Sleepiness Scale	Maintenance of wakefulness test
• Epworth Sleepiness Scale	HLA subtypes
• Pediatric Daytime Sleepiness Scale	CSF hypocretin-1 levels
Sleep questionnaires	
• Childhood Sleep Habits Questionnaire	
• Pediatric Sleep Questionnaire	

Table 24.4 Pediatric Daytime Sleepiness Scale (PDSS) [28]

The PDSS is an eight-item questionnaire developed to measure EDS in younger school age populations.

Items
1. How often do you fall asleep or get drowsy during class periods?
2. How often do you get sleepy or drowsy while doing your homework?
3. *Are you usually alert most of the day?
4. How often are you ever tired and grumpy during the day?
5. How often do you have trouble getting out of bed in the morning?
6. How often do you fall back to sleep after being awakened in the morning?
7. How often do you need someone to awaken you in the morning?
8. How often do you think that you need more sleep?*

* Reverse score this item.
Total score: Normal <15; Sleepy 20.

are two extensively used sleep scales to assess sleepiness in adults. PDSS is a recently introduced validated measure for assessing sleepiness in children. It was developed to measure excessive sleepiness in younger children. Scores ranged from 0 to 32. Mean normal score values in the original study [28] were 15.3 ± 6.2. Higher scores indicate greater sleepiness. By using this scale, daytime sleepiness was found to be related to lower school grades and other negative school-related outcomes [29]. Please refer to Table 24.4 for further details on the PDSS.

3. Sleep questionnaires

The two most widely used questionnaires in children are the Childhood Sleep Habits Questionnaire [30], and the Pediatric Sleep Questionnaire [31].

The Childhood Sleep Habits Questionnaire is a detailed 35-item questionnaire assessing sleep problems, habits, and practices [30]. It is normed for middle-class suburban white children 4–10 years old.

The Pediatric Sleep Questionnaire involves a 22-item sleep-related breathing disorder subscale, a 4-item daytime sleepiness subscale, and a 6-item inattention/hyperactive behavior subscale normed for children 2–18 years old [31].

Both questionnaires have reliable internal consistency and test–retest reliability.

The development of valid self-report measures of daytime sleepiness in younger populations is important because the available ones used in the adult population are not as useful for children. For example, although common experiences such as watching television may unmask sleepiness in a sleep-deprived adult, a child may be aroused by the television [32]. Questionnaires should also be directed towards minority populations. A recent validated questionnaire has also been developed in adolescents [33].

Objective measures of EDS

1. Actigraphy

As indicated by several recent reviews and the newly updated practice parameters of the American Academy of Sleep Medicine (AASM), [34, 35] actigraphy has been widely recognized as a low-cost alternative to conventional PSG for the screening of sleep disorders, with special emphasis on sleep–wake cycles and, more specifically, insomnia. Although actigraphy provides much less information than a full PSG and serves only as a surrogate marker of sleep–wake function in the form of movements, there are a number of situations in which it is particularly suitable because of its low cost and non-invasive characteristics [36]. In particular, actigraphy is a viable tool for assessing insomnia and circadian rhythm disorders. Sleep parameters most closely estimated by actigraphy include sleep duration, sleep efficiency, and waking time after initial sleep onset. The major advantage of this technique is the ability to obtain longitudinal data about sleep–wake function over many days, its portability, and its application in an ambulatory setting [37]. A concomitantly maintained sleep log provides important supplemental data for accurate interpretation of actigraphy [34]. Limitations of actigraphy are the incapability to differentiate the sleep stages, the difficulty for accurate measure of sleep–wake periods if the patient has a concurrent movement disorder, and the underestimation of wakefulness if the patient lies quietly awake without movement [38].

Actigraphy was used to determine the sleep–wake patterns of healthy 1- to 5-year-old children and was reliable when compared with parental diaries of sleep times [39]. It has also been used in children with intellectual disability and autism spectrum disorders to determine sleep disruption in these populations, correlating with parental report [40]. Actigraphy may be a useful tool in objectively assessing a child's sleep in cases where highly unusual sleep patterns are reported by parents [41]. Actigraphic analysis proved to be useful in detecting sleep/wake problems in children with chronic fatigue syndrome [42], and provides a reasonably good estimate of TST in adolescents without sleep disordered breathing (SDB) [43]. Recently, Sitnick *et al.* [44] compared actigraphy with videosomnography in preschool-aged children, with special emphasis on the accuracy of detection of nighttime awakenings. Fifty-eight participants wore an actigraph for 1 week and were videotaped for 2 nights while wearing the actigraph. One group ($n = 22$) was diagnosed with autism, another group ($n = 11$) had developmental delays without autism, and a third group ($n = 25$) were normally developing children. Actigraphy had poor agreement for detecting nocturnal awakenings, compared with video-observations, in preschool-aged children.

2. Multiple Sleep Latency Test (MSLT)

The MSLT is a validated measure of the ability or tendency to fall asleep. It is considered the de-facto standard for objective measurement of sleepiness and in combination with the nocturnal polysomnography forms the gold standard in the objective assessment of the EDS [45]. The AASM has provided specific recommendations for conducting the MSLT that are designed to exclude common sleep disorders and minimize environmental and test protocol-related factors known to affect sleep latency [45].

MSLT is generally performed on the following day of PSG to assess the degree of sleepiness and the timing of rapid eye movement (REM) sleep onset. The MSLT is performed by allowing 5 nap opportunities lasting 20 min each at 2-h intervals. Details of the protocol have been recently described [45]. Sleep stages are recorded with particular attention to REM sleep onset. For each nap opportunity, sleep latency is defined as the time from lights out to stage 1 of sleep. Sleep-onset REM periods (SOREMPs) are characterized by onset within 15 min of sleep onset [45]. The mean sleep latency (MSL; arithmetic mean of sleep latency of all naps) is an index of severity of sleepiness.

Test properties and available normative data have recently been extensively reviewed [46]. Prepubertals (and geriatric patients) have longer MSL, whereas adolescents and young adults have the shortest MSL. Gozal et al. [47] and Palm et al. [48] found a mean sleep latency of 23.7 and 26.4 min, respectively, in prepubertal children. For these reasons, 30-min naps in children have been proposed on a research basis [49]. A sleep latency of 5–10 min indicates moderate daytime sleepiness, whereas <5 min indicates severe daytime sleepiness.

MSLTs in children are indicated in patients with suspected narcolepsy and idiopathic hypersomnia. Patients with narcolepsy usually have MSL of less than 8 min, whereas healthy children show an MSL of 15–20 min [45]. The presence of 2 or more SOREMPs with an MSL <8 min is considered diagnostic for narcolepsy [2]. However, the reliability of the MSLT for the diagnosis of narcolepsy has been questioned by recent evidence showing that similar results can occur in up to 15% of the normal population [46, 50, 51]. In adults, the combination of 2 SOREMPs and an MSL <5 min is estimated to have a sensitivity of 70% and a specificity of 97% for narcolepsy [46, 50, 51]. However, 30% of patients with this combination did not have narcolepsy [51]. Comparable data are not available for children and adolescents.

Based on the observation that the sensitivity for the identification of ≥2 SOREMPs in patients is 70%, the AASM [45] recommends repeating MSLT testing when the patient is suspected to have narcolepsy, but earlier MSLT evaluation(s) did not provide polygraphic confirmation to increase the likelihood of recording ≥2 SOREMPs. Another indication for a repeat MLST is the possible alteration of the initial test by extraneous circumstances or the lack of the appropriate study conditions during the initial testing. Antidepressants are withdrawn for 2 weeks before and stimulants on the day of performing the MSLT. Urine for toxicology may also be performed in teenagers to detect abuse of alerting drugs. The MSLT is associated with good to excellent interrater and intra-rater reliability and excellent test–retest reliability [52]. The test–retest reliability of MSLT was 0.97 [53]. The intra-rater reliability coefficient for the mean MSLT score was 0.87, and the interrater reliability was 0.90. Similar values for SOREM were 0.90 and 0.81, respectively [54].

Limitations of the MSLT are the lack of normative data in pediatric patients, the last nap effect (increased arousal because of the anticipation of going home on completion of this extensive testing!), and motivation (to remain awake or attempt to sleep). In our experience, MSLTs can be performed satisfactorily in children above 4–6 years of age.

3. The Maintenance of Wakefulness Test

The MWT is indicated to assess the efficacy of treatment in patients with narcolepsy and for safety issues regarding driving [45]. The MWT, the mirror image of the MSLT, is a validated objective measure of the ability to stay awake for a defined time [55]. A detailed protocol has recently been published [45]. Normal values of MWT are more than 30 min, whereas the test is considered abnormal when it is less than 12 min [45, 46]. Motivation of the patient to stay awake is the key for the interpretation of the results [45]. Pediatric normative values are not available.

4. Nocturnal polysomnography

Polysomnography (PSG), the gold standard for evaluating sleep disorders, measures multiple physiological variables during sleep and is an integral component of all sleep laboratory testing [56]. It provides information about a variety of disturbances associated with daytime sleepiness in children [57, 58].

The PSG report contains data regarding the total sleep time, sleep efficiency (total sleep time divided by time in bed, normal being >85%), sleep latency (time to go into sleep from wakefulness), REM latency (time to go into REM after falling asleep), arousal index (arousals/h; normal <10/h), apnea hypopnea index, periodic leg movement index (PLMI), periodic leg movement arousal index (PLMA), average and nadir of pulse oximetry data; end-tidal CO_2 ($ETCO_2$) trends; and abnormality in EEG, electrocardiogram, and sleep staging (non-REM 1, 2, 3 (slow-wave sleep), and REM sleep).

Nocturnal PSG is the only diagnostic technique shown to quantify the ventilatory and sleep abnormalities associated with sleep-disordered breathing and is currently the gold standard [59]. PSG rules out causes of daytime sleepiness such as OSAS (PSG is considered positive for OSAS when the numbers of obstructive apnea plus hypopnea per hour are more than 1 per hour (apnea hypopnea index >1/h) [2,60]), upper-airway resistance syndrome, obstructive hypoventilation, periodic limb movements of sleep, bruxism, gastroesophageal reflux, and seizures. PSG must be performed before the MSLT to ensure at least 75% of normal sleep requirement for age on the previous night. Moreover, continuous polysomnography can also be performed for 24 h or more to assess the degree of sleepiness, especially in younger children incapable of undergoing MSLTs. This may also help in evaluating circadian variations in sleepiness. Pediatric PSGs should be performed in child-friendly sleep laboratories with equipment to simultaneously monitor $ETCO_2$ during the sleep study [61]. PSG suffers from several drawbacks: it is costly and labor-intensive, usually performed in a sleep laboratory and, because of the many sensors and wires placed on the patient, can disrupt the very sleep architecture it is designed to measure (the so-called "first night effect"). A parent usually sleeps in a separate bed in the same room during the study.

5. Pupillometry

Pupillometry is an infrared video-recording system to gauge sleepiness on the basis of changes in pupillary size or stability in a dark environment based on the premise that size and stability are inversely related to degree of sleepiness. McLaren et al. [62] assessed hypersomnolent patients and normal volunteers by using pupillometry and found the usefulness of this technique in the diagnosis of pathologic sleepiness in individual patients. It is mainly a research tool with no pediatric normative data available.

6. Cerebrospinal fluid hypocretin-1 levels

Narcolepsy with cataplexy in humans has been shown to be associated with low levels of CSF hypocretin-1 in many but not all patients, and the measurement of CSF hypocretin-1 levels is now being considered as an important diagnostic tool [63]. CSF orexin levels <110 pg/ml have >95% specificity in diagnosing narcolepsy with cataplexy and >50% specificity in narcolepsy without cataplexy [64, 65]. In children, in whom symptoms of cataplexy may be delayed, low CSF orexin levels in a narcoleptic child may be predictive of cataplexy developing in the future. CSF orexin level measurement is particularly helpful when the patient is already receiving antidepressants/stimulants, which may be unsafe to discontinue for the purpose of obtaining the MSLT, and when MSLTs cannot be performed in children below 4–6 years of age. Values in post-traumatic hypersomnia and Kleine–Levine syndrome are not known.

7. HLA subtypes

Genetic studies have indicated a strong association between narcolepsy and HLA DQ antigens, specifically DQB1*0602 and DQA1*0102. HLA DQB1*0602 appears in narcolepsy with cataplexy (76–90%), narcolepsy without cataplexy (40–57%), and also in the normal population (12–38%) [67]. Lower CSF levels of hypocretin-1 (<110 pg/ml) have been shown to correlate with HLA DQB1*0602 antigen positivity or symptoms of cataplexy [65, 66].

8. Miscellaneous studies

Other studies include spectral electroencephalographic analysis for the assessment of sleepiness [67, 68]. Greneche et al. [68] showed that in a sustained wakefulness paradigm, higher activity in delta, theta, and beta bands was associated with patients suffering from OSAS showing marked signs of higher sleepiness and stronger efforts than controls to stay awake, even though they tended to underestimate their sleepiness.

Sangal et al. have shown prolongation of long latency evoked potentials such as P300 in hypersomnias and also predict treatment response to modafinil in patients with narcolepsy [69].

In addition, every sleepy child needs to be screened for subclinical hypothyroidism, especially in obese children with sleep disordered breathing (SDB) [70, 71].

Genetic testing for Prader-Willi syndrome [72], myotonic dystrophy [73], and Niemann-Pick C disease [74] can lead to hypersomnias and secondary narcolepsy, and should be screened in appropriate sleepy children.

Functional-magnetic resonance imaging (f-MRI) and positron emission tomography (PET) studies have been performed in adults to assess regional differences in blood flow in patients with hypersomnia as compared with controls [75]. Similar data in children are as yet unavailable.

Neurocognitive and behavioral consequences of sleep loss in children

It must be noted that excessive daytime sleepiness can result from reduction in sleep duration, disturbed and fragmented sleep at night, or from a primary hypersomnia syndrome such as narcolepsy. However, whatever the cause, this daytime sleepiness in children has been shown to be associated with hyperactivity, inattention, aggressive outburst, irritability, anxiety, and depression [76–81]. It has also been shown that it is fully reversible, once sleep recovery occurs. In a study of sleep and daytime behavior in young children, 36% of those children with global reports of sleep problems had significant sleep problems [82]. In adults, sleep disruption has been associated with deficits in attention, concentration, memory, and verbal and non-verbal intelligence [83]. Executive function is defined as "the ability to plan and coordinate a willful action in the face of alternatives, to monitor and update action as necessary and suppress distracting material by focusing attention on the task at hand" [84]. There is evidence that sleep deprivation in adults and children affects prefrontal cortex-related executive attention and working memory abilities [85]. In addition, Thomas *et al.* have shown in an imaging study using PET scans, that the areas of deficits also extend to the thalamus, anterior cingulate cortex, and inferior and posterior parietal and temporal cortices [86, 87]. Gozal *et al.* have shown in children as well as in animal models that during obstructive sleep apnea, the sleep fragmentation with increased arousals leads to more inattention in the daytime, while the acute intermittent hypoxemia during these episodes leads to more memory deficits, which in animal models has been shown to be secondary to neuronal loss in the hippocampus [88–90]. The effect of intermittent hypoxia may involve activation of inflammatory cascades, and apolipoprotein E modulation, thus inducing further neuronal loss [91]. Besides executive dysfunction seen with OSAS in children, other domains affected are expressive language skills, visual perception, and working memory [92]. Carskadon *et al.* have shown that higher cognitive functions that involve verbal creativity and abstract thinking may be more sensitive to sleep restriction in children [93, 94]. In general, sleep deprivation rather than sleep restriction appears to be associated with more prominent decrements in cognition and academic performances [95].

These deficits in neurocognitive functioning secondary to sleep loss make common sense, since sleep is essential to human life, and involves both physiological and behavioral processes [96]. Sleep is recognized not simply as a resting state, but also a state that involves intense brain activity. An essential process involved in brain maturation is "brain plasticity", which is the genetically determined ability of the young and developing brain of a child to change its structure and function in response to the environment. Studies have shown that when young animals are REM and non-REM sleep-deprived, there is a loss of brain plasticity; this loss is characterized by smaller brains, diminished learning, and negative long-term behavioral effects [97]. "Endogenous stimulation" refers to discharges from neurons within the neurosensory system that may not be related to the immediate environmental circumstances of the child but may appear to be essential for axon growth and targeting [98]. These discharges create various connections between sensory organs and essential brain structures. Healthy development depends on endogenous stimulation, and it occurs only during REM sleep. Interference with REM sleep can lead to abnormal development of these sensory systems and structures in animal models. Similarly, K-complexes and sleep-spindles are also essential for normal brain maturation, especially in processes of memory and learning [99].

Hence any loss or disruption of both REM and non-REM sleep in early childhood may predispose to abnormal brain development.

Treatment of EDS in children

I   Treatment options of EDS in children and adolescents due to insufficient/adequate sleep and fragmented sleep are summarized in Table 24.5 [11, 13, 99, 100].
II Treatment of EDS in children due to narcolepsy and other hypersomnias of central origin.

Management of disorders that may coexist with hypersomnia of central origin such as obstructive sleep apnea, periodic limb movements, insufficient sleep, psychiatric disorders, medications, and circadian rhythm disorders will require specific therapeutic interventions, but need to be done for optimal outcome in children with narcolepsy [101].

The general approach to the treatment of childhood narcolepsy and other hypersomnias of central

Table 24.5 Treatment of EDS in children and adolescents due to insufficient sleep or sleep fragmentation [11, 13, 99,100]

Causes of EDS	Treatment
Insufficient or inadequate sleep	Address sleep needs and **appropriate sleep hygiene** with all family members
	Behavioral contracts may be effective in helping children and their families target sleep behaviors that need to change and the steps that are needed to achieve these goals
Delayed sleep phase syndrome	Difference between the actual and desired bedtime : <3 h: **phase advancement** (the adolescent is not to go to bed until the delayed bedtime and then advance his bedtime by 15 min every few nights); >3 h phase delay (**chronotherapy**) (the bedtime and wake time are shifted 2–3 h later every day until the desired sleeping time is reached). **Light-therapy** (10 000 lux light source); strict sleep hygiene; last resort: working with the school system.
	Melatonin promotes sleep initiation and maintenance. Hypnotic when given 1 h prior to sleep onset; phase-advancing when given 5.5–6 h prior to sleep onset.
	In *resistant* cases, use of a sedative at night and stimulant in the day may be tried to break the cycle over a three-month period.
Sleep-disordered breathing	70% of children with symptoms of OSA are alleviated with **tonsillectomy and/or adenoidectomy**. A follow-up overnight PSG post-surgery is recommended. For overweight children, **weight loss** is the recommended treatment.
	Pharmacological approaches may be indicated for children who have chronic nasal congestion.
	In children in whom tonsillectomy or adenoidectomy is contraindicated or unsuccessful, **nasal continuous positive airway pressure** (CPAP) may be appropriate.
Disorders of arousals	**Providing the family with information** about creating a safe sleep environment, education about the events, and how to interact with the child appropriately during the event. Medications rarely used (only when very frequent events, or arousal and awakenings are highly disruptive to the family).
Restless Legs Syndrome and Periodic Limb Movement Disorder	**Iron replacement** therapy; **levodopa** 50–100 mg/d; **bromocriptine** 7.5 mg/d; **oxycodone HCl** 10–15 mg/d; **clonazepam** 0.5–4 mg/d; **carbamazepine** 100–300 mg/d; **clonidine** HCl 0.1–0.3 mg/d, **ropinarole** 0.1–1.0 mg in the evening, **pramipexole** 0.1–5 mg in the evening, **gabapentin** 10 mg/kg in the evening.

origin is based on the adult experience. Recently, the American Academy of Sleep Medicine (AASM) published the practice parameters for the treatment of these disorders [102].

i. Non-pharmacological treatment (lifestyle changes)

Education support and counseling of both family and especially school officials are cornerstones of management in children with narcolepsy. According to the AASM, "scheduled naps can be beneficial to combat sleepiness but seldom suffice as primary therapy to narcolepsy (guideline)" [102]. In our experience, short naps during school time (e.g. during lunch break) have been effective in improving daytime functioning [103]. The combination of regular bedtimes and two 15-min regularly scheduled naps reduced unscheduled daytime sleep episodes and sleepiness when compared to stimulant therapy alone [104].

ii. Pharmacological treatment (Table 24.6)

CNS-alerting or CNS neuromodulator agents are the mainstay of treatment of narcolepsy and other hypersomnias of central origin. Co-administration of two or more classes of compounds may be needed in some patients to adequately address their symptoms [102, 105].

Stimulant medications are used with the goal of providing optimal alertness during school hours and other social situations. Most clinicians initially prescribe methylphenidate or amphetamines, with dosage titration based on side-effects and clinical response [102, 106, 107].

Modafinil, a non-amphetamine wakefulness-promoting medication is now considered the first-line treatment for excessive sleepiness in adults with narcolepsy [108]. It is chemically unrelated to central nervous system stimulants, and although its exact mechanism of action remains unknown, its action may be related to dopaminergic or histaminergic pathways [108].

24. Sleepiness in children

Table 24.6 Pharmacological treatment options for narcolepsy and other hypersomnias of central origin [101–110]

	Stimulants	Modafinil	Sodium oxybate	TCAs	SSRIs
Symptoms — Daytime sleepiness	+ (G)	+ (S)	+ (S)	–	–
Cataplexy	–	–	+ (S)	+ (G)	+ (G)
Hypnagogic hallucinations	–	–	+ (O)	+ (O)	+ (O)
Sleep paralysis	–	–	+ (O)	+ (O)	+ (O)
Disrupted sleep	–	–	+ (S)	–	–
Mode of action	Indirect sympathomimetics, dopamine reuptake inhibitors	Unknown; partial dopamine reuptake inhibitor	Unknown; GABA$_B$ receptor agonist	Block the presynaptic reuptake of catecholamines	Block the presynaptic reuptake of catecholamines (serotonin)
Daily dosage	Methyphenidate 10–30 mg/day Amphetamine 10–30 mg/day	100–400 once daily or in two divided doses	6–9 g divided nightly in two doses	Clomipramine: 3 mg/kg/d (10–200 mg) Imipramine 1.5–5 mg/kg/d (max 100 mg)	Fluoxetine: 10–40 mg/day
Side-effects	Headache, anxiety/irritability, increased BP, appetite suppression, tremor, insomnia, tics	Insomnia, headache, nausea, anxiety, irritability	Sedation, nausea, bad taste, enuresis, night terror, lingering sluggishness, respiratory depression	Nausea, anorexia, dry mouth, urinary retention, tachycardia	Headache, nausea, weight gain, dry mouth
Pediatric issues	Not recommended in pts <3 years (amphetamine) and <6 years (methyphenidate)	Pediatric use not systematically studied	Safety and effectiveness in pts <16 years not established	Safety and efficacy of clomipramine in children younger than 10 years of age have not been established	Safety and effectiveness assessed in children aged 8–18 years with major depressive disorder and 7–18 yrs with OCD

American Academy Sleep Medicine levels of recommendation: S stands for Standard (generally accepted patient-care strategy that reflects a high degree of clinical certainty), G for Guideline (patient-care strategy that reflects a moderate degree of clinical certainty), O for Option (patient-care strategy that reflects uncertain clinical use) [68].
TCAs, tricyclic antidepressants; SSRIs, selective serotonin reuptake inhibitors; BP, blood pressure; OCD, Obsessive–Compulsive Disorder.

Rapid eye movement suppressant medications such as tricyclic antidepressants or serotonin reuptake inhibitors can be added to control cataplexy or hypnagogic hallucinations [103, 106]. Recently, we have demonstrated that the treatment with modafinil and serotonin reuptake inhibitors provided amelioration of hypersomnia and reduced concomitant REM intrusion in wakefulness and sleep in 10 of 12 children with narcolepsy [103].

Sodium oxybate is a γ-aminobutyric acid (GABA) B receptor agonist currently approved by the Food and Drug Administration for the treatment of narcolepsy with cataplexy in patients aged >16 years [108–110]. According to the AASM practice parameters, "sodium oxybate is effective for treatment of cataplexy, daytime sleepiness and disrupted sleep due to narcolepsy and may be effective for treatment of hypnagogic hallucinations and sleep paralysis" [107]. Although the administration of sodium oxybate is associated with a modulation of serotoninergic, dopaminergic, and opioid activity, along with an increase in slow-wave sleep, its pharmacologic action on cataplexy remains unknown [108]. When used for the treatment of narcolepsy, one-half of a therapeutic dose of sodium oxybate is administered at bedtime and repeated 2.5–4.0 h later, providing effective plasma concentrations throughout the night while ensuring that the majority of the drug has been eliminated when the patient awakens in the morning [108]. Even though it is indicated for narcolepsy above 16 years of age, we and others have shown that it can be used safely in the pediatric population.

Conclusion

We have attempted to provide the causes, the measures of assessing EDS, the consequences and the treatment options in a child with sleepiness in the clinic setting. The most common cause of daytime sleepiness in children is insufficient sleep. Narcolepsy and other hypersomnias are uncommon lifelong conditions which are often underrecognized, especially in children, and are associated with significant impairment in quality of life. Several methods have been developed to assess hypersomnia; however, various methodological issues need to be addressed. The genetic basis of individual differences in sleep–wake regulation remains largely unknown. Gene expression using microarray technology for "sleepy genes" may be available in the future [111, 112]. The microarray technology may provide insights into physiological processes and facilitate the identification of novel biological markers for diagnostic, prognostic, and pharmacologic treatments for a number of diseases including those associated with EDS. Even though a number of different drug therapies are available, the treatment options are still supportive and not curative. There is a pressing need for research into future treatment strategies, such as hypocretin replacement regimens which would mostly benefit patients with narcolepsy and other hypersomnias of central origin.

References

1. **Carkadon M A**, **Dement W C**. Normal human sleep: an overview. In: Kryger M H, Roth T, Dement W C, Eds. *Principles and Practice of Sleep Medicine*. Philadelphia, PA: Harcourt Brace Jovanich, Inc., 1989: 3–13.
2. **American Academy of Sleep Medicine**. *International Classification of Sleep Disorders* (2nd Ed). Diagnostic and Coding Manual. Westchester, IL: American Academy of Sleep Medicine, 2005.
3. **Kotagal S**, **Pianosi P**. Sleep disorders in children and adolescents. *BMJ*, 2006; **332**:828–32.
4. **Blunden S**, **Lushington K**, **Lorenzen B**, et al. Are sleep problems under-recognised in general practice? *Arch Dis Child*, 2003; **89**:708–12.
5. **Calamaro C J**, **Mason T B**, **Ratcliffe S J**. Adolescents living the 24/7 lifestyle: effects of caffeine and technology on sleep duration and daytime functioning. *Pediatrics*, 2009; **123**:e1005–10.
6. **Saarenpaa O S**, **Laippala P**, **Koivikko M**. Subjective sleepiness in children. *Fam Pract*, 2000; **17**:129–33.
7. **Gaina A**, **Sekine M**, **Hamanishi S**, et al. Daytime sleepiness and associated factors in Japanese school children. *J Pediatr*, 2007; **151**:518–22.
8. **Gibson E S**, **Powles A C**, **Thabane L**, et al. "Sleepiness" is serious in adolescence: two surveys of 3235 Canadian students. *BMC Public Health*, 2006; **6**:116.
9. **Blunden S**, **Hoban T F**, **Chervin R D**. Sleepiness in children. *Sleep Med Clin*, 2006; **1**:105–18.
10. **Roffwarg H P**, **Muzio J N**, **Dement W C**. Ontogenetic development of the human sleep-dream cycle. *Science*, 1966; **152**:604–19.
11. **Maletzer L J**, **Mindell J A**. Sleep and sleep disorders in children and adolescents. *Psychiatr Clin North Am*, 2006; **29**:1059–76.
12. **Kothare S V**, **Kaleyias J**. The clinical and laboratory assessment of the sleepy child. *Semin Pediatr Neurol*. 2008; **15**:61–69.
13. **Givan D C**. The sleepy child. *Pediatr Clin North Am*, 2004; **51**:15–31.
14. **Kotagal S**. Sleep disorders in childhood. *Neurol Clin*, 2003; **21**:961–81.
15. **Ivanenko A**, **McLaughlin Crabtree V**, et al. Sleep in children with psychiatric disorders. *Pediatr Clin North Am*, 2004; **51**:51–68.
16. **Liu X**, **Buysse D**, **Gentzler A**, et al. Insomnia and hypersomnia associated with depressive phenomenology and comorbidity in childhood depression. *Sleep*, 2007; **30**:83–90.
17. **LeBourgeois M K**, **Avis K**, **Mixon M**, et al. Snoring, sleep quality, and sleepiness across attention-deficit/hyperactivity disorder subtypes. *Sleep*, 2004; **27**:520–25.
18. **Cortese S**, **Konofal E**, **Yateman N**, et al. Sleep and alertness in children with attention-deficit/hyperactivity disorder: a systematic review of the literature. *Sleep*, 2006; **29**:504–11.
19. **Caroli M**, **Argentieri L**, **Cardone M**, et al. Role of television in childhood obesity prevention. *Int J Obes Relat Metab Disord*, 2004; **28**(Suppl 3):S104–08.
20. **Adad V C**, **Guilleminault C**. Sleep and psychiatry. *Dialog Clin Neurosci*, 2005; **7**:291–303.

21. **Owens J A**, **Dalzell V**. Use of the "BEARS" sleep screening tool in a pediatric residents' continuity clinic: a pilot study. *Sleep Med*, 2005; **6**:63–69.

22. **Flint J**, **Kothare SV**, **Zihlif M**, *et al*. Association between inadequate sleep and insulin resistance in obese children. *J Pediatr*, 2007; **150**:364–69.

23. **Martin S K**, **Eastman C I**. Sleep logs of young adults with self-selected sleep times predict the dim light melatonin onset. *Chronobiol Int*, 2002; **19**:695–707.

24. **Westermeyer J**, **Sutherland R J**, **Freerks M**, *et al*. Reliability of sleep log data versus actigraphy in veterans with sleep disturbance and PTSD. *Anxiety Disord*, 2007; **2**:966–75.

25. **Bradshaw D A**, **Yanagi M A**, **Pak E S**, *et al*. Nightly sleep duration in the 2-week period preceding multiple sleep latency testing. *Clin Sleep Med*, 2007; **15**:613–19.

26. **Hoddes E**, **Zarcone V**, **Smythe H**, *et al*. Quantification of sleepiness: a new approach. *Psychophysiology*, 1973; **10**:431–36.

27. **Johns M W**. A new method for measuring daytime sleepiness: the Epworth Sleepiness Scale. *Sleep*, 1991; **14**:540–45.

28. **Drake C**, **Nickel C**, **Burduvali E**, *et al*. The paediatric daytime sleepiness scale (PDSS): sleep habits and school outcomes in middle-school children. *Sleep*, 2003; **26**:455–58.

29. **Perez-Chada D**, **Perez-Lloret S**, **Videla A J**, *et al*. Sleep disordered breathing and daytime sleepiness are associated with poor academic performance in teenagers. A study using the pediatric daytime sleepiness scale (PDSS). *Sleep*, 2007; **30**:1698–703.

30. **Ivanenko A**, **Crabtree V M**, **O'Brien L M**, *et al*. Sleep complaints and psychiatric symptoms in children evaluated at a pediatric mental health clinic. *J Clin Sleep Med*, 2006; **2**:42–48.

31. **Chervin R D**, **Hedger K**, **Dillon J E**, *et al*. Pediatric sleep questionnaire (PSQ): validity and reliability of scales for sleep-disordered breathing, snoring, sleepiness, and behavioral problems. *Sleep Med*, 2000; **1**:21–32.

32. **Carskadon M A**, **Dement W C**. Daytime sleepiness: quantification of a behavioral state. *Neurosci Biobehav Rev*, 1987; **11**:307–11.

33. **Spilsbury J C**, **Drotar D**, **Rosen C L**, *et al*. The Cleveland adolescent sleepiness questionnaire: a new measure to assess excessive daytime sleepiness in adolescents. *J Clin Sleep Med*, 2007; **3**:603–12.

34. **Morgenthaler T**, **Alessi C**, **Friedman L**, *et al*. Standards of Practice Committee of the American Academy of Sleep Medicine. Practice parameters for the use of actigraphy in the assessment of sleep and sleep disorders: an update for 2007. *Sleep*, 2007; **30**:519–29.

35. **Ancoli-Israel S**, **Cole R**, **Alessi C**, *et al*. The role of actigraphy in the study of sleep and circadian rhythms. *Sleep*, 2003; **26**:342–92.

36. **Ancoli-Israel S**. Actigraphy. In: Kryger M H, Roth T, Dement W C Eds. *Principles and Practice of Sleep Medicine*. Philadelphia, PA: Saunders, 2000: 1295–301.

37. **Kotagal S**, **Goulding P M**. The laboratory assessment of daytime sleepiness in childhood. *Clin Neurophysiol*, 1996; **13**:208–18.

38. **Sadeh A**, **Hauri P J**, **Kripke D**, *et al*. The role of actigraphy in the evaluation of sleep disorders. *Sleep*, 1995; **18**:288–302.

39. **Acebo C**, **Sadeh A**, **Seifer R**, *et al*. Sleep/wake patterns derived from activity monitoring and maternal report for healthy 1- to 5-year-old children. *Sleep*, 2005; **28**:1568–77.

40. **Wiggs L**, **Stores G**. Sleep patterns and sleep disorders in children with autistic spectrum disorders: insights using parental report and actigraphy. *Dev Med Child Neurol*, 2004; **46**:372–80.

41. **Applebee G A**, **Bingham P M**, **Attarian H P**. Using actigraphy to evaluate parental report of abnormal sleep patterns in children. *Clin Pediatr (Phil)*, 2009; **48**:558–60.

42. **Ohinata J**, **Suzuki N**, **Araki A**, *et al*. Actigraphic assessment of sleep disorders in children with chronic fatigue syndrome. *Brain Dev*, 2008; **30**:329–33.

43. **Johnson N L**, **Kirchner H L**, **Rosen C L**, *et al*. Sleep estimation using wrist actigraphy in adolescents with and without sleep disordered breathing: a comparison of three data modes. *Sleep*, 2007; **30**:899–905.

44. **Sitnick S L**, **Goodlin-Jones B L**, **Anders T F**. The use of actigraphy to study sleep disorders in preschoolers: some concerns about detection of nighttime awakenings. *Sleep*, 2008; **31**:395–401.

45. **Littner M R**, **Kushida C**, **Wise M**, *et al*. Standards of Practice Committee of the American Academy of Sleep Medicine Practice parameters for clinical use of the multiple sleep latency test and the maintenance of wakefulness test. *Sleep*, 2005; **28**:113–21.

46. **Arand D**, **Bonnet M**, **Hurwitz T**, *et al*. The clinical use of the MSLT and MWT. *Sleep*, 2005; **28**:123–44.

47. **Gozal D**, **Wang M**, **Pope D W**. Objective sleepiness measures in pediatric obstructive sleep apnea. *Pediatrics*, 2001; **108**:693–97.

48. **Palm L**, **Persson E**, **Elmquist D**, *et al*. Sleep and wakefulness in normal preadolescents. *Sleep*, 1989; **12**:299–308.

49. **Fallone G**, **Owens J A**, **Deane J**. Sleepiness in children and adolescents: clinical implications. *Sleep Med Rev*, 2002; **6**:287–306.

50. **Singh M**, **Drake C L**, **Roth T**. The prevalence of multiple sleep-onset REM periods in a population-based sample. *Sleep*, 2006; **29**:890–95.

51. **Aldrich M S**, **Chervin R D**, **Malow B A**. Value of the multiple sleep latency test (MSLT) for the diagnosis of narcolepsy. *Sleep*, 1997; **20**:620–29.

52. **Wise M S**. Objective measures of sleepiness and wakefulness: application to the real world? *J Clin Neurophysiol*, 2006; **23**:39–49.

53. **Zwyghuizen-Doorenbos A**, **Roehrs T**, **Schaefer M**, et al. Test–retest reliability of the MSLT. *Sleep*, 1988; **11**:562–65.

54. **Drake C L**, **Rice M F**, **Roehrs T A**, et al. Scoring reliability of the multiple sleep latency test in a clinical population. *Sleep*, 2000; **23**:911–13.

55. **Mitler M M**, **Doghramji K**, **Shapiro C**. The Maintenance of Wakefulness Test. Normative data by age. *J Psychosom Res*, 2000; **49**:363–65.

56. **Kushida C A**, **Littner M R**, **Morgenthaler T**, et al. Practice parameters for the indications for polysomnography and related procedures: an update for 2005. *Sleep*, 2005; **28**:499–521.

57. **Chesson A L Jr**, **Ferber R A**, **Fry J M**, et al. The indications for polysomnography and related procedures. A review. *Sleep*, 1997; **20**:423–87.

58. **Montgomery-Downs H E**, **O'Brien L M**, **Gulliver T E**, et al. Polysomnographic characteristics in normal preschool and early school-aged children. *Pediatrics*, 2006; **117**:741–53.

59. **American Academy of Pediatrics, Section on Pediatric Pulmonology, Subcommittee on Obstructive Sleep Apnea Syndrome**. Clinical practice guideline: diagnosis and management of childhood obstructive sleep apnea syndrome. *Pediatrics*, 2002; **109**:704–12.

60. **American Thoracic Society**. Cardiorespiratory sleep studies in children: establishment of normative data and polysomnographic predictors of morbidity. *Am J Respir Crit Care Med*, 1999; **160**:1381–87.

61. **Zaremba E K**, **Barkey M E**, **Mesa C**, et al. Making polysomnography more "child friendly": a family-centered care approach. *J Clin Sleep Med*, 2005; **1**:189–98.

62. **McLaren J W**, **Hauri P J**, **Lin S C**, et al. Pupillometry in clinically sleepy patients. *Sleep Med*, 2002; **3**:347–52.

63. **Heier M S**, **Evsiukova T**, **Vilming S**, et al. CSF hypocretin-1 levels and clinical profiles in narcolepsy and idiopathic CNS hypersomnia in Norway. *Sleep*, 2007; **30**:969–73.

64. **Nishino S**, **Ripley B**, **Overeem S**, et al. Hypocretin (orexin) deficiency in human narcolepsy. *Lancet*, 2000; **355**:39–40.

65. **Nishino S**, **Ripley B**, **Overeem S**, et al. Low cerebrospinal fluid hypocretin (orexin) and energy homeostasis in human narcolepsy. *Ann Neurol*, 2001; **50**:381–88.

66. **Mignot E**, **Young T**, **Lin L**, **Finn L**. Nocturnal sleep and daytime sleepiness in normal subjects with HLA-DQB1*0602. *Sleep*, 1999; **22**:347–52.

67. **Alloway C E**, **Ogilvie R D**, **Shapiro C M**. EEG spectral analysis of the sleep-onset period in narcoleptics and normal sleepers. *Sleep*, 1999; **22**:191–203.

68. **Greneche J**, **Krieger J**, **Erhardt C**, et al. EEG spectral power and sleepiness during 24 h of sustained wakefulness in patients with obstructive sleep apnea syndrome. *Clin Neurophysiol*, 2008; **119**:418–28.

69. **Sangal R B**, **Sangal J M**, **Balisle C**. Visual P300 latency predicts treatment response in patients with narcolepsy. *Clin Neurophysiol*, 1999; **110**:1041–47.

70. **Resta O**, **Pannacciulli N**, **Di Gioia G**, et al. High prevalence of previously unknown subclinical hypothyroidism in obese patients referred to a sleep clinic for sleep disordered breathing. *Nutr Metab Cardiovasc Dis*, 2004; **14**:248–53.

71. **Misiolek M**, **Marek B**, **Namyslowski G**, et al. Sleep apnea syndrome and snoring in patients with hypothyroidism with relation to overweight. *Physiol Pharmacol*, 2007; **58**(Suppl 1):S77–85.

72. **Manni R**, **Politini L**, **Nobili L**, et al. Hypersomnia in the Prader Willi syndrome: clinical–electro-physiological features and underlying factors. *Clin Neurophysiol*, 2001; **112**:800–05.

73. **Ciafaloni E**, **Mignot E**, **Sansone V**, et al. The hypocretin neurotransmission system in myotonic dystrophy type 1. *Neurology*, 2008; **70**:226–30.

74. **Smit L S**, **Lammers G J**, **Catsman-Berrevoets C E**. Cataplexy leading to the diagnosis of Niemann–Pick disease type C. *Pediatr Neurol*, 2006; **35**:82–84.

75. **Kjaer T W**, **Law I**, **Wiltschiotz G**, et al. Regional cerebral blood flow during light sleep – a $H_2(^{15})O$-PET study. *J Sleep Res*, 2002; **11**:201–07.

76. **Touchette E**, **Petit D**, **Segui JR**, et al. Association between sleep duration patterns and behavioral/cognitive functioning at school entry. *Sleep*, 2007; **30**:1213–19.

77. **Dahl R E**. The impact of inadequate sleep on children's daytime cognitive function. *Semin Pediatr Neurol*, 1996; **3**:44–50.

78. **Lam P, Hiscock H, Wake M.** Outcomes of infant sleep problems: a longitudinal study of sleep, behavior and maternal well-being. *Pediatrics*, 2003; **111**:e203–07.

79. **Gottleib D J, Chase C, Vezina R M,** *et al.* Sleep disordered breathing symptoms are associated with poorer cognitive function in 5-year old children. *J Pediatric*, 2004; **145**:458–64.

80. **Wake M, Morton-Allen E, Poulakis Z,** *et al.* Prevalence, stability and outcomes of cry-fuss and sleep problems in the first two years of life: prospective community based study. *Pediatrics*, 2006; **117**:836–42.

81. **Hiscock H, Canterford L, Ukoumunne OC,** *et al.* Adverse association of sleep problems in Australian pre-schoolers: national population study. *Pediatrics*, 2007; **119**:836–42.

82. **Smedje H, Broman J E, Hetta J.** Association between disturbed sleep and behavioral difficulties in 635 children aged six to eight years: a study based on parent's perception. *Eur J Child Adolesc Psychiatry*, 2001; **10**:1–9.

83. **Chugh D K, Weaver T E, Dinges D F.** Neurobehavioral consequences of arousals. *Sleep*, 1996; **19**:S198–201.

84. **Jones K, Harrison Y.** Frontal lobe function, sleep loss, and fragmented sleep. *Sleep Med Rev*, 2001; **5**:463–75.

85. **Goel N, Rao H, Durmer J S,** *et al.* Neurocognitive consequences of sleep deprivation. *Sem Neurol*, 2009; **29**:320–34.

86. **Thomas M, Sing H, Belenky G,** *et al.* Neural basis of alertness and cognitive performance impairments during sleepiness. I. Effect of 24 h of sleep deprivation on waking human regional brain activity. *J Sleep Res*, 2000; **9**:335–52.

87. **Thomas M, Sing H, Belenky G,** *et al.* Neural basis of alertness and cognitive performance impairment during sleepiness. II. Effect of 48 and 72 h of sleep deprivation on waking human regional brain activity. *Thalamus Relat Syst*, 2003; **2**:199–229.

88. **Gozal D.** Obstructive sleep apnea in children: implications for the developing central nervous system. *Sem Pediatr Neurol*, 2008; **15**:100–06.

89. **Gozal D, Kheirandish-Gozal L.** Neurocognitive and behavioral morbidity in children with sleep disorders. *Curr Opin Pulm Med*, 2007; **13**:505–09.

90. **Gozal E, Gozal D, Pierce WM,** *et al.* Proteomic analysis of CA1 and CA3 regions of rat hippocampus and differential susceptibility to intermittent hypoxia. *J Neurochem*, 2002; **83**:331–45.

91. **Row B W, Liu R, Xu W,** *et al.* Intermittent hypoxia is associated with oxidant stress and spatial learning deficits in the rat. *Am J Respir Crit Care Med*, 2003; **167**:1548–53.

92. **Beebe D W.** Neurobehavioral morbidity associated with disordered breathing during sleep in children: a comprehensive review. *Sleep*, 2006; **29**:1115–34.

93. **Carskadon M A, Harvey K, Dement W C.** Sleep loss in young adolescents. *Sleep*, 1981; **4**:299–312.

94. **Carskadon M A, Harvey K, Dement W C.** Acute restriction of nocturnal sleep in children. *Percept Motor Skills*, 1981; **53**:103–12.

95. **Eliasson A, Eliasson A, King J,** *et al.* Association of sleep and academic performance. *Sleep Breath*, 2002; **6**:45–48.

96. **Ednick M, Cohen A P, McPhail G L,** *et al.* A review of the effects of sleep during the first year of life on cognition, psychomotor, and temperament development. *Sleep*, 2009; **32**:1149–58.

97. **Maquet P, Smith C, Stickgold R.** Introduction. In: Maquet P, Smith C, Stickgold R, Eds. *Sleep and Brain Plasticity*. New York, NY: Oxford University Press, 2003: 1–13.

98. **Penn A A, Shatz C J.** Principles of endogenous and sensory activity dependent brain development. The visual system. In: Lagercrantz H, Hanson M, Evrard P, Eds. *The Newborn Brain: Neuroscience and Clinical Applications*. New York, NY: Cambridge University Press, 2002: 204–25.

99. **Timofeev I, Contreras D, Steriade M.** Synaptic responsiveness of cortical and thalamic neurons during various phases of slow sleep oscillation in cat. *J Physiol*, 1996; **494**:265–78.

100. **Bonnet M H, Arand D L.** Performance and cardiovascular measures in normal adults with extreme MSLT scores and subjective sleepiness levels. *Sleep*, 2005; **28**:685–93.

101. **Kothare S V, Kaleyias J.** Narcolepsy and other hypersomnias in children. *Curr Opin Pediatr*, 2008; **20**:666–75.

102. **Morgenthaler T I, Kapur V K, Brown T,** *et al.* Standards of Practice Committee of the American Academy of Sleep Medicine. Practice parameters for the treatment of narcolepsy and other hypersomnias of central origin. *Sleep*, 2007; **30**:1705–11.

103. **Vendrame M, Havaligi N, Matadeen-Ali C,** *et al.* Narcolepsy in children: a single-center clinical experience. *Pediatr Neurol*, 2008; **38**:314–20.

104. **Rogers A E, Aldrich M S, Lin X.** A comparison of three different sleep schedules for reducing daytime sleepiness in narcolepsy. *Sleep*, 2001; **24**:385–91.

105. **Wise M S, Arand D L, Auger R,** *et al.* American Academy of Sleep Medicine. Treatment of narcolepsy and other hypersomnias of central origin. *Sleep*, 2007; **30**:1712–27.

106. **Wise M S**, **Lynch J**. Narcolepsy in children. *Semin Pediatr Neurol*, 2001; **8**:198–206.

107. **Bassetti C**, **Aldrich M S**. Idiopathic hypersomnia. A series of 42 patients. *Brain*, 1997; **120**:1423–35.

108. **Thorpy M**. Therapeutic advances in narcolepsy. *Sleep Med*, 2007; **8**:427–40.

109. **Robinson D M**, **Keating G M**. Sodium oxybate: a review of its use in the management of narcolepsy. *CNS Drugs*, 2007; **21**:337–54.

110. **Murali H**, **Kotagal S**. Off-label treatment of severe childhood narcolepsy–cataplexy with sodium oxybate. *Sleep*, 2006; **29**:1025–29.

111. **Gottlieb D J**, **O'Connor G T**, **Wilk J B**. Genome-wide association of sleep and circadian phenotypes. *BMC Med Genet*, 2007; **8** (Suppl 1):S9.

112. **Viola A U**, **Archer S N**, **James L M**, *et al.* PER3 polymorphism predicts sleep structure and waking performance. *Curr Biol*, 2007; **17**:613–18.

Section 3: Medical, Psychiatric and Neurological Causes of Sleepiness

Section 3 Chapter 25

Medical, Psychiatric and Neurological Causes of Sleepiness

Depression and sleepiness: a chronobiological approach

Sarah Laxhmi Chellappa and Christian Cajochen

Introduction

Excessive Daytime Sleepiness (EDS) consists of the propensity to fall asleep despite volitional attempts to remain vigilant. Major underlying reasons for EDS encompass numerous sleep disorders, such as obstructive sleep apnea (OSA), narcolepsy, and psychiatric disorders, most importantly depression. Depressive states are associated with comorbid insomnia in approximately 80% of cases, which are related or unrelated to EDS [1]. Depressed patients exhibit a plethora of complaints interconnected to daytime energy levels. However, despite the fact that depressed subjects often exhibit sleep complaints, patients do not necessarily have an increased likelihood of falling asleep during the day, but rather experience a subjective state of sleepiness [1]. This difference in sleepiness states sharply contrasts with what is observed in clinical conditions, such as in narcolepsy, whereby subjects experience EDS as short and recurrent periods of sleep in daytime, regardless of the prior amount or quality of night sleep.

Within the framework of psychiatric disorders, there is consistent evidence in favor of a relationship between moderate to severe depression and EDS [2]. Therefore, it is of significant clinical relevance to unearth how EDS and depression are linked, and knowledge on the inter-relation between these conditions may assist in the management of depression.

In order to achieve a holistic comprehension of EDS and depression, one should keep in mind that circadian rhythms play a pivotal role in this association. Indeed, depression is intertwined with biological rhythms on a wide array of dimensions [3]. This rhythmicity can manifest as an intra-episodic expression, with diurnal variation of mood and early morning awakening, and/or as an inter-episodic expression, characterized by clinical depression or its remittance after therapeutic management. Disorders of the human circadian system per se can result in circadian misalignment, leading to sleep disturbances (namely, insomnia and/or EDS), reduced attention and impaired daytime alertness, lack of energy, low performance and negative mood. Major depression, bipolar depression and seasonal affective disorder are defined as being both episodic and recurrent, thus possibly reflecting a chronobiological disorder [4].

The application of chronobiological concepts in the treatment of depressive disorder has led to effective therapeutic strategies, like bright light therapy and sleep deprivation [3]. The circadian system has been implicated in pharmacological treatment mechanisms, such as lithium therapy for bipolar depression. Lithium can modify the phase angle between temperature and rest–activity cycle and lengthens the period of circadian rhythms, by increasing the period of firing rate rhythms of SCN neurons in concentration-dependent manner [5], which suggests that stabilization of circadian rhythms is an effective mood-stabilizing treatment.

In this chapter, we highlight studies on EDS and depression within the framework of human sleep and chronobiology, and we provide an outlook of chronobiological underpinnings of this relationship in order to provide insights and candidates for chronobiological management.

Sleepiness: Causes, Consequences and Treatment, ed. Michael J. Thorpy and Michel Billiard. Published by Cambridge University Press. © Cambridge University Press 2011.

Clinical findings

Depression and excessive daytime sleepiness

Excessive daytime sleepiness is a frequent complaint in medical practice, with several limitations on daily activities, and is viewed as a cardinal sign of disturbed sleep directly linked to depression [2]. In a recent study conducted with a large-scale American population sample, 8.7% had EDS [6], which was strikingly associated with depressive symptoms. Furthermore, we observed a significant association between EDS and suicidal ideation in depressed patients, presumably due to the fact that patients with severe depressive disorder rank daytime sleepiness in line with other major depressive symptoms [7, 8].

Despite the significant evidence linking EDS to depression, the pathophysiological mechanisms underlying this relationship remain uncertain. One important line of research builds upon findings in which approximately 20% of depressed patients exhibit undiagnosed sleep-disordered breathing, mostly obstructive sleep apnea [9]. This goes in line with the link between metabolic syndrome, obesity and diabetes or insulin resistance, together with elevated inflammatory markers, to both sleep-disordered breathing and depression [10]. Given that several hormonal and inflammatory variables undergo a clear circadian-driven modulation, the next logical question arises as to whether changes in circadian rhythms can underlie the pathophysiology of depression. In the next section, we address how depression can be underpinned by the circadian clock.

Depression, sleepiness and circadian rhythms

Diurnal variations of mood and sleep disturbances pertain to the core of classical symptoms that link depression to the circadian system [11], with substantial improvement of mood in the evening, in contrast to the morning after sleep. Shortening of REM sleep latency and an abnormal distribution of REM sleep throughout the night may typically occur in depression [12]. Given that REM sleep is under strong circadian control, these sleep alterations may reflect disturbances in the circadian system. Another illustration as to how daytime sleepiness in depressed patients can result from dampened circadian rhythm of sleep

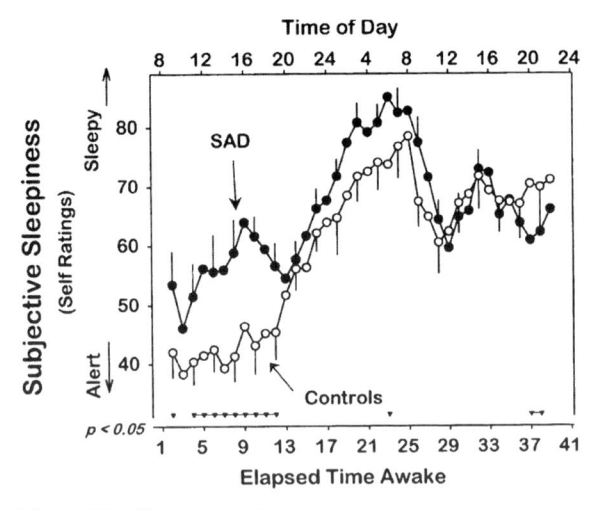

Figure 25.1 Time course of subjective sleepiness ratings as assessed on a visual analogue scale (VAS) during extended wakefulness in seasonal affective disorder (SAD) patients ($n = 8$, filled symbols) and control subjects ($n = 9$, open symbols). Hourly mean values ±1 SEM. Triangles near the abscissa indicate significant differences between SAD and control subjects ($p < .05$, least significant difference test). Higher numbers indicate greater sleepiness (with permission from Cajochen et al., 2000 [14]).

propensity occurs in seasonal affective disorder (SAD). In SAD, the alteration between the external light–dark cycle (i.e. photoperiod) and circadian rhythms may elicit depression. This usually leads the vast majority of SAD patients to become depressed during winter because of the later dawn, which in turn leads their circadian rhythms to delay with respect to both clock time and to the sleep–wake cycle [13]. Subjective sleepiness appears to differ in SAD patients in comparison to healthy controls, such that the former are sleepier under stringent laboratory conditions, as illustrated in Figure 25.1 [14].

Abnormalities in the circadian rhythm are observed in non-seasonal depressed patients, with changes, for instance, in the circadian phase and amplitude of core body temperature [11]. Although the results may be conflicting, chronobiological studies in which sleep timing and/or total amount of sleep were rescheduled in patients provide evidence for the implication of circadian rhythms in depression [15]. However, it is still unclear whether these observations represent functional changes of the circadian system itself or are due to the influence of other factors downstream. Major depression has been consistently associated with hyperactivity of the hypothalamus–pituitary–adrenal (HPA) axis, which, in turn, reflects a stress response and/or abnormality of cortisol rhythm [16]. Usually, the acrophase of the cortisol rhythm occurs early in the morning, while the nadir is at night, shortly after initiating sleep [17]. However, in depressive states, HPA hyperactivity leads to sustained high levels of cortisol resulting in insomnia.

Considering the substantial body of evidence in favor of disruption of circadian rhythms as a very likely candidate for depression, a new question arises: How can changes in circadian rhythms result in EDS in depression?

From a conceptual point of view, EDS can be considered to result from the biological need for sleep as characterized by a complex interaction between circadian and homeostatic processes. Briefly, the master pacemaker driving circadian rhythms, the suprachiasmatic nuclei (SCN), is synchronized to the external light–dark cycle through retinal light input (light being the main synchronizer or "zeitgeber") [18]. A specialized non-visual retinohypothalamic tract provides direct neuronal connection to the SCN from novel photoreceptors in the retinal ganglion cells that measure illuminance [19]. Although the SCN is the so-called master clock, circadian oscillators have been found in practically every cell; therefore, the SCN would act in a manner to organize an internal temporal conjunction of several peripheral oscillators. The homeostatic component is dependent on the duration of prior wakefulness, and is dissipated during sleep, reinitiating its build-up during the following wake period [20]. The two-process model of sleep regulation has unified these two components in order to understand the timing and architecture of sleep [21]. This model can also be utilized to describe possible disturbances in either process during depression. The clinical sleep disturbance with early morning awakening could arise from an impaired build-up of S during waking (diminished sleep pressure), or an earlier timing of process C. Another possible hypothesis builds-up from the Process S-Deficiency model, whereby a deficient build-up of process S (i.e. sleep need) can occur in depression, with process C remaining unaffected [20].

Two important protocols can dissect out the relative contributions of circadian and sleep homeostatic processes in humans: constant routine and forced desynchrony protocols. In the former, the phase and amplitude of circadian rhythms can be unravelled without masking effects of motor activity, meals, and lighting conditions. In the last, participants live on artificially very long or very short days, so that the circadian system is no longer entrained to the imposed sleep–wake cycle. The desynchronized subjects sleep at different circadian phases of the entire 24-h cycle, and subsequent analyses can differentiate the contribution of the sleep homeostat or the biological clock to a given variable. Both factors are deemed to substantially contribute in subjective measures as mood, sleepiness, and neurobehavioral performance [14, 22]. However, few studies have used these techniques to unmask the relative contribution of the circadian clock in depression. Table 25.1 provides an overview of studies using constant routine and forced desynchrony protocols in depressed patients.

Pathophysiology of depression and sleepiness

The neurobiological substrates of sleepiness are fairly unknown. Sleepiness may reflect the waning of processes maintaining wakefulness and/or may result from distinct neural systems acting to promote sleep. According to the "flip-flop" model of sleep and wakefulness (depicted in Figure 25.2) [23], monoaminergic nuclei, including locus coeruleus, serotonergic dorsal, median raphe nuclei and histaminergic tuberomammillary neurons, promote wakefulness by direct excitatory effects on the cortex and by inhibition of sleep-promoting neurons of the ventrolateral preoptic nucleus. During sleep, the last inhibits monoaminergic-mediated arousal regions through GABAergic and galaninergic projections. Orexin-containing neurons seem to play an important stabilizing role in the proposed "flip-flop" mechanism. On the other hand, the accumulation of a sleep-promoting substance that enhances the activity of sleep-promoting cells and reduces the activity of wake-promoting neurons may be a potential mechanism for homeostatic sleep regulation. However, it remains to be determined how these and other brain structures act and interact to generate EDS in various disorders.

Some of the emerging concepts of sleepiness neurophysiology are consistent with the cholinergic–aminergic imbalance hypothesis of mood disorders, which proposes that depression may be linked with an increased ratio of central cholinergic to aminergic neurotransmission [24]. Accordingly, sleep abnormalities associated with depression, particularly insomnia associated or not to EDS, may reflect a relative predominance of cholinergic activity in the lateral dorsal

3. Medical, Psychiatric and Neurological Causes

Table 25.1 Constant routine (CR) and forced desynchrony (FD) protocols with depressed patients (with permission from Chellappa et al., [40])

	Type of study	Subjects	Depression diagnosis	Protocol procedure	Circadian marker	Phase/amplitude/ phase angle changes in depressed
Dahl et al. [65]	CR	6 SD[1] 6 CT[2]	SAD	27h CR	DLMO[3] CBT[4]	DLMO & CBT phase-delay
Buysse et al. [66]	CR	26 UP[5] 17 CT	DSM-IV unipolar depression	36h CR	CBT Melatonin Cortisol	No differences
Wirz-Justice et al. [67]	CR	11 SD 8 CT	SAD	40h CR	CBT Melatonin	No differences
Avery et al. [68]	CR	6 SD 6 CT	SAD	27h CR	CBT Cortisol	CBT & Cortisol phase-delay
Koorengevel et al. [69]	FD	7 SD 7 CT	SAD	120-h FD (six 20-h days)	CBT Melatonin	CBT amplitude ↓
Koorengevel et al. [22]	FD	7 SD 7 CT	SAD	120-h FD (six 20-h days)	CBT Melatonin	CBT amplitude ↓

[1] Seasonal depressed.
[2] Control subjects.
[3] Dim light melatonin onset.
[4] Core body temperature.
[5] Uipolar Depression.

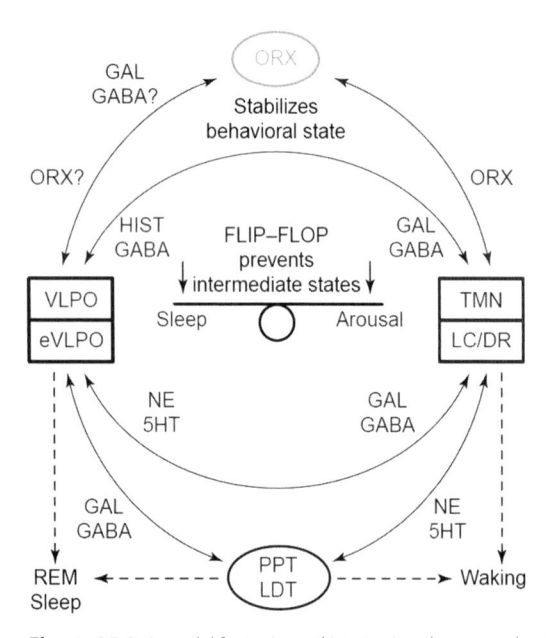

Figure 25.2 A model for reciprocal interactions between sleep- and wake-promoting brain regions. Abbreviations: DR, dorsal raphe nucleus; HIST, histamine; LC, locus coeruleus; LDT, laterodorsal tegmental nuclei; PPT, pedunculopontine tegmental nuclei; REM, rapid eye movement; TMN, tuberomammillary nucleus; VLPO, ventrolateral preoptic nucleus (modified from Saper et al., 2003 [23]).

tegmental and pedunculopontine tegmental regions, in relation to noradrenergic and serotonergic activity in the locus coeruleus, and the dorsal raphe nucleus, respectively. This imbalance can be targeted by antidepressant medications which presumably reduce REM sleep either by their anticholinergic properties or by enhancing aminergic neurotransmission.

Recent imaging studies have shed new light on the neurobiological basis of depression. The increased magnitude of ultradian (i.e. within-day) mood variability in depressed patients can be linked to regional cerebral metabolic changes in the evening relative to morning and may reflect functional variations in the ventral and dorsal emotion neural systems [25]. Similarly, diurnal mood variations can be underpinned by differential patterns of diurnal changes in regional cerebral metabolic rate of glucose (rCMRglc) in depressed subjects. rCMRglc morning-to-evening variations fluctuate with respect to the wake-promoting brain systems, such that in healthy individuals, relative rCMRglc increases during evening as compared to morning in wake-promoting brainstem and hypothalamic regions [26]. This pattern can be triggered by the circadian timing system to promote wake despite increasing homeostatic sleep pressure.

Given that circadian rhythms can be blunted in depression, rCMRglc diurnal variations in brainstem and hypothalamic areas may be, therefore, attenuated in depressed individuals.

Could the physiological underpinnings of sleepiness in depression involve genetic control? In other words, is it likely that the molecular clock machinery be implicated with depression, and its comorbid sleepiness? If so, how and to what extent is its role? In the following section, we will address some novel ideas that are going on in this field.

Genetics on depression and sleepiness

Epidemiologic studies of individuals aged as young as 15 years to 100 years show a significant association between increased daytime sleepiness and diagnostic depression [6]. Furthermore, longitudinal investigations show evidence that sleep disturbances, most commonly insomnia and hypersomnia, predict later depression/depressive symptomatology [2]. Both daytime sleepiness and depressive symptomatology are moderately heritable, with heritability coefficients on the order of 38–48% for daytime sleepiness [27] and 16–55% for depressive symptoms. Despite the fact that not all studies yielded a strong association between sleepiness and depressed mood, a substantial body of evidence suggests at least a modest association between the two phenomena, with significant heritability for both phenotypes.

The accepted model for the molecular machinery that generates circadian rhythms involves a number of clock genes and their products, which provide the mechanism for the regulation of circadian and seasonal rhythms, with allelic variants influencing individual rhythms at a behavioral and cellular level [28]. Deregulation of the circadian system is suspected to be involved in the pathogenesis of depression, and several candidate genes in the circadian rhythm pathway, namely *BmaL1*, *Timeless*, and *Period3*, seem to be associated with specific depressive states, such as bipolar disorder [29]. Genotypic variants of clock genes could then influence core features of mood disorders. The Period (*PER*) gene family is a central component of the biological clock. The coding region of *PER3* gene contains a variable-number tandem-repeat (VNTR) polymorphism in which a motif encoding 18 amino acids is repeated either four (*PER3*[4]) or five (*PER3*[5]) times [30]. Studies investigating circadian phenotypes showed that in healthy subjects, *PER3*[5] was associated with increased slow-wave activity in non-rapid eye movement (non-REM) sleep and theta and alpha activity during wakefulness and REM sleep, with greater decrement of cognitive performance in response to sleep loss [31]. These findings have lead to the assumption that variants of *PER3* can act as potentially useful endophenotypes of bipolar disorder like other components of the molecular clock, as indicated by haplotypes in *PER3* that are significantly associated with bipolar disorder via single-gene permutation tests [32].

Furthermore, genetic sleep disorders, including familial advanced sleep phase syndrome (FASPS), in which individuals have shifted circadian rhythms where they fall asleep and wake up earlier than needed, or delayed sleep phase syndrome (DSPS), which has the opposite phenotype, are both highly comorbid with depression [33]. Interestingly, even individuals genetically predisposed towards "eveningness" (preference for the evening) versus "morningness" (preference for the morning) are more susceptible to develop depression [34]. Genetic variations in the circadian genes appear to be associated with these sleep disorders and diurnal preference measures including an association between certain variants of clock genes, such as *Per2* with FASPS; *Per3*, and *Clock* with DSPS; and *Per1*, *Per2*, *Per3* and *Clock* with diurnal preference [29].

Although the physiological mechanisms that underlie depression and circadian rhythms remain uncertain, one assumption postulates that the influence of the molecular clock on certain neurotransmitters and their receptors might play a key role in depression. This can be illustrated by neurotransmitters implicated in mood regulation, namely serotonin, norepinephrine and dopamine, which all appear to exhibit a clear circadian rhythmicity in their levels, release, and synthesis-related enzymes [35]. For instance, associations have been reported between depressive symptoms and serotonin, which is known to play an important part in sleep regulation, particularly prefrontal cortical serotonin. The key associations between depressive symptomatology and serotonin include variations in the serotonin receptor 2a gene (*5-HTR2A*), in the tryptophan hydroxylase gene (*TPH*) responsible for serotonin synthesis, in the vesicular monoamine transporter 2 gene (*VMAT2*) responsible for serotonin transport, and in the monoamine oxidase A gene (*MAO-A*) responsible for serotonin degradation [35]. Taken together, these inter-relationships have been conceptualized in a dual model whereby circadian rhythms and serotonin [36] together are involved in a system vulnerable to depression – through genetic, hormonal, and light exposure factors.

Furthermore, expression and activity of several receptors that bind these neurotransmitters also undergo circadian rhythmicity, which suggests that the entire synaptic circuitry might be under circadian control [37]. Part of this modulation seems to occur through connections between the SCN and other brain regions, as in the case of the indirect projection from the SCN to the locus coeruleus, which regulates the circadian rhythm in noradrenergic neuronal activity [38]. Taken together, these aspects point towards a strong association between mood regulation and a functioning circadian clock. Given that mood and sleep/wake regulation mutually impact upon each other, it could be speculated that deregulation of the circadian rhythmicity at the molecular level might have clear repercussions on depression and comorbid excessive daytime sleepiness.

Diagnosis of depression and excessive daytime sleepiness

Clinical rating scales measuring depression often inquire about fatigue and tiredness. Instruments probing on such phenomena include the Schedule for Affective Disorders and Schizophrenia (tiredness), Beck Depression Inventory (tiredness), Montgomery–Åsberg Rating Scale for Depression (lassitude), Hamilton Rating Scale for Depression (component of somatic symptoms), the Depression Scale of the Symptom Check-List 90 (low energy), Centres for Epidemiologic Studies Depression Scale (CES-D) ("could not get going"), Zung Depression Scale (fatigue), and diagnostic major depressive disorder (fatigue and sleep problems). Although somewhat varied in the nature of the behaviors that they assess, none of these instruments specifically inquire about the tendency to feel sleepy during normal waking hours of the day or excessive daytime sleepiness (EDS) [39]. EDS is considered to be conceptually and operationally independent from fatigue and tiredness that characterize depression, which makes it mandatory to make the distinction between tiredness and sleepiness. A first-step approach includes probing questions concerning the patient's actual need for naps, their capacity to doze when subjected to passive or active situations, and time to usually fall asleep, among others. This set of questions enable clinicians to discern between sleepiness and less-specific complaints [1]. Together with this initial clinical assessment, a wide array of tools has been developed to assess sleepiness, which includes subjective scales and performance tests [1]. For instance, subjective scales, such as the Stanford Sleepiness Scale and the Karolinska Sleepiness Scale, track down individual perception of alertness/sleepiness by providing an appropriate assessment of the *temporary* alertness/sleepiness level [40]. On the other hand, the Epworth Sleepiness Scale offers a better method for assessing *global* sleepiness, since it covers sleepiness over a one-month period, during active and passive behavioral situations of sleepiness [40]. Performance tests, such as the PVT which involves a 5-min visual reaction time (RT) performance test in which the subject is required to maintain the fastest possible RTs to a simple visual stimulus, have been frequently utilized to measure sustained attention [41], and have been demonstrated to be sensitive to circadian variation and sleep loss. As can be noticed, the diagnosis of daytime sleepiness can be a challenge. For instance, the assessment of subjective sleepiness (e.g. the Epworth scale or the Stanford scale) does not always correlate with objective quantifications. Objective tests of daytime sleepiness rely on measurement of physiological parameters, the most extensively used objective test of sleepiness being the multiple sleep latency test (MSLT) [42]. The MSLT is performed after an overnight polysomnogram, in order to assess sleep during the prior night and to control for obvious reasons of nocturnal sleep disruption, which could account for daytime symptoms, such as OSA. Briefly, this test consists of four or five chances to nap that are spaced across the day at 2-h intervals. Standardized conditions are employed, in which the patient is placed in a quiet, dark, comfortable room and asked to sleep, and monitored by EEG, EMG, and eye movements. Besides sleep latency, the MSLT assesses sleep onset rapid eye movement sleep periods (SOREMPs), a diagnostic criterion for narcolepsy. On the MSLT, a mean sleep latency >10 min is considered normal, the 5–10 min range is considered as a gray zone and <5 min as severe daytime sleepiness. For EDS in narcolepsy or idiopathic hypersomnia, the necessary diagnostic cut-off threshold lies currently at 8 min.

Objective assessment of sleep may also be provided by electroencephalographic (EEG) sleep (polysomnography) measurement, which consists in

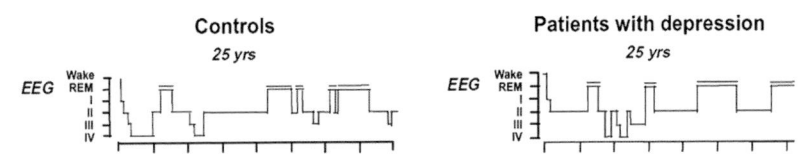

Figure 25.3 Differences in sleep architecture between healthy controls and depressed patients. Abbreviations: I, NREM stage 1, II, NREM stage 2, III NREM stage 3, and IV, NREM stage 4 (drawn by authors).

an established method of studying sleep architecture [43]. Figure 25.3 illustrates an example of differences in sleep architecture between healthy and depressed conditions.

The range of differences in sleep architecture during depression is both wide and conflicting. For instance, a previous study which compared depressed subjects with healthy controls indicated that the former group exhibited prolonged sleep latency, reduced total sleep time, and reduced sleep efficiency [44]. Rapid eye movement (REM) sleep may also be affected, such that REM latency is shortened and the duration of the first REM period is increased. The REM density over the whole night is increased and the same applies to the percentage of REM (%REM) sleep over the total sleep time. While it is estimated that short REM latency and increased wakefulness are present in 40–70% of depressed outpatients, it is also very likely that depressed patients may not exhibit any of these sleep-related differences [4]. This can be illustrated by changes in non-REM sleep patterns.

Classically, overall NREM sleep, slow-wave sleep (SWS), dissipation rate of slow-wave activity and the percentage of SWS over the total sleep time can be substantially reduced in depressed patients [45]. However, the direction of changes in this sleep stage may be diametrically different. For instance, identification and scoring of the cyclic alternating pattern (CAP) during sleep allows a different approach to investigating NREM sleep [46]. CAP is formed by electrocortical events that recur at regular intervals in the range of seconds during NREM sleep [47]. These events are clearly distinguishable from the background electroencephalographic (EEG) rhythm as abrupt frequency shifts or amplitude changes. Two phases (A and B) are present that are part of a CAP cycle and recur within 2–60 s. Phase A is identified by transient events typically observed in NREM sleep, and includes EEG patterns of higher-voltage, slower-frequency and lower-voltage, faster-frequency than the background EEG. Phase B follows Phase A, and is defined by decreased EEG amplitude with EEG features of stages 1–2 NREM sleep. In a study purported to explore whether CAP analysis can unearth more information on NREM sleep in major depressive patients, results clearly indicated that there was an abnormally high CAP rate and CAP time during NREM sleep in depressive patients as compared to controls [46]. The calculation of CAP rate, CAP time, and CAP cycles per sleep stage showed a significantly higher CAP rate during SWS when, physiologically, it should have been less than in stages 1 and 2. CAP time and CAP cycle were significantly higher during stage 2 NREM sleep in comparison to controls, indicating a difficulty evolving toward further NREM sleep stages, that is, to stages 3 and 4 (SWS) as habitually described in healthy subjects. This demonstrates the importance of the NREM sleep disruption that involved all stages of NREM sleep. The disruption underlines the interruption of the normal passage to the hypersynchronization phase, translated in the central EEG leads by high-amplitude slow waves. If this normal progression is impaired, there will be interruption of the normal development of the slow-wave process with the presence of a CAP rate in a larger amount than expected from normal control data. Taken together, CAP analysis demonstrates the presence of more important NREM sleep disturbances in depressed patients than does conventional sleep staging, suggesting the involvement of SWS in the sleep impairment in depression. Within the framework of sleepiness, it is crucial to unravel which are the correlates of electrophysiological sleep associated with the depressive episode. By establishing this aspect in a *first step* – if sleep differences encompass either REM and/or NREM sleep – it is possible to suggest the *next step*, the appropriate therapeutic strategy to counteract depression and sleepiness. While both subjective and objective measurements may be very useful in tracking the course of the illness and the treatment effects (as well as offering prognostic indicators for outcome and relapse), they often overlap in what they measure [43]. What is not very well established is how they relate to each other; in other words, whether the

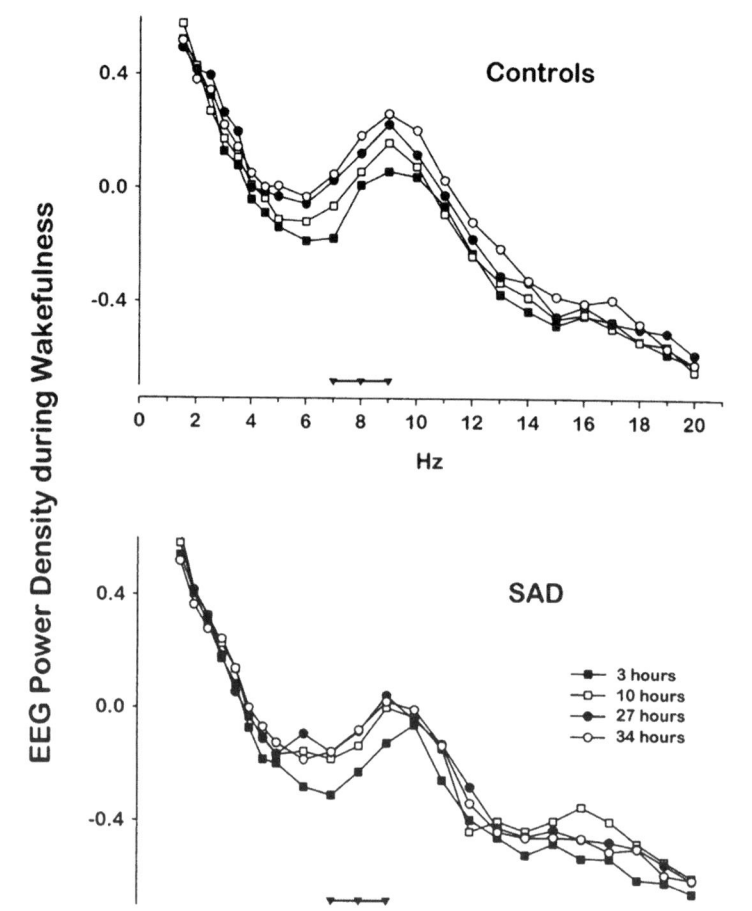

Figure 25.4 Electroencephalogram power density (μV^2/Hz, log transformed) in single frequency bins (1.5–20 Hz) recorded after 3, 10, 27, and 34 h of elapsed time awake for seasonal affective disorder patients ($n = 8$) and control subjects ($n = 9$). Triangles above the abscissa indicate frequency bins for which significant changes over time were present (with permission from Cajochen et al., 2000 [14]).

subjective sleep complaints correspond to discernible alterations of sleep structure, and vice versa. For instance, comparison of the prevalence of subjective and objective sleep disturbances in depressed patients indicates that the former may be more common than the latter. Indeed, it is not unusual in clinical practice to see patients complaining of poor sleep without any abnormal polysomnography findings, such that depressed patients experienced more "sleep distress" than healthy individuals, even though their estimates of sleep disturbance were similar to those of controls [43].

Differences in waking EEG may also provide insight into the state of sleepiness in depression. In a 40-h constant routine study looking at the EEG and subjective sleepiness in seasonal affective disorder (SAD), the progressive build-up of sleepiness was considerably reduced in SAD patients [14], as depicted in Figure 25.4 [14]. The time course of waking EEG theta-alpha activity showed a rapid increase during the first 10 h which then remained constant, in contrast to control subjects who showed a slower continuous exponential increase in the course of the 40-h episode of sustained wakefulness. Given that this pattern was independent of clinical state or season, SAD patients may have a trait deficiency in the homeostatic build-up of sleep pressure.

Management: therapeutical strategies for depression and EDS

Pharmacological management

On a pharmacological domain, there is emerging evidence that the circadian system is implicated in some of the treatment mechanisms, such as lithium therapy for bipolar depression. Lithium may modify the phase angle between the circadian temperature rhythm and the rest–activity cycle [5], and may lengthen the period of circadian rhythms, by increasing the circadian period of firing rate rhythms of SCN neurons in a concentration-dependent manner. Thus, the stabilization of circadian rhythms may play a key action of clinically effective mood-stabilizing medications.

The use of modafinil, a wake-promoting agent, has been recently suggested in the treatment of EDS and depression. In a previous study, modafinil was investigated as an adjunctive treatment of depressed patients with EDS. Subjects were assessed at 2-week intervals for improvement using standard depression scales, sleepiness scales and a neuropsychological battery. Significant improvements were seen across all the measures, thus suggesting that modafinil may be a useful and a well-tolerated adjunctive treatment of major depression [48]. Furthermore, it is a particularly attractive alternative to other stimulants because of its low abuse potential. However, data on modafinil use in depression present some conflicting evidence. As an illustration, in a double-blind placebo-controlled study, no significant improvements for daytime sleepiness, depression scores or overall clinical state were found [49]. Therefore, caution should be kept in mind with regard to the use of modafinil in this clinical condition.

With respect to antidepressant intake, the therapeutic properties of selective serotonin (5-HT) reuptake inhibitor (SSRI) drugs can be related to the 5-HT$_{2C}$ receptor subtype, and it is interesting to observe that 5-HT$_{2C}$ receptor agonists in the rat SCN mimic the effects of light. Serotonergic drugs may, thus, improve entrainment. Most recently, unique antidepressant drugs such as agomelatine – a melatonin agonist and 5-HT$_{2c}$ antagonist – target both the circadian system and mood. Agomelatine has identical physiological actions to melatonin when administered in the evening, to advance circadian phase and promoting a rapid sleep onset without after-effects on the following day [50]. Indeed, unlike other antidepressants, notably SSRIs, agomelatine does not lead to insomnia, fragmentation of SWS, and nightmares, but rather improves the quality of sleep, with increases in both SWS and, to a lower extent, REM sleep in depressed patients. The interesting aspect of this treatment is that its core action is aimed at the circadian rhythms, and it has been shown to be especially useful for synchronizing circadian rhythms of body temperature, cortisol, thyroid-stimulating hormone and growth hormone secretion. Agomelatine may be particularly indicated for the management of depression associated with insomnia and/or EDS [51]. Indeed, a recent study focusing on the agomelatine use in depression has led to an impressive response, which in turn has been directly linked to the action of this medication on the melatoninergic and serotonergic systems [52].

Orexin-antagonists of OX1 and OX2 receptors have been recently tested in the treatment of insomnia. Orexins are hypothalamic peptides that play a critical role in consolidating wakefulness. When administered during the active period of the circadian cycle, a dual antagonist of both orexin OX1 and OX2 receptors was shown to increase subjective and objective EEG sleep in humans [53]. Despite the fact that this study focused on narcolepsy, these results may shed new light in the investigation of endogenous orexins in sleep–wake regulation. Considering that orexins play a key role in regulating sleep–wake cycles, it has been suggested that several sleep disorders may be associated with maladaptive orexinergic tone [53]. Whether orexin-antagonists can be utilized for other types of sleep disturbances, such as insomnia in depressed patients, however, remains to be answered.

Non-pharmacological management

On a non-pharmacological domain, the circadian rhythm and sleep research have led to promising therapies of depression. The rationale for aiming to resynchronize disturbed phase relationships between the "biological clock" and sleep is the concomitant improvement in mood. Furthermore, a chronobiological approach may address some of the unmet needs in the treatment of depression, such as diminishing the latency of onset of antidepressant action, reducing residual symptoms, and preventing relapse in the long term [54].

Sleep-deprivation therapy challenges the sleep–wake homeostat and exerts rapid, although short-lasting, mood improvement in the majority of depressed patients. One night total sleep deprivation (TSD) appears to improve depressive symptoms in 40–60% of treatments [55] and the degree of clinical variations spans a continuum from complete remission to worsening. After recovery sleep, 50–80% of first-day responders suffer a complete or partial relapse; nevertheless, improvement can last for weeks. Partial sleep deprivation (PSD) in the second half of the night has been shown to be similarly effective as compared to TSD. Sleep deprivation may hasten the action onset of antidepressant medication and repeated SD can also be an efficient treatment strategy in drug refractory depression [55]. Given that insomnia associated or not with EDS is such a prominent feature of depression, further investigations may consider tracking EDS as an outcome measure of sleep deprivation therapy for depression.

Light therapy has been applied as stand-alone therapy or as adjunct to antidepressant pharmacotherapy to a wide range of mood disorders [54]. Light exerts powerful, non-visual effects on a wide range of biological functions including the modulation of human alertness levels. Factors such as the dose (illuminance levels), exposure duration, timing and wavelength of light have important repercussions on the alerting response to light in humans and can lead to a substantial decrement in sleepiness [56]. Bright light therapy is characterized by a fast onset of antidepressant action and by additive properties to antidepressant medication. Bright light therapy, beginning in the morning after partial sleep deprivation, has been demonstrated to prevent the depressive relapse after recovery sleep in sleep deprivation responders [57]. Regarding non-seasonal depression, there is evidence in support of the efficacy of bright light therapy as an adjuvant treatment to antidepressant pharmacotherapy [58]. Taking into account the insufficient remission rate of depression solely with pharmacotherapy and the favorable risk-to-benefit ratio of light therapy, it can offer a promising, non-pharmacological, biologically oriented treatment approach. None the less, investigations on the exclusive efficacy of bright light therapy have yielded inconsistent results to date, mostly due to the inclusion of several types of non-seasonal depression in the same study sample [59]. To tackle this problem, future therapeutic studies should target homogeneous subgroups of non-seasonal depressed patients. This selection could be based on predictors of response to light therapy previously identified in SAD. On the other hand, since bright light therapy modulates its antidepressant effect through the circadian system, subgroups of patients could be selected in respect to their chronobiological characteristics. These could either be clinically defined, such as chronotypes, or based on their circadian phase position according to physiological parameters, such as the dim light melatonin onset.

However, further research is needed to conclude more accurately in what way bright light therapy can act as an adjuvant treatment for depression and its concomitant sleep disorders, such as insomnia and EDS.

The combination of these two chronobiological treatment strategies has led to very promising results. For instance, one combination encompasses TSD together with phase advance [15]. Accordingly, after a successful sleep deprivation, evading recovery sleep during a hypothesized critical early morning time period may prevent sleep deprivation associated relapses, with a concomitant improvement in both mood and subjective sleepiness. This combination strategy could provide an interesting therapeutical approach for the management of depression and sleepiness.

On a different dimension, there is recent evidence in favor of transcranial magnetic stimulation (TMS) in major depression as a potentially non-pharmacological therapy [60]. This technique enables a non-invasive electrical stimulation of the cerebral cortex through magnetic fields generated by a handheld coil, which act as a vector that goes unimpeded across the human skull, and then converting into an electrical field within the brain [61]. One of its positive aspects is the possibility to target the cortical stimulation area with extreme precision, reliability, and reproducibility over the treatment. The efficacy of rTMS in major depression has showed significant effects for active stimulation when it was delivered to the left dorso-lateral prefrontal cortex (DLPFC) after 4 weeks of treatment in depressive patients [62]. Similar results were observed in a recent study whereby patients with bipolar depression, non-responsive to prior pharmacological treatment, underwent three weeks of rTMS [60]. Accordingly, augmentative low-frequency rTMS of the right DLPFC combined with brain navigation was effective and well tolerated in these bipolar depressive patients, with an enhancement of depressive symptoms as indexed by clinical scales, such as the Hamilton Depression Rating Scale, Montgomery–Åsberg Depression Rating Scale, and Clinical Global Impression Scale of severity. One possible underlying reason for this mood improvement may stem from the fact that there appears to be a contrasting role in mood regulation between right and left hemispheres. For instance, it has been hypothesized that right DLPFC stimulation at low frequency may produce the same antidepressant effect as left DLPFC stimulation at high frequency [63]. Furthermore, longer duration of treatment (3 weeks) was used in the present trial in comparison to the standard duration (2 weeks) of most acute clinical trials with rTMS, which goes in line with the concept that any antidepressant treatment, either pharmacological or non-pharmacological, with the exception of ECT, has a latency of efficacy not shorter than 3 weeks [64]. Within the scope of depression and sleepiness, it is of great interest to unravel if concomitant sleepiness can be substantially reduced after 3 weeks or more of rTMS in patients with major depression, unresponsive to other types of pharmacological treatments.

Conclusions

Excessive daytime sleepiness is a complaint frequently encountered in clinical scenarios, such as depression; however, the theoretical underpinnings of this relationship remain fairly unknown. Considering that depression is intertwined with circadian rhythms on a wide array of dimensions, a chronobiological approach may lead to insights on the complex interaction of EDS and depression, despite the wide gaps of uncertainty. Knowledge on how the circadian system can be deregulated in depression, thus leading to depressive symptoms and sleepiness, may help to unravel the pathophysiology of this disorder. The theoretical framework for this relationship is under intense investigation. New data on genetics and molecular expression, like clock gene polymorphisms and neurotransmitters, may shed new light on the interindividual differences associated with sleep architecture, and their implication in depression. Insights on the link among EDS, depression and chronobiology can provide a better comprehension of this sleep–wake disturbance, together with promising therapeutic managements.

References

1. **Fava M**. Daytime sleepiness and insomnia as correlates of depression. *J Clin Psychiatry*, 2004; **65**:27–32.
2. **Breslau N**, **Roth T**, **Rosenthal L**, et al. Sleep disturbance and psychiatric disorders: a longitudinal epidemiological study of young adults. *Biol Psychiatry*, 1996; **39**:411–18.
3. **Wirz-Justice A**. Chronobiology and mood disorders. *Dial Clinl Neurosci*, 2003; **5**:223–33.
4. **Cano-Lozano M**, **Espinosa-Fernandez L**, **Miro E**, et al. A review of sleep disorders in depression. *Rev Neurol*, 2003; **36**:366–75.
5. **Nagayama H**. Chronic administration of imipramine and lithium changes the phase-angle relationship between the activity and core body temperature circadian rhythms in rats. *Chronobiol Int*, 1996; **13**:251–59.
6. **Bixler E O**, **Vgontzas A N**, **Lin H M**, et al. EDS in a general population sample: the role of sleep apnea, age, obesity, diabetes, and depression. *J Clin Endocrinol Metab*, 2005; **90**:4510–15.
7. **Chellappa S L**, **Araujo J F**. Sleep disorders and suicidal ideation in patients with depressive disorder. *Psychiatr Res*, 2007; **153**:131–36.
8. **Chellappa S L**, **Araújo J F**. Excessive daytime sleepiness in patients with depressive disorder. *Rev Bras Psiquiatr*, 2006; **28**:126–30.
9. **Sharafkhaneh A**, **Giray N**, **Richardson P**, et al. Association of psychiatric disorders and sleep apnea in a large cohort. *Sleep*, 2005; **28**:1405–11.
10. **Schuster S R**, **Tabba M**, **Sahota P**. Relationship between the cardiometabolic syndrome and obstructive sleep apnea. *J Cardio Metabol Syndr*, 2006; **1**:204–08.
11. **Boivin D B**. Influence of sleep–wake and circadian rhythm disturbances in psychiatric disorders. *J Psychiatry Neurosci*, 2000; **25**:446–58.
12. **Thase M E**, **Fasicka A L**, **Berman S R**, et al. Electroencephalographic sleep profiles in single-episode and recurrent unipolar forms of major depression: comparison during acute depressive states. *Biol Psychiatry* 1995; **38**:99–108.
13. **Lewy A J**, **Lefler B J**, **Emens J S**, et al. The circadian basis of winter depression. *Proc Natl Acad Sci USA*, 2006; **103**:7414–19.
14. **Cajochen C**, **Brunner D P**, **Kräuchi K**, et al. EEG and subjective sleepiness during extended wakefulness in seasonal affective disorder: circadian and homeostatic influences. *Biol Psychiatry*, 2000; **47**:610–17.
15. **Berger M**, **Vollmann J**, **Hohagen F**, et al. Sleep deprivation combined with consecutive sleep phase advance as a fast-acting therapy in depression: an open pilot trial in medicated and unmedicated patients. *Am J Psychiatry*, 1997; **154**:870–72.
16. **Steiger A**. Sleep and the hypothalamo–pituitary–adrenocortical system. *Sleep Med Rev*, 2002; **6**:125–38.
17. **Stokes P E**. The potential role of excessive cortisol induced by HPA hyperfunction in the pathogenesis of depression. *Eur Neuropsychopharmacol*, 1996; **5**:77–82.
18. **Klein D C**, **Moore R Y**, **Reppert S M**. *Suprachiasmatic Nucleus: The Mind's Clock*. New York, NY: Oxford University Press, 1991.

19. **Provencio I**, **Rodriguez I R**, **Jiang G**, *et al.* A novel human opsin in the inner retina. *J Neurosci*, 2000; **20**:600–05.

20. **Borbély A A**, **Wirz-Justice A**. Sleep, sleep deprivation and depression. A hypothesis derived from a model of sleep regulation. *Hum Neurobiol*, 1982; **1**:205–10.

21. **Daan S**, **Beersma D G M**, **Borbély A A**. Timing of human sleep: recovery process gated by a circadian pacemaker. *Am J Physiol Regulatory Integr Comp Physiol*, 1984; **246**:R161–78.

22. **Koorengevel K M**, **Beersma D G M**, **den Boer J A**, *et al.* Mood regulation in seasonal affective disorder patients and healthy controls studied in forced desynchrony. *Psychiatry Res*, 2003; **117**:57–74.

23. **Saper C B**, **Chou T C**, **Scammell T E**. The sleep switch: hypothalamic control of sleep and wakefulness. *Trends Neurosci*, 2001; **24**:726–31.

24. **Riemann D**, **Berger M**, **Voderholzer U**. Sleep and depression – results from psychobiological studies: an overview. *Biol Psychol*, 2001; **57**:67–103.

25. **Phillips M L**, **Drevets W C**, **Rauch S L**, *et al.* Neurobiology of emotion perception I: The neural basis of normal emotion perception. *Biol Psychiatry*, 2003; **54**:504–14.

26. **Buysse D J**, **Nofzinger E A**, **Germain A**, *et al.* Regional brain glucose metabolism during morning and evening wakefulness in humans: preliminary findings. *Sleep*, 2004; **27**:1245–54.

27. **Watson N F**, **Goldberg J**, **Arguelles L**, *et al.* Genetic and environmental influences on insomnia, daytime sleepiness, and obesity in twins. *Sleep*, 2006; **29**:645–49.

28. **Reppert S M**, **Weaver D R**. Coordination of circadian timing in mammals. *Nature*, 2002; **418**:935–41.

29. **McClung C A**. Circadian genes, rhythms and the biology of mood disorders. *Pharmacol Therap*, 2007; **114**:222–32.

30. **Ebisawa T**, **Uchiyama M**, **Kajimura N**, *et al.* Association of structural polymorphisms in the human period 3 gene with delayed sleep phase syndrome. *EMBO Rep*, 2001; **2**:342–46.

31. **Viola A U**, **Archer S N**, **James L M**, *et al.* PER3 polymorphism predicts sleep structure and waking performance. *Curr Biol*, 2007; **17**:613–18.

32. **Artioli P**, **Lorenzi C**, **Pirovano A**, *et al.* How do genes exert their role? Period 3 gene variants and possible influences on mood disorder phenotypes. *Eur Neuropsychopharmacol*, 2007; **17**:587–94.

33. **Xu Y**, **Padiath Q S**, **Shapiro R E**, *et al.* Functional consequences of a CKI mutation causing familial advanced sleep phase syndrome. *Nature*, 2005; **434**:640–44.

34. **Chelminski I**, **Ferraro F R**, **Petros T V**, *et al.* An analysis of the "eveningness–morningness" dimension in depressive college students. *J Affect Disord*, 1999; **52**:19–29.

35. **Weber M**, **Lauterburg T**, **Tobler I**, *et al.* Circadian patterns of neurotransmitter related gene expression in motor regions of the rat brain. *Neurosci Lett*, 2004; **358**:17–20.

36. **Lam R W**, **Tam E M**, **Yatham L N**, *et al.* Seasonal depression. The dual vulnerability hypothesis revisited. *J Affect Disord*, 2001; **63**:123–32.

37. **Akhisaroglu M**, **Kurtuncu M**, **Manev H**, *et al.* Diurnal rhythms in quinpirole-induced locomotor behaviors and striatal D2/D3 receptor levels in mice. *Pharmacol Biochem Behav*, 2005; **80**:371–77.

38. **Aston-Jones G**, **Chen S**, **Zhu Y**, *et al.* A neural circuit for circadian regulation of arousal. *Nature Neurosci*, 2001; **4**:732–38.

39. **Lessov-Schlaggar C N**, **Bliwise D L**, **Krasnow R E**, *et al.* Genetic association of daytime sleepiness and depressive symptoms in elderly men. *Sleep*, 2008; **31**:1111–17.

40. **Chellappa S L**, **Schröder C**, **Cajochen C**. Chronobiology, excessive daytime sleepiness and depression: is there a link? *Sleep Med*, 2009; **10**:505–14.

41. **Doran S M**, **Van Dongen H P A**, **Dinges D F**. Sustained attention performance during sleep deprivation: evidence of state instability. *Arch Ital Biol*, 2001; **139**:253–67.

42. **Carskadon M A**, **Dement W C**, **Mitler M M**, *et al.* Guidelines for the multiple sleep latency test (MSLT): a standard measure of sleepiness. *Sleep*, 1986; **9**:519–24.

43. **Argyropoulos S V**, **Hicks J A**, **Nash J R**, *et al.* Correlation of subjective and objective sleep measurements at different stages of the treatment of depression. *Psychiatr Res*, 2003; **120**:179–90.

44. **Armitage R**, **Hoffmann R**, **Fitch T**, *et al.* A comparison of period amplitude and power spectral analysis of sleep EEG in normal adults and depressed outpatients. *Psychiatry Res*, 1995; **56**:245–56.

45. **Armitage R**, **Hoffmann R**, **Madhukar T**, *et al.* Slow-wave activity in NREM sleep: sex and age effects in depressed outpatients and healthy controls. *Psychiat Res*, 2000; **95**:201–13.

46. **Lopes M C**, **Quera-Salva M A**, **Guilleminault C**. Non-REM sleep instability in patients with major depressive disorder: subjective improvement and improvement of non-REM sleep instability with treatment (Agomelatine). *Sleep Med*, 2007; **9**:33–41.

47. **Terzano M G**, **Mancia D**, **Salati M R**, *et al.* The cyclic alternating pattern as a physiologic component of normal NREM sleep. *Sleep*, 1985; **8**:137–45.

48. **DeBatista C, Lambke A, Solvason H B**. A prospective trial of modafinil as an adjunctive treatment of major depression. *J Clin Psychopharm*, 2004; **24**:87–90.

49. **DeBatista C, Doghramji K, Menza M A**. Adjuvant modafinil for the short-term treatment of fatigue and sleepiness in patients with major depressive disorder: a preliminary double-blind, placebo-controlled study. *J Clin Psychiatry*, 2003; **64**:1057–64.

50. **Cajochen C, Kräuchi K, Möri D**, *et al*. Melatonin and S-20098 increase REM sleep and wake-up propensity without modifying NREM sleep homeostasis. *Am J Physiol Regul Integr Comp Physiol*, 1997; **272**:R1189–96.

51. **Wirz-Justice A**. Biological rhythm disturbances in mood disorders. *Int Clin Psychopharmacol*, 2006; **21**(Suppl 1):S11–15.

52. **Loo H, D'Haenen H, Hale A**. Determination of the dose of agomelatine, a melatoninergic agonist and selective 5-HT2c antagonist, in the treatment of major depressive disorder: a placebo-controlled dose range study. *Int J Neuropsychopharmacol*, 2002; **17**:239–47.

53. **Brisbare-Roch C, Dingemanse J, Koberstein R**, *et al*. Promotion of sleep by targeting the orexin system in rats, dogs and humans. *Nature*, 2007; **12**:150–55.

54. **Wirz-Justice A**. Circadian disturbances in depression: therapeutic perspectives. *Medicographia*, 2003; **25**:29–36.

55. **Giedke H, Schwärzler F**. Therapeutic use of sleep deprivation in depression. *Sleep Med Rev*, 2002; **6**:361–77.

56. **Cajochen C**. Alerting effects of light. *Sleep Med Rev*, 2007; **11**:453–64.

57. **Loving R T, Kripke D F, Shuchter S R**. Bright light augments antidepressant effects of medication and wake therapy. *Depress Anxiety*, 2002; **16**:1–3.

58. **Martiny K, Lunde M, Unden M**, *et al*. Adjunctive bright light in non-seasonal major depression: results from clinician-rated depression scales. *Acta Psychiatr Scand*, 2005; **112**:117–25.

59. **Even C, Schröder C M, Friedman S**, *et al*. Efficacy of light therapy in nonseasonal depression: a systematic review. *J Affect Disord*, 2008; **108**:11–23.

60. **Dell'Osso B, Mundo E, D'Urso N**, *et al*. Augmentative repetitive navigated transcranial magnetic stimulation (rTMS) in drug-resistant bipolar depression. *Bipolar Disord*, 2009; **11**:76–81.

61. **Sparing R, Buelte D, Meister I G**, *et al*. Transcranial magnetic stimulation and the challenge of coil placement: a comparison of conventional and stereotaxic neuronavigational strategies. *Hum Brain Mapp*, 2008; **29**:82–96.

62. **O'Reardon J P, Solvason H B, Janicak P G**, *et al*. Efficacy and safety of transcranial magnetic stimulation in the acute treatment of major depression: a multisite randomized controlled trial. *Biol Psychiatry*, 2007; **62**:1208–16.

63. **Loo C K, Mitchell P B**. A review of the efficacy of transcranial magnetic stimulation (TMS) treatment for depression, and current and future strategies to optimize efficacy. *J Affect Disord*, 2005; **88**:255–67.

64. **Stassen H H, Delini-Stula A, Angst J**. Time course of improvement under antidepressant treatment: a survival–analytical approach. *Eur Neuropsychopharmacol*, 1993; **3**:127–35.

65. **Dahl K, Avery D H, Lewy A J**, *et al*. Dim light melatonin onset and circadian temperature during a constant routine in hypersomnic winter depression. *Acta Psychiatr Scand*, 1993; **88**:60–66.

66. **Buysse D J, Monk T H, Kupfer D J**, *et al*. Circadian patterns of unintended sleep episodes during a constant routine in remitted depressed patients. *J Psychiat Res*, 1995; **29**:407–16.

67. **Wirz-Justice A, Kräuchi K, Brunner D P**, *et al*. Circadian rhythms and sleep regulation in seasonal affective disorder. *Acta Neuropsychiatr*, 1995; **7**:41–43.

68. **Avery D H, Dahl K, Savage M V**, *et al*. Circadian temperature and cortisol rhythms during a constant routine are phase-delayed in hypersomnic winter depression. *Biol Psychiatry*, 1997; **41**:1109–23.

69. **Koorengevel K M, Beersma D G, den Boer J A**, *et al*. A forced desynchrony study of circadian pacemaker characteristics in seasonal affective disorder. *J Biol Rhythms*, 2002; **17**:463–75

Section 3 Chapter 26

Medical, Psychiatric and Neurological Causes of Sleepiness

Aging, Alzheimer's disease and sleepiness

Jennifer L. Martin and Sonia Ancoli-Israel

Daytime sleepiness is a construct that is at times difficult to measure. In general, in the majority of research studies, daytime sleepiness is objectively measured either by the ability to quickly fall asleep during the day with the Multiple Sleep Latency Test (MSLT), or by recording inadvertent napping behavior with wrist actigraphy. Daytime sleepiness can also be estimated from reports of daytime napping or a subjective report of "sleepiness". Therefore, daytime napping, particularly inadvertent napping, has become synonymous with daytime sleepiness in many studies. A third measure of daytime sleepiness is self-report questionnaires, most commonly the Epworth Sleepiness Scale (ESS), which measures the likelihood of dosing off in different situations [1]. Although used with older adults, the ESS has never been validated in this population, and as pointed out in Martin and Ancoli-Israel, some older adults may not engage in one or more of the eight activities examined, creating some ambiguity around the validity of this measure in frail older adults [2]. This chapter will attempt to make a distinction between studies of sleepiness and studies of napping and will present data on both.

Prevalence of daytime sleepiness among older adults

It is a common belief that daytime napping and dozing are "normal" among older adults, yet rates of daytime sleepiness vary widely across studies, suggesting that daytime napping is not limited to the older individual. Increases in rates of daytime sleepiness across the lifespan are not linear. In one large population-based study of adults aged 20–100 years, rates of self-reported excessive daytime sleepiness (EDS) were highest among those over age 90 years (12%) and those aged 20–25 years (10%) [3]. The study also described an "inverted U" pattern in which the lowest rates of sleepiness were among those in the age range of 50–80 years (approximately 6%). In that study, depression was the strongest predictor of EDS, but the strength of that relationship decreased with advancing age. In a second study spanning 10 countries around the world, adults over the age of 65 were less likely to report daytime sleepiness than adults under age 65 (8.6 vs. 10.7%); however, older adults did report more difficulties with functioning during the day than younger adults [4]. In a study of older US adults carried out in 2003 by the National Sleep Foundation, 14.8% of adults aged 55–84 years reported EDS and those with EDS reported more overall sleep disturbance, poorer self-rated health, more insomnia, and more symptoms of sleep apnea and restless legs syndrome [5]. Taken together, studies suggest that approximately 10–15% of older adults report excessive daytime sleepiness. Table 26.1 reviews studies which have examined rates of daytime sleepiness among older adults.

To date, there have been no studies of objectively measured daytime sleepiness among large samples of older adults. Hoch *et al.* compared adults in their 20s ($n = 46$) to adults in their 80s ($n = 52$) and found no difference between age groups in daytime sleepiness based on the MSLT. Importantly, there was also no difference between groups in self-reported sleepiness and there was no relationship between sleepiness and performance on cognitive tasks among young or old participants. The study also showed that, after a night of sleep deprivation, younger adults were sleepier (based on the MSLT) than older adults [6]. These findings suggest that older adults are not necessarily predisposed to daytime sleepiness due to age alone; rather, daytime sleepiness in an older adult likely reflects an underlying problem with sleep, health or both.

Sleepiness: Causes, Consequences and Treatment, ed. Michael J. Thorpy and Michel Billiard. Published by Cambridge University Press. © Cambridge University Press 2011.

Table 26.1 Selected recent studies of self-reported excessive daytime sleepiness (EDS) among older adults

Reference	Study sample N (women)/age	Methods	Prevalence/findings among older adults
Bixler et al., 2005 [3]	Penn State Cohort subsample 1741 (1000 W) aged 20–100 years	2-question EDS screening	• EDS decreased through age 70, then increased • 5–12% for age groups 65–90 years
Soldatos et al., 2005 [4]	International survey 35 327 (17 734 W) aged 15–99 years	Epworth Sleepiness Scale	• 9% for those over 65 years
Chasens et al., 2009 [13]	National Sleep Foundation Poll, 2003 1506 (872 W) aged 55–84 years	1 question on daytime sleepiness that impacts functioning "a few days a month" or more	• 15% of total respondents had EDS • 13% of those without diabetes • 20% of those with diabetes
Foley et al., 2007 [33]	National Sleep Foundation Poll, 2003 1506 (872 W) aged 55–84 years	1 question on napping, "4–7 days per week"	• 15% of total respondents were regular nappers • 10% for age 55–64 years • 25% for age 75–84 years

Causes of daytime sleepiness

In considering difficulties with excessive daytime sleepiness among older adults, one key factor is poor-quality nighttime sleep. Studies show that older adults suffer from a disproportionately high degree of nighttime sleep disturbance, and while a full discussion of the topic is beyond the scope of this chapter, one cannot ignore the role of poor nighttime sleep in increasing the risk for excessive daytime sleepiness among older people.

Compared to younger adults, older adults are more likely to suffer from sleep apnea [7, 8], restless legs syndrome and periodic limb movements in sleep [9, 10], insomnia [11], or more than one of these conditions. As a result, any older adult complaining of daytime sleepiness should be queried about symptoms of nighttime sleep disorders.

Many studies have found that depression is associated with EDS, with some of those studies focusing specifically on older adults. In one study, depression (indicated by use of antidepressant medications) was the strongest predictor of EDS in a model including age, sleep duration, diabetes, body mass index (BMI), and sleep apnea [3]. In a second study, those with EDS (based on ESS $\geq$ 10) reported more symptoms of depression based on the geriatric depression scale compared to those without EDS (based on ESS $<$ 10) [12]. In a third study among older adults with self-reported diabetes, depressive symptoms were associated with EDS after controlling for age, BMI and comorbidities [13]. One limitation of these cross-sectional studies is that the direction of the relationship between EDS and depression cannot be established. Prospective studies are needed to address the question of whether depression causes EDS, whether EDS predisposes people to subsequent depression, or whether EDS and depression may share common underlying mechanisms.

Finally, there are several aspects of lifestyle that may predispose an older adult to daytime sleepiness. In particular, retirement from the workforce may have a tremendous impact on daytime routines and nighttime sleep habits. Unfortunately, little work has been done to explore how sleep changes with retirement in recent decades; however, a study in the 1980s found that retirees slept more on weeknights and napped less than working comparison subjects aged 50–70 years [14]. It is unclear whether this pattern may have changed in recent decades, as many older people delay retirement to a later age, and may retire with greater health concerns than their counterparts in the 1980s. Additional research is needed in this area.

Consequences of daytime sleepiness

Among older adults, daytime sleepiness may not be benign. Studies show that daytime sleepiness is associated with elevated disease risk and mortality. In a cohort of 5888 elderly subjects aged 65–100 years, Newman et al. observed a significant association between daytime sleepiness complaints and mortality, with an unadjusted Cox hazard ratio of 1.71 [15]. Women reporting both daytime sleepiness and frequent nocturnal awakening had a multivariate adjusted hazard ratio of 2.34 for incident congestive heart failure, compared to women with daytime sleepiness but without frequent nocturnal awakenings.

Studies also show that daytime sleepiness is associated with increased blood pressure among older adults. Goldstein *et al.* found that, among adults aged 55–80 years, those with more sleepiness (measured by self-report) had higher blood pressure both during wakefulness and during sleep [12].

Daytime sleepiness may also contribute to functional impairment among older adults. In a survey study of US adults, those with self-reported diabetes were more likely to report EDS [13], and the EDS was associated with lower self-rated health and higher degrees of functional impairment [5]. In a recent study of older adults receiving inpatient post-acute care (i.e. physical, occupational, and kineseotherapy) after hospitalization, Alessi *et al.* reported that patients who slept more during the daytime hours showed less functional improvement during their rehabilitation stay, even after controlling for mental status, hours of rehabilitation therapy received, rehospitalization, and reason for admission [16]. This study suggests that daytime sleepiness may be an independent risk factor for declining health among older people.

Treatment considerations for older adults

Few studies have examined direct treatment of daytime sleepiness among older adults; however, several themes emerge from the literature. One key treatment consideration in the management of daytime sleepiness among older adults is to address primary sleep disorders that disrupt nighttime sleep. One such example is a randomized controlled trial of the effect of treatment of sleep apnea on daytime functioning in patients with Alzhiemer's disease. Three weeks of sleep apnea treatment resulted in a decrease in daytime sleepiness, as reported by the patient and/or the patient's caregiver, as compared to sham treatment [17].

A second important consideration is the use of sedating medications during the daytime hours. Often adjusting the timing of the sedating medication or the dose of the medication can result in less daytime sleepiness [11]. To our knowledge, there have been no studies of pharmacotherapy specifically for treating daytime sleepiness among older adults. There is a need for studies of wake-promoting agents (e.g. armodafinil, modafinil) as a treatment for daytime sleepiness among older adults, particularly among those whose sleepiness cannot be managed in other effective ways and where the sleepiness leads to impairment in daytime functioning.

Daytime sleepiness in dementia

Studies show that patients with dementia, particularly with Alzheimer's disease (AD), commonly suffer from daytime sleepiness. In a study using wrist actigraphy in over 200 nursing home residents, Ancoli-Israel *et al.* found that those with severe dementia spent 29% of the day napping, while those with mild-moderate dementia slept for 15% of the day [18]. In a study of 492 nursing home patients, Martin *et al.* found that 69% slept excessively during the day (based on being observed asleep >15% of the time from 9am to 5pm) and that 60% of this same group had disturbed sleep at night [19].

Causes of daytime sleepiness in dementia

In general, many of the causes of daytime sleepiness among patients with dementia are the same as those for older adults without dementia, such as primary sleep disorders, depression, and medical conditions and their treatments. Among patients with dementia, however, there are additional considerations. In particular, psychotropic medications used to manage behavioral symptoms (e.g. sedating antipsychotics, anxiolytics) can cause severe daytime sleepiness. Lack of social engagement can lead to daytime napping and dozing that perpetuates a cycle of excessive sleepiness during the daytime hours. All these factors need to be considered when treating patients with dementia living in institutional settings.

Consequences of daytime sleepiness in dementia

Perhaps one of the most noticeable consequences of daytime sleepiness among patients with dementia is the disruption of the sleep/wake cycle, due in part to increased daytime napping/dozing. Unlike older adults without dementia, patients with dementia, and particularly patients with AD, may confuse day and night, sleep for extended periods during the daytime hours, and therefore spend extended periods awake at night. This can then become a circular phenomenon where daytime sleepiness is increased by the fragmentation of nighttime sleep, leading to nighttime confusion, wandering, and increased caregiver burden at night.

Daytime sleepiness among AD patients is also associated with functional limitations. Among patients with AD, EDS appears to be independent of the degree of cognitive decline, but is related to functional limitations [20]. This is particularly important as functional impairment results in higher caregiver burden, and may contribute to institutionalization or increase the need for home-based services for persons with AD.

Treatment of daytime sleepiness in dementia

Studies show that increased exposure to bright light, particularly when combined with efforts to reduce time in bed during the day, may be an effective method for decreasing daytime sleepiness. To date, most studies of bright light therapy have been carried out in institutional settings, primarily nursing homes. In one randomized controlled trial of a multi-component non-pharmacological intervention on sleep in nursing homes, Alessi *et al.* found that the intervention reduced daytime sleeping (based on behavioral observations of sleep) by 11% with an increase of 2% in the usual-care control condition [21]. Other randomized controlled trials of light exposure, however, have not found improvements in daytime sleepiness among older adults in nursing homes [22–25].

Napping

A full discussion of daytime sleepiness among older adults must consider age-related changes in napping behavior. The general trends show that napping frequency and duration increase with age [26–30]. Reported prevalence rates for habitual daytime napping in elderly populations range from 22 to 61%, with some studies showing gender differences in napping patterns among older adults [31, 32]. In one survey of over 1500 older adults over the age of 55 years, 15% of respondents reported regular napping, ranging from 10% among those 55–64 years to 25% among those 75–84 years. Older age was strongly associated with EDS, as was depression, bodily pain, and nocturia [33].

In a study comparing daytime napping and 24-h sleep–wake patterns in healthy elderly (mean age 83 years) and young adults (mean age 25 years), elderly subjects reported a significantly greater mean number of daytime naps over a 2-week period (3.4 vs. 1.1 among young subjects; $p < 0.004$) with 64% of the elderly group, but only 45% of the younger group taking any naps during the 2-week study period [29]. Furthermore, the elderly subjects took naps most frequently around 2:30 pm, whereas young adults showed no distinct pattern. Results of studies examining napping patterns in "old old" and "young old" subjects indicated that napping tendency continued to increase with age [34]. The 2003 National Sleep Foundation survey found that 10% of respondents aged 55–64 years reported taking naps regularly (4–7 times/week), compared with 24% of respondents aged 75–84 years [26].

Clearly, napping may simply be a lifestyle choice based upon changes in daily work habits and family responsibilities, and studies are mixed in terms of the relationship between daytime napping and nighttime sleep disruption. Some studies have found a relationship between napping and symptoms of insomnia [32, 35, 36], sleep fragmentation [37, 38], poor sleep quality [39], and circadian rhythm disturbances [37, 40]. In a study of over 200 older men and women, those with more sleep fragmentation (as measured with actigraphy) were at greater risk for taking a nap the following day [41], suggesting that naps may indeed be a reflection of daytime sleepiness associated with poor nighttime sleep. Nonetheless, other studies failed to find a relationship between daytime napping and sleep disruption at night [29, 31, 42–45]. Some of the studies that failed to find a relationship, however, were small, and statistical power may have limited the ability to detect a relationship statistically.

Taken together, these findings support the relationship between nocturnal sleep disruption and daytime napping, with napping representing an attempt to compensate for problematic daytime sleepiness; however, given the correlational nature of most studies, this conclusion cannot be firmly drawn, and napping itself is not sufficient evidence to assume an older adult suffers from nighttime sleep disturbance or pathological daytime sleepiness.

The napping controversy

Negative consequences of napping

While napping might be seen as a normal behavior, at times it could be a sign of pathology with negative health consequences. Several studies have found a relationship between daytime napping and negative health outcomes such as hypertension, cardiovascular disease, diabetes, falls, and mortality.

In a large epidemiological study of over 8000 older women, those who reported napping daily had significantly higher odds of suffering two or more falls during the subsequent year than women who did not nap daily, even after adjusting for multiple other confounders [46]. Xu et al. studied over 10,000 older adults and found that longer naps were associated with a higher risk of diabetes [47]. A case-control study in a middle-aged Costa Rican population (mean age 57 years) found a significant trend toward taking long daily siestas (defined as afternoon nap or rest) and increased risk of myocardial infarction (MI), compared with taking a siesta less than once per week, even after adjusting for cardiovascular disease risk factors (including lipids, smoking, body mass index, light physical activity, night sleep, and history of diabetes, hypertension, and angina) [48]. The prevalence of daily siestas among MI survivors was 44%, compared with 35% in controls. This study, however, did not analyze the association between actual daytime sleep (i.e. naps) and MI risk, and did not control for depression or dementia, both of which may be confounding variables.

On the other hand, Trichopoulos et al. reported a 30% reduction in incidence of non-fatal coronary heart disease (CHD) events in association with 30-min naps [49], and Kalandidi et al. reported that the duration of siesta (afternoon rest or sleep) was negatively related to risk of CHD events [50]. However, the latter study did not establish a clear association between napping and CHD risk.

There have been several large-scale prospective studies that specifically examined the risk of mortality associated with daytime napping in the elderly. These studies showed a significant increase in risk of mortality in subjects who napped. Hays et al. reported a 4-year mortality rate of 24% among frequent nappers versus 15% among infrequent nappers [51]. The 4-year mortality risk was higher particularly in frequent nappers with moderate or severe cognitive impairment, relative to infrequent nappers or non-nappers (Odds Ratio, 1.73; 95% CI, 1.24–2.41). Three other studies using the same prospective dataset found a twofold increase in risk of mortality among nappers relative to non-nappers, even after adjusting for traditional cardiovascular disease risk factors and after 12 years of follow-up [52–55]. In this series of studies, napping (siestas) appeared to be uniquely associated with mortality, with a stronger association in men than women. There was a higher prevalence of napping among MI survivors (78% vs. 58% among those without previous MIs; $p = 0.009$), and after controlling for the presence/absence of previous MIs, napping was still associated with increased mortality risk (Odds Ratio, 1.78; 95% CI, 1.0–3.2). The association remained significant (and double that of non-nappers) in multivariate analysis. When subjects were stratified according to daytime napping, daytime resting without napping (i.e. ceased strenuous activity without sleeping), or no daytime napping or resting, the 6-year mortality rate for those who napped was more than double the rate for those who neither napped nor rested without sleeping (19.0% vs. 9.5%, respectively); the rate for those who only rested was 10.9% ($p < 0.02$). Furthermore, the mortality risk for those who napped more than 1 h was more than twice as high as those who only rested (Odds Ratio, 2.6; 95% CI, 1.14–6.23), and almost 4 times higher than those who neither napped nor rested (Odds Ratio, 3.68; 95% CI, 1.36–9.92). The mortality rate in men who napped for less than 1 h was 14%, compared with 28% in men who napped for 1 h or more ($p = 0.02$). In multivariate analysis incorporating conventional risk factors, duration of daytime sleep was significantly associated with mortality for men ($p = 0.02$). Although duration of naps as a continuous variable was not predictive of mortality for women, women who napped for less than 1 h and those who napped for 1–2 h had over 4 times and 5 times, respectively, increases in mortality risk (Odds Ratios of 4.67 and 5.57, respectively). After 12-years of follow-up, results showed that 74% of those not napping regularly survived compared to only 64% who regularly took naps ($p < 0.01$). These results extended the finding of the 6-year observations.

As part of the large epidemiological studies by Stone et al. described above, napping was also associated with increased risk of shorter survival. Women who reported napping daily were 44% more likely to die from any cause, 58% more likely to die from cardiovascular causes and 59% more likely to die from non-cardiovascular non-cancer causes than women who did not nap daily [56]. In another cohort of 5888 elderly subjects, Newman et al. observed a significant association between daytime sleepiness complaints and mortality (unadjusted hazard ratio of 1.71) [15].

The mortality findings associated with daytime napping have been interpreted in several ways. First, the association between mortality and daytime napping suggests that napping may be a marker of excessive daytime sleepiness, a problem associated with negative outcomes [54], rather than as a simple compensatory strategy for a restricted night's sleep. Consequently, some have hypothesized that excessive daytime sleepiness may result from the presence of an underlying sleep disorder [53]. As mentioned above, conventional wisdom suggests that a number of older individuals with excessive daytime sleepiness may have undetected sleep apnea, a condition with a clear age- and gender-related differential prevalence that is linked strongly to increased cardiovascular risk [57, 58]. While this may partially explain the relationship between daytime napping and mortality, some studies found no association between snoring (a cardinal symptom of sleep apnea) or body mass index (a risk factor for sleep apnea) and napping-related mortality [52, 53].

One causal hypothesis suggests that the increased heart rate and blood pressure observed directly after the onset of daytime napping is similar to the changes seen upon morning awakening [59]. These morning heart-related changes have been linked to increased MI and other acute cardiovascular events [59, 60]. Increased heart rate and blood pressure result in increased myocardial oxygen demand, which subsequently may act as a trigger for cardiovascular events in the morning after awakening and in the afternoon after napping cessation. Bursztyn et al. further hypothesized that arousal from afternoon napping may result in an abrupt surge of sympathetic nervous system activity [53], triggering hemodynamic changes (e.g. increased myocardial oxygen demand and brain vascular shear stress precipitated by abrupt elevation of blood pressure and heart rate upon awakening), as well as thrombogenic changes that may contribute to cardiovascular events [61]. Further, the rapid increase in myocardial oxygen demand immediately after a 2-h rest (not necessarily resulting in sleep) appears similar in magnitude to the increase observed after morning awakening in healthy young adults [60, 62]. This finding suggests that arousal from afternoon napping, like morning arousal, may result in a period of increased cardiovascular risk [60]. There is preliminary evidence, however, that the changes in heart rate upon arousal from napping are negligible, suggesting lesser potential for ischemia compared with the morning hours soon after arousal [59, 60]. It is difficult to determine, however, whether napping-related hemodynamic changes directly contribute to mortality risk or whether the overlap in risk factors for these two conditions accounts for the observed relationships. Daytime sleepiness and napping may be directly caused by medical illnesses (and medications used to manage cardiovascular risk factors), resulting in the observed link between napping and mortality. Further research using objective measures of both sleep apnea and daytime sleepiness are needed.

On the other hand, it is plausible that long daytime sleep may play a direct role in enhancing the risk of mortality by, for example, changing the secretion of hormones, altering inflammatory mechanisms, and creating a mismatch across biological systems. If a causal relationship between napping and mortality exists, then napping would represent a lifestyle factor that could be modified with interventions similar to diet, exercise, or smoking. To date, however, possible mechanisms suggesting a causal relationship between daytime sleeping and mortality have not been established.

Beneficial effects of napping

Whether napping is beneficial or detrimental for older adults is controversial, as both positive and negative effects have been reported. To date, research with younger adults (e.g. shift workers, long-distance drivers) has suggested beneficial effects of napping on performance and alertness [63, 64]. In elderly adults, beneficial effects of napping include improvement in objective [63], and subjective evening sleepiness [64], as well as in performance [62]. One study found that an afternoon nap (1.30–3.00pm, average of 57 min of sleep per nap) was associated with a significant increase in mean sleep latency on the Multiple Sleep Latency Test (from 11.5 to 15.6 minutes; $p < 0.01$), indicating a significant decrease in objective evening sleepiness. However, napping had no effect on subjective evening alertness or on measures of evening performance (visual vigilance, manual dexterity, and response time), relative to no napping [63]. In a second study, Tamaki et al. found that a short nap (30 min) decreased subjective sleepiness among habitual nappers [65]. In a polysomnographic laboratory study of naps in 32 healthy older adults, Campbell et al. found that an afternoon nap (mean nap time 81 min) had no negative effect on subsequent nighttime sleep, but did result in a significant increase in total sleep time per 24-h and enhanced cognitive and psychomotor performance immediately after the nap and throughout the next day [62].

Conclusion

Studies suggest that a significant minority of older adults suffer from excessive daytime sleepiness. The causes of this sleepiness are likely to differ across individuals, with nighttime sleep disorders, medical conditions, and medications likely culprits. Few studies have attempted to directly treat daytime sleepiness among older adults; however, available research suggests that treatment of nighttime sleep disorders leads to a decrease in daytime sleepiness, and there is some evidence that the lifestyle changes associated with retirement may increase daytime sleeping among older people. Among individuals with dementia, daytime sleepiness is an even more significant problem, and treatment remains a challenge, although behavioral interventions do show some promise. It remains controversial whether napping is a cause or consequence of daytime sleepiness, and results are mixed in terms of whether napping is harmful or beneficial for older persons. Further research is needed to examine the underlying pathways linking daytime sleepiness to increased mortality, poor health and functional decline among older adults and to explore treatments that will reduce sleepiness and improve quality of life.

Acknowledgment

Supported by NIA AG08415 (SAI); NIA K23 AG028452 (Martin).

References

1. **Johns M W**. Daytime sleepiness, snoring, and obstructive sleep apnea. The Epworth Sleepiness Scale. *Chest*, 1993; **103**:30–36.
2. **Martin J L, Ancoli-Israel, S**. Napping in older adults. *Sleep Med Clin*, 2006; **1**:177–86.
3. **Bixler E O, Vgontzas A N, Lin H M**, et al. Excessive daytime sleepiness in a general population sample: the role of sleep apnea, age, obesity, diabetes, and depression. *J Clin Endocrinol Metab*, 2005; **90**:4510–15.
4. **Soldatos C R, Allaert F A, Ohta T**, et al. How do individuals sleep around the world? Results from a single-day survey in ten countries. *Sleep Med*, 2005; **6**:5–13.
5. **Chasens E R, Sereika S M, Weaver T E**, et al. Daytime sleepiness, exercise, and physical function in older adults. *J Sleep Res*, 2007; **16**:60–65.
6. **Hoch C C, Reynolds C F I, Jennings R J**, et al. Daytime sleepiness and performance among healthy 80 and 20 year olds. *Neurobiol Aging*, 1992; **13**:353.
7. **Ancoli-Israel S, Kripke D F, Klauber M R**, et al. Sleep disordered breathing in community-dwelling elderly. *Sleep*, 1991; **14**:486–95.
8. **Mehra R, Stone K L, Blackwell T**, et al. Prevalence and correlates of sleep-disordered breathing in older men: MrOS sleep study. *J Am Geriatr Soc*, 2007; **55**:1356–64.
9. **Ancoli-Israel S, Kripke D F, Klauber M R** et al. Periodic limb movements in sleep in community-dwelling elderly. *Sleep*, 1991; **14**:496–500.
10. **Claman D M, Redline S S, Blackwell T**, et al. Prevalence and correlates of periodic limb movements in older women. *J Clin Sleep Med*, 2006; **2**:438–45.
11. **Ancoli-Israel S**. Insomnia in the elderly: a review for the primary care practitioner. *Sleep*, 2000; **23**:S23–30.
12. **Goldstein I, Ancoli-Israel S, Shapiro D**. Relationship between daytime sleepiness and blood pressure in healthy older people. *Am J Hypertens*, 2004; **17**:787–92.
13. **Chasens E R, Sereika S M, Burke L E**. Daytime sleepiness and functional outcomes in older adults with diabetes. *Diabetes Educ*, 2009; **35**:455–64.
14. **Webb A R, Aber W R**. Relationship between sleep and retirement–nonretirement status. *Int J Human Devpt*, 1985; **20**:13–19.
15. **Newman A B, Spiekerman C F, Enright P**, et al. Daytime sleepiness predicts mortality and cardiovascular disease in older adults. The Cardiovascular Health Study Research Group. *J Am Geriatr Soc*, 2000; **48**:115–23.
16. **Alessi C A, Martin J L, Webber A P**, et al. More daytime sleeping predicts less functional recovery among older people undergoing inpatient post-acute rehabilitation. *Sleep*, 2008; **31**:1291–300.
17. **Chong M S, Ayalon L, Marler, M**, et al. Continuous positive airway pressure reduces subjective daytime sleepiness in patients with mild to moderate Alzheimer's disease with sleep disordered breathing. *J Am Geriatr Soc*, 2006; **54**:777–81.
18. **Ancoli-Israel S, Klauber M R, Jones D W**, et al. Variations in circadian rhythms of activity, sleep and light exposure related to dementia in nursing home patients. *Sleep*, 1997; **20**:18–23.
19. **Martin J L, Webber A P, Alam T**, et al. Daytime sleeping, sleep disturbance, and circadian rhythms in the nursing home. *Am J Geriatr Psychiatry*, 2006; **14**:121–29.
20. **Lee J H, Bliwise D L, Ansari F P**, et al. Daytime sleepiness and functional impairment in Alzheimer disease. *Am J Geriatr Psychiatry*, 2007; **15**:620–26.
21. **Alessi C A, Martin J L, Webber A P**, et al. Randomized, controlled trial of a nonpharmacological intervention to improve abnormal sleep/wake patterns

in nursing home residents. *J Am Geriatr Soc*, 2005; **53**:803–10.

22. **Ancoli-Israel S, Martin J L, Gehrman P**, *et al*. Effect of light on agitation in institutionalized patients with severe Alzheimer's disease. *Am J Geriatr Psychiatry*, 2003; **11**:194–203.

23. **Ancoli-Israel S, Martin J L, Kripke D F**, *et al*. Effect of light treatment on sleep and circadian rhythms in demented nursing home patients. *J Am Geriatr Soc*, 2002; **50**:282–89.

24. **Hale T S, Hariri A R, McCracken J T**. Attention-deficit hyperactivity disorder: perspectives from neuroimaging. *Mental Retard Devptl Disabil Res Rev*, 2000; **6**:214–19.

25. **Sloane P D, Williams C S, Mitchell C M**, *et al*. High-intensity environmental light in dementia: effect on sleep and activity. *J Am Geriatr Soc*, 2007; **55**:1524–33.

26. **National Sleep Foundation** 2003 Sleep in America Poll. Retrieved from: http://www.sleepfoundation.org/site/c.huIXKjM0IxF/b.2422247/k.146C/2003_Sleep_in_America_Poll.htm.

27. **Metz M E, Bunnell D E**. Napping and sleep disturbance in the elderly. *Fam Pract Res J*, 1990; **10**:47–56.

28. **Ancoli-Israel S, Klauber M R, Gillin J C**, *et al*. Sleep in non-institutionalized Alzheimer's disease patients. *Aging Clin Exp Res*, 1994; **6**:451–58.

29. **Buysse D J, Browman K E, Monk T H**, *et al*. Napping and 24-hour sleep/wake patterns in healthy elderly and young adults. *J Am Geriatr Soc*, 1992; **40**:779–86.

30. **Dinges D F**. Napping patterns and effects in human adults. In: Dinges D F, Broughton R J, Eds. *Sleep and Alertness: Chronobiological, Behavioral and Medical Aspects of Napping*. New York, NY: Raven Press, 1989: 171–204.

31. **Mallon L, Hetta J**. A survey of sleep habits and sleeping difficulties in an elderly Swedish population. *Upsala J Med Sci*, 1997; **102**:185–97.

32. **Gislason T, Reynisdottir H, Kristbjarnarson H**, *et al*. Sleep habits and sleep disturbances among the elderly – an epidemiological survey. *J Intern Med*, 1993; **234**:31.

33. **Foley D J, Vitiello M V, Bliwise D L**, *et al*. Frequent napping is associated with excessive daytime sleepiness, depression, pain, and nocturia in older adults: findings from the National Sleep Foundation '2003 Sleep in America' poll. *Am J Geriatr Psychiatry*, 2007; **15**:344–50.

34. **Reynolds C F I, Jennings R J, Hoch C C**, *et al*. Daytime sleepiness in the healthy "old old": a comparison with young adults. *J Am Geriatr Soc*, 1991; **39**:957–62.

35. **Carskadon M A, Brown E D, Dement W C**. Sleep fragmentation in the elderly: relationship to daytime sleep tendency. *Neurobiol Aging*, 1982; **3**:321–27.

36. **Frisoni G B, De Leo D, Rozzini R**, *et al*. Napping in the elderly and its association with night sleep and psychological status. *Int Psychogeriatr* 1996; **8**:477–87.

37. **Ancoli-Israel S, Kripke D F**. Prevalent sleep problems in the aged. *Biofeedb Self-Regul*, 1991; **16**:349–59.

38. **Ohayon M M, Caulet M, Philip P**, *et al*. How sleep and mental disorders are related to complaints of daytime sleepiness. *Arch Intern Med*, 1997; **157**:2645–52.

39. **Pilcher J J, Schoeling S E, Prosansky C M**. Self-report sleep habits as predictors of subjective sleepiness. *Behav Med*, 2000; **25**:161–68.

40. **Yoon I Y, Kripke D F, Youngstedt S D**, *et al*. Actigraphy suggests age-related differences in napping and nocturnal sleep. *J Sleep Res*, 2003; **12**:87–93.

41. **Goldman S E, Hall M, Boudreau R**, *et al*. Association between nighttime sleep and napping in older adults. *Sleep*, 2008; **31**:733–40.

42. **Asplund R**. Sleep disorders in the elderly. *Drugs Aging*, 1999; **14**:91–103.

43. **Wauquier A, Van Sweden B, Lagaay A M**, *et al*. Ambulatory monitoring of sleep wakefulness patterns in healthy elderly males and females (>88 years): The "Senieur" protocol. *J Am Geriatr Soc*, 1992; **40**:109–14.

44. **Morin C M, Gramling S E**. Sleep patterns and aging: comparison of older adults with and without insomnia complaints. *Psychol Aging*, 1989; 4:290–94.

45. **Bliwise N G**. Factors related to sleep quality in healthy elderly women. *Psychol Aging*, 1992; **7**:83–88.

46. **Stone K L, Ewing S K, Lui L Y**, *et al*. Self-reported sleep and nap habits and risk of falls and fractures in older women: the study of osteoporotic fractures. *J Am Geriatr Soc*, 2006; **54**:1177–83.

47. **Xu Q, Song Y, Hollenbeck A**, *et al*. Day napping and short night sleeping are associated with higher risk of diabetes in older adults. *Diabetes Care*, 2010; **33**:78–83.

48. **Campos H, Siles X**. Siesta and the risk of coronary heart disease: results from a population-based, case-control study in Costa Rica. *Int J Epidemiol*, 2000; **29**:429–37.

49. **Trichopoulos D, Tzonou A, Christopoulos C**, *et al*. Does a siesta protect from coronary heart disease? *Lancet*, 1987; **2**:269–70.

50. **Kalandidi A, Tzonou A, Toupadaki N**, *et al*. A case-control study of coronary heart disease in Athens, Greece. *Int J Epidemiol*, 1992; **21**:1074–80.

51. **Hays J C, Blazer D G, Foley D J**. Risk of napping: excessive daytime sleepiness and mortality in an older

community population. *J Am Geriatr Soc*, 1996; **44**:693–98.

52. **Bursztyn M**, **Ginsberg G**, **Stessman J**. The siesta and mortality in the elderly: effect of rest without sleep and daytime sleep duration. *Sleep*, 2002; **25**:187–91.

53. **Bursztyn M**, **Ginsberg G**, **Hammerman-Rozenberg R**, *et al*. The siesta in the elderly: risk factor for mortality? *Arch Intern Med*, 1999; **159**:1582–86.

54. **Bursztyn M**, **Stressman J**. The siesta and mortality: twelve years of prospective observations in 70-year-olds. *Sleep*, 2005; **28**:345–47.

55. **Burazeri G**, **Gofin J**, **Kark J D**. Siesta and mortality in a Mediterranean population: a community study in Jerusalem. *Sleep*, 2003; **26**:578–84.

56. **Stone K L**, **Ewing S K**, **Ancoli-Israel S**, *et al*. Self-reported sleep and nap habits and risk of mortality in a large cohort of older women. *J Am Geriatr Soc*, 2009; **57**:604–11.

57. **Wroe S J**, **Sandercock P**, **Bamford J**, *et al*. Diurnal variation in incidence of stroke – Oxfordshire community stroke project. *BMJ*, 1992; **304**:155.

58. **Behar S**, **Halabi M**, **Reicher-Reiss H**, *et al*. Circadian variation and possible external triggers of onset of myocardial infarction. *Am J Med*, 1993; **94**:395–400.

59. **Somers V K**, **Dyken M E**, **Mark A L**, *et al*. Sympathetic-nerve activity during sleep in normal subjects. *N Engl J Med*, 1993; **328**:303–07.

60. **Mulcahy D**, **Wright C**, **Sparrow J**, *et al*. Heart rate and blood pressure consequences of an afternoon SIESTA (Snooze-Induced Excitation of Sympathetic Triggered Activity). *Am J Cardiology*, 1993; **7**:611–14.

61. **Bursztyn M**, **Mekler J**, **Ben-Ishay D**. The siesta and ambulatory blood pressure: is waking up the same in the morning and the afternoon? *J Human Hypertens*, 1996; **10**:287–92.

62. **Campbell S S**, **Murphy P J**, **Stauble T N**. Effects of a nap on nighttime sleep and waking function in older subjects. *J Am Geriatr Soc*, 2005; **53**:48–53.

63. **Monk T H**, **Buysse D J**, **Carrier J**, *et al*. Effects of afternoon "siesta" naps on sleep, alertness, performance, and circadian rhythms in the elderly. *Sleep*, 2001; **24**:680–87.

64. **Tamaki M**, **Shirota A**, **Tanaka H**, *et al*. Effects of a daytime nap in the aged. *Psychiatry Clin Neurosci*, 1999; **53**:273–75.

65. **Tamaki M**, **Shirota A**, **Hayashi M**, *et al*. Restorative effects of a short afternoon nap (<30 min) in the elderly on subjective mood, performance and EEG activity. *Sleep Res On Line* 2000; **3**:131–39.

Section 3 Chapter 27

Medical, Psychiatric and Neurological Causes of Sleepiness

Excessive daytime sleepiness in Parkinson's disease

David B. Rye

Excessive sleepiness in PD

Dopamine cell death attending Parkinson's disease (PD) profoundly alters the sleep–wake state which can be classified into disturbances of: (1) nocturnal movement, and (2) thalamocortical arousal state. The former includes periodic limb movements of sleep (PLMS) and rapid-eye-movement (REM) sleep behavior disorder (RBD) [1]. The latter includes loss of sleep-spindles and slow-wave sleep, long sleep periods, microsleeps, excessive daytime sleepiness, and intrusion of REM sleep into daytime naps (sleep onset REM sleep (SOREMs)) [2, 3]. The initial report of dose-related "sleep attacks" with pramipexole and ropinirole was interpreted as a novel, idiosyncratic response unique to non-ergot D_2/D_3 receptor agonists [4]. This report heightened awareness to complaints of sleepiness in PD patients and has prompted a critical reappraisal of the underlying contributing factors, including the potential role of medications. Sleepiness in PD is common, real, increasingly recognized, and has garnered significant attention and investigation as detailed in multiple reviews [5–9]. By self-report, 10–75% of PD patients experience unintended sleep episodes or sleepiness that interfere with activities of daily living [10–14]. Nearly half of these meet physiological criteria for the prototypical disorder of sudden-onset of sleep – narcolepsy [3]. Clinical experience and more comprehensive assessments agree that sleepiness has long been under-recognized in PD and that it is a phenomenon not restricted to a specific class of dopaminomimetics [10, 15–17].

In community-based samples of PD patients, sleepiness affects from 7 to 14% as compared to 1–2% of healthy, elderly controls [11, 18], and increases at a rate of ~6% per year [19]. In specialized movement disorder clinic-based samples, the rate is much higher (20–76%) [10, 12, 15, 20, 21]. Employing the multiple sleep latency test (MSLT; see below), a standardized measure of physiological sleep tendency across five daytime nap opportunities, "pathological" sleepiness has been documented in 20–50% of patients, and a narcolepsy-like phenotype in 15–50% of these (mean sleep latency (MSL) <8 min and ≥2 daytime naps with REM sleep) [2, 3, 22–26]. In the majority, but not all [23], studies, physiological impairments in arousal state bear little relationship to the primary *motor* manifestations of disease (e.g. disease and treatment duration, and disability scales), or sleep architecture measures (e.g. total sleep time, stage %, etc.). In several studies impaired arousal (namely, "sleepiness") is associated with a greater dopaminergic drug load, thereby confirming empirical clinical experience [22, 23, 27]. Contrary to what one would expect based upon the demands of sleep homeostatic mechanisms, poor nocturnal sleep in PD is typically associated with greater, rather than lesser, degrees of daytime alertness. Simply stated, sleepiness in PD is unlikely reflective of inadequate sleep amounts or quality, but rather, it is intrinsic to the disease and its treatment. This point is best made by continuous electrophysiological recordings of PD subjects complaining of sleepiness. These paint a more naturalistic picture that includes "microsleeps", daytime napping, and excessive 24-h total sleep times [28–30]. It therefore appears that parkinsonian-related daytime sleepiness occurs against a backdrop of genuine "hypersommnia", quite in-line with the phenotypes observed in several animal models in which dopaminergic signaling is disrupted (see below).

Dissociation of arousal state from the motor manifestations of disease and homeostatic sleep drives (namely, sleep propensity should be inversely rather than positively correlated with the quantity and quality of prior night's sleep) in PD has several implications.

Sleepiness: Causes, Consequences and Treatment, ed. Michael J. Thorpy and Michel Billiard. Published by Cambridge University Press. © Cambridge University Press 2011.

First, it emphasizes that the integrity of dopaminergic pathways or exogenous dopaminomimetic drugs interfere with normal homeostatic sleep mechanisms. Second, it points to the pathophysiological basis of impaired thalamocortical arousal state residing outside of the nigrostriatal circuits traditionally thought to underlie parkinsonian *motor* disabilities. A threshold of 60–90% of dopamine loss in the sensorimotor putamen is necessary for the emergence of waking clinical manifestations [31], and then proceeds in an orderly fashion through associative (i.e. caudate), and eventually limbic (i.e. nucleus accumbens) striatal subcircuits. Thus, it is loss of dopamine in these latter circuits, most characteristic of advanced disease, that is a potential factor in the narcolepsy-like phenotype discussed above.

Dopamine and behavioral state control: insights from basic science

As cell loss in the dopamine-rich substantia nigra is the pathological hallmark of parkinsonian conditions, a brief discussion of dopamine's modulation of wake–sleep states is a prerequisite to considerations of the pathophysiological basis of the sleepiness that attends parkinsonism. A comprehensive accounting in a recent volume includes a more in-depth discussion and complete bibliography [32].

Dopamine's physiological effects are best characterized as "neuromodulatory". Rather than eliciting excitatory or inhibitory post-synaptic potentials, dopamine gates inputs via altering membrane properties and specific ion conductances [33]. This manifests as different intensities, durations, and timings of neural output commensurate with environmental and homeostatic demands. Dopamine acts by way of five subtypes of seven transmembrane domain G-protein coupled receptors (D1–D5) which based upon similarities in pharmacology, biochemistry, and amino acid homology are divided into two classes, D_{1-like} (D_1, D_5) and D_{2-like} (D_2, D_3, D_4) [34]. Ligand binding studies estimate the average K_d of dopamine for its receptors to be (in nM); D_3, 55; D_4, 209; D_2, 892; and D_1, 6500 (and hence, the order of affinity for endogenous dopamine is $D_3 > D_4 > D_2 \gg D_1$) [average of values obtained from references provided by a search of http://pdsp.cwru.edu/stestw.asp]. Both D_{1-like} and D_{2-like} receptors are found post-synaptically on neurons targeted by dopaminergic axons. D_{2-like} receptors are also localized presynaptically on dendrites and soma, and the terminals of dopaminergic cells, functioning as autoreceptors that regulate neural firing and the synthesis and release of dopamine, respectively [35]. Each receptor subtype has a unique pattern of brain localization. Indirect effects upon arousal may occur via receptors present on endothelial cells where dopamine promotes vasoconstriction of the brain's microvasculature.

The mesocortical, mesolimbic, and mesostriatal systems are the most conspicuous of the brain's dopamine circuits, and are thought to govern cognition, emotion, and movement, respectively. Historically, state-related mean discharge rates of mesencephalic dopaminergic neurons were thought to vary little across state and this dealt a blow to considerations of dopamine as a player in arousal state regulation. As previously detailed [32], these studies failed to appreciate variances in interspike intervals (e.g. a burst firing pattern) recently rediscovered in ventral tegmental area (VTA) neurons prior to and during REM sleep [36]. Synaptic dopamine release is more efficiently driven by such "burst firing" [37], and is modulated by afferents from brain regions intimately involved in thalamocortical arousal (i.e. wake and REM sleep) [38]. Additional anatomical and physiological evidence highlight that midbrain dopamine neurons do indeed mediate thalamocortical arousal. Excitatory inputs originate from the bed nucleus of the stria terminalis and central nucleus of the amygdala, hypothalamic hypocretin (i.e. orexin) neurons, glutamatergic and cholinergic pedunculopontine tegmental (PPN) neurons, medullary, noradrenergic A1 and A2, and pontine A4–A5 (locus coeruleus; LC) neurons, and act via multiple glutamate receptor subtypes, hypocretin-2, muscarinic, nicotinic, and α_1-adrenoreceptors. Serotonergic inputs from the dorsal raphe have complex effects that are generally inhibitory and predominate in mesocorticolimbic versus nigrostriatal dopamine neurons. Dopaminergic "tone" is also influenced by local GABA-ergic neurons that themselves appear to modulate wake and REM sleep [39].

Outputs from midbrain dopaminergic neurons are diverse and can affect thalamocortical arousal both directly and indirectly. An extensive set of thalamic collaterals originate from traditional nigrostriatal and mesocorticolimbic pathways. Because at least half of A8–A9–A10 neurons simultaneously target the thalamus and striatum, the spectrum of disorders thought to arise from midbrain dopamine neuron dysfunction should have an accompanying disturbance of thalamocortical arousal (i.e. sleep/wake state), albeit yet to be extensively characterized or universally appreciated (see [40]). The effects of dopamine upon thalamic physiology are little studied and include both D_{1-like} excitatory effects, D_{2-like} receptor-mediated presynaptic and GABA-ergic interneuron inhibition, and D_4-mediated inhibition of GABA release in the thalamic reticular nucleus where it is strategically positioned to gate all thalamocortical transmission and spindle generation. Indirect effects of midbrain dopamine neurons upon thalamocortical arousal state might also occur by way of output pathways to the ventral forebrain, perifornical hypocretin/orexin and adjacent hypothalamic neurons, and the LC (amongst others). The physiological and behavioral effects of these interactions are incompletely defined and include putative direct and indirect, excitatory and inhibitory effects upon magnocellular cholinergic and perifornical hypocretin/orexin neurons. Dopaminergic innervation of the LC originates from the hypothalamic A11 and A13, and midbrain VTA A10 cell groups, and has been implicated in inhibiting REM sleep and enhancing muscle tone in REM sleep, as well as enhancing slow-wave and REM sleep via α_2-adrenoreceptors [41].

Diurnal rhythms in the content, turnover, release and behavioral responsiveness of the brain's principal dopamine systems are well established. While we are far from a comprehensive understanding of what drives these rhythms, dopamine synthesis, release, and signaling peak early during the active, wake period and nadir early on in sleep. Circadian influences are conveyed in part via melatonin as pinealectomy dampens striatal dopamine rhythms [42], as well as by circadian-related gene products. Increased expression and phosphorylation of tyrosine hydroxylase, and commensurate enhancements in A10 dopaminergic neural activity and associated behaviors, for example, are observed in mice expressing an inactive *Clock* protein [43]. Sleep and REM sleep deprivation also lead to robust changes in the availability of dopamine and the density and affinity of its various receptors in mesotelencephalic circuits.

The most direct assessments of dopaminergic "tone" come from microdialysates collected from the behaving organism. Striatal and prefrontal cortical dopamine rise in anticipation of, and are maintained throughout, the major wake period of the rat in concert with declines in dopamine metabolites. This pattern is mirrored by tissue contents of: (1) whole brain, striatal, cerebellar, cortical, hippocampal, midbrain, and brainstem dopamine contents; (2) tyrosine hydroxylase and tetrahydrobiopterin (both necessary for dopamine synthesis); and (3) the dopamine transporter (DAT) (a principal determinant of synaptic dopamine availability). These rhythms appear to be more pronounced in "limbic" as opposed to "motor" subcircuits, although this remains somewhat controversial. Time of day also influences the kinetics of L-DOPA metabolism (clearance being highest early in wake), and receptor activation in species as diverse as fruit flies [44] and humans [45].

In non-human primates and humans, diurnal dopamine rhythms are present in the brain, cerebrospinal fluid (CSF), plasma, and urine, and are generally concordant with those observed in rodents. Seminal studies of post-mortem hypothalamic tissue reveal a peak in dopamine content during the active period, 1500–1800 h, with a nadir in the early morning hours. Dopamine content in the lumbar CSF [46], urine, and plasma peak at 0800–1000 h and nadir at 0400–0600 h. Similar patterns are evident for extracellular dopamine in dialysates from the amygdala and adjacent limbic cortex of humans and the putamen of non-human primates [47]. Afternoon and end-of-day dips in extracellular dopamine coincide with 10–20% reductions in D_{1-like} receptor density in the putamen and frontal cortex in humans. The functional significance of these rhythms remains to be determined. More comprehensive analyses that include sleep deprivation and constant environmental conditions are needed in order to tease out the interrelationships between dopamine and homeostatic and circadian alerting signals.

There is a paucity of data on the release of dopamine during specific sleep states. Negative findings are difficult to interpret given the temporal and spatial limitations of microdialysis, and the real possibility for species and regional brain differences in dopamine release. Dopamine in the feline caudate assessed by voltammetry – whose temporal resolution is superior to that of microdialysis – fluctuates between sleep states, while microdialysates from the feline amygdala and locus coeruleus are unrevealing. Dopamine release in the more densely innervated medial prefrontal cortex and nucleus accumbens of the rat is highest in wake and REM sleep. In the rhesus monkey putamen and human limbic brain regions, discernable fluctuations in dopamine in relation to specific sleep stages are undetectable by microdialysis.

The regional and molecular substrates mediating dopamine's effects upon the sleep–wake continuum derive from: (1) the systemic administration of receptor-specific agents; (2) focal pharmacological manipulations and lesioning paradigms; (3) molecular engineering in flies and mice; and (4) animal models of disease. The proportion of time spent awake or asleep is greatly influenced by pharmacological agents that target molecules that modulate dopamine signaling. Because of differential regional expression in the central *and* peripheral nervous systems, and binding affinities of the dopamine receptor subtypes, and their pre- versus post-synaptic localizations, the effects of dopaminomimetics upon sleep–wake state are complex. Strategies to untangle this complexity have included systemic, intracerebroventricular, or focal brain delivery of pharmacological agents that activate or inactivate, more or less selectively, the individual pharmacologically and molecularly defined dopamine receptors. More recent paradigms include genetic engineering of some of the molecules involved in dopamine signaling. These studies tell a compelling story that dopamine is essential to normal arousal and rest–activity patterns.

Pharmacological agents that interfere with the primary route of removal of dopamine, namely, presynaptic reuptake via DAT, enhance wake and alpha power in the EEG in proportion to their binding affinities for DAT [48]. Genetically engineered mice lacking DAT exhibit increased activity levels and wake bout lengths, and are immune to the wake-promoting effects of DAT blockers [49]. A genetically engineered lesion rendering DAT inactive in *Drosophila melanogaster* [50] yields a hyperactive mutant appropriately named fumin, whose literal translation from Japanese is "sleepless" [51]. These flies, as well as those with allelic DAT variants [52], spend an increased amount of time in the active (waking) phase. Blockade of dopamine synthesis in wild-type flies either pharmacologically or via genetic manipulation renders them unresponsive to methamphetamine-induced increases in wake-like activity [53].

The wake-promoting actions of dopamine signaling are further supported by consideration of the effects of systemic and focally applied dopaminomimetics upon sleep–wake state. These effects are dose- and receptor-dependent and describe a biphasic dose–response relationship also manifest in many other physiological and behavioral outputs such as locomotion, pain sensitivity, blood pressure, prolactin secretion, oxytocin release, and heart rate [54]. A more detailed discussion of the effects of receptor-specific dopaminomimetics is presented elsewhere [32]. In summary, $D_{1\text{-like}}$ receptors promote wake and suppress slow-wave and REM sleep, while $D_{2\text{-like}}$ receptors promote sleep *and* wake, at low and high levels of endogenous dopamine, respectively. Sleep is mediated via $D_{2\text{-like}}$ inhibitory autoreceptors on the cell bodies or terminal axonal fields of dopaminergic VTA neurons. Local applications of $D_{2\text{-like}}$ receptor antagonists in the VTA, for example, block the sedation provoked by systemic agonists. Wake is promoted by the same VTA and contiguous dopaminergic neurons since amphetamine administered into their ventral forebrain targets initiates and maintains alert waking, and their selective lesioning disrupts wakefulness (see below).

Molecular engineering of murine dopamine receptors provides additional details. Dopamine by way of D_2 receptor modulation of non-visual photic responses in the retina is necessary for light to disrupt circadian rest–activity rhythms (i.e. light "masking" of endogenous circadian rhythms) [55]. Mice lacking a functional D_3 receptor exhibit marked increases in wake (at the expense of slow-wave *and* REM sleep), suggesting that this receptor is necessary for normal sleep and sleep stages [56]. This observation is particularly relevant because low doses of the D_3-preferring agonists promote sleep in rats and humans, and the D_3 receptor is most sensitive to endogenous dopamine (*vide supra*). Wakefulness attributable to dysfunctional D_3 receptors may alternatively be an epiphenomenon of a heightened response to novelty, or decrements in the gating of spinal sensorimotor and autonomic excitability. As wake is a prerequisite for locomotion, and a paucity of locomotion conducive to sleep, dissociating dopamine receptor effects upon arousal state as distinct from those upon locomotion will continue to necessitate simultaneous recording of related behaviors and careful interpretation.

Clinicians have long relied upon the wake-promoting effects of dopaminomimetics inclusive of traditional psychostimulants. Work in mice, rats, non-human primates, and humans are consistent in pointing to dopaminergic neurons of the medial aspects of the midbrain (i.e. the VTA and periaqueductal midline regions) as critical in modulating the quality, quantity, and timing of thalamacortical arousal states – both wake and REM sleep. Excess sleep time with increases in both non-REM and REM sleep lacking observable decrements in locomotion follow selective destruction of dopaminergic midbrain periaqueductal gray neurons [57], whereas lesions of the dopaminergic VTA and the adjacent substantia nigra yield a similar phenotype accompanied by a "non-dipping" heart rate and blood pressure pattern, without the enhancement of REM sleep [58]. These state changes are unique to mesolimbic versus nigrostriatal projections to the striatum (e.g. the nucleus accumbens vs. caudate/putamen) with enhancement of REM sleep being notably robust following selective lesioning of dopaminergic terminal fields [59, 60]. A narcolepsy-like phenotype (i.e. sleepiness and REM sleep intrusion into daytime naps) also occurs in methyl,4-phenyl-1,2,3,6-tetrahydropyridine (MPTP)-induced parkinsonism in non-human primates [5, 61]. Distinct from genuine narcolepsy, however, decrements in alertness encountered with damage to midbrain dopamine cells in the MPTP-treated primate manifests as a genuine hypersomnia – i.e. increased sleep time over 24 h [62]. Temperature, activity, and neuroendocrine rhythms are generally unaffected by "chronic" parkinsonism induced by MPTP in murine and non-human primate models of parkinsonism, and emphasize that midbrain dopaminergic cell groups are intimately involved in homeostatic sleep–wake mechanisms (e.g. process S) as opposed to circadian (C) processes.

Determinants of sleepiness in PD

Consistent with what has been gleaned from the experimental studies reviewed above, findings in a small number of newly diagnosed, unmedicated or young PD patients [2, 63] emphasize that excessive sleepiness with SOREMs are intrinsic to the parkinsonian phenotype. While reductions in striatal DAT binding correlate with subjective measures of sleepiness in early stage PD [64], the precise cellular and subcellular substrates underlying these disease-related signs and symptoms remain enigmatic. These phenomena may reflect loss of dopamine's effects upon neural excitability in any one of a number of brain regions beyond the striatum that are necessary for maintaining normal states of thalamocortical excitability. One plausible substrate, given the narcolepsy-like phenotype seen in nearly half of "sleepy" PD patients, is hypocretin-containing neurons in the lateral hypothalamus known to degenerate in primary narcolepsy with cataplexy [65]. Other plausible neural substrates deserving of future investigation as potential contributors to sleepiness and SOREMs in the setting of dopamine depletion include targets of VTA dopamine neurons such as the prefrontal cortex, the cholinergic magnocellular basal forebrain, and midline thalamic nuclei. Alternatively, sleepiness and SOREMs may reflect extranigral pathology [66], e.g. in nuclei comprising the ascending reticular activating system such as the hypothalamic hypocretin (orexin) system, dorsal raphe, LC, and PPN. Impairments in central release of hypocretins might seem a parsimonious explanation for the narcolepsy-like phenotype seen in a subset of PD patients; however, in the majority of PD cases with a variety of comorbidities such as sleepiness, sudden onset of sleep, or dementia, cerebrospinal fluid hypocretin-1 levels are normal [24, 67–70]. That being said, neuropathological investigations have documented hypocretin cell loss that increases with disease severity [71], and changing out D_3 receptor preferring agonists for alternate dopaminergics in four PD patients with sudden sleep episodes normalized CSF hypocretin levels in tandem with resolution of their sleepiness [70]. Alternatively, dysregulation of the brainstem PPN region, an area known to promote the thalamocortical aroused states of wake and REM sleep, may be as important a mediator of impaired alertness and SOREM expression in PD. The PPN region is not only the principal brainstem target of pathological basal ganglia outflow, it is sometimes involved by synuclein pathology in parkinsonism [72]. The most recent experiences with low-frequency stimulation of the PPN to treat medically refractory parkinsonism are supportive and promise exciting future insights into the modulation of daytime alertness and nocturnal sleep in PD [9, 73, 74].

Apart from the neurobiological substrates governing PD, genetic and disease factors may also influence expression of sleepiness and SOREMs (Table 27.1). Alleles of catechol-O-methyltransferase (COMT; a degradative enzyme of dopamine) confer a greater risk for sleepiness [75], as do variants of the D_4 dopamine receptor [76] and preprohypocretin polymorphisms [77]. Advanced disease or disease duration are also potential contributing factors [2, 17, 19], as are predominance of involvement of the non-dominant hemisphere by disease [78], benzodiazepine use [2] (see, however, [26]), male sex [15], comorbid dementia or psychosis [19], and autonomic failure (e.g. orthostatic

Table 27.1 Factors associated with excessive sleepiness in PD

Genetic factors in dopamine or arousal signaling pathways [75–77]

Male sex [15]

Disease duration [2, 15]

Advanced disease [15, 17, 19, 21]

Non-dominant hemisphere predominance in asymmetry of initial symptoms [78]

Benzodiazepine use [2]

Comorbid dementia or psychosis [19]

Autonomic failure (e.g. orthostatic hypotension) [20]

---

hypotension) [20]. Many of these features characterize patients exhibiting dementia with Lewy bodies (DLB), suggesting that sleepiness may be a phenotypic characteristic of this disease subtype (also, see [7, 24]). This is further supported by a longitudinal study finding that nearly two-thirds of PD patients with sleepiness went on to develop dementia [19]. As REM sleep behavior disorder can presage PD by years and is a supportive criteria for a diagnosis of DLB, it is tempting to speculate that sleepiness may also be a "subclinical" harbinger of PD, or PD variants such as DLB. Support for this tenet comes from a longitudinal study of the large Honolulu–Asia Aging cohort [79].

There has been a veritable explosion over the past decade in the number of reports of sleepiness and more specifically, unintended sleep episodes (i.e. "sleep attacks"), associated with dopaminomimetic use [4, 80–85]. Sleepiness or unintended sleep associated with dopaminomimetics in a subset of PD patients appear dose-related, but are not clearly related to specific class of agent (e.g. levodopa vs. ergot and non-ergot derived D_2/D_3 receptor agonists) [10, 15, 17]. Most reports are largely anecdotal and those that have documented or investigated the physiological correlates of sleepiness and unintended sleep suggest that: (a) it indeed occurs [86]; (b) it is a relatively stable trait when assessed over two days [87]; (c) conventional sleep laboratory assessments cannot distinguish between subjects reporting sleepiness or "sleep attacks" and those that do not [25, 26]; and (d) unintended sleep likely represents an extreme and rare event on a continuum that includes both excess sleep and sleepiness [25, 28–30, 88, 89]. What remain open questions are how often dopaminomimetic use in PD contributes to sleepiness and unintended sleep episodes, and how much of a contributing factor it is. The D_2 and D_3 receptor agonists ropinirole [90] and pramipexole [91], for example, cause demonstrable sleepiness *and* excessive sleep even in drug-naive, healthy subjects. Sleepiness is not as severe or as consistently observed with less selective dopaminomimetics such as levodopa or bromocriptine [91, 92], again highlighting the prominent role of D_2 and D_3 receptor activation in mediating sleepiness.

It has been suggested that obstructive sleep apnea (OSA) and periodic leg movements of sleep (PLMS) coexisting with PD may also contribute to sleepiness and SOREMs [3, 7]. Yet, this is controversial since sleepiness in *nonparkinsonian* patients is not completely explained by the severity of OSA and PLMS. One recent study suggests that the frequency and severity of sleep-disordered breathing in PD is modest, at best, and unlikely to be a significant contributor to excessive sleepiness [93]. A final important determinant of sleepiness in PD is a premorbid sleepiness level which is increasingly recognized to be a heritable trait in the general population. One survey of sudden onset of sleep in several large movement disorders clinics, in fact, found that 20% of PD patients reporting sudden sleep while driving experienced similar events *prior to* the diagnosis of PD being made [10]. In summary, the pathophysiological bases underlying the spectrum of PD-related changes in sleep–wake tendencies are complex and unique to the individual patient. Until more data are forthcoming, the most prudent clinical approaches and experimental considerations should proceed from the assumption that the parkinsonian state reflects an underlying diathesis to daytime sleepiness with SOREMs expression that can be exaggerated by numerous coexistent factors including use of D_2, and particularly, D_3 preferring dopamine receptor agonists and levodopa, sedative-hypnotic and potentially other medications, primary sleep disorders, and potentially comorbid conditions such as dementia.

Measurement of sleepiness

The utility of the MSLT and other objective (e.g. the maintenance of wakefulness test (MWT)), and subjective measures of sleepiness in PD has been reviewed [94]. In interpreting an MSLT, one should keep in mind that the reported mean latency to fall asleep in minutes reflects an operationally defined "sleepiness" collected in a unique environmental setting. The

MSLT, for example, does not distinguish between an increased homeostatic drive for sleep as occurs following sleep deprivation, from decrements in the ability to remain awake, as might be conceptualized to occur with insults to the reticular activating system. To this end, as reflected by the MWT, PD patients appear to exhibit less of a problem with maintaining alertness in a soporific testing environment when instructed to stay wake [22, 23].

The Epworth Sleepiness Scale (ESS) has been widely used as a time- and cost-effective means of screening for subjective daytime sleepiness and sudden onset of sleep in PD and other populations [3, 10, 11, 14–17, 20, 21, 95, 96]. The results of Tan et al. [11] demonstrate that ESS scores of greater than 10 out of a maximal 24 in PD are 71% sensitive and 88% specific for the occurrence of "sudden, irresistible, and overwhelming sleepiness that occurs without warning and not preceded by feeling sleepy". Another survey found a similar sensitivity, but only ~50% specificity for ESS > 7 [10]. While near-pathological levels of sleepiness have been documented by the MSL in a large group of "sleepy" PD patients (mean MSL <6.5 min) [3], self-reported sleepiness was not accurately reflected by the ESS (10% false-negative and 20% false-positive rates). Overall, the ESS scores here and elsewhere [22, 26] do not correlate significantly with MSL, consistent with reports in other sleep-disorder populations. Taken together, these results argue that the ESS should not be used as the sole indicator, or as a substitute, for the MSLT. This is not to imply that the ESS should not play a role in the clinical assessment of sleepiness in PD. Sleep propensity in real-life situations (e.g. while driving), as assessed by the scale, can differ significantly from physiologic sleep tendency measured in a soporific environment. To this end, higher ESS scores in PD have been shown to be somewhat predictive of sleepiness while driving [12, 97]. Discrepancies between subjective and objective measures may reflect the insidious nature/chronicity of sleepiness, poor insight into sleepiness and sleep episodes as has been documented in PD [98], or preference for different terms – e.g. "fatigue", "tired", or "lack of energy" – to describe physiological sleep tendency. This highlights the critical importance of careful clinical assessment and actual observation of daytime sleep behaviors in PD patients by clinicians and family members. A validated, user-friendly instrument for PD patients to enhance recognition and treatment of sleepiness awaits development.

General approach and management

Daytime sleepiness experienced by idiopathic PD patients is real, common, and potentially as severe as that manifest by narcoleptics. An MSL <5 min is present in one-half of PD patients with sleepiness [3], a level deemed "pathological" because it has been associated with cognitive and motor performance impairments in other sleep-disorder populations. Proper treatment can dramatically enhance quality of life and prevent the significant morbidity and mortality that attends pathological sleepiness. Physicians treating PD should therefore educate patients and their families on the potential detrimental effects of this disease and its treatment not only upon motor symptoms but also upon the ability to maintain an active, awake state. Patients should be informed about the potential dangers of driving. Administration of the ESS – possibly completed by the caregiver or significant other – and queries about unintended sleep episodes, particularly while driving, should be routine. Anywhere from 11 to 22% of PD patients experience sleepiness while driving, and this risk tends to correlate with higher ESS scores [10, 12, 15, 88, 97]. The frequency of sudden onset of sleep while driving is reported to be ~3.8% [10], with the majority of these preceded by drowsiness or warning signs (~85%). If significant or unpredictable sleepiness is suspected, driving should be temporarily restricted until the sleepiness resolves. This being said, the clinician should appreciate that self-reported sleepiness and MSLT are not predictive of driving performance/increased MVA rates in other sleep-disorder populations [99].

The first step in effecting resolution of parkinsonian-related sleepiness demands a careful review of medications and defining any temporal relationship between dosing and symptoms, as dosage reduction or discontinuation of dopaminomimetics, particularly agonists, or long-lasting benzodiazepines might ameliorate sleepiness. Switching to an equivalent dose of the extremely long-lasting agonist cabergoline at night has met with some success in nine patients on dopamine agonist monotherapy suffering from excessive sleepiness [100]. Nightly benzodiazepine use intended to improve daytime alertness by lengthening total sleep time and preventing nocturnal arousals seems unwarranted given the inverse correlation of parkinsonian sleepiness with the quantity or quality of the prior night's sleep. If medication adjustments are ineffectual, the diagnostic yield for polysomnography and MSLT evaluation of PD patients is considerable (15% prevalence of PLMS, 20% prevalence of OSA, 40% prevalence of "secondary" narcolepsy) [7]. Treatment strategies might then need to be targeted at alleviating PLMs and OSA, if present. If sleepiness persists, treatments that until now have focused primarily on minimizing waking motor disability should include agents specifically designed to promote daytime alertness. Prescribing wake-promoting agents such as modafinil, bupropion or traditional psychostimulants seems justified upon identification of a narcolepsy-like phenotype or an MSL <8 min. Initial open-label experiences with modafinil in PD patients with drug-related drowsiness were encouraging [101–104]. Two double-blind, randomized, placebo-controlled studies demonstrate improvements in a subset of patients [105, 106] that could not be corroborated by objective MWT testing [107].

Selection of the most appropriate drug and its dosing for maximizing wakefulness in PD will require future clinical trials. In the non-human MPTP primate model of PD, sleepiness and SOREMs have been reversed with the dopamine precursor levodopa, the dopamine reuptake blocker bupropion [108], but not the $D_{2\text{-like}}$ receptor agonist pergolide [61]. Levodopa and bupropion require presynaptic integrity to enhance synaptic availability of dopamine by promoting its synthesis, or by blockade of dopamine transporter, respectively. Thus, the abilities of these agents to reverse sleepiness and SOREMs likely reflects actions upon surviving mesocorticolimbic dopamine circuits which are less vulnerable to MPTP and affected only later in the course of idiopathic PD. Enhancement of synaptic dopamine availability in mesocorticolimbic circuits, in fact, may underly the success of amphetamines in the treatment of PD described nearly 30 years ago [109, 110] – providing beneficial alerting effects in truly "sleepy" patients.

Treatment strategies

The clinician treating sleepiness in the parkinsonian patient is in the unenviable position of weighing the potential positive impact of dopaminomimetics upon sleep as it relates to daytime motor function (namely, the phenomenon of "sleep benefit" [111]), against the real possibility of adverse effects upon daytime alertness. This being said, it cannot be understated that much of parkinsonian-related sleepiness is reflective of the disease process itself. Therefore, a low-threshold for use of supplemental wake-promoting agents to optimize daytime alertness seems appropriate. These goals appear critical to the well-being of not only the parkinsonian patient, but also the primary caregiver and family. Treatment should be tailored to the individual patient so that they can actively participate in activities which they enjoyed prior to receiving a diagnosis of PD. Despite maximal treatment, it should be expected that a certain amount of residual sleepiness will remain and that scheduled naps not be perceived as a treatment failure. As the problem of PD-related sleepiness has only recently been recognized, there is a paucity of studies on how it might best be reversed. The following suggestions largely reflect personal experience gathered from a Sleep Disorders clinic within a Neurology department with a large Movement Disorders section.

Non-pharmacologic

The effects of diet and lifestyle upon parkinsonian-related sleepiness have not been comprehensively addressed. This being said, it is common clinical experience that post-prandial sleepiness appears exaggerated in PD and can present as sudden onset of sleep on the backdrop of sleepiness. This phenomenon is not well understood, but also manifests as a worsening of parkinsonian-related disability scores [112]. These phenomena likely reflect lessening of synaptic dopamine release known to attend baroreceptor unloading [113] as would be expected to occur with venous pooling attending meals. For this reason, careful screening for, and treatment of, orthostatic hypotension seems reasonable, as well as smaller-sized, more frequent meals (Table 27.2).

Pharmacologic

Pharmacologic treatment is employed only for those patients in whom identification and treatment of other causes of daytime sleepiness has proved ineffectual (see Table 27.2). Modafinil is a novel wake-promoting agent with FDA approval for treatment of narcolepsy/cataplexy. Modafinil appears to promote wakefulness by improving dopaminergic transmission [49], although its precise mechanism of action is unknown. Experience and success with modafinil for parkinsonian-related sleepiness includes several case reports [101, 103, 104], one open-label trial in 10 patients [102], and two larger double-blind,

Table 27.2 Treatment of sleepiness in PD

Medication adjustments
  Reduce OTC sleeping aids or antidepressants with anti-histaminergic activity
  Minimize benzodiazepine use
  Minimize "sedating" antidepressant use
  Dopaminomimetic dose adjustment if dosing temporally associated with sleepiness

Treat documented sleep or other disturbance
  Continuous positive airway pressure (CPAP) for sleep apnea
  Nighttime dosing of dopaminomimetics, opiates, or gabapentin for periodic limb movements of sleep.
  Consider treatment of orthostatic hypotension

Treat "residual" daytime sleepiness
  Hygiene measures:
    Scheduled naps
    More frequent, smaller meals

  Pharmacologic measures:
    Bupropion (75–150 mg BID or TID)
    Modafinil (100–200 mg QAM and noon)
    Dextroamphetamine sulfate (5–30 mg QAM and noon) – combination of sustained-release and regular tablets.
    Sodium Oxybate (3–4.5 g QHS and again, 4 h later)

placebo-controlled trials [105, 106]. Modafinil is well-tolerated by older patients, has no apparent interactions with antiparkinsonian medications, and adverse effects upon the clinical severity of PD have not been reported. The most common adverse events noted include suboccipital headache which can be avoided with dosage titration in increments of 100 mg every 5–7 days to a maximal divided (morning and noon) daily dosage of 400 mg. Patients should be advised that prolonged absorption and distribution times delay beneficial effects until 90–120 min after dosing.

Bupropion is marketed for depression and smoking cessation, but has additional wake-promoting effects [61, 114], likely due to its ability to increase synaptic dopamine via blockade of the dopamine transporter. There are no published data on bupropion for parkinsonian-related sleepiness. One study in PD has reported 30% improvement of parkinsonian-related disability which is heavily weighted upon motor dysfunction [115]. In non-human primate models of PD, bupropion while having little benefit upon motor deficits, improves "alertness and posture accompanied by head checking movements" [116]. Reversal of daytime sleepiness in this same animal model has been verified objectively [61]. Bupropion (225–450 mg/day in divided doses) is generally well-tolerated by PD patients, and adverse effects upon the clinical severity of PD have not been reported [115]. The most common adverse events noted are nausea/vomiting and restlessness/hyperexcitability in ~50%, and hallucinations in 15% of PD patients also taking carbidopa/levodopa [115]. Beneficial effects upon comorbid depression have been noted in ~25% of PD patients prescribed bupropion [115]. The most troublesome side-effect related to its use is seizure (0.4% risk at 450 mg/day) [117].

Traditional psychostimulants are reserved for patients who have failed modafinil and bupropion. Our preferred agent is dextroamphetamine administered at the lowest effective dose (initiate at 5–10 mg BID) (Table 27.2). Sustained-release formulations are favored as they are less likely to result in rebound hypersomnolence in the wearing-off stage. Evening dosing should be avoided so as to prevent against insomnia. Such agents necessitate avoidance of co-administration of monoamine oxidase inhibitors which can lead to marked irritability/restlessness, headaches, and frank hypertensive crises. While tolerance and psychological dependence are real possibilities in the non-parkinsonian patient population, these potential complications are unusual in the PD patient.

A novel treatment awaiting further development and testing attempts to take advantage of the relative survival of wake-promoting, histaminergic, tuberomamillary neurons in PD. Tiprosilant, an inverse agonist of the histamine H(3) receptor [118], has shown some early promise in alleviating sleepiness in PD [119].

Surgical

Surgical treatments for PD are advocated when faced with refractoriness to traditional treatment and/or undesirable medical-related dyskinesias. Routine, objective assessments of sleepiness have not been incorporated into these treatment algorithms. Effects of surgical intervention upon parkinsonian-related sleep and sleepiness are therefore limited. Bilateral subthalamic stimulation improves sleep quality [120–122], yet in our experience with two well-studied patients (unpublished observations) and subjective assessment by others [122], has little benefit upon daytime alertness. It remains to be established whether subsequent reductions in dopaminomimetic medication load afforded by surgery in this unique patient population resolves presurgical sleepiness. Bilateral subthalamic nucleus stimulator placement [123] and pallidotomy [124] have improved daytime alertness in two isolated cases. The field awaits objective testing of daytime alertness and nighttime sleep with deep brain stimulation of the PPN which preliminary experience suggests may have rather striking positive benefits [9, 73, 74].

Follow-up management

Utilizing the ESS to determine response to treatment or disease progression seems prudent. Since self-reported sleepiness in PD is not accurately reflected by the ESS (10% false-negative and 20% false-positive rates), it is preferable to have the ESS completed by the primary caregiver or a close family member or co-worker. At follow-up careful attention should be paid to medication changes that might account for changes in sleepiness state, and defining any coincident change in PD-related symptomatology that might have developed (e.g. "on"–"off" phenomena; disrupted sleep, periodic limb movements of sleep, witnessed apneas, cognitive problems, psychosis, or REM sleep behavior disorder). The emergence of any of these symptoms call for their own tailored treatments, and possibly polysomnographic evaluation, before escalating the dose of wake-promoting agents. As progression of PD is the rule, the clinician is constantly presented with a changing face of sleep disturbances and daytime sleepiness. Longitudinal studies are sorely needed to better define the natural history of this progression and thereby guide clinicians with regards to management.

Conclusions

The majority of formal, objective, physiological assessments, clinical experience, and experimental animal studies concur that parkinsonism itself, and not simply medication, accounts for much of the sleepiness that attends the disease. Male patients with advanced disease, cognitive impairment, drug-induced psychosis, and orthostatic hypotension appear most at risk. While sleepiness observed with levodopa and dopamine agonists in PD has been increasingly publicized and believed to be dose-dependent, even at low doses, dopaminergic agents showing preference for D_3 receptors cause significant sleepiness in drug-naive, healthy subjects. Thus, the extent to which drug use in PD contributes further to sleepiness remains unresolved.

Dopamine pathways promote arousal, maintenance of sleep/wake homeostasis, and are responsible for the wake-promoting effects of psychostimulants. Rodents and non-human primates rendered parkinsonian by dopamine depletion exhibit altered sleep/wake architecture and excessive sleep that mimics what is encountered in the human condition. Therefore, as captured by Oliver Sacks' familiar memoir *Awakenings*, the sleepiness of the parkinsonian patient transcends the metaphor. It is undeniably verifiable, and likely as much a consequence of the disease as its treatment. Intrinsic sleepiness therefore represents an important target in disease management.

Acknowledgments

Dr. Rye's work is supported by USPHS grants NS055015.

References

1. **Rye D**, **Bliwise D**, Movement disorders specific to sleep and the nocturnal manifestations of waking movement disorders. In: Watts R, Koller W, Eds. *Movement Disorders: Neurologic Principles and Practice* (2nd Ed.). New York: McGraw-Hill, 2004: 855–90.
2. **Rye D B**, **Bliwise D L**, **Dihenia B**, *et al.* FAST TRACK: daytime sleepiness in Parkinson's disease. *J Sleep Res*, 2000; **9**:63–69.
3. **Arnulf I**, **Konofal E**, **Merino-Andreu M**, *et al.* Parkinson's disease and sleepiness: an integral part of PD. *Neurology*, 2002; **58**:1019–24.
4. **Frucht S**, **Rogers J**, **Greene P**, *et al.*, Falling asleep at the wheel: motor vehicle mishaps in persons taking pramipexole and ropinirole. *Neurology*, 1999; **52**:1908–10.
5. **Rye D**, **Daley J**, **Freeman A**, *et al.*, Daytime sleepiness and sleep attacks in idiopathic Parkinson's disease. In: Bedard M-A, *et al.*, Eds. *Mental and Behavioral Dysfunction in Movement Disorders* : Totawa, NJ: Humana Press, 2003: 527–38.
6. **Schapira A**. Excessive daytime sleepiness in Parkinson's disease. *Neurology*, 2004; **63**(8 Suppl 3):S24–27.
7. **Arnulf I**. Excessive daytime sleepiness in parkinsonism. *Sleep Med Rev*, 2005; **9**:185–200.
8. **Arnulf I**, **Leu S**, **Oudiette D**. Abnormal sleep and sleepiness in Parkinson's disease. *Curr Opin Neurol*, 2008; **21**:472–77.
9. **Arnulf I**, **Leu-Semenescu S**. Sleepiness in Parkinson's disease. *Parkinsonism Relat Disord*, 2009; **2009**:S101–04.
10. **Hobson D E**, **Lang A E**, **Martin W R W**, *et al.* Excessive daytime sleepiness and sudden-onset sleep in Parkinson disease. *JAMA*, 2002; **287**:455–63.

11. **Tan E K**, **Lum S Y**, **Fook-Chong S M C**, *et al.* Evaluation of somnolence in Parkinson's disease: comparison with age and sex matched controls. *Neurology*, 2002; **58**:465–68.

12. **Brodsky M**, **Godbold J**, **Roth T**, *et al.* Sleepiness in Parkinson's disease: a controlled study. *Mov Disord*, 2003; **18**:668–72.

13. **Ghorayeb I**, **Loundou A**, **Auquier P**, *et al.* A nationwide survey of excessive daytime sleepiness in Parkinson's disease in France. *Mov Disord*, 2007; **22**:1567–72.

14. **Suzuki K**, **Miyamoto T**, **Miyamoto M**, *et al.* Excessive daytime sleepiness and sleep episodes in Japanese patients with Parkinson's disease. *J Neurol Sci*, 2008; **271**:47–52.

15. **Ondo W G**, **Vuong K V**, **Khan H**, *et al.* Daytime sleepiness and other sleep disorders in Parkinson's disease. *Neurology*, 2001; **57**:1392–96.

16. **Sanjiv C C**, **Schulzer M**, **Mak E**, *et al.* Daytime somnolence in patients with Parkinson's disease. *Parkinsonism Relat Disord*, 2001; **7**:283–86.

17. **O'Suilleabhain P E**, **Dewey R B**. Contributions of dopaminergic drugs and disease severity to daytime sleepiness in Parkinson disease. *Arch Neurol*, 2002; **59**:986–89.

18. **Tandberg E**, **Larsen J**, **Karlsen K**. Excessive daytime sleepiness and sleep benefit in Parkinson's disease: a community based study. *Mov Disord*, 1999; **14**:922–27.

19. **Gjerstad M D**, **Aarsland D**, **Larsen J P**. Development of daytime somnolence over time in Parkinson's disease. *Neurology*, 2002; **58**:1544–46.

20. **Montastruc J-L**, **Brefel-Courbon C**, **Senard J-M**, *et al.* Sleep attacks and antiparkinsonian drugs: a pilot prospective pharmacoepidemiologic study. *Clinical Neuropharmacol*, 2001; **24**:181–83.

21. **Kumar S**, **Bhatia M**, **Behari M**. Sleep disorders in Parkinson's disease. *Mov Disord*, 2002; **17**:775–81.

22. **Razmy A**, **Lang A**, **Shapiro C**. Predictors of impaired daytime sleep and wakefulness in patients with Parkinsons disease treated with older (ergot) vs newer (nonergot) dopamine agonists. *Arch Neurol*, 2004; **61**:97–102.

23. **Stevens S**, **Comella C**, **Stepanski E**. Daytime sleepiness and alertness in patients with Parkinson disease. *Sleep*, 2004; **27**:967–72.

24. **Baumann C**, **Ferini-Strambi L**, **Waldvogel D**, *et al.* Parkinsonism with excessive daytime sleepiness-a narcolepsy like disorder? *J Neurol*, 2005; **252**:139–45.

25. **Roth T**, **Rye D**, **Borchert L**, *et al.* Assessment of sleepiness and unintended sleep in Parkinson's disease patients taking dopamine agonists. *Sleep Med*, 2003; **4**:275–80.

26. **Shpirer I**, **Miniovitz A**, **Klein C**, *et al.* Excessive daytime sleepiness in patients with Parkinson's dease: a polysomnographic study. *Mov Disord*, 2006; **21**:1432–38.

27. **Kaynak D**, **Kiziltan G**, **Kaynak H**, *et al.* Sleep and sleepiness in patients with Parkinson's disease before and after dopaminergic treatment. *Eur J Neurol*, 2005; **12**:199–207.

28. **Ulivelli M**, **Rossi S**, **Lombard C**, *et al.* Polysomnographic characterization of pergolide-induced "sleep attacks" in an idiopathic PD patient. *Neurology*, 2002; **58**:462–65.

29. **Manni R**, **Terzaghi M**, **Sartori I**, *et al.* Dopamine agonists and sleepiness in PD: a review of the literature and personal findings. *Sleep Med*, 2004; **5**:189–93.

30. **Pacchetti C**, **Martignoni E**, **Terzaghi M**, *et al.* Sleep attacks in Parkinson's disease: a clinical and polysomnographic study. *Neurol Sci*, 2003; **24**:195–96.

31. **Agid Y**. Parkinson's disease: pathophysiology. *Lancet*, 1991; **337**:1321–24.

32. **Freeman A**, **Rye D**. Dopamine in behavioral state control. In: Sinton C, Perumal P, Monti J, Eds. *The Neurochemistry of Sleep and Wakefulness*. Cambridge: Cambridge University Press, 2008: 179–223.

33. **Nicola S**, **Surmeier J**, **Malenka R**. Dopaminergic modulation of neuronal excitability in the striatum and nucleus accumbens. *Ann Rev Neurosci*, 2000; **23**:185–215.

34. **Missale C**, **Nash S R**, **Robinson S W**, *et al.* Dopamine receptors: from structure to function. *Physiol Rev*, 1998; **78**:189–225.

35. **Cragg S**, **Greenfield S**. Differential autoreceptor control of somatodendritic and axon terminal dopamine release in substantia nigra, ventral tegmental area and striatum. *J Neurosci*, 1997; **17**:5738–46.

36. **Dahan L**, **Astier B**, **Vautrelle N**, *et al.* Prominent burst firing of dopaminergic neurons in the ventral tegmental area during paradoxical sleep. *Neuropsychopharmacology*, 2007; **32**:1232–41.

37. **Floresco S B**, **West A R**, **Ash B**, *et al.* Afferent modulation of dopamine neuron firing differentially regulates tonic and phasic dopamine transmission. *Nat Neurosci*, 2003; **6**:968–73.

38. **Kitai S T**, **Shepard P D**, **Callaway J C**, *et al.* Afferent modulation of dopamine neuron firing patterns. *Curr Opin Neurobiol*, 1999; **9**:690–97.

39. **Lee R S**, **Steffensen S C**, **Henriksen S J**. Discharge profiles of ventral tegmental area GABA neurons during movement, anesthesia, and the sleep–wake cycle. *J Neurosci*, 2001; **21**:1757–66.

40. **McCormick D A**. Are thalamocortical rhythms the Rosetta Stone of a subset of neurological disorders? *Nat Med*, 1999; **5**:1349–51.

41. **Keating G L**, **Rye D B**. Where you least expect it: dopamine in the pons and modulation of sleep and REM-sleep. *Sleep*, 2003; **26**:788–89.

42. **Khaldy H**, **Leon J**, **Escames G**, et al. Circadian rhythms of dopamine and dihydroxyphenyl acetic acid in the mouse striatum: effects of pinealectomy and of melatonin treatment. *Neuroendocrinology*, 2002; **75**:201–08.

43. **McClung C**, **Sidiropoulou K**, **Vitaterna M**, et al. Regulation of dopaminergic transmission and cocaine reward by the *Clock* gene. *Proc Natl Acad Sci USA*, 2005; **102**:9377–81.

44. **Andretic R**, **Hirsh J**. Circadian modulation of dopamine receptor responsiveness in *Drosophila melanogaster*. *Proc Natl Acad Sci USA*, 2000; **97**:1873–78.

45. **Garcia-Borreguero D**, **Larrosa O**, **Granizo J**, et al. Circadian variation in neuroendocrine response to L-dopa in patients with restless legs syndrome. *Sleep*, 2004; **27**: 669–73.

46. **Poceta J**, **Parsons L**, **Engelland S**, et al. Circadian rhythm of CSF monoamines and hypocretin-1 in restless legs syndrome and Parkinson's disease. *Sleep Med*, 2009; **10**:129–33.

47. **Daley J T**, **Turner R S**, **Freeman A**, et al. Prolonged assessment of sleep and daytime sleepiness in unrestrained *Macaca mulatta*. *Sleep*, 2006; **29**:221–31.

48. **Nishino S**, **Mao J**, **Sampathkumaran R**, et al. Increased dopaminergic transmission mediates the wake-promoting effects of CNS stimulants. *Sleep Res Online*, 1998; **1**:49–61.

49. **Wisor J**, **Nishino S**, **Sora I**, et al. Dopaminergic role in stimulant-induced wakefulness. *J Neurosci*, 2001; **21**:1787–94.

50. **Porzgen P**, **Park S K**, **Hirsh J**, et al. The antidepressant-sensitive dopamine transporter in *Drosophila melanogaster*: a primordial carrier for catecholamines. *Mol Pharmacol*, 2001; **59**:83–95.

51. **Kume K**, **Kume S**, **Park S K**, et al. Dopamine is a regulator of arousal in the fruit fly. *J Neurosci*, 2005; **25**:7377–84.

52. **Wu M N**, **Koh K**, **Yue Z**, et al. A genetic screen for sleep and circadian mutants reveals mechanisms underlying regulation of sleep in *Drosophila*. *Sleep*, 2008; **31**:465–72.

53. **Andretic R**, **Shaw P J**. Essentials of sleep recordings in *Drosophila*: moving beyond sleep time. *Meth Enzymol*, 2005; **393**:759–72.

54. **Calabrese E J**. Dopamine: biphasic dose responses. *Crit Rev Toxicol*, 2001; **31**:563–83.

55. **Davidson S**, **Miller K A**, **Dowell A**, et al. A remote and highly conserved enhancer supports amygdala specific expression of the gene encoding the anxiogenic neuropeptide substance-P. *Mol Psychiatry*, 2006; **11**:323.

56. **Hue G**, **Decker M**, **Solomon I**, et al. Increased wakefulness and hyper-responsivity to novel environments in mice lacking functional dopamine D3 receptors. Society for Neuroscience (Abstr); Program Number 616.16, 2003.

57. **Lu J**, **Jhou T C**, **Saper C B**. Identification of wake-active dopaminergic neurons in the ventral periaqueductal gray matter. *J Neurosci*, 2006; **26**:193–202.

58. **Sakata M**, **Sei H**, **Toida K**, et al. Mesolimbic dopaminergic system is involved in diurnal blood pressure regulation. *Brain Res*, 2002; **928**:194–201.

59. **Decker M J**, **Keating G L**, **Freeman A**, et al. Focal depletion of dopamine in the sensorimotor striatum of the rat recapitulates parkinsonian-like sleep/wake disturbances. *Sleep*, 2000; **23**(Suppl 2):A136.

60. **Decker M**, **Hue G**, **Caudle W**, et al. Episodic neonatal hypoxia evokes executive dysfunction and regionally specific alterations in markers of dopamine signaling. *Neurosci*, 2003; **117**:417–25.

61. **Daley J**, **Turner R**, **Bliwise D**, et al. Nocturnal sleep and daytime alertness in the MPTP-treated primate. *Sleep*, 1999; **22**(Suppl):S218–19.

62. **Barraud Q**, **Lambrecq V**, **Forni C**, et al. Sleep disorders in Parkinson's disease: the contribution of the MPTP non-human primate model. *Exp Neurol*, 2009; **219**:574–82.

63. **Rye D**, **Johnston L**, **Watts R**, et al. Juvenile Parkinson's disease with REM sleep behavior disorder, sleepiness and daytime REM-onset. *Neurology*, 1999; **53**:1868–70.

64. **Happe S**, **Baier P**, **Helmschmied K**, et al. Association of daytime sleepiness with nigrostriatal dopaminergic degeneration in early Parkinson's disease. *J Neurol*, 2007; **254**:1037–43.

65. **Silber M H**, **Rye D B**. Solving the mysteries of narcolepsy. *Neurology*, 2001; **56**:1616–18.

66. **Jellinger K**. Pathology of Parkinson's disease. Changes other than the nigrostriatal pathway. *Mol Chem Neuropathol*, 1991; **14**:153–97.

67. **Overeem S**, **van Hilten J J**, **Ripley B**, et al. Normal hypocretin-1 levels in Parkinson's disease patients with excessive daytime sleepiness. *Neurology*, 2002; **58**:465–68.

68. **Drouot X**, **Moutereau S**, **Nguten J**, *et al.* Low levels of ventricular CSF orexin/hypocretin in advanced PD. *Neurology*, 2003; **61**:540–43.

69. **Compta Y**, **Santamaria J**, **Ratti L**, *et al.* Cerebrospinal hypocretin, daytime sleepiness and sleep architecture in Parkinson's disease dementia. *Brain*, 2009; **132**:3308–17.

70. **Asai H**, **Hirano M**, **Furiya Y**, *et al.* Cerebrospinal fluid-orexin levels and sleep attacks in four patients with Parkinson's disease. *Clin Neurol Neurosurg*, 2009; **111**:341–44.

71. **Thannickal T**, **Lai Y-Y**, **Siegel J**. Hypocretin (orexin) cell loss in Parkinson's disease. *Brain*, 2007; **130**: 1586–95.

72. **Rye D**. Contributions of the pedunculopontine region to normal and altered REM sleep. *Sleep*, 1997; **20**:757–88.

73. **Lim A**, **Moro E**, **Lozano A**, *et al.* Selective enhancement of rapid eye movement sleep by deep brain stimulation of the human pons. *Ann Neurol*, 2009; **66**:110–14.

74. **Alessandro S**, **Ceravolo R**, **Brusa L**, *et al.* Non-motor functions in parkinsonian patients implanted in the pedunculopontine nucleus: focus on sleep and cognitive domains. *J Neurol Sci*, 2010; **289**:44–48.

75. **Frauscher B**, **Hogl B**, **Maret S**, *et al.* Association of daytime sleepiness with COMT polymorphism in patients with parkinson disease: a pilot study. *Sleep*, 2004; **27**:733–36.

76. **Paus S**, **Seeger G**, **Brecht H**, *et al.* Association study of dopamine D2, D3, D4 receptor and serotonin transporter gene polymorphisms with sleep attacks in Parkinson's disease. *Mov Disord*, 2004; **19**: 507–09.

77. **Rissling I**, **Korner Y**, **Geller F**, *et al.* Preprohypocretin polymorphisms in Parkinson disease patients reporting "sleep attacks". *Sleep*, 2005; **28**:871–75.

78. **Stavitsky K**, **McNamara P**, **Durso R**, *et al.* Hallucinations, dreaming, and frequent dozing in Parkinson disease: impact of right-hemisphere neural networks. *Cogn Behav Neurol*, 2008; **21**:143–49.

79. **Abbott R D**, **Ross G W**, **White L R**, *et al.* Excessive daytime sleepiness and subsequent development of Parkinson disease. *Neurology*, 2005; **65**:1442–46.

80. **Frucht S**, **Rogers J**, **Greene P**, *et al.* Falling asleep at the wheel: motor vehicle mishaps in people taking pramipexole and ropinirole – letters to the editor. *Neurology*, 2000; **54**:274–77.

81. **Olanow C**, **Schapira A**, **Roth T**. Waking up to sleep episodes in Parkinson's disease. *Mov Disord*, 2000; **15**:212–15.

82. **Ryan M**, **Slevin J**, **Wells A**. Non-ergot dopamine agonist-induced sleep attacks. *Pharmacotherapy*, 2000; **20**:724–26.

83. **Hauser R A**, **Gauger L**, **Anderson W M**, *et al.* Pramipexole-induced somnolence and episodes of daytime sleep. *Mov Disord*, 2000; **15**:658–63.

84. **Ferreira J**, **Galitzky M**, **Montastruc J**, *et al.* Sleep attacks and Parkinson's disease treatment. *Lancet*, 2000; **355**:1333–34.

85. **Bares M**, **Kanovsky P**, **Rektor I**. Excessive daytime sleepiness and 'sleep attacks' induced by entacapone. *Fundam Clin Pharmacol*, 2003; **17**:113–16.

86. **Tracik F**, **Ebersbach G**. Sudden daytime sleep onset in Parkinson's disease: polysomnographic recordings. *Mov Disord*, 2001; **16**:500–06.

87. **Trotti L**, **Rye D**, **Bliwise D**. Comment on Shpirer *et al.* ("Excessive daytime sleepiness in patients with Parkinson's disease: a polysomnographic study"). *Mov Disord*, 2007; **22**:1520.

88. **Moller J C**, **Stiasny K**, **Hargutt V**, *et al.* Evaluation of sleep and driving performance in six patients with Parkinson's disease reporting sudden onset of sleep under dopaminergic medication: a pilot study. *Mov Disord*, 2002; **17**:474–81.

89. **Contin M**, **Provini F**, **Martinelli P**, *et al.* Excessive daytime sleepiness and levodopa in Parkinson's disease: polygraphic, placebo-controlled monitoring. *Clin Neuropharmacol*, 2003; **26**:115–18.

90. **Ferreira J J**, **Galitzky M**, **Thalamas C**, *et al.* Effect of ropinirole on sleep onset: a randomized placebo controlled study in healthy volunteers. *Neurology*, 2002; **58**:460–62.

91. **Micallef J**, **Rey M**, **Eusebio A**, *et al.* Antiparkinsonian drug-induced sleepiness: a double-blind placebo controlled study of L-dopa, bromocriptine and pramipexole in healthy subjects. *Br J Clin Pharmacol*, 2009; **67**:333–40.

92. **Andreau N**, **Chale J**, **Senard J**, *et al.* L-dopa induced sedation: a double-blind cross-over controlled study versus triazolam and placebo in healthy volunteers. *Clin Neuropharmacol*, 1999; **22**:15–23.

93. **De Cock V**, **Abouda M**, **Leu S**, *et al.* Is obstructive sleep apnea a problem in Parkinson's disease? *Sleep Med*, 2010; **11**:247–52.

94. **Santamaria J**. How to evaluate excessive daytime sleepiness in Parkinson's disease. *Neurology*, 2004; **63**(Suppl 3): S21–23.

Section 3 Chapter 28

Medical, Psychiatric and Neurological Causes of Sleepiness

Myotonic dystrophy and sleepiness

Luc Laberge and Yves Dauvilliers

History

Myotonic dystrophy type I (DM1, MIM160900), or Steinert's disease, is the most common adult-onset form of muscular dystrophy [1]. The worldwide prevalence of DM1 ranges from 2.1 to 14.3 per 100 000, but reaches 189 per 100 000 in the relatively isolated and homogeneous population of the Saguenay–Lac-Saint-Jean (SLSJ) region located in the eastern part of the province of Quebec (Canada) [2]. DM1 is a slowly progressive and pleiotropic disorder caused by an expansion of a CTG repeat of the myotonic dystrophy protein kinase (*DMPK*) gene on chromosome 19 [3]. DM1 is one of the most variable of all human disorders, with virtually all body systems affected in some way, and age at disease onset varies from fetal life to old age [1]. Clinical characteristics include weakness of limb, facial and respiratory muscles, myotonia, cardiomyopathy, endocrinopathies, frontal balding, neuropsychological deficits, and cataracts. Three different clinical phenotypes are generally recognized in DM1 according to the age of onset: (1) the congenital form, mainly consisting of hypotonia at birth, mental retardation, and progressive muscular dystrophy, (2) the childhood onset, characterized by mild facial weakness, myotonia, and learning difficulties, and (3) the adult onset (classical) form,[1] displaying considerable heterogeneity in symptoms but consistently showing myotonia and progressive loss of muscle strength. Life expectancy is greatly reduced, more so in patients with early disease onset and proximal muscle involvement [4].

Rohrer was the first to note apathy and excessive somnolence in patients with DM1 [5]. Thomasen later identified fatigue and adynamia as prominent symptoms of DM1 patients and underlined the difficulty to distinguish between true fatigue and lack of initiative characteristic of mental change [6]. Excessive daytime sleepiness (EDS)[2] has been referred to as DM1 patients' most frequent non-muscular symptom [7], the slowing of muscle relaxation (myotonia) being the hallmark of the condition.

Clinical findings

Clinical presentation of EDS

DM1 is undoubtedly the one chronic neuromuscular disease entailing the highest prevalence of EDS. According to liberal estimates, EDS may be present in up to 70–80% of patients affected by DM1 [7]. In childhood-onset DM1, EDS complaints are present in about 50% of patients [8]. A recent study has found that subjective and/or objective EDS, as assessed by the Epworth Sleepiness Scale (ESS) and the Multiple Sleep Latency Test (MSLT), respectively, was present in about 70% of a sample of DM1 patients recruited with no selection or referral bias as regards daytime sleepiness complaints [9]. However, Hilton-Jones et al. advanced that the widely used ESS may not be the most sensitive or appropriate tool to assess EDS in DM1 [10]. In this respect, a reliability study has shown that the ESS possesses weak internal consistency in patients with DM1, indicating poor correlation

---

[1] Although there are other rare genetic forms of myotonic dystrophy, this chapter deals exclusively with adult forms of DM1 unless otherwise specified. Also, we shall use the convenient term DM1 throughout the text even though earlier studies performed before the advent of DNA-based diagnosis may have included some, if any, type 2 patients.

[2] The term excessive daytime sleepiness (and its abbreviation, EDS) rather than (diurnal) hypersomnia, hypersomnolence or (daytime) somnolence will be used throughout, even when the original source of data uses these latter terms.

Sleepiness: Causes, Consequences and Treatment, ed. Michael J. Thorpy and Michel Billiard. Published by Cambridge University Press. © Cambridge University Press 2011.

between ESS items [11]. More precisely, all 27 DM1 patients estimated that they would never doze in 3 of 8 of the real-life situations depicted by the ESS (e.g. when "sitting and talking to someone"). Yet, falling asleep in such situations is uncharacteristic of DM1-related EDS. The Daytime Sleepiness Scale (DSS) was specifically devised to assess the level of daytime sleepiness in patients with DM1 [12]. Its five items are consistent with the clinical features most commonly noted in association with DM1-related EDS and correlate with the degree of muscular impairment. Principal component analysis revealed that the DSS measured a single factor and its internal consistency and test–retest reliability was also demonstrated [11, 12].

The character of DM1-related EDS is that of a persistent sleepiness unaffected by naps, the latter being long, unrefreshing and without any associated dream [13]. The DM1 sleepiness per se seems unrelated to the duration and the quality of the nighttime sleep. Sleepiness is believed to occur when attention is not being held or in monotonous situations as compared to that of narcolepsy which rather occurs in an episodic fashion and tends to arise during activity [1, 14, 15]. EDS may be apparent as one of the earlier symptoms of DM1, with many patients having manifestations for years before DM1 is diagnosed [13, 14, 16, 17]. In our experience, and as noted by many others [1, 7, 15, 18], DM1 patients often do not report spontaneously EDS and it may first be mentioned by family members. Leygonie-Goldenberg and colleagues posited that the early appearance of EDS prompts the patients to consider it as a constitutional oddness rather than as a pathologic phenomenon [15]. More generally, Dement advanced a semantic explanation that some would be unwilling to describe their subjective state as sleepy because of the perception that need for sleep is a sign of personal weakness or lack of initiative, but would otherwise describe it as tired because it is perceived to be the result of effort or hard work, thus making it more acceptable [19]. Similar to EDS, fatigue is more common in DM1 than in other neuromuscular disorders and can reportedly be salient in some patients with only mild muscular impairment [1, 20]. In his early description, Thomasen had observed that some patients with relatively mild physical disability exhibited excessive fatigue such that they were unable to perform even light work, and this was considered as far exceeding what might have been expected from their degree of muscle dystrophy [6]. Also, it was recently observed that the relatives rated the level of fatigue experienced by DM1 patients lower than did the patient himself [21], giving support to Dement's position.

Table 28.1 Sociodemographic and clinical characteristics of 200 DM1 patients with and without EDS

Variable	EDS (n = 61)	Non-EDS (n = 139)
Mean (SD) Age (years)	43.5 (10.6)***	48.6 (8.1)
Mean (SD) Age at onset of symptoms[a]	19.1 (6.4)**	23.5 (10.9)
Mean (SD) Educational level (years)	9.5 (2.3)	10.1 (2.8)
Currently working, % (n)	11.5 (7)*	23.7 (33)
Social assistance, % (n)	52.5 (32)	38.1 (53)
Mean (SD) BMI (kg/m^2)	27.3 (6.7)	25.5 (5.1)
Mean (SD) MIRS (grade)	3.8 (0.9)*	3.4 (1.1)
Mean (SD) CTG repeats (n)	893 (476)	772 (549)

*$P<0.05$; **$P<0.01$; ***$P<0.001$; Excessive Daytime Sleepiness (EDS) was defined by a Daytime Sleepiness Scale (DSS) score ≥ 7 [12]; MIRS: Muscular Impairment Rating Scale; [a] data available for 142 patients.

EDS, functional disability, and quality of life

Tables 28.1 to 28.3 present sociodemographic, clinical, personality, cognitive, and sleep–wake characteristics of a series of 200 DM1 patients (79 men, 121 women). Further details regarding this sample as well as the design and survey instruments used are published elsewhere [22, 23]. It must first be mentioned that a total of 61 DM1 patients (30.5%) reported EDS, as assessed by the DSS, but no gender difference was observed for this symptom [23]. Table 28.1 first reveals that DM1 patients with EDS are younger ($P<0.001$) and have a younger age at disease onset ($P<0.01$) than patients without EDS. Moreover, DM1 patients with EDS show a greater muscular impairment ($P<0.05$) than those without EDS but do not differ as regards BMI and the number of CTG trinucleotide repeat expansions. These latter results concur with previous observations in another series of 157 adult DM1 patients [12]. In addition, while both DM1 patients with and without EDS have completed about 10 years of schooling, 11.5% of DM1 patients with EDS hold a job as compared to 23.7% of those without EDS

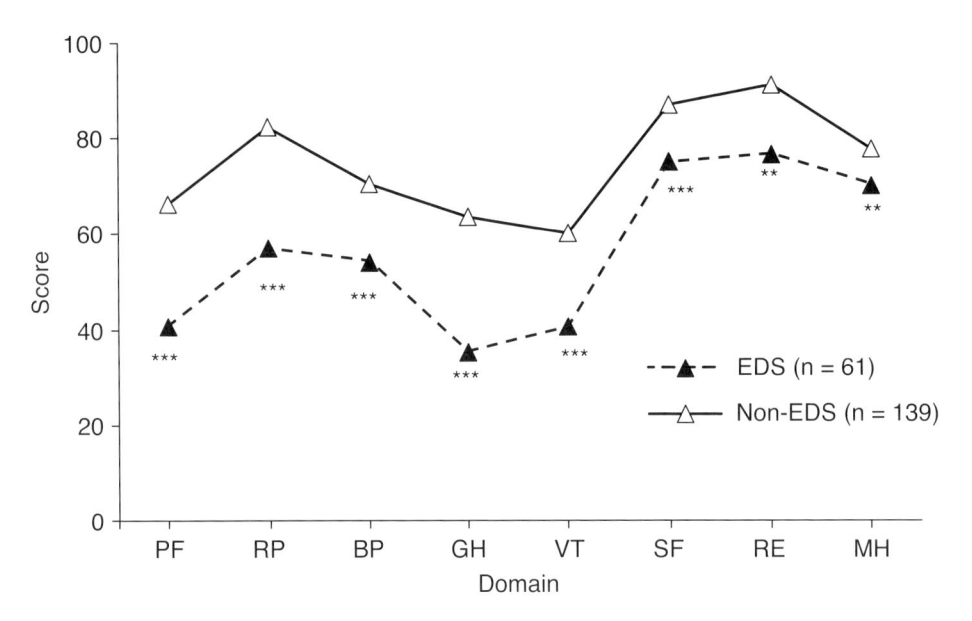

Figure 28.1 Health-related quality of life in 200 patients with myotonic dystrophy type 1 with and without excessive daytime sleepiness (EDS).
**$P < 0.01$; ***$P < 0.001$; PF: physical functioning, RP: role limitations due to physical problems, BP: bodily pain, GH: general health, VT: vitality; SF: social functioning, RE: role limitations due to emotional problems, MH: mental health. Health-related quality of life was measured by the Short-Form 36 (SF-36) subscales; EDS was defined by a the Daytime Sleepiness Scale (DSS) Score ≥ 7 [12].

($P < 0.05$). Also, a tendency for DM1 patients with EDS to rely more often on social welfare was noted ($P = 0.059$).

Figure 28.1 presents scores of DM1 patients with and without EDS on the eight Short-Form 36-item Health Survey (SF-36) subscales, a frequently used generic health-related quality of life (HRQoL) questionnaire. More particularly, it shows that DM1 patients with EDS report significantly lower scores than patients without EDS on all subscales, namely physical functioning ($P < 0.001$), role limitations due to physical problems ($P < 0.001$), bodily pain ($P < 0.001$), general health ($P < 0.001$), vitality ($P < 0.001$), social functioning ($P < 0.001$), role limitations caused by emotional problems ($P < 0.01$), and mental health ($P < 0.01$). Social deterioration has long been noted in patients affected by DM1 [6]. More particularly, the present sample of 200 DM1 patients was previously characterized as showing poor academic achievement, high unemployment, low family income, and high reliance on social assistance compared with the general reference population [22]. In agreement with two previous research findings on the relationship of EDS to functional disability, the present results suggest that EDS impinges upon social functioning of DM1 patients and is associated with a significantly worsened HRQoL [16, 24]. While Rubinsztein and co-workers hypothesized that EDS may either follow the course of the illness more closely in the later phase or that it may be independently associated with the extent of disability [16], Phillips and colleagues emphasized the possibility that the degree of disability affects the level of daytime sleepiness [24]. In our opinion, this latter possibility appears very unlikely, since onset of EDS predates any muscular involvement in many cases. Longitudinal assessments are needed to verify these assumptions, as well as to determine how the degree of muscular impairment mediates the relationship between EDS and HRQoL.

EDS, personality, and cognitive dysfunction

Table 28.2 presents personality and cognitive characteristics of 200 DM1 patients with and without EDS. Unsurprisingly, Table 28.2 first indicates that DM1 patients with EDS report higher levels of fatigue than those without EDS. In this respect, a recent study assessing the relationship of EDS to fatigue

Table 28.2 Personality and cognitive characteristics of 200 DM1 patients with and without EDS

Variable	EDS (n = 61)	Non-EDS (n = 139)
Mean (SD) Krupp Fatigue Severity Scale score	5.7 (1.2)***	4.1 (1.6)
Mean (SD) SCL-90-R depression score[b]	56.7 (8.1)***	50.9 (9.2)
Mean (SD) NEO-FFI score[a]		
Neuroticism	55.5 (9.9)***	47.2 (9.1)
Extraversion	43.9 (8.5)*	50.3 (9.6)
Openness	37.5 (5.2)***	42.8 (7.4)
Agreeableness	44.9 (9.2)*	49.9 (9.2)
Conscientousness	44.3 (8.1)***	50.3 (8.3)
Mean (SD) WAIS full-scale IQ score[c]	80.9 (7.1)	83.3 (8.9)

*$P < 0.05$; ***$P < 0.001$; Excessive Daytime Sleepiness (EDS) was defined by a Daytime Sleepiness Scale score ≥ 7 [12]; NEO-FFI: NEO Five-Factor Inventory; SCL-90-R: Symptom Check-List-90-Revised; WAIS: Wechsler Adult Intelligence Scale; [a]data available for 172 patients, [b]110 patients, and [c]188 patients.

conversely showed that DM1 patients with excessive fatigue, as assessed by the standardized Krupp's Fatigue Severity Scale, report higher levels of daytime sleepiness [23]. Also, DM1 patients with excessive fatigue are characterized by greater muscular impairment, higher CTG repeat number, more frequent sleep-related complaints, and higher depressive symptoms as compared to DM1 patients with neither fatigue nor EDS [23]. It was concluded that a moderate overlap exists between these symptoms in DM1 and suggested that clinicians should systematically consider both, since EDS and fatigue are associated to lower scores on SF-36 subscales than fatigue alone [23]. If EDS and fatigue truly coexist as distinct clinical entities in DM1, it is likely that currently available rating scales do not permit one to systematically distinguish them.

Consistent with the results of Phillips *et al.* [24], DM1 patients with EDS present higher depressive symptoms than those without EDS (Table 28.2). There are still unresolved differences of opinions as to whether depression in DM1 is a direct result of brain dysfunction or a secondary reaction to the physical disability or a combination of both. Phillips *et al.* contended that depression in DM1 may be largely ascribed to the additional life stresses caused by disability [24]. Our results of increased muscular impairment, fatigue and depression levels in DM1 patients with EDS support this view. In addition, the widely acknowledged peculiar personality of DM1 patients regarding temperament and character is even more evident in patients with EDS. Indeed, Table 28.2 indicates that DM1 patients with EDS are characterized by more proneness to psychological distress, and tend to be less sociable, optimistic, active, empathetic, persistent, organized, and motivated in goal-directed behaviors than those without EDS. In view of these results, it is not coincidental that EDS is often confounded with apathy of central origin [10]. However, the study by Rubinsztein and colleagues using standardized rating scales of daytime sleepiness and apathy in 36 patients established that EDS is an independent feature of apathy in DM1 [16]. Table 28.2 further indicates that a majority of DM1 patients are below average full scale IQ range (90–109), a finding indicating that social deterioration in DM1 is not only due to physical disability but also to mental cause with deterioration of intelligence [6]. Winblad and colleagues have shown that DM1 patients had lower performances than controls on tests measuring speed and attention as well as executive, visuospatial, and arithmetic ability [25]. However, DM1 patients with and without EDS appeared comparable in term of intellectual functioning. Altogether, these results suggest that EDS imposes an additional burden on quality of life and activities of daily living of DM1 patients. Further studies are thus needed to assess whether EDS is associated with specific neurocognitive sequelae, such as decrements in attention, vigilance, and memory.

EDS, habitual sleep–wake schedule, and sleep-related complaints

In the first article dedicated to EDS in DM1, Phemister and Small mentioned an unmanageable liability to oversleep at night [14]. Since then, many research reports have documented longer than habitual nocturnal sleep in DM1 patients than in controls [12, 18, 24]. Table 28.3 presents habitual sleep–wake schedule and sleep-related complaints of 200 DM1 patients with and without EDS. In a study by Manni *et al.*, all 10 DM1 patients (half of whom had daytime sleepiness complaints) reported sleeping each night for ≥ 8 h [26]. The mean habitual time in bed (TIB) of 9.3 h observed in our cohort (data not shown) is consistent with this latter observation by Manni *et al.* [26]. However, no difference was observed between DM1 patients with and

Table 28.3 Habitual sleep–wake schedule and sleep-related complaints of 200 DM1 patients with and without EDS

Variable	EDS (n = 61)	Non-EDS (n = 139)
Habitual sleep–wake schedule[a], (hr:min)		
Mean (SD) habitual bedtime	23:39 (1:35)	23:37 (1:38)
Mean (SD) habitual wake time	9:17 (1:55)	8:46 (1:45)
Mean (SD) habitual time in bed	9:37 (1:50)	9:08 (1:43)
Sleep-related complaints, % (n)		
Non-restorative sleep[a]	45.0 (27)**	28.9 (40)
Sleep inertia upon morning awakening[b]	63.9 (39)*	40.6 (56)
Difficulty staying awake after meals[c]	73.8 (45)***	32.4 (44)
Pain following nocturnal awakenings	36.1 (22)*	15.1 (21)
Cataplexy	9.8 (6)	3.6 (5)
Sleep paralysis[b]	6.6 (4)	1.4 (2)
Hypnagogic hallucinations	4.9 (3)	2.2 (3)
Leg restlessness at bedtime	19.7 (12)	10.1 (14)
Feeling of weariness or pain in the legs upon morning awakening	34.4 (21)*	13.7 (19)

*$P < 0.05$; **$P < 0.01$; ***$P < 0.001$; Excessive Daytime Sleepiness (EDS) was defined by a Daytime Sleepiness Scale (DSS) score ≥ 7 [12]; [a]data available for 198 patients, [b]199 patients, and [c]197 patients.

without EDS as regards habitual bedtime, wake time, and TIB (Table 28.3).

Discrepancies in the quality of nocturnal sleep in DM1 have long been documented, with self-reports of either sleep disruption [15, 27, 28] or deep, restorative sleep [17, 18, 24, 26, 29]. In a previous study, it was shown that more DM1 patients than control subjects report difficulty falling asleep in 30 min, non-restorative sleep, and sleep inertia upon morning awakenings [12]. Such findings raise the question of whether sleep disturbances are the prerogative of DM1 patients with EDS. Table 28.3 further shows that DM1 patients with EDS more frequently experience non-restorative sleep at night ($P < 0.01$) and sleep inertia upon morning awakenings ($P < 0.05$) than DM1 patients without EDS. We may add also that leg pain following nocturnal awakenings ($P < 0.05$) and in the morning ($P < 0.05$) was more frequent in DM1 patients with EDS compared to those without. Interestingly, van der Meché and colleagues described the clinical picture of their 17 DM1 patients with daytime sleepiness complaints as long, quiet sleepers difficult to arouse in the morning, with most patients needing either more than one alarm bell or to be shaken by their partner to arise in the morning [17]. As noted by many authors [12, 17, 26, 30], the persistent daytime sleepiness, long nocturnal sleep, morning sleep inertia, and long unrefreshing naps documented in DM1 [14, 17, 18, 24, 26, 29] closely resemble the complaints of patients with idiopathic hypersomnia (IH).

Symptoms of sleep paralysis and hypnagogic hallucinations were occasionally reported in DM1 patients [14, 15, 29], but their frequency is not different from that of control subjects [12]. Table 28.3 shows that relatively few DM1 patients report symptoms of sleep paralysis and hypnagogic hallucinations, irrespective of the presence or absence of EDS. The presence of possible cataplexy as sometimes pinpointed by questionnaires needs face-to-face interviews to be further validated and to exclude the presence of pseudo-cataplexy due to muscle weakness or myotonia [9]. Finally, feelings of pain during the night may relate to the peripheral vascular symptoms such as coldness and episodic pallor of hands and feet that are commonly found in DM1 [1].

Laboratory investigations

Polysomnographic studies

Sleep continuity and sleep architecture

To the best of our knowledge, three studies have compared and reported polysomnographic (PSG) data of DM1 patients with those of healthy control subjects recorded under identical conditions. Using data from the second night in three distinct groups of seven subjects, Gilmartin and colleagues first showed that DM1 patients presented a normal sleep architecture and a similar total sleep time (TST) than both control subjects and patients with non-myotonic muscle weakness [27]. Later, van der Meché *et al.* and Giubilei *et al.* equally noted normal sleep stage distribution in samples of 10 DM1 patients, but found that sleep duration was higher in DM1 patients than in control subjects [17, 31]. Sleep fragmentation or sleep disruption was reported in neither these latter studies nor in several other uncontrolled series of patients with DM1 [9, 17, 18, 26, 27, 31, 32]. Yet, some uncontrolled studies have reported disturbed sleep and abnormal sleep structure in DM1 patients [15, 33, 34]. We may explain such discrepancies by populations sampled (sample sizes, age ranges, disease severity, differences in the referral patterns, etc.), and ascertainment methods used.

Very few studies have compared sleep continuity and sleep architecture of DM1 patients with and without subjective EDS, even though it was repeatedly suggested that EDS might be attributable to sleep fragmentation consecutive to abnormalities of breathing during sleep. In this respect, the PSG study by Gilmartin and colleagues revealed no difference in the distribution of sleep stages between DM1 patients with and without EDS, evaluated using a simple sleep questionnaire [27]. More recently, our group investigated contributors to EDS in an unbiased sample of 43 DM1 patients as regards daytime sleepiness. Details regarding study design as well as patients and methods are described elsewhere [9]. Our PSG parameters acquired on the second night in the sleep laboratory in these DM1 patients with and without subjective EDS, as assessed by the DSS, reveal that sleep continuity (sleep latency, TST, sleep efficiency) and sleep architecture were comparable between groups with the exception of stage 2 sleep, which was lower in DM1 patients with EDS than in those without (31.9 vs. 39.9, $P < 0.05$) (data not shown).

Objective EDS

A study by Giubilei *et al.* reported that the mean sleep latency (MSL) on the MSLT was lower in DM1 patients than in controls (13.5 vs. 18.3), but defined MSL < 14.7 min as pathological EDS, making study comparisons difficult [31]. Gibbs and colleagues have found that 12 of their 13 DM1 patients with subjective complaints of EDS exhibited a pathological MSL on the MSLT as defined by a MSL $\leq$ 8 min [30]. Martinez-Rodriguez *et al.* have also documented such pathological MSL in their 6 DM1 patients with complaints of EDS [35]. In a prospective cohort of DM1 patients, Ciafaloni and colleagues more recently reported that 7 of 13 DM1 patients (53.8%) showed a MSL $\leq$ 8 min [32]. In our study of 43 DM1 patients without selection bias, 44.2% had a MSL $\leq$ 8 min [9]. Also, we found, in a random subsample of 23 DM1 patients who completed a 10-min psychomotor vigilance task (PVT-192, CWE Inc, Ardmore, PA) 30 min prior to each nap of the MSLT, that DM1 patients with MSL $\leq$ 8 min presented longer mean median reaction times than those with MSL > 8 min [36].

While objective EDS was positively related to the degree of muscular impairment in DM1 patients, it was not associated with age, BMI, and CTG repeat number [9]. Moreover, there is no relationship between the DSS and the MSLT ($r = -0.03$, n.s., $n = 42$) (data not shown). These findings echo data from previous studies in DM1 patients which acknowledged the problem of confirming subjective EDS with the MSLT [9, 18, 33]. Moreover, it should be mentioned that no relationship was found between the MSL and the Krupp's Fatigue Severity Scale ($r = -0.14$, n.s., $n = 42$) (data not shown). Therefore, altogether, these results suggest that subjective rating scales and objective measurement instruments such as the MSLT address different aspects of daytime sleepiness in DM1 as also reported in many neurological disorders (e.g. Parkinson's disease). In addition, the lack of relationship between either the DSS or the ESS and the MSLT cannot be merely explained in terms of a putative inability of DM1 patients to perceive correctly daytime sleepiness symptoms as opposed to fatigue symptoms.

In the study by Gibbs *et al.*, 11 of the 12 DM1 patients with pathological MSL had a sleep efficiency $\geq 80\%$ and a TST greater than 360 min [30]. Our results in 43 DM1 patients corroborate these findings. Indeed, patients with ($n = 19$) and without ($n = 24$) objective EDS demonstrated no difference as regards sleep continuity and sleep architecture, with the exception of patients with objective EDS showing a greater percentage of stage 4 sleep compared with patients without EDS (16.7 vs. 9.7) [9]. Hence, the presence of EDS in DM1 patients as assessed by the DSS, the ESS, a simple sleep questionnaire or the MSLT seems unrelated to objective evidence of sleep disruption [9, 27].

Sleep-onset REM periods

The presence of sleep-onset rapid eye movement (REM) periods (SOREMPs) on the MSLT is frequently reported in DM1. More particularly, DM1 patients referred to a sleep disorders clinic or recruited on the basis of EDS complaints presented 2 or more SOREMPs in 33–60% of cases [13, 30, 35]. In DM1 patients unselected for EDS, the proportion of patients with 1 SOREMP and 2 or more SOREMPs is about 40% and 25%, respectively [9, 32]. Also, DM1 patients with 2 or more SOREMPs were found to have higher muscular impairment and lower MSL than DM1 patients with 1 or no SOREMP [9].

Periodic leg movements in sleep

Ciafaloni and colleagues have found periodic leg movements (PLM) not to be prominent in DM1 [32], the mean PLM index in their cohort being 7.2/h with all 13 patients having a PLM index below 21. In our study of 43 DM1 patients, the mean PLM awake (5.3/h) and in sleep (10.5/h) were relatively low [9]. We may add that 10 DM1 patients (23.3%) had a PLM index above 15/h, including 7 of them having neither complaint of EDS nor abnormal MSL on the MSLT (data not shown). Moreover, in childhood-onset DM1, 8 of 21 patients (38%) were characterized as having a PLM index > 5/h (mean total PLM index = 15.5/h) [8]. However, the PLM group did not differ from patients in the Sleep Apnea Syndrome (SAS) group and in the non-SAS group as regards sleep continuity and objective EDS [8]. In summary, PLM in sleep is not a rare occurrence in DM1 but probably constitutes a minor contributor to EDS.

Sleep-related breathing disorders

Sleep-disordered breathing (SDB), hypercapnia, and nocturnal desaturation are all frequent in DM1 [27, 33, 37, 38]. SDB is explained by a dual mechanism: involvement of respiratory muscles (weakness and myotonia) and abnormalities of central control of ventilation. A high prevalence of mild chronic hypercapnia increasing in relation with the severity of muscular disability is observed in DM1 [38]. More particularly, chronic hypercapnia is present in about 25% of DM1 patients with minimal disease and in 77% of those with severe proximal weakness [38]. Inspiratory muscle weakness, increased respiratory elastance, and presumably low central ventilatory drive are likely to be involved in the pathogenesis of chronic hypercapnia in this condition. Chronic hypercapnic DM1 patients though have a relative preservation of vital capacity and maximum breathing capacity, supporting the view that abnormalities of central ventilatory control mechanisms participate to chronic alveolar hypoventilation in DM1 [38]. Also, this hypothesis is supported by findings of neuronal loss in various medullary nuclei linked to respiratory function in DM1 patients with alveolar hypoventilation [39]. However, hypercapnia does not necessarily relate to EDS, since DM1 patients without CO_2 retention may exhibit EDS [27, 33]. Inversely, correction of the alveolar hypoventilation does not always lead to the elimination of EDS [40]. To summarize, alveolar hypoventilation participates in the production of EDS in a minority of cases [1].

In addition, DM1 patients are characterized by a variable but generally high prevalence of apneas–hypopneas and episodic hypoxemia. Also, the relative prevalence of central [17, 33, 34] versus obstructive apnea [9, 37, 41] in DM1 patients varies considerably among studies. In a review of the medical literature, 57% of 86 DM1 patients with EDS had some degree of sleep apnea identified and 10% had alveolar hypoventilation documented [13]. In a study of 43 DM1 patients without selection bias, it was found that 86.0% of patients showed at least a mild apnea–hypopnea index (AHI ≥ 5)[3] and 27.9% showed severe apnea–hypopnea (AHI > 30), 86.6% of apnea events being of the obstructive type [9]. In another study comparing DM1 patients and a group of patients with a comparable degree of thoracic muscle weakness, DM1 patients showed greater AHI and nocturnal oxygen desaturation [27]. It was concluded that respiratory muscle weakness alone does not provide an adequate explanation for abnormalities of breathing during sleep in DM1.

Sleep-related ventilatory deficit in DM1 patients may cause transient nocturnal hypoxemia and episodes of desaturation that precipitate arousals and sleep fragmentation, ultimately resulting in EDS. However, there is substantial evidence that EDS in DM1 patients may occur in the absence of any identified sleep apnea and, conversely, that significant sleep apnea is not systematically accompanied by EDS [9, 17, 18, 26, 30]. In a series by van der Meché et al., DM1 patients exhibited central sleep apneas with

---

[3] The term apnea-hypopnea index (and its abbreviation, AHI) rather than respiratory disturbance index (RDI) will be used throughout, even when the original source of data uses the latter term.

minor fluctuations in oxygen saturation that, in the authors' opinion, were insufficient to lead to EDS [17]. Also, Gibbs and colleagues were unable to explain the objective EDS observed in 14 of their 19 DM1 patients based solely on respiratory abnormalities (AHI > 15 and/or upper airway resistance syndrome) [30]. Kiyan and colleagues more recently reported that 16 of 17 DM1 patients (94.1%) without subjective EDS (ESS score ≤ 10) had an AHI ≥ 5 [41]. Moreover, it was found in our series of 43 DM1 patients that AHI and nocturnal desaturation did not vary with subjective or objective EDS [9] and that PSG measures of sleep continuity and sleep architecture did not differ between DM1 patients with (AHI ≥ 15) and without moderate to severe sleep apneas (data not shown), hence confirming the recent findings by Kumar *et al.* [42].

Finally, there is generally low agreement between daytime pulmonary function parameters and nocturnal parameters [28]. As regards EDS, no relationship was found between daytime respiratory function tests results and subjective EDS [9, 24, 38]. In our series of 43 DM1 patients, we found though that DM1 patients with objective EDS were characterized by more severe respiratory muscle weakness, lung volume restriction and daytime hypercapnia [9]. Although AHI was found to significantly correlate with total lung capacity and vital capacity, these latter lung volume measurements could account for only 16% of AHI variance.

Metabolic abnormalities

Metabolic-endocrine dysfunctions in DM1 include hypogonadism, insulin resistance, and dysregulation of the hypothalamic–pituitary–adrenal (HPA) axis [1], but the most relevant to EDS and sleep disturbances probably are the findings of an impaired growth hormone (GH) secretion and hypercytokinemia. While the largest bursts of GH secretion normally occur in association with slow-wave sleep (SWS), plasma GH elevation was reported to be either absent or markedly decreased in the majority of DM1 patients [43]. Also, DM1 is characterized by a clearly abnormal regulation of cytokines, with namely increased levels of interleukin-6 (IL-6) and tumor-necrosis factor-α (TNF-α) in comparison with controls [44]. These immunoendocrine abnormalities were hypothesized to be of importance for sleepiness and fatigue in DM1.

Genetics

Myotonic dystrophy is an autosomal dominant disorder characterized by an amplified trinucleotide CTG repeat in the 3-prime untranslated region of the *DMPK* gene on chromosome 19q13 [3]. Disease severity varies with the number of CTG repeats: normal subjects have 5–30 repeats, mildly affected subjects have 50–80 repeats, and severely affected subjects have 2000 or more copies [3]. Amplification is frequently observed after parent-to-child transmission, defined as each subsequent generation demonstrating worsening manifestations and presenting at earlier ages, but extreme amplifications are only transmitted through the female line. This mechanism explains genetic anticipation and the occurrence of the severe congenital form almost exclusively in the offspring of affected women. The mechanism by which the expanded CTG repeat in the *DMPK* gene leads to the clinical features is unclear. However, several lines of evidence support a model in which nuclear accumulation of RNA from the expanded allele contributes to pathogenesis through a trans-dominant toxic effect of CUG-repeat RNA on RNA processing by altering the function of CUG-binding proteins [45]. Also, mutant *DMPK* transcripts were found to be widely expressed in cortical and subcortical neurons in postmortem DM1 brain tissue, with neuronal pre-mRNAs showing abnormal regulation of alternative splicing [46]. Hence, sleep regulatory dysfunctioning in DM1 may result from a toxicity of CNS expanded *DMPK* mRNA on alternative splicing regulation.

Pathogenesis

Although EDS is a prominent feature of DM1, its pathogenesis remains unclear. Available clinical, neurophysiological and histopathologic evidence supports the hypothesis that EDS in DM1 patients most often stems from a primary CNS disturbance, and possibly from a central dysfunction of sleep regulation. Among evidence suggesting that DM1 affects sleep regulatory circuits are the fact that EDS predates muscular weakness in many cases, there is not a coherent relationship between PSG abnormalities and evidence of SDB, and EDS sometimes persists even after treatment that greatly improved the blood gas values.

Metabolic-endocrine dysfunctions, especially disturbance of the HPA axis with disruption of the pulsatile secretion of cortisol and GH, are likely to affect sleep regulatory circuits in the CNS of DM1 patients

[43, 47]. In addition, van Hilten *et al.* previously reported a complex, widespread malfunction of the circadian and ultradian timing system in 10 patients with DM1 [18], results that need to be replicated in a larger sample of patients.

Some authors proposed to conceive DM1 as a brain disorder [48]. First, a substantial number of reports on brains of DM1 patients have delineated histopathological abnormalities. Culebras *et al.* was the first to note a high incidence of intracytoplasmic inclusions bodies in the anterior and dorsomedial thalamic nuclei of DM1 patients and suggested it related to the presence of EDS, apathy, and mental decline [49]. Also, the landmark series of studies by Ono and colleagues have notably described severe neuronal loss and gliosis in the reticular formation and in the midbrain and pontine raphe in association with EDS as well as a lower density of serotonin-containing neurons in the raphe of DM1 patients with EDS as compared to that of DM1 patients without EDS and control subjects [39, 50, 51]. Second, magnetic resonance imaging (MRI) studies have identified many brain regions affected in DM1, the most common structural abnormalities being white matter lesions and global cerebral atrophy with dilated ventricles [1]. However, no relationship was found between objective sleepiness and either cerebral atrophy or white matter hyperintense areas [26, 31]. However, one may reasonably argue that the sample size in these latter studies was not large enough ($n = 10$) to confidently exclude effects where no significant correlations were detected.

Finally, as DM1 is frequently associated with severe EDS and SOREMPs, similar to that observed in narcolepsy, several groups looked for an association with HLA and CSF hypocretin-1 levels [26, 32, 35, 52]. A previous study failed to report an association between DM1 with objective EDS and HLA DQB1*0602 as in narcolepsy, but reported a higher frequency of DQw1 and particularly of DRw6-DQw1 haplotypes [26]. Moreover, CSF hypocretin-1 levels have been measured in more than 40 DM1 patients with or without EDS, with results mainly showing normal levels [32, 35, 52]. In addition, one study revealed normal splicing of hypocretin receptor 1 and 2 mRNAs in postmortem samples of temporal cortex of DM1 patients [32]. Non of these results favor any relationship between sleep–wake disturbances characteristic of DM1 and that found in narcolepsy–cataplexy. However, one may expect the presence of other alternative splicing involved in CNS sleep regulatory mechanisms in DM1.

Management

In 1997, Hilton-Jones affirmed that most patients with DM1 were "badly managed or, to be more precise, not managed at all" [7]. With the exception of specialized neuromuscular clinics, it is likely that the situation has not changed substantially in the last decade. In view of the heavy toll that EDS likely exacts upon physical and social functioning of DM1 patients, it is mandatory to identify and treat those affected by this incapacitating symptom accordingly.

Identification of EDS

DM1 patients should be routinely assessed for EDS and SDB since these are treatable problems that may help alleviate an otherwise progressive condition. In order to do so, clinicians should thoroughly inquire about sedentary activities, sleep schedules, and functional limitations and ask the opinion of the spouse or significant other regarding the complaint of EDS [1]. An approach to quantify EDS or assess various treatment modalities may then include sleep logs and/or actigraphy, daytime sleepiness, fatigue, and depression rating scales, sleep disorder questionnaire, disability indexes as well as HRQoL scales. Also, PSG remains the gold standard to evaluate the nature and severity of sleep disorders in DM1 patients, and the MSLT for assessment of daytime sleepiness.

Assisted nocturnal ventilation

Since EDS may be the result of a potentially correctable sleep respiratory abnormality in some instances, various forms of ventilation have been used in patients with DM1 (intermittent positive pressure breathing, continuous positive airway pressure (CPAP), and bilevel positive airway pressure (BiPAP)) [13, 28, 53]. However, only the latter was shown to effectively treat EDS in 3 of 6 DM1 patients [28]. More recently, domiciliary non-invasive assisted ventilation (NIAV) was used in 13 DM1 patients [54]. Although compliance with NIAV was lower in DM1 patients than in a group of age- and sex-matched postpoliomyelitis patients, Nugent and colleagues observed that its use was associated with a sustained improvement in arterial blood gas tensions and prolonged survival. Also, they deemed symptoms to have improved in 8 of 9 survivors experiencing EDS [54]. A recent study in DM1 patients unselected for EDS recorded for two consecutive nights has shown that about 30% of patients exhibited severe sleep apneas [9]. More importantly, it was demonstrated in this cohort that a single night of PSG monitoring would have failed to identify severe sleep apneas (AHI > 30) in about 25% of patients with DM1 [55]. A consensus statement by Loube *et al.* had recommended that obstructive sleep apnea syndrome (OSAS) patients with an AHI > 30 should automatically be treated with nocturnal ventilation regardless of symptoms or associated conditions [56]. A high suspicion for the presence of respiratory disorders thus needs to be maintained in the DM1 patient population. Targeted sleep monitoring in DM1 patients with multiple symptoms suggestive of SDB is needed. Interestingly, a recent study reported that home unattended oximetry was well tolerated and offers a practical screening tool in this patient population [42]. Still, EDS in DM1 is not completely controlled with appropriate treatment of SDB [28]. Independent of underlying dysfunction, EDS may persist after treatment of SDB and stimulant medication may constitute a helpful adjunct [28].

CNS stimulant drugs

Psychostimulant drugs are increasingly used to treat EDS in DM1. The latest American Academy of Sleep Medicine (AASM) Practice Parameters for the Treatment of Narcolepsy and other Hypersomnias of Central Origin [57] stated that methylphenidate may be effective for treatment of EDS due to myotonic dystrophy [17]. In an updated Cochrane review, Annane and co-workers considered all well-designed trials that have assessed any type of psychostimulants in children and adults with proven DM1 and EDS [58]. They reported no evidence to support the routine use of psychostimulants to treat EDS in DM1 [58], but noted some evidence from two studies that modafinil may improve EDS [59, 60]. However, a recent multicenter French study conducted in 28 DM1 patients reported that modafinil had no significant effects on EDS as measured using the objective maintenance of wakefulness test (MWT) [61]. Yet the authors mentioned that their study might be underpowered (13 DM1 patients in the modafinil group) and stressed the importance of larger controlled studies to confirm these findings. It should nonetheless be added that some authors suggested that modafinil may play a role in such indications as OSAS already treated by nasal CPAP but persisting EDS [62].

Conclusions (including future directions)

DM1 entails prominent EDS but with different phenotypes that can mimic symptoms of primary sleep disorders, namely IH, narcolepsy, and OSAS. Also, DM1 patients are highly prone to associate sleep-related disorders. Despite a presumed multifactorial etiology for EDS, most authors are of the opinion that it is primarily caused by a dysfunction of brain areas regulating sleep patterns. Moreover, the possibility that two or more types of abnormalities coexist in a given DM1 patient and participate in the production of EDS should not be excluded. In order to further clarify the phenotype of EDS in DM1, it is essential that researchers utilize standardized methods for measuring EDS, and preferably for both subjective and objective EDS. Future studies may use the maintenance of wakefulness test (MWT) or follow PSG and the MSLT by a 24-h continuous PSG on an ad-lib sleep–wake protocol. Those studies are also warranted to elucidate the mechanisms underlying the production of EDS or SOREMPs.

The high prevalence of EDS, SOREMPs and SDB found in this patient population emphasizes the need for routine use of clinical sleep interviews assessing for both EDS and SDB and for systematic investigation of both diurnal and nocturnal sleep. The general lack of relationship between results of self-assessed instruments and pulmonary function tests, on the one hand, and those of objective assessment of EDS and assessment of sleep-related respiratory disorders, on the other, underpins the importance of taking into account several outcome measures and offering DM1 patients adapted sleep treatment to augment their HRQoL. Also, there still is a need [10] for properly structured trial of assisted nocturnal ventilation and further randomized trials of CNS stimulant drugs in large samples of DM1 patients without selection bias. Indeed, the literature in both areas is scarce, and numerous questions remain unanswered as to the best form of treatment and the best ways to evaluate the severity and consequences of EDS. Future research must namely clarify the indications for PSG and MSLT, and determine the optimal timing for commencing NIAV to treat SDB in this condition.

References

1. **Harper P S**. *Myotonic Dystrophy* (3rd Ed). Philadelphia: W.B. Saunders, 2001.

2. **Mathieu J, De Braekeleer M, Prévost C**. Genealogical reconstruction of myotonic dystrophy in the Saguenay–Lac-Saint-Jean area (Quebec, Canada). *Neurology*, 1990; **40**:839–42.

3. **Harley H G, Brook J D, Rundle S A**, et al. Expansion of an unstable DNA region and phenotypic variation in myotonic dystrophy. *Nature*, 1992; **355**:545–46.

4. **Mathieu J, Allard P, Potvin L**, et al. A 10-year study of mortality in a cohort of patients with myotonic dystrophy. *Neurology*, 1999; **52**:1658–62.

5. **Rohrer K**. Ueber myotonia atrophica (dystrophia myotonica). *Dtsch Z Nervenheilkd*, 1916; **55**:242–304.

6. **Thomasen E**. *Myotonia*. Denmark: Aarhuus Universitetsforlaget, 1948.

7. **Hilton-Jones D**. Myotonic dystrophy – forgotten aspects of an often neglected condition. *Curr Opin Neurol*, 1997; **10**:399–401.

8. **Quera Salva M A, Blumen M, Jacquette A**, et al. Sleep disorders in childhood-onset myotonic dystrophy type 1. *Neuromuscul Disord*, 2006; **16**:564–70.

9. **Laberge L, Bégin P, Dauvilliers Y**, et al. A polysomnographic study of daytime sleepiness in myotonic dystrophy type 1. *J Neurol Neurosurg Psychiatry*, 2009; **80**:642–46.

10. **Hilton-Jones D, Damian M S, Meola G**. Somnolence and its management. In: Harper P, van Engelen B, Eymard B, et al., Eds. *Myotonic Dystrophy: Present Management, Future Therapy*. Oxford: Oxford University Press, 2004: 135–49.

11. **Laberge L, Gagnon C, Jean S**, et al. Fatigue and daytime sleepiness rating scales in myotonic dystrophy: a study of reliability. *J Neurol Neurosurg Psychiatry*, 2005;**76**:1403–05.

12. **Laberge L, Bégin P, Montplaisir J**, et al. Sleep complaints in patients with myotonic dystrophy. *J Sleep Res*, 2004; **13**:95–100.

13. **Park J D, Radtke R A**. Hypersomnolence in myotonic dystrophy: demonstration of sleep onset REM sleep. *J Neurol Neurosurg Psychiatry*, 1995; **58**:512–13.

14. **Phemister J C, Small J M**. Hypersomnia in dystrophia myotonica. *J Neurol Neurosurg Psychiatry*, 1961; **24**:173–75.

15. **Leygonie-Goldenberg F, Perrier M, Duizabo P**, et al. [Disturbances of wakefulness, sleep and respiratory function in Steinert's disease]. *Rev Neurol (Paris)*, 1977; **133**:255–70.

16. **Rubinsztein J S, Rubinsztein D C, Goodburn S**, et al. Apathy and hypersomnia are common features of myotonic dystrophy. *J Neurol Neurosurg Psychiatry*, 1998; **64**:510–15.

17. **van der Meché F G, Bogaard J M, van der Sluys H C**, et al. Daytime sleep in myotonic dystrophy is not caused by sleep apnoea. *J Neurol Neurosurg Psychiatry*, 1994; **57**:626–28.

18. **van Hilten J J, Kerkhof G A, van Dijk J G**, et al. Disruption of sleep–wake rhythmicity and daytime sleepiness in myotonic dystrophy. *J Neurol Sci*, 1993; **114**:68–75.

19. **Dement W C**. Tiredness versus sleepiness: semantics or a target for public education? *Sleep*, 2003; **26**:485–86.

20. **Kalkman J S, Schillings M L, van der Werf S P**, et al. Experienced fatigue in facioscapulohumeral dystrophy, myotonic dystrophy, and HMSN-I. *J Neurol Neurosurg Psychiatry*, 2005; **76**:1406–09.

21. **Kalkman J S, Schillings M L, Zwarts M J**, et al. Influence of relatives on fatigue experienced by patients with facioscapulohumeral dystrophy, myotonic dystrophy and HMSN-I. *Eur Neurol*, 2006; **56**:24–30.

22. **Laberge L, Veillette S, Mathieu J**, et al. The correlation of CTG repeat length with material and social deprivation in myotonic dystrophy. *Clin Genet*, 2007; **71**:59–66.

23. **Laberge L, Dauvilliers Y, Bégin P**, et al. Fatigue and daytime sleepiness in patients with myotonic dystrophy type 1: to lump or split? *Neuromuscul Disord*, 2009; **19**:397–402.

24. **Phillips M F, Steer H M, Soldan J R**, et al. Daytime somnolence in myotonic dystrophy. *J Neurol*, 1999; **246**:275–82.

25. **Winblad S, Lindberg C, Hansen S**. Cognitive deficits and CTG repeat expansion size in classical myotonic dystrophy type 1 (DM1). *Behav Brain Funct*, 2006; **2**:16.

26. **Manni R, Zucca C, Martinetti M**, et al. Hypersomnia in dystrophia myotonica: a neurophysiological and immunogenetic study. *Acta Neurol Scand*, 1991; **84**:498–502.

27. **Gilmartin J J, Cooper B G, Griffiths C J**, et al. Breathing during sleep in patients with myotonic dystrophy and non-myotonic respiratory muscle weakness. *Q J Med*, 1991; **78**:21–31.

28. **Guilleminault C, Philip P, Robinson A**. Sleep and neuromuscular disease: bilevel positive airway pressure by nasal mask as a treatment for sleep disordered breathing in patients with neuromuscular disease. *J Neurol Neurosurg Psychiatry*, 1998; **65**:225–32.

29. Kilburn K H, Eagen J T, Heyman A. Cardiopulmonary insufficiency associated with myotonic dystrophy. *Am J Med*, 1959; **26**:929–35.

30. Gibbs J W, 3rd, Ciafaloni E, Radtke R A. Excessive daytime somnolence and increased rapid eye movement pressure in myotonic dystrophy. *Sleep*, 2002; **25**:672–75.

31. Giubilei F, Antonini G, Bastianello S, et al. Excessive daytime sleepiness in myotonic dystrophy. *J Neurol Sci*, 1999; **164**:60–63.

32. Ciafaloni E, Mignot E, Sansone V, et al. The hypocretin neurotransmission system in myotonic dystrophy type 1. *Neurology*, 2008; **70**:226–30.

33. Cirignotta F, Mondini S, Zucconi M, et al. Sleep-related breathing impairment in myotonic dystrophy. *J Neurol*, 1987; **235**:80–85.

34. Broughton R, Stuss D, Kates M, et al. Neuropsychological deficits and sleep in myotonic dystrophy. *Can J Neurol Sci*, 1990; **17**:410–15.

35. Martinez-Rodriguez J E, Lin L, Iranzo A, et al. Decreased hypocretin-1 (orexin-A) levels in the cerebrospinal fluid of patients with myotonic dystrophy and excessive daytime sleepiness. *Sleep*, 2003; **26**:287–90.

36. Laberge L, Lacroix G, Bégin P, et al. Psychomotor vigilance performance is associated with objective daytime sleepiness in myotonic dystrophy. *J Sleep Res*, 2004; **13**(Suppl 1):421.

37. Finnimore A J, Jackson R V, Morton A, et al. Sleep hypoxia in myotonic dystrophy and its correlation with awake respiratory function. *Thorax*, 1994; **49**:66–70.

38. Bégin P, Mathieu J, Almirall J, et al. Relationship between chronic hypercapnia and inspiratory-muscle weakness in myotonic dystrophy. *Am J Respir Crit Care Med*, 1997; **156**:133–39.

39. Ono S, Kanda F, Takahashi K, et al. Neuronal loss in the medullary reticular formation in myotonic dystrophy: a clinicopathological study. *Neurology*, 1996; **46**:228–31.

40. Coccagna G, Martinelli P, Lugaresi E. Sleep and alveolar hypoventilation in myotonic dystrophy. *Acta Neurol Belg*, 1982; **82**:185–94.

41. Kiyan E, Okumus G, Cuhadaroglu C, et al. Sleep apnea in adult myotonic dystrophy patients who have no excessive daytime sleepiness. *Sleep Breath*, 2010; **14**:19–24.

42. Kumar S P, Sword D, Petty R K, et al. Assessment of sleep studies in myotonic dystrophy. *Chron Respir Dis*, 2007; **4**:15–18.

43. Culebras A, Podolsky S, Leopold N A. Absence of sleep-related growth hormone elevations in myotonic dystrophy. *Neurology*, 1977; **27**:165–67.

44. Johansson A, Carlstrom K, Ahren B, et al. Abnormal cytokine and adrenocortical hormone regulation in myotonic dystrophy. *J Clin Endocrinol Metab*, 2000; **85**:3169–76.

45. Timchenko L T. Myotonic dystrophy: the role of RNA CUG triplet repeats. *Am J Hum Genet*, 1999; **64**:360–64.

46. Jiang H, Mankodi A, Swanson M S, et al. Myotonic dystrophy type 1 is associated with nuclear foci of mutant RNA, sequestration of muscleblind proteins and deregulated alternative splicing in neurons. *Hum Mol Genet*, 2004; **13**:3079–88.

47. Johansson A, Henriksson A, Olofsson B O, et al. Adrenal steroid dysregulation in dystrophia myotonica. *J Intern Med*, 1999; **245**:345–51.

48. Ashizawa T. Myotonic dystrophy as a brain disorder. *Arch Neurol*, 1998; **55**:291–93.

49. Culebras A, Feldman R G, Merk F B. Cytoplasmic inclusion bodies within neurons of the thalamus in myotonic dystrophy. A light and electron microscope study. *J Neurol Sci*, 1973; **19**:319–29.

50. Ono S, Kurisaki H, Sakuma A, et al. Myotonic dystrophy with alveolar hypoventilation and hypersomnia: a clinicopathological study. *J Neurol Sci*, 1995; **128**:225–31.

51. Ono S, Takahashi K, Jinnai K, et al. Loss of catecholaminergic neurons in the medullary reticular formation in myotonic dystrophy. *Neurology*, 1998; **51**:1121–24.

52. Dauvilliers Y, Baumann C R, Carlander B, et al. CSF hypocretin-1 levels in narcolepsy, Kleine–Levin syndrome, and other hypersomnias and neurological conditions. *J Neurol Neurosurg Psychiatry*, 2003; **74**:1667–73.

53. Coccagna G, Mantovani M, Parchi C, et al. Alveolar hypoventilation and hypersomnia in myotonic dystrophy. *J Neurol Neurosurg Psychiatry*, 1975; **38**:977–84.

54. Nugent A M, Smith I E, Shneerson J M. Domiciliary-assisted ventilation in patients with myotonic dystrophy. *Chest*, 2002; **121**:459–64.

55. Beaudry M, Laforte M, Bégin P, et al. Is a 2-night polysomnographic study necessary to diagnose moderate to severe sleep apnea in myotonic dystrophy type 1? *Sleep Med*, 2006; **7**:S121–22.

56. Loube D I, Gay P C, Strohl K P, et al. Indications for positive airway pressure treatment of adult obstructive

sleep apnea patients: a consensus statement. *Chest* 1999; **115**: 863–6.

57. **Morgenthaler T I**, **Kapur V K**, **Brown T**, et al. Practice parameters for the treatment of narcolepsy and other hypersomnias of central origin. *Sleep*, 2007; **30**:1705–11.

58. **Annane D**, **Moore D H**, **Barnes P R**, et al. Psychostimulants for hypersomnia (excessive daytime sleepiness) in myotonic dystrophy. *Cochrane Database Syst Rev*, 2006; **3**:CD003218.

59. **MacDonald J R**, **Hill J D**, **Tarnopolsky M A**. Modafinil reduces excessive somnolence and enhances mood in patients with myotonic dystrophy. *Neurology*, 2002; **59**:1876–80.

60. **Talbot K**, **Stradling J**, **Crosby J**, et al. Reduction in excess daytime sleepiness by modafinil in patients with myotonic dystrophy. *Neuromuscul Disord*, 2003; **13**:357–64.

61. **Orlikowski D**, **Chevret S**, **Quera-Salva M A**, et al. Modafinil for the treatment of hypersomnia associated with myotonic muscular dystrophy in adults: a multicenter, prospective, randomized, double-blind, placebo-controlled, 4-week trial. *Clin Ther*, 2009; **31**:1765–73.

62. **Banerjee D**, **Vitiello M V**, **Grunstein R R**. Pharmacotherapy for excessive daytime sleepiness. *Sleep Med Rev*, 2004; **8**:339–54.

Section 3 Medical, Psychiatric and Neurological Causes of Sleepiness

Chapter 29

Post-traumatic sleepiness

Christian R. Baumann

Terminology

Traumatic brain injury (TBI) is caused by an outside force traumatically injuring the brain. External mechanical forces include rapid acceleration or deceleration, blast waves from an explosion, direct impact, and penetration. Non-traumatic brain injuries such as stroke, tumors, and inflammation, which do not involve external mechanical force, must be clearly distinguished from TBI. Common causes of TBI include vehicle and sport accidents, falls, and any form of violence. The classification of TBI is based either on the mechanism (closed versus penetrating TBI), the severity (as assessed by scales such as the Glasgow Coma Scale, or by neuroimaging of the brain), or the localization of the trauma (e.g. localized in a specific brain area versus widespread). TBI is one of the major causes of death and disability throughout the world, particularly amongst children and young adults. In the literature, the annual incidence rate of department visits for TBI has been reported to be around 400/100 000 [1]. An estimated number of 1.6 million people sustain TBI each year in the USA, accounting for 52 000 deaths and 80 000 patients suffering from irreversible neurological impairment [2, 3]. Data from Europe indicate an annual incidence of hospitalized and fatal TBI of 235 per 100 000 [4].

In the acute stage of TBI, loss of consciousness or retrograde/post-traumatic amnesia or both are the hallmark symptoms. The diagnosis of TBI (as opposed to head injury) is established on the basis of these clinical symptoms. Other symptoms are dependent on the type, severity and localization of TBI. Typical symptoms of all forms of TBI include headache, nausea and vomiting, disturbed motor coordination, dizziness, cognitive disturbances, mood changes, blurred vision, tinnitus, fatigue, and changes in sleep patterns.

With increasing TBI severity, symptoms become more severe and last longer. Depending on the localization of trauma and of mass lesions such as intracranial hemorrhage, other symptoms such as anisokoria, coma, epileptic seizures, abnormal posturing, and focal neurological deficits can occur. An important contributor to fatal outcome after TBI is the increase of intracranial pressure. Signs of elevated intracranial pressure include sopor and coma, paralysis of limbs, dilated pupils, and autonomic failure with bradycardia, increased arterial blood pressure, and respiratory depression. These symptoms develop over hours to days after trauma, which necessitates treatment and monitoring in an intensive care unit.

Improvement of neurological function usually occurs for two or more years after the trauma but is fastest during the first six months. Most patients with TBI have milder injuries, but residual deficits in these patients are not infrequent either [5]. Residual symptoms after TBI include impaired consciousness, hyposmia and other focal neurological deficits, post-traumatic epilepsy and movement disorders, hormonal disturbances, cognitive deficits, psychiatric disorders, and sleep–wake disturbances including post-traumatic sleepiness. The last can be defined as the presence of excessive daytime sleepiness (EDS) caused by TBI.

Post-traumatic sleep–wake disturbances have been widely neglected by the scientific literature for many years. Accordingly, medical textbooks and internet encyclopedias provide a long list of complications and sequelae after TBI, but most still fail to mention sleep–wake problems after TBI. In the next section, this chapter will give a short overview on post-traumatic sleep–wake disturbances, particularly post-traumatic sleepiness.

Sleepiness: Causes, Consequences and Treatment, ed. Michael J. Thorpy and Michel Billiard. Published by Cambridge University Press. © Cambridge University Press 2011.

Clinical findings

Although there are not many studies systematically dealing with post-traumatic sleep–wake disturbances, there is growing evidence that sleep and wakefulness are often disturbed after TBI. Two prospective studies on post-traumatic sleep–wake disturbances identified EDS as the most common symptom after TBI, but other symptoms also frequently occur [6, 7]. Therefore, this chapter will give a short overview on other sleep symptoms than EDS before focusing on post-traumatic sleepiness.

The most disparate epidemiological findings have been published on *post-traumatic insomnia*. A prospective study based on sleep questionnaires found a high prevalence (30%) of insomnia and poor sleep quality in 50 patients after TBI [8]. In a retrospective study comprising a heterogeneous population of 184 somnolent subjects suffering from TBI or head–neck trauma (whiplash injury), 45% of the patients reported insomnia ("disturbed nocturnal sleep"), mostly due to nocturnal pain [9]. In a questionnaire study, more than 50% of 452 TBI patients reported insomnia symptoms [10]. In another study by the same group, using subjective and objective measures of sleep quality, 14 TBI patients were compared to 14 healthy good sleepers [11]. The authors found that TBI patients with insomnia have a tendency to overestimate their sleep disturbance compared to polysomnographic measures of sleep, indicating that insomnia symptoms may be overestimated after TBI. In the same line, our prospective study which included actigraphy and polysomnography studies 6 months after trauma revealed insomnia in only 5% of 65 consecutive patients [6]. Insomnia has been shown to persist 3 years after TBI [12], and insomnia symptoms are associated with concomitant headache, depressive symptoms, and irritability [13].

The findings pertaining to *post-traumatic circadian sleep–wake disorders* are sparse and rather inconclusive. Anecdotal reports on post-traumatic delayed sleep phase syndrome have been published, but a study of 10 patients using questionnaires, sleep diaries, polysomnography, and saliva melatonin measurements failed to provide evidence of any shift in circadian timing of sleep subsequent to TBI [14, 15]. However, in a recent study, 42 TBI patients with complaints of insomnia, examined by actigraphy, saliva melatonin, and oral temperature measurements, the authors found circadian sleep–wake disorders in 36% [16]. Two types of circadian sleep–wake disorders were observed: delayed sleep phase syndrome and irregular sleep–wake pattern. The observation of frequent circadian sleep–wake disorders following TBI misinterpreted as insomnia by the patients themselves further supports the assumption that post-traumatic insomnia might be overestimated.

The assessment of the frequency of *post-traumatic fatigue* is difficult because there are no objective measurements of the complaint, and the few available studies used a multitude of different assessment scales that have not been validated properly. Furthermore, the definition of fatigue is inconsistent and vague: it can be defined as a subjective experience, and includes such symptoms as rapid inanition, persisting lack of energy, exhaustion, physical and mental tiredness, and apathy [17]. Therefore, definite conclusions regarding fatigue after TBI cannot be drawn.

The terms "hypersomnia" and "excessive daytime sleepiness" are often used synonymously, even in official classifications. However, in a strict sense, hypersomnia is defined by increased sleep need per 24 h, whereas EDS refers to increased daytime sleep propensity, i.e. difficulty fighting sleep during daytime. Studies on *post-traumatic hypersomnia* are sparse. In our own prospective study in 65 TBI patients, we defined post-traumatic hypersomnia as increased sleep need ≥ 2 hours per 24 hours compared to pre-TBI conditions [6]. Six months after trauma, we found hypersomnia in 22% of our patients, and most patients with post-traumatic sleep–wake disturbances suffered either from hypersomnia or from EDS/fatigue [6]. TBI patients on a job with strict working schedules and TBI patients with young children more often suffered from EDS, whereas students, adults without a job, and elderly patients more often suffered from hypersomnia. Furthermore, an association between severity of TBI and the presence of hypersomnia was found. In the light of these findings, it could be hypothesized whether the primary sleep–wake disorder after TBI may be hypersomnia. Thus, patients whose psychosocial environment allows extended sleeping times per 24 h may avoid increased sleep propensity during the daytime, whereas in patients who cannot compensate for the increased sleep need, EDS may occur.

Finally, *post-traumatic sleepiness* has been examined in several studies. However, the assessment of EDS is hampered by methodological issues, despite the presence of so-called objective tests. Excessive daytime sleepiness can be assessed with questionnaires such as the Epworth sleepiness scale (subjective EDS), and with sleep laboratory tests, such as the multiple sleep latency test (MSLT) (objective EDS). However, it has been shown that there is no statistically or clinically significant association between Epworth scores and mean sleep latency on the MSLT [18]. One possible explanation is that the subjective Epworth sleepiness scale and the objective MSLT may evaluate different, complementary aspects of sleepiness. Unfortunately, studies in heterogeneous samples of TBI patients used different subjective and objective measures, which makes comparisons between populations impossible. Furthermore, there is still no consensus on which diagnostic test should be used for the measurement of excessive daytime sleepiness. Many authors doubt the accuracy of the MSLT to diagnose and quantify EDS, whereas questionnaires are limited by their subjective character [18, 19].

In 1983, based on a polygraphic study, Guilleminault and colleagues alluded to the importance of recognizing EDS as a residual symptom after TBI, and they found an association of post-traumatic sleepiness with sleep apnea in a significant portion of their patients [20]. Others measured EDS with the MSLT and found post-traumatic sleepiness in almost 50% (33 of 71) of their patients with different types of brain injury (traumatic, ischemic, hemorrhagic, anoxic) [21]. In a small study using polysomnography and MSLT in 10 patients with TBI and EDS, underlying sleep–wake disorders such as sleep apnea and periodic limb movement syndrome were found in all tested patients [22]. Our own prospective data, however, suggested that in most TBI patients, the majority of cases with post-traumatic sleepiness cannot be explained by underlying sleep–wake, neurological or other disorders [6]. Alternatively, these data suggest that post-traumatic EDS is directly related to the neuronal injury itself. Subjective post-traumatic sleepiness (as assessed with the Epworth sleepiness scale) was found in 28% of 65 consecutive TBI patients, objective post-traumatic sleepiness (as assessed by the MSLT) in 25%. Subjective and/or objective post-traumatic sleepiness were found in 38%, the concurrence of both subjective and objective post-traumatic sleepiness was found in only 9 patients. Similarly, there was no significant correlation between mean sleep latency on MSLT and ESS. Another recent prospective clinical and sleep laboratory study in 87 patients at least 3 months after trauma, however, confirmed the high frequency of post-traumatic sleepiness [7]. The authors found sleep–wake disturbances in 46% of the examined population, with post-traumatic sleepiness as the most common finding (25%).

Natural history

TBI patients often ask their doctors whether or not their enhanced sleep drive and their increased sleep need will ameliorate over time. Unfortunately, scientific evidence on the evolution of post-traumatic sleepiness is extremely sparse. To better understand the natural history of post-traumatic sleepiness and other sleep–wake disturbances after TBI, we extended the observation period of our prospective study from 6 months to 3 years (unpublished results). Fifty-one of the 65 TBI patients of the original study were included and examined by the means of interviews and questionnaires including the Epworth sleepiness scale (ESS) and the Fatigue severity scale (FSS). Compared to 6 months after trauma, the prevalence of (subjective) post-traumatic sleepiness decreased markedly from 28% to 12%. On the other hand, we identified more patients suffering from fatigue: 35% of TBI patients were diagnosed with fatigue, as compared to 17% 6 months after trauma. Therefore, at least in TBI, there might be a continuum of fatigue and sleepiness: in the course after TBI, sleep propensity during daytime might fade, giving way to a rather unspecific tiredness which may become more prominent.

Diagnostic investigations

Table 29.1 gives an overview on suggested tests to assess post-traumatic sleepiness. The interview and scales should consist not only of sleepiness questions, but should also include questions on fatigue and hypersomnia, because these symptoms may be related (see above).

Pathology

The etiology of post-traumatic sleepiness is not known, nor are the underlying pathological causes. In general, sleep–wake disturbances likely result from and contribute to multiple factors associated with the brain injury, all of which complicate recovery and resolution of symptoms. In this respect, impaired alertness may be related to physical disability and increased exhaustion, and also to psychiatric symptoms such as depression and anxiety. Furthermore, it is unknown whether or not increased sleep need after TBI is

Table 29.1 Suggested diagnostic work-up in TBI patients with suspected post-traumatic sleepiness

Interview	Following trauma
	– are you often unable to stay awake, which leads to unintended lapses into sleep?
	– have you had car accidents due to sleepiness or short attacks of sleep?
	– do you often perform daytime naps?
	– do you often feel a lack of energy, or physical and mental tiredness?
	– are you easily exhausted?
	– how many hours do you sleep per 24 h (including daytime naps)?
	– do you need at least 2 hours more sleep than before trauma?
Questionnaires	e.g. Epworth sleepiness scale, Fatigue severity scale
Sleep laboratory tests	Suggested tests (can be adapted according to suspected causes and diagnosis)
	– actigraphy study (to rule out hypersomnia and chronic sleep deprivation)
	– polysomnography (to rule out other causes of sleepiness than the trauma)
	– multiple sleep latency test
	– maintenance of wakefulness test (can be performed to test treatment effects)

linked to neuroplasticity processes which are important for the post-traumatic recovery process. Last but not least, it is unknown whether injury to specific brain regions might be responsible for the evolution of post-traumatic sleepiness. For instance, it is conceivable that lesions in wake-promoting brain areas might contribute to sleepiness after TBI. Descriptions of injury in TBI often focus on the midbrain and subthalamus, but hypothalamic and brainstem injury is also common: one early study showed damage to the hypothalamus in 42% of deceased TBI patients, and brainstem regions are also commonly involved [23, 24]. Similarly, there is evidence of pituitary and hypothalamic dysfunction after TBI [25, 26].

The exact pathophysiology of traumatic damage to these midbrain structures is unknown. In general, there are two types of traumatic brain damage [27]. Primary damage relates to external forces, as a consequence of rapid acceleration or deceleration, direct impact, penetrating objects, or blast waves. Primary damage includes shearing injuries of white-matter tracts leading to diffuse axonal injury, focal contusions, hematomas, and edema. On a cellular level, primary damage contains membrane and ion channel dysfunction as well as conformational protein changes. Each type of TBI can initiate a variety of pathophysiological mechanisms, leading to secondary brain damage. These secondary cascades include free-radical generation, gene activation, neurotransmitter release, calcium-mediated damage, mitochondrial dysfunction, and inflammatory responses. Combinations of these mechanisms may lead to cellular damage not only in the region of direct impact, but also in neighboring and more distant brain areas.

In the acute period after TBI, low and undetectable cerebrospinal fluid levels of the wake-promoting neurotransmitter hypocretin (orexin) have been observed [28]. Hypocretins are produced by a small and distinct population of neurons in the posterior hypothalamus. Six months after TBI, hypocretin levels recovered. However, in a subset of patients, this recovery was only partial [6]. Furthermore, in the same patients, there was an association between low hypocretin levels and post-traumatic sleepiness. Together with the early reports on hypothalamic damage in TBI, this finding led to the hypothesis of hypocretin neuronal loss in TBI. The first preliminary study confirmed this assumption and revealed a 30% loss of hypocretin neurons in deceased TBI patients (Figure 29.1) [29]. This injury, on the other hand, was not limited to the hypocretin neurons as there was a partial loss of neighboring neurons producing melanin concentrating hormone and gliosis throughout the hypothalamus of TBI patients. These findings confirmed that TBI can injure the hypothalamus and suggested that, maybe together with lesions in other wake-promoting neurotransmitter systems in the brainstem, reduced hypocretin signaling may contribute to the persistent sleepiness often seen in TBI patients.

Management

Despite the high prevalence of post-traumatic sleepiness, and despite the fact that post-traumatic sleepiness impairs daytime functioning and quality of life of TBI patients, there are no larger studies on its management. Before considering treatment with stimulants, other causes for sleepiness than the trauma, e.g. obstructive sleep apnea or sleep-related movement disorders, must be searched for and treated.

A recent randomized questionnaire-based trial in more than 50 TBI patients with post-traumatic EDS did not reveal a beneficial effect of 400 mg modafinil on post-traumatic sleepiness [30]. In this study, however,

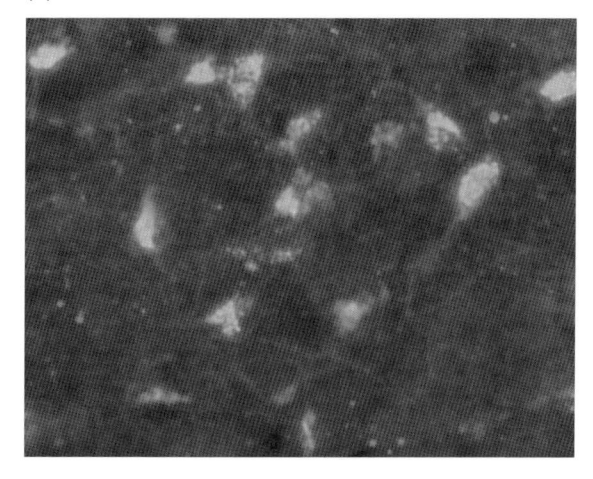

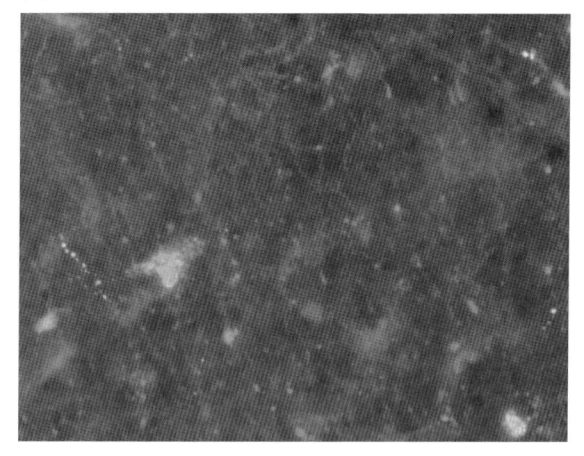

Figure 29.1 Photomicrographs depicting the relationship between the number of hypocretin neurons and gliosis (glial fibrillary acidic protein=GFAP staining of astrocytes). Double immunofluorescence staining shows that along with the reduction in the number of hypocretin neurons (green), there is an increase in red GFAP-labeled astrocytes and fibers in TBI (Figure 29.1B) compared to a control subject (Figure 29.1A) [29]. (See color plate section).

electrophysiological sleep laboratory studies including polysomnography (PSG) and vigilance tests have not been performed, and other possible causes of vigilance impairment have not been excluded by actigraphy. In our center, we performed a first double-blind, randomized, placebo-controlled study which included electrophysiological sleep laboratory tests in 20 TBI patients with post-traumatic sleepiness and fatigue (unpublished results). We found that 100–200 mg modafinil is effective and well tolerated in the treatment of post-traumatic excessive daytime sleepiness but not of fatigue. Epworth sleepiness scale values decreased significantly, and mean sleep latencies on the maintenance of wakefulness test increased by more than 8 min. In addition, we observed that modafinil-treated patients were almost 2 h more awake per day.

In summary, all treatments for post-traumatic sleepiness are still off-label. The first results on modafinil are promising, showing not only an improvement of post-traumatic sleepiness, but possibly also of post-traumatic hypersomnia. To create stronger evidence, larger multicenter trials are currently being undertaken to study the effect of modafinil and armodafinil on post-traumatic sleepiness. Other stimulants such as methylphenidate have not been examined systematically either. In addition, it is unknown whether sleep hygiene ameliorates post-traumatic sleepiness. Considering the hypothesis that post-traumatic sleepiness might also result from an increased sleep need per 24 h, it seems conceivable that sleep extension might be helpful.

Conclusions

In the field of sleep medicine, there is growing interest in post-traumatic sleep–wake disturbances, particularly post-traumatic sleepiness. However, there is still a lack of studies regarding the pathophysiology, epidemiology, clinical characteristics, and treatment of post-traumatic sleepiness. Current evidence suggests that post-traumatic sleepiness is common amongst TBI patients, probably somehow related to an increased sleep need per 24 h and to fatigue, caused by a multitude of factors including a loss of wake-promoting hypothalamic hypocretin neurons, and can be treated with modafinil and possibly also other stimulants. Several larger studies to better understand and manage post-traumatic sleepiness are ongoing.

References

1. **Langlois J A, Rutland-Brown W, Thomas K E.** *Traumatic Brain Injury in the United States: Emergency Department Visits, Hospitalizations, and Deaths.* Atlanta, GA: Centers for Disease Control and Prevention, National Center for Injury Prevention and Control, 2006.
2. **Sosin D M, Sniezek J E, Thurman D J.** Incidence of mild and moderate brain injury in the United States, 1991. *Brain Inj*, 1996; **10**:47–54.

3. **Bruns J Jr, Hauser W A**. The epidemiology of traumatic brain injury: a review. *Epilepsia*, 2003; **44**:2–10.

4. **Tagliaferri F, Compagnone C, Korsic M**, et al. A systematic review of brain injury epidemiology in Europe. *Acta Neurochir (Wien)*, 2006; **148**:255–68.

5. **Thornhill S, Teasdale G M, Murray G D**, et al. Disability in young people and adults one year after head injury: prospective cohort study. *BMJ*, 2000; **320**:1631–35.

6. **Baumann C R, Werth E, Stocker R**, et al. Sleep–wake disturbances 6 months after traumatic brain injury: a prospective study. *Brain*, 2007; **130**:1873–83.

7. **Castriotta R J, Wilde M C, Lai J M**, et al. Prevalence and consequences of sleep disorders in traumatic brain injury. *J Clin Sleep Med*, 2007; **3**:349–56.

8. **Fichtenberg N L, Zafonte R D, Putnam S**, et al. Insomnia in a post-acute brain injury sample. *Brain Inj*, 2002; **16**:197–206.

9. **Guilleminault C, Yuen K M, Gulevich M G**, et al. Hypersomnia after head-neck trauma: a medicolegal dilemma. *Neurology*, 2000; **54**:653–59.

10. **Ouellet M C, Beaulieu-Bonneau S, Morin C M**. Insomnia in patients with traumatic brain injury: frequency, characteristics, and risk factors. *J Head Trauma Rehabil*, 2006; **21**:199–212.

11. **Ouellet M C, Morin C M**. Subjective and objective measures of insomnia in the context of traumatic brain injury: a preliminary study. *Sleep Med*, 2006; **7**:486–97.

12. **Kaufman Y, Tzischinsky O, Epstein R**, et al. Long-term sleep disturbances in adolescents after minor head injury. *Pediatr Neurol*, 2001; **24**:129–34.

13. **Chaput G, Giguère J F, Chauny J M**, et al. Relationship among subjective sleep complaints, headaches, and mood alterations following a mild traumatic brain injury. *Sleep Med*, 2009; **10**:713–16.

14. **Quinto C, Gellido C, Chokroverty S**, et al. Posttraumatic delayed sleep phase syndrome. *Neurology*, 2000; **54**:250–52.

15. **Steele D L, Rajaratnam S M, Redman J R**, et al. The effect of traumatic brain injury on the timing of sleep. *Chronobiol Int*, 2005; **22**:89–105.

16. **Ayalon L, Borodkin K, Dishon L**, et al. Circadian rhythm sleep disorders following mild traumatic brain injury. *Neurology*, 2007; **68**:1136–40.

17. **Valko P O, Bassetti C L, Bloch K E**, et al. Validation of the Fatigue Severity Scale in a large Swiss cohort. *Sleep*, 2008; **31**:1601–07.

18. **Benbadis S R, Mascha E, Perry M C**, et al. Association between the Epworth sleepiness scale and the multiple sleep latency test in a clinical population. *Ann Intern Med*, 1999; **130**:289–92.

19. **Johns M W**. Sensitivity and specificity of the multiple sleep latency test (MSLT), the maintenance of wakefulness test and the Epworth sleepiness scale: failure of the MSLT as a gold standard. *J Sleep Res*, 2000; **9**:5–11.

20. **Guilleminault C, Faull K F, Miles L**, et al. Posttraumatic excessive daytime sleepiness: a review of 20 patients. *Neurology*, 1983; **33**:1584–89.

21. **Masel B E, Scheibel R S, Kimbark T**, et al. Excessive daytime sleepiness in adults with brain injuries. *Arch Phys Med Rehabil*, 2001; **82**:1526–32.

22. **Castriotta R J, Lai J M**. Sleep disorders associated with traumatic brain injury. *Arch Phys Med Rehabil*, 2001; **82**:1403–06.

23. **Crompton M R**. Hypothalamic lesions following closed head injury. *Brain*, 1971; **94**:165–72.

24. **Crompton M R**. Brainstem lesions due to closed head injury. *Lancet*, 1971; **1**:669–73.

25. **Karavitaki N, Wass J, Henderson Slater J D**, et al. A case of post-traumatic isolated ACTH deficiency with spontaneous recovery 9 months after the event. *J Neurol Neurosurg Psychiatry*, 2006; **77**:276–77.

26. **Schneider H J, Aimaretti G, Kreitschmann-Andermahr I**, et al. Hypopituitarism. *Lancet*, 2007; **369**:1461–70.

27. **Maas AI, Stocchetti N, Bullock R**. Moderate and severe traumatic brain injury in adults. *Lancet Neurol*, 2008; **7**:728–41.

28. **Baumann C R, Stocker R, Imhof H G**, et al. Hypocretin-1 (orexin A) deficiency in acute traumatic brain injury. *Neurology*, 2005; **65**:147–49.

29. **Baumann C R, Bassetti C L, Valko P O**, et al. Loss of hypocretin (orexin) neurons with traumatic brain injury. *Ann Neurol*, 2009; **66**:555–59.

30. **Jha A, Weintraub A, Allshouse A**, et al. A randomized trial of modafinil for the treatment of fatigue and excessive daytime sleepiness in individuals with chronic traumatic brain injury. *J Head Trauma Rehabil*, 2008; **23**:52–63.

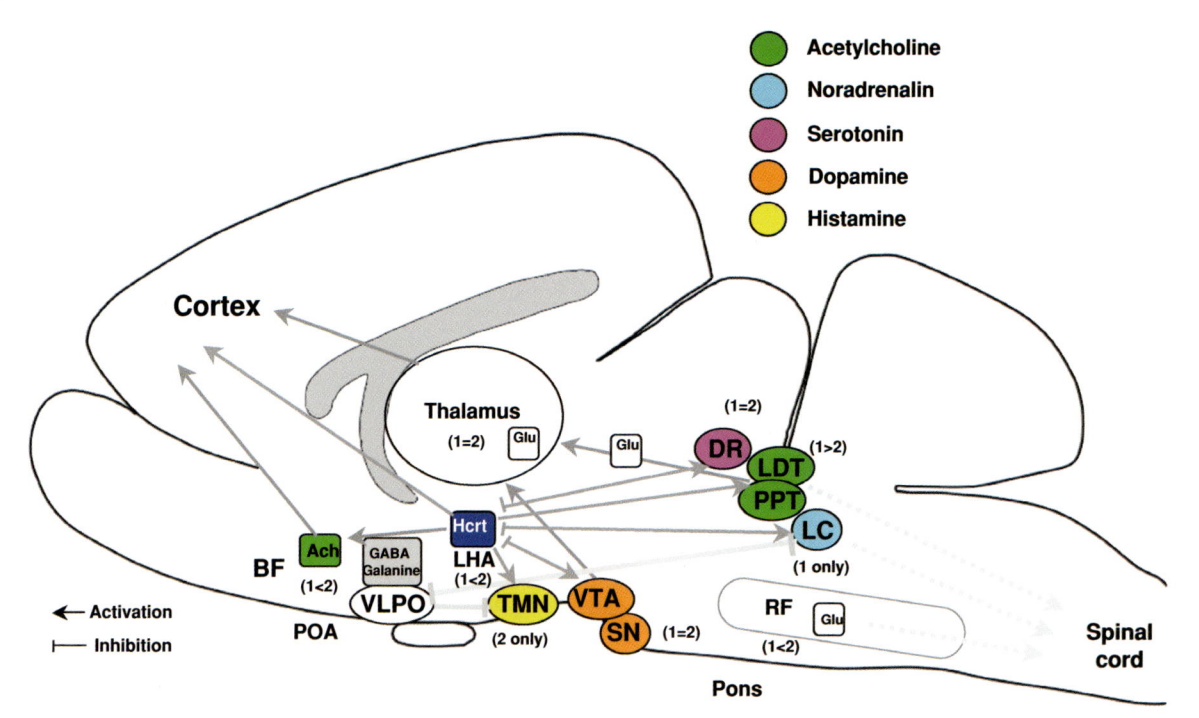

Figure 2.2 (a) Structures of mature hypocretin-1 (orexin-A) and hypocretin-2 (orexin-B) peptides. (b) Schematic representation of the hypocretin (orexin) system. (c) Projections of hypocretin neurons in the rat brain and relative abundances of hypocretin receptor 1 and 2. (a) The topology of the two intrachain disulfide bonds in orexin-A is indicated in the above sequence. Amino acid identities are indicated by shaded areas. (b) The actions of hypocretins are mediated via two G-protein-coupled receptors named hypocretin receptor-1 (Hcrtr1) and hypocretin receptor-2 (Hcrtr2), also known as orexin-1 (OX$_1$R) and orexin-2 (OX$_2$R) receptors, respectively. Hcrtr1 is selective for hypocretin-1, whereas Hcrtr2 is non-selective for both hypocretin-1 and hypocretin-2. Hcrtr1 is coupled exclusively to the G$_q$ subclass of heterotrimeric G proteins, whereas in-vitro experiments suggest that Hcrtr2 couples with G$_i$/G$_o$, and/or G$_q$ (adapted from [25]). (c) Hypocretin-containing neurons project to these previously identified monoaminergic and cholinergic and cholinoceptive regions where hypocretin receptors are enriched. The relative abundance of Hcrtr1 vs. Hcrtr2 in each brain structure was indicated in parenthesis (data from [4]). Impairments of hypocretin input may thus result in cholinergic and monoaminergic imbalance and generation of narcoleptic symptoms. Most drugs currently used for the treatment of narcolepsy enhance monoaminergic neurotransmission and adjust these symptoms. VTA, ventral tegmental area; SN, substantia nigra; LC, locus coeruleus; LDT, laterodorsal tegmental nucleus; PPT, pedunculopontine tegmental nucleus; RF, reticular formation; BF, basal forebrain; VLPO, ventrolateral preoptic nucleus; LHA, lateral hypothalamic area; TMN, tuberomamillary nucleus; DR, dorsal raphe; Ach, acetylcholine; Glu, glutamate; GABA, gamma-aminobutyric acid; HI, histamine; DA, dopamine; NA, noradrenalin, 5-HT, serotonin.

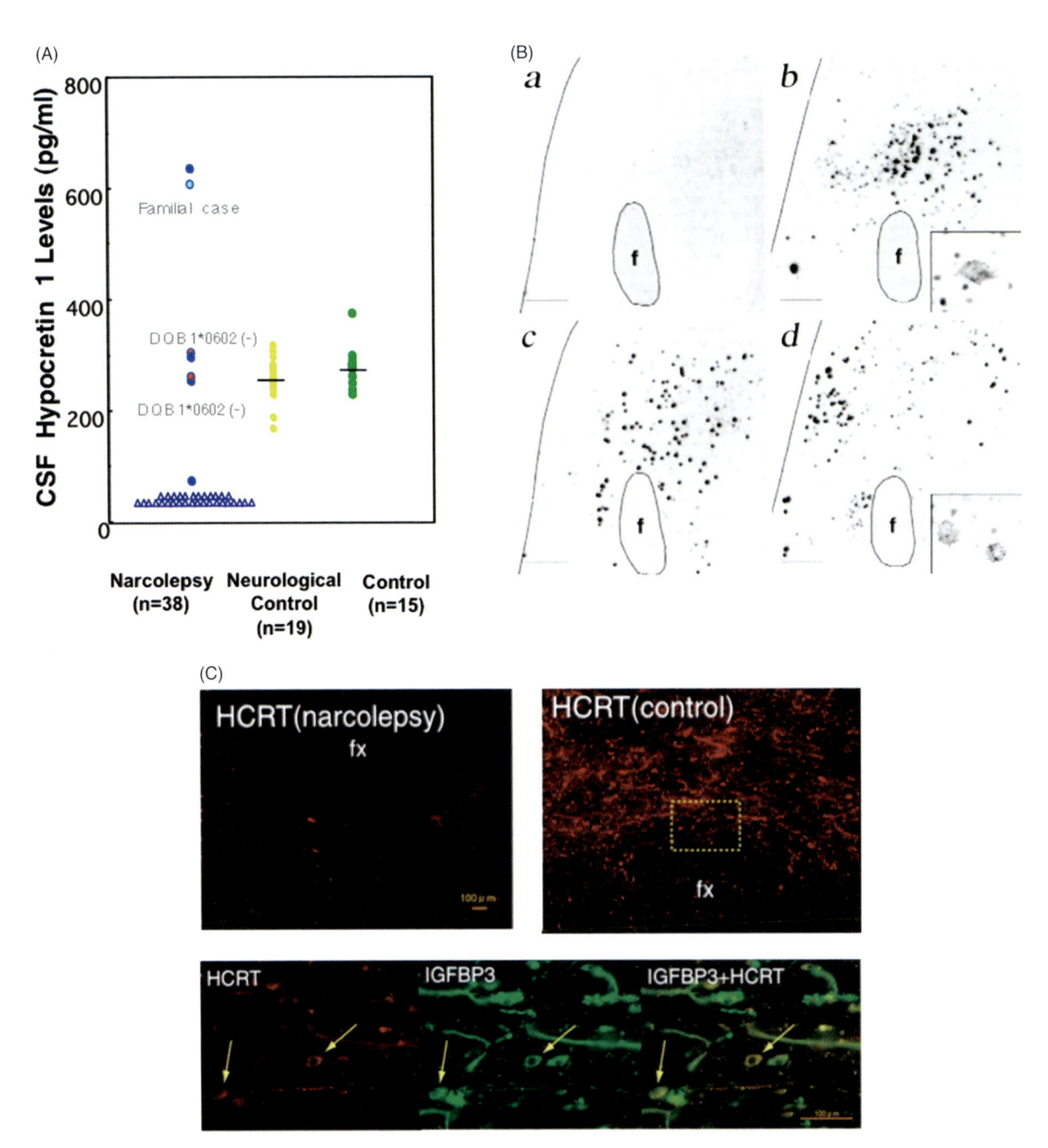

Figure 2.3 Hypocretin deficiency in narcoleptic subjects. (A) CSF hypocretin-1 levels are undetectably low in most narcoleptic subjects (84.2%). Note that two HLA DqB1*0602-negative and one familial case have normal or high CSF hypocretin levels. (B) Preprohypocretin transcripts are detected in the hypothalamus of control (b) but not in narcoleptic subjects (a). Melanin-concentrating hormone (MCH) transcripts are detected in the same region in both control (d) and narcoleptic (c) sections. (C) Colocalization of IGF BP3 in HCRT cells in control and narcolepsy human brain. Upper panel: Distribution of hypocretin cells and fibers in the perifornical area of human hypothalamus. (e) In control brains, HCRT cells and fibers were densely stained by an anti-HCRT monoclonal antibody (red fluorescence: VectorRed), while in narcolepsy brains, staining was markedly reduced. (f) Lower panel: HCRT immunoreactivity (g: red fluorescence) and IGF BP3 immunoreactivity (h: green fluorescence; Q-dot525) and a composite picture (i) arrows indicate HCRT cells colocalized with IGF BP3). Note non-neuronal autofluorescent elements. f and fx, fornix. Scale bar represents 10 mm (a–d), 500 mm in e and f, 100 mm in g–i (adapted from [17] and [21]).

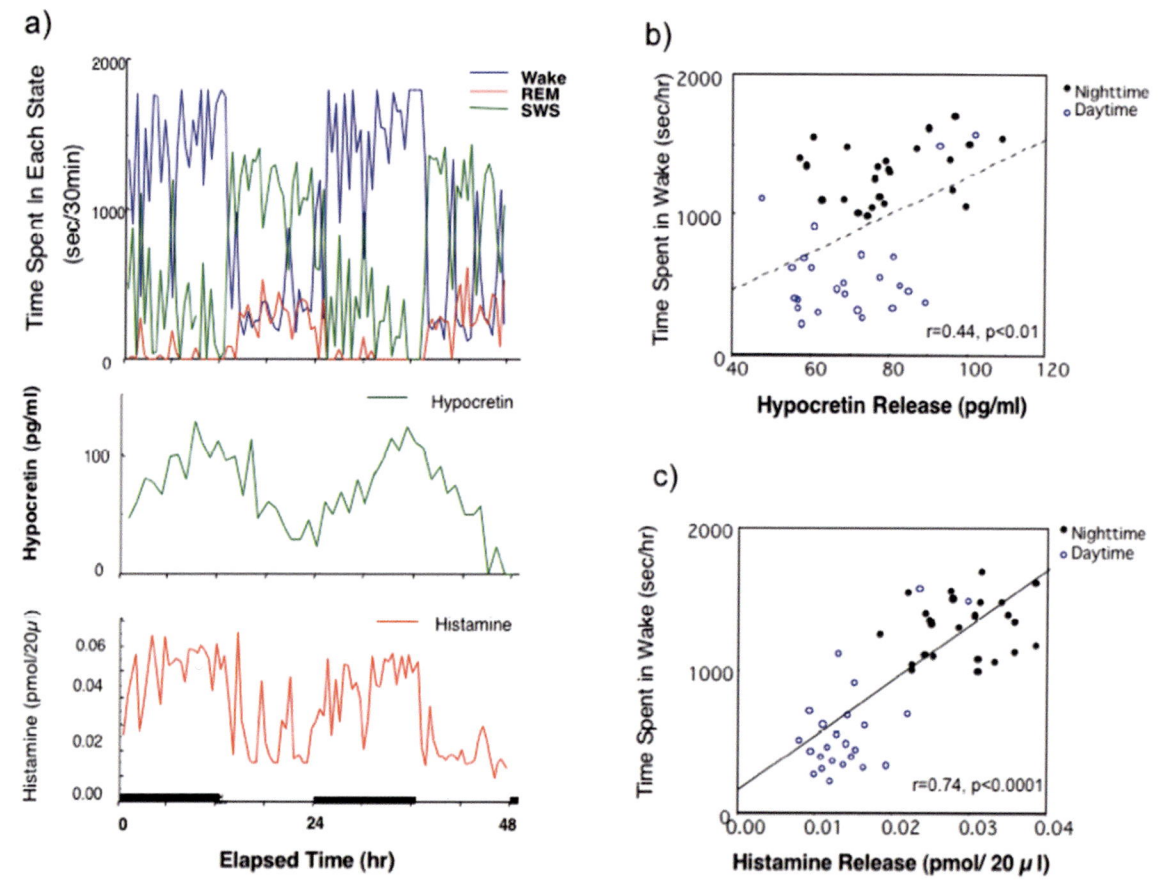

Figure 2.5 Fluctuation of extracellular hypocretin and histamine levels with changes in amount of wakefulness. Extracellular hypocretin and histamine levels simultaneously monitored in rats with sleep recordings under freely moving conditions using special floor-rotating rat chambers [30]. Changes in amount of wakefulness, hypocretin, and histamine levels were analyzed in 1-h time bins (the hypocretin levels were measured in 1-h time bins, while the mean of two consecutive 30-min bins were used for the histamine levels, see the Method). The dark periods are indicated by filled bars. (a) Typical data from one animal. Amount of wakefulness is displayed as s/h, while hypocretin and histamine concentrations are shown as pg/ml and pmol/20μl, respectively. (b, c) Correlations between time spent in wake and hypocretin/histamine releases in 4 rats. Filled symbols indicate data collected during dark periods. Extracellular histamine levels (c) are significantly (and positively) correlated with time spent in wakefulness across 24 h, while hypocretin levels (b) were clustered in light and dark periods, and the overall correlation between hypocretin levels and time spent in wakefulness is less significant.

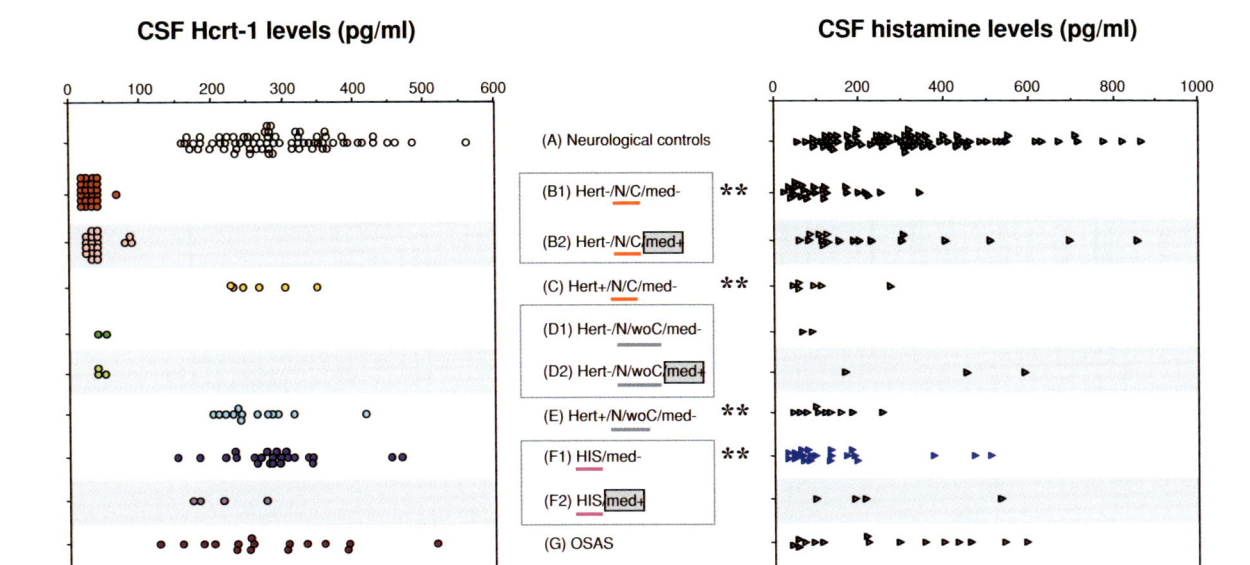

Figure 2.6 CSF Hcrt1 and histamine values for each individual with sleep disorders. CSF Hcrt1 (i: left panel) and histamine (ii: right panel) values for each individual are plotted. The patient groups are indicated as Group A to Group G from above. The results of the subjects with CNS stimulants (shadowed) and without CNS stimulants medication are presented separately in the figure. The vertical lines show mean values. The cut off value of CSF hypocretin-1 level (less than or equal to 110 pg/ml) clearly segregated hypocretin deficiency from non-deficiency. None of the patients with idiopathic hypersomnia and OSAS showed hypocretin deficiency. We found significant reductions in CSF histamine levels in hypocretin-deficient (B: 176 ± 25.8 pg/ml) and non-deficient narcolepsy with cataplexy (C: 97.8 ± 38.4 pg/ml), hypocretin non-deficient narcolepsy without cataplexy (E: 113.6 ± 16.4 pg/ml) and IHS (F: 161.0 ± 29.3 pg/ml), while those in hypocretin-deficient narcolepsy without cataplexy (D: 273.6 ± 105 pg/ml) and OSAS (G: 259.3 ± 46.6 pg/ml) were not statistically different from those in the control range (A: 333.8 ± 22.0 pg/ml). The low CSF histamine levels were mostly observed in non-medicated patients, and significant reductions in histamine levels were observed only in non-medicated patients with hypocretin-deficient narcolepsy with cataplexy (B1: 112.1 ± 16.3 pg/ml) and IHS (F1: 143.3 ± 28.8 pg/ml). The levels in the medicated subjects are in the normal range (B2: 256.6 ± 51.7 pg/ml and F2: 259.5 ± 94.9 pg/ml). Non-medicated subjects had a tendency for low CSF histamine levels in hypocretin-deficient narcolepsy without cataplexy (D1: 77.5 ± 11.5 pg/ml) (adapted from [6]).

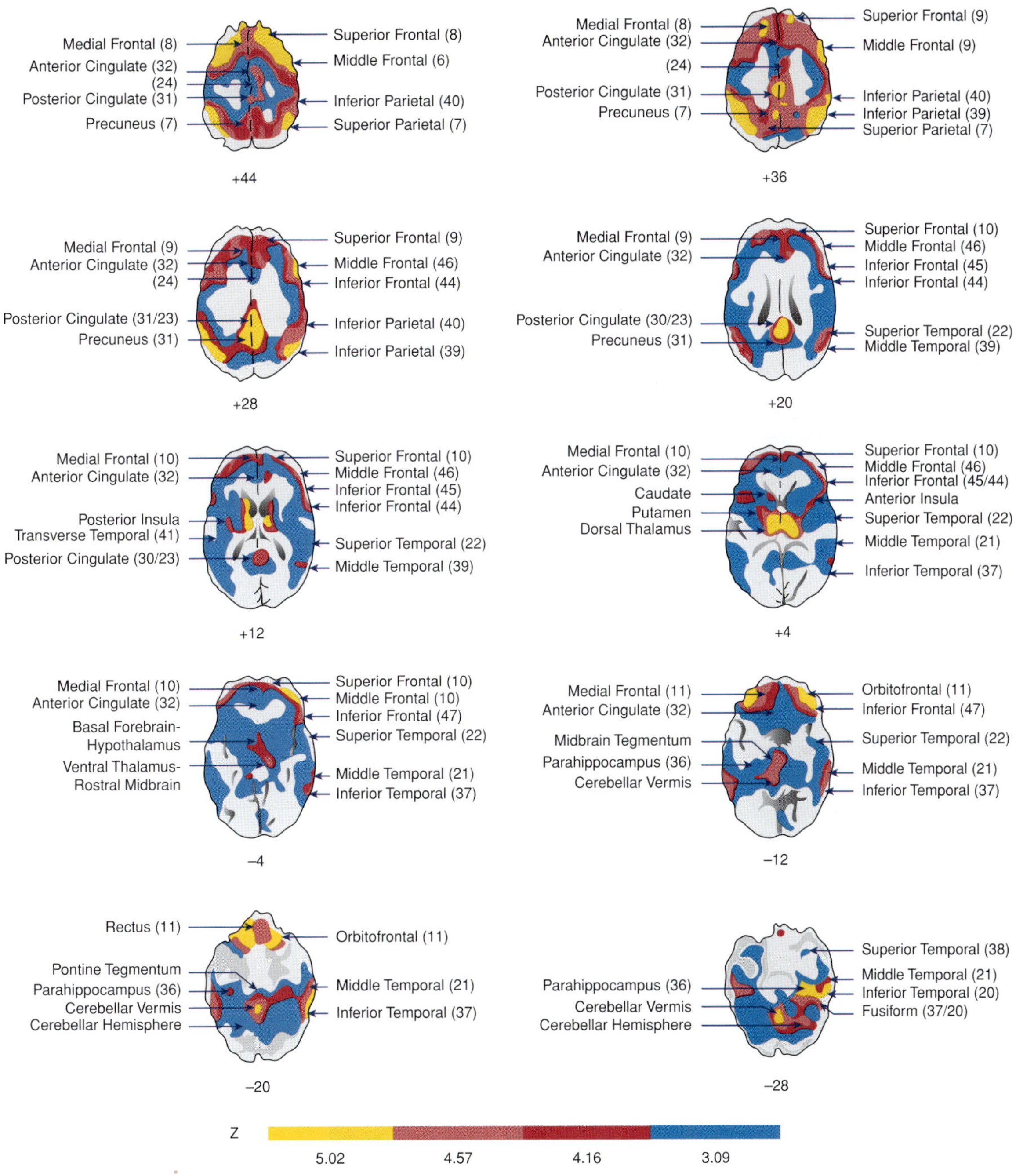

Figure 3.1 Significant decreases from baseline in absolute regional CMRglu during wakefulness and cognitive task performance after 24 h of sleep deprivation across 17 subjects. Deactivations are superimposed on a single subject's magnetic resonance imaging (MRI) template. Axial images are oriented in millimeters relative to the anterior commissure–posterior (AC–PC) plane. The left/right hemispheres appear as the left/right sides of each image. Significant regions are color-coded to reflect thresholds for statistical probability levels: $5.02 = 0.001$ corrected, $4.57 = 0.01$ corrected, $4.16 = 0.05$ corrected, $3.09 = 0.001$ uncorrected. Thresholds for statistical significance are $Z \geq 3.09$ for regions predicted to decrease a priori (thalamus and prefrontal cortex) and/or previously published for short-term sleep deprivation effects on regional CMRglu (temporal cortex, thalamus, and cerebellum [18]), and $Z \geq 4.16$ for non-hypothesized regions. Statistically significant regions are neuroanatomically labeled and approximate Brodmann areas (BAs) are noted in parenthesis ( ).

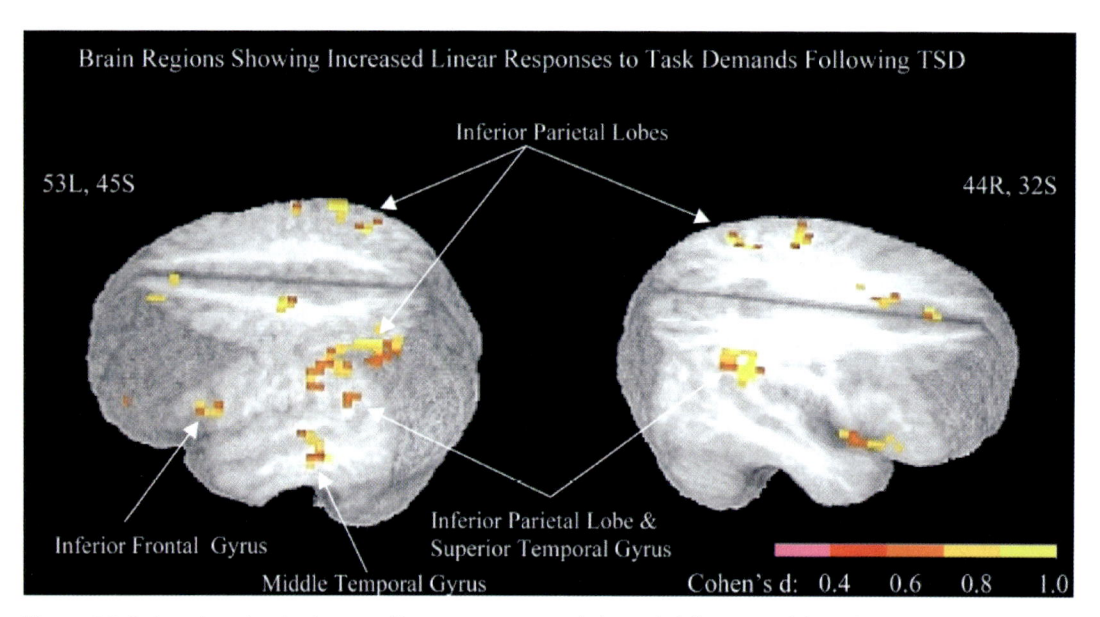

Figure 3.2 Brain regions showing increased linear responses to task demands following total sleep deprivation. Picture depicts the anatomic image averaged across all subjects as an underlay and the results of the main effect of total sleep deprivation (TSD) on the linear response to increasing task demands as the overlay. Functional data are color-coded per voxel by the effect size, Cohen's d, associated with the increased linear response following TSD compared to normal sleep. Only those voxels surviving our cluster threshold α protection method are shown. Each three-dimensional brain image has two slices removed. Left image: 53 mm left and 45 mm superior of the anterior commissure–posterior commissure line (AC–PC). Right image: 44 mm right and 32 mm superior of the AC–PC line.

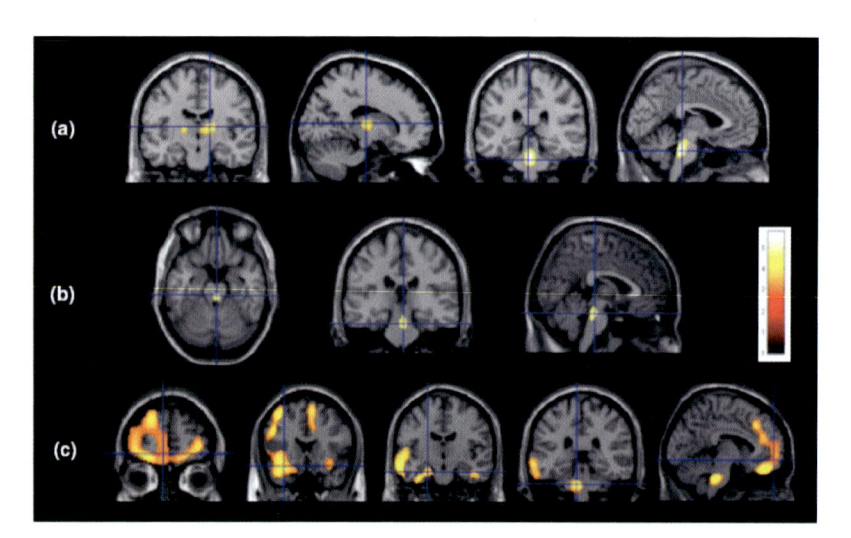

Figure 3.3 Brain regions showing significant rCBF changes after modafinil or placebo administration in healthy volunteers. (a) *On modafinil vs. Off modafinil*: Modafinil increased rCBF in bilateral thalami and in mid- and dorsal pons of the brainstem on T1 template overlaid MR coronal and sagittal images. (b) *On placebo vs. Off placebo*: Placebo increased rCBF in smaller regions in the mid- and dorsal pons of the brainstem on axial, coronal and sagittal images. (c) *On modafinil vs. On placebo*: Modafinil increased rCBF in bilateral orbitofrontal cortices, left dorsolateral prefrontal cortex (first imaging session from left side), left superior/middle frontal gyri, bilateral anterior insular gyri (second imaging session), left lateral and basal temporal areas (third imaging session), and in left anterior cingulate cortex, left mid- and dorsal pons of the brainstem (fourth and fifth imaging sessions in right side). Left to right panel order represents coronal images of the brain taken in the anterior to posterior direction. Left sides of images represent brain left sides. (a)–(c) were all significant at the uncorrected $P < 0.001$. (c) was also significant at FDR corrected $P < 0.05$.

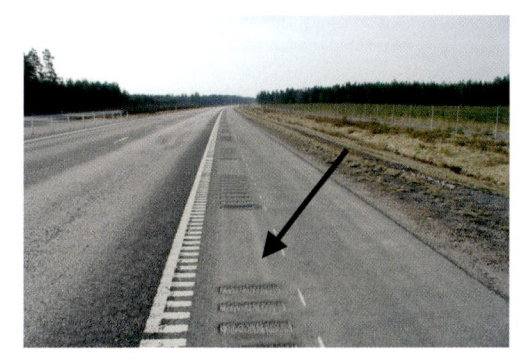

Figure 8.3 Rumble strip milled into the road surface at the shoulder.

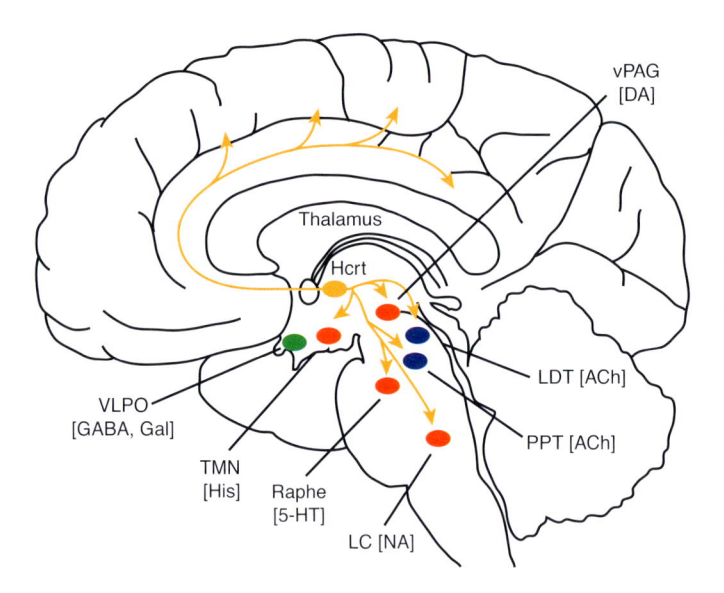

Figure 11.2 Projections of hypocretin. Hypocretin neurons, located in the lateral hypothalamus, innervate all nuclei of the AAS and the entire cerebral cortex. *Abbreviations:* VLPO, ventrolateral preoptic nucleus; GABA, γ-aminobutyric acid; Gal, galanin; TMN, tuberomammillary nuclei; His, histamine; LH, lateral hypothalamus; Hcrt, hypocretin; vPAG, ventral periaqueductal gray matter; DA, dopamine; Raphe, dorsal and median raphe nuclei; 5-HT, serotonin; LDT, laterodorsal tegmental nuclei; PPT, pedunculopontine tegmental nuclei; ACh, acetylcholine; LC, locus coeruleus; NA, noradrenalin.

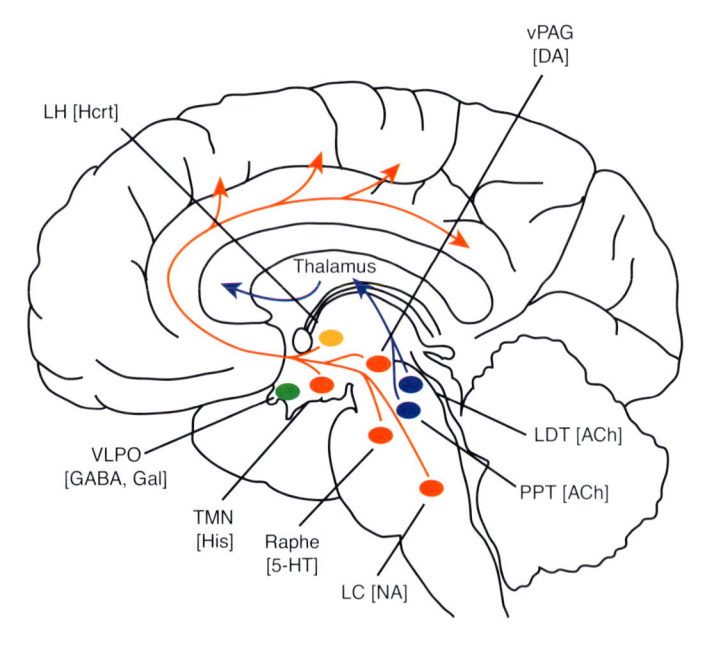

Figure 11.3 Ascending arousal system (AAS). The AAS comprises two pathways: (1) *Monoaminergic branch (red)*; the locus coeruleus (LC), dorsal and median raphe nuclei (Raphe), tuberomammillary nuclei (TMN) and ventral periaqueductal gray matter (vPAG) project diffusely to the cortex of the entire hemisphere. This pathway receives also contribution from peptidergic neurons in the lateral hypothalamus (LH) containing hypocretin (Hcrt). (2) *Cholinergic branch (blue)*; the pedunculopontine and laterodorsal tegmental nuclei (PPT, LDT), project to the thalamic reticular nucleus via thalamic relay neurons and activate the cerebral cortex. *Abbreviations:* VLPO, ventrolateral preoptic nucleus; GABA, γ-aminobutyric acid; Gal, galanin; His, histamine; DA, dopamine; 5-HT, serotonin; ACh, acetylcholine; NA, noradrenalin.

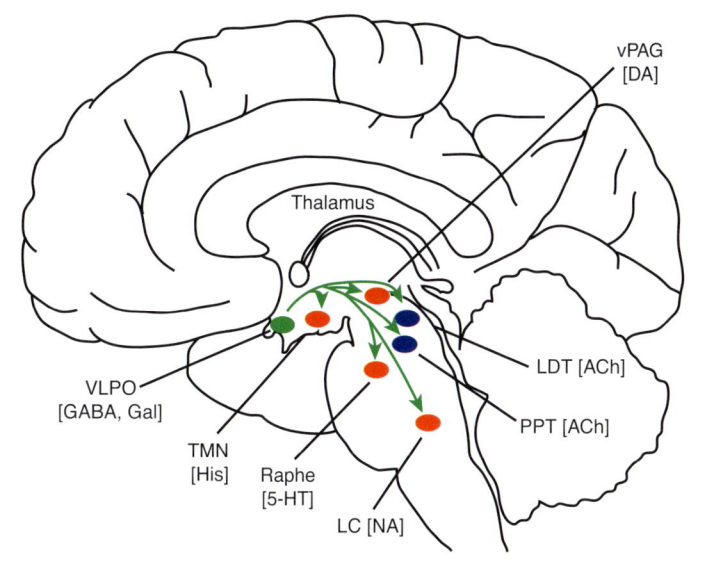

Figure 11.4 Projections of the ventrolateral preoptic nucleus (VLPO). The VLPO has projections to the nuclei of both the monoaminergic branch (red) and the cholinergic branch (blue).
Abbreviations: GABA, γ-aminobutyric acid; Gal, galanin; TMN, tuberomammillary nuclei; His, histamine; vPAG, ventral periaqueductal gray matter; DA, dopamine; Raphe, dorsal and median raphe nuclei; 5-HT, serotonin; LDT, laterodorsal tegmental nuclei; PPT, pedunculopontine tegmental nuclei; ACh, acetylcholine; LC, locus coeruleus; NA, noradrenalin.

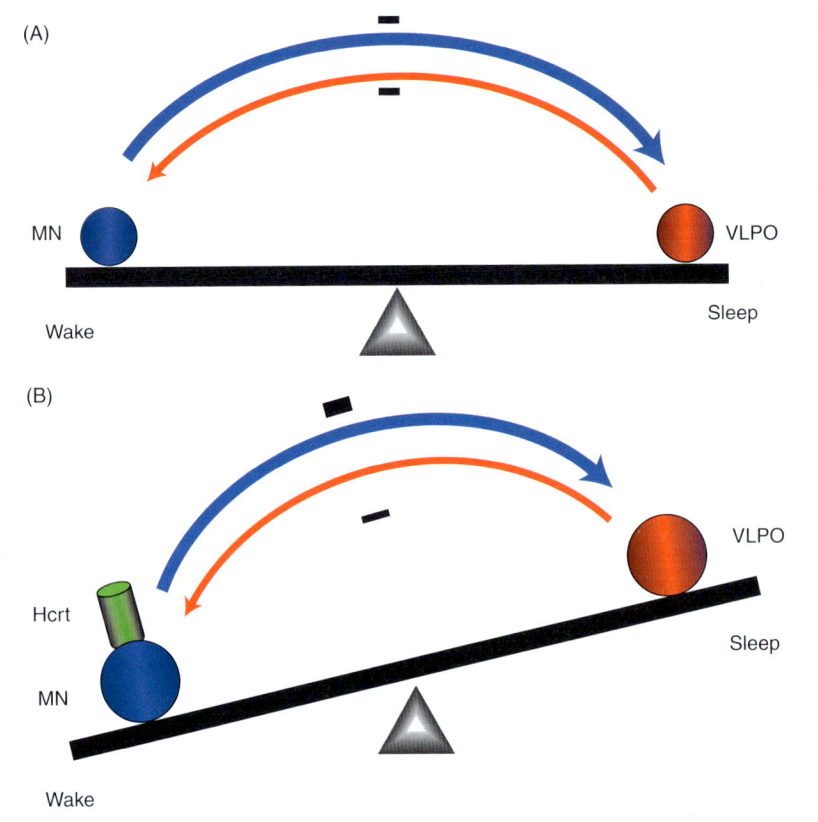

Figure 11.5 The "sleep-switch". The sleep-switch describes a feedback loop with a self-reinforcing firing pattern resulting in two possible states: sleep and wake. (A) The reciprocal inhibition of the ventrolateral preoptic nucleus (VLPO) and the monoaminergic nuclei (MN). It prevents the occurrence of intermediate states: if there is a transition, it is abrupt and complete. (B) A disadvantage of the sleep-switch is its instability; minor disturbances may lead to abrupt switches. During wakefulness the VLPO is inhibited by the monoaminergic nuclei and hypocretin (Hcrt) reinforces the arousal systems, stabilizing the switch in the waking state.

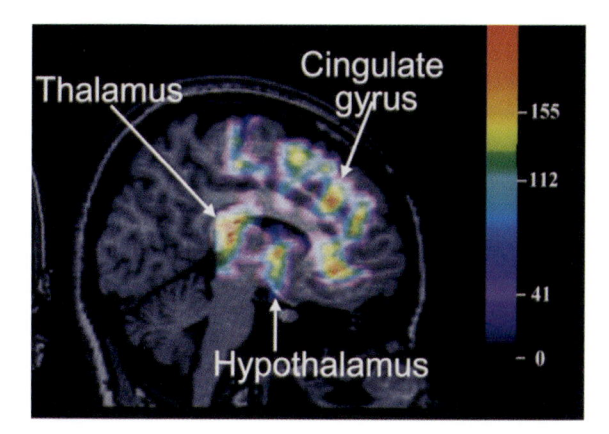

Figure 13.3 Brain scintigraphy during vs. after an episode, coregistered to MRI. Thalamic, hypothalamic, cingulate and frontal area are hypoactivated (in yellow and red) during the episode. Figure reproduced with the authorization of the *Sleep* journal [41].

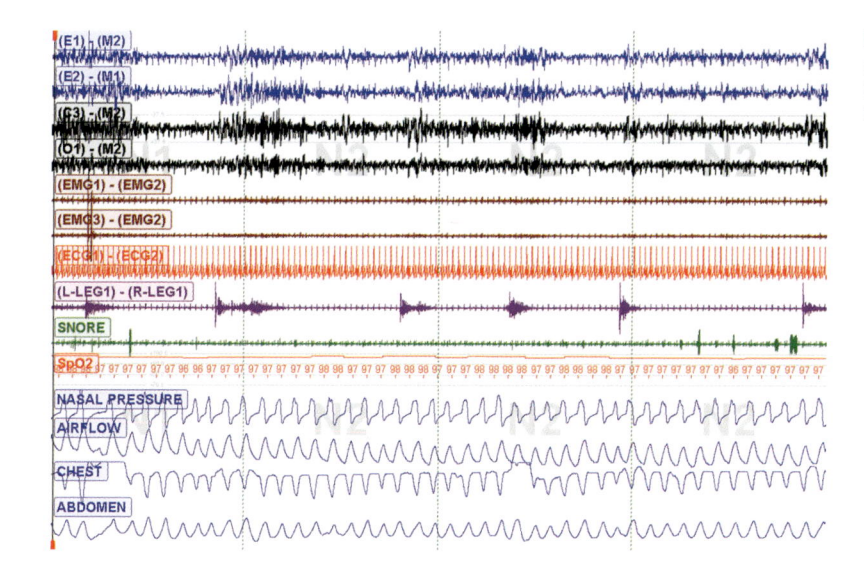

Figure 22.1 The 120-s polysomnography epoch demonstrates periodic movements of sleep associated with cortical arousals.

(A)

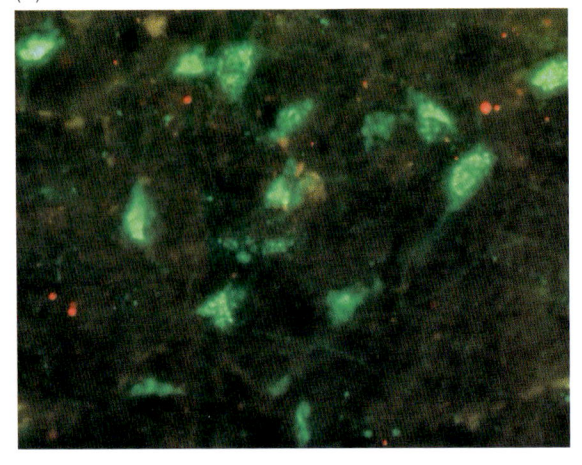

(B)

Figure 29.1 Photomicrographs depicting the relationship between the number of hypocretin neurons and gliosis (glial fibrillary acidic protein=GFAP staining of astrocytes). Double immunofluorescence staining shows that along with the reduction in the number of hypocretin neurons (green), there is an increase in red GFAP-labeled astrocytes and fibers in TBI (Figure 29.1B) compared to a control subject (Figure 29.1A) [29].

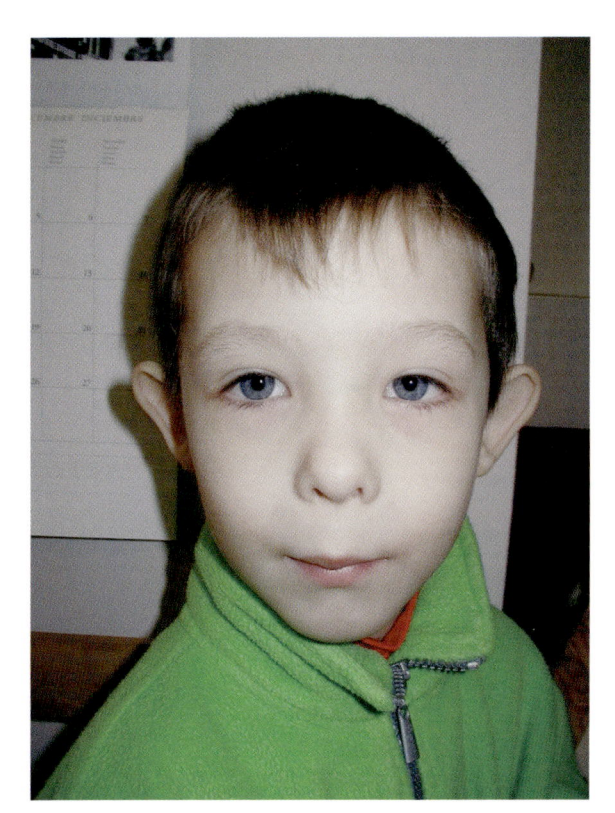

Figure 30.1 A 3-year-old boy with fragile X chromosome. Note his typical elongated face with large ears and protruding jaw.

(A)

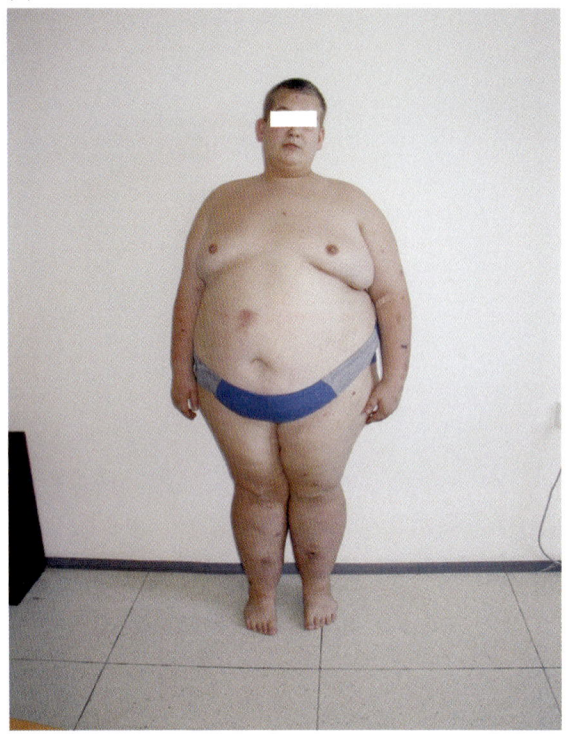

Figure 30.2a A 16-year-old boy with a typical Prader–Willi phenotype.

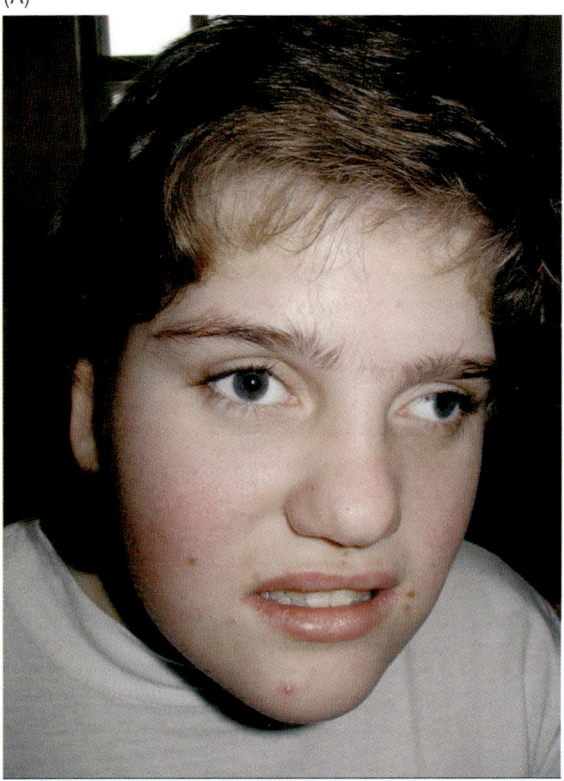

Figure 30.3a A 13-year-old girl with Smith–Magenis syndrome. Note her craniofacial dysmorphic features with brachycephaly, midface hypoplasia and prognathism.

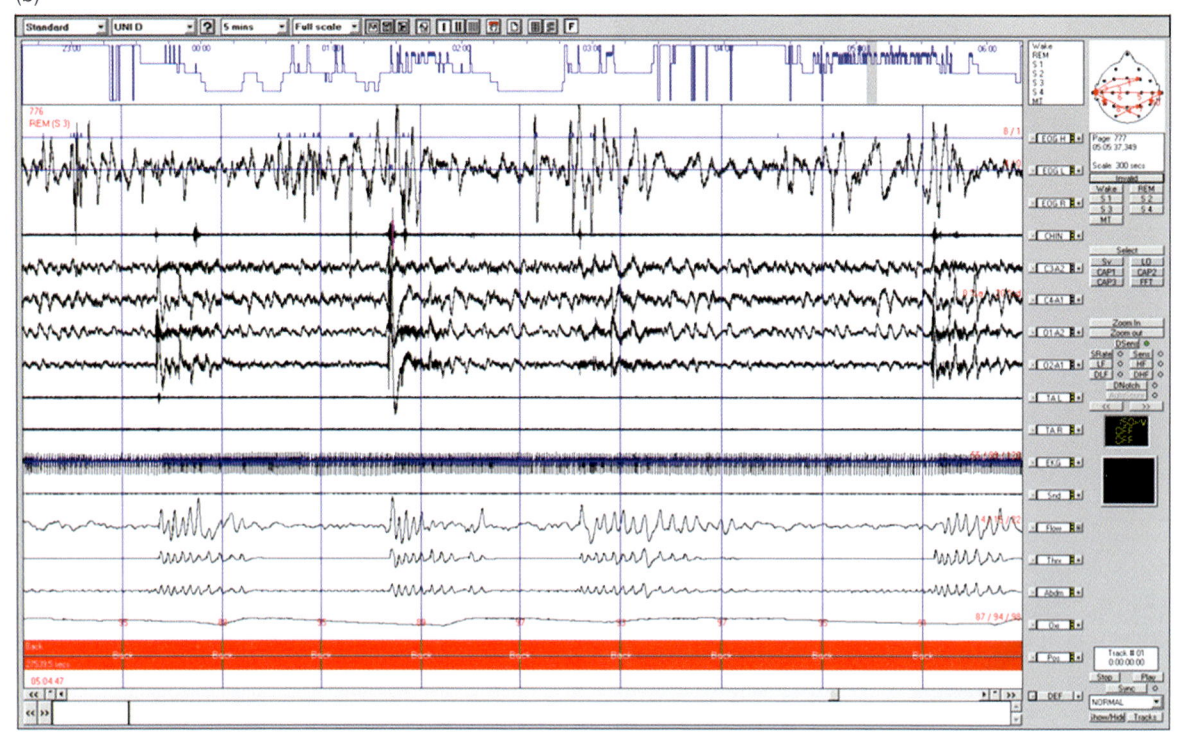

Figure 30.5b A compressed polysomnographic record illustrating a number of central sleep apnea episodes during REM sleep accompanied by awakenings.

Section 3 Chapter 30

Medical, Psychiatric and Neurological Causes of Sleepiness

Genetic disorders and sleepiness

Sona Nevsimalova

Introduction

Sleep problems are highly prevalent in patients suffering from diverse genetic syndromes, not only nocturnal sleep complaints but also daytime functioning – tiredness or even excessive daytime sleepiness (EDS). EDS can be a result of nocturnal breathing disorder and/or primary vigilance dysfunction. Most of the patients affected by genetic syndromes are children, in whom sleep quality is extremely important for brain development and synaptic plasticity during further life. There is a close relationship between the degree of brain abnormality and impaired ability to generate physiological sleep–wake cycles and normal sleep architecture. There is also considerable evidence that different sleep stages have a role in learning and memory and in the development of neuronal plasticity. The consequences of nocturnal sleep disorders not only include EDS, but are clearly connected with school performance worsening and mood changes such as irritability, aggression, and depression, as well as leading to hyperactivity and conduct problems. Severe and prolonged sleep disturbance may also result in impaired growth and depressed immune system functioning. Pediatric sleep problems have a major impact not only on the child, but on the whole family, and consequences for parenting can be serious [1].

This chapter reviews the type and prevalence of sleep problems including daytime sleepiness in a range of commonly presenting genetic syndromes and diseases, and covers (1) chromosomal abnormalities and genetic programming malformations of the nervous system, (2) inherited metabolic disorders and heredodegenerative diseases (not included in the previous chapters), (3) neurodevelopmental syndromes with genetic compound, and marginally also (4) genetically based neuromuscular diseases.

Chromosomal abnormalities and genetic programming malformations of the nervous system

The main chromosomal aberration features include mentally or neurologically handicapped phenotype with multiple congenital abnormalities. Since more than 30 000 genes are expressed in the human brain, it is not surprising that impaired brain function is the most common symptom of chromosomal anomalies. Using marker chromosome screening detection, pathological features were found on amniocentesis in up to 1.2 of 1000 newborns and in up to 1.5 of 1000 fetuses [2]. Sleep disorders and daytime sleepiness can be detected in (1) autosomal abnormalities, (2) sex chromosome abnormalities, and (3) chromosomal anomalies in various dysmorphic syndromes (usually called microdeletion syndrome).

Autosomal abnormalities

Down syndrome, the most common autosomal abnormality, occurs in 0.9 per 1000 live births, its probability being directly proportional to increasing maternal age. Three chromosomal abnormalities cause Down syndrome: (a) trisomy 21, (b) translocation of the long arm of an extra chromosome 21 to chromosome 14 or 22, and (c) mosaicism of trisomy 21. Single transverse crease on the palm, craniofacial features including a small head, almond-shaped eyes, maxillary hypoplasia, a small nose, an enlarged tongue and a short neck are characteristic signs. The prevalence of congenital heart disease is increased, and the patients have delayed psychomotor development with generalized hypotonia and impaired cognitive performance with selective deficits in verbal short-term memory and

---

Sleepiness: Causes, Consequences and Treatment, ed. Michael J. Thorpy and Michel Billiard. Published by Cambridge University Press. © Cambridge University Press 2011.

delayed recall. At around 50 years of age, Alzheimer's disease emerges in at least half of Down syndrome patients [3], in the presence of common pathological features (amyloid plaques).

Sleep problem prevalence is between 35 and 45% of the affected subjects. The leading complaints are sleep maintenance and sleep-related breathing disorders. The prevalence of obstructive sleep apnea (OSA) in Down syndrome is higher than 50%; the obstruction being caused by an anatomically narrow upper airway due to midfacial and mandibular hypoplasia, relative macroglossia, glossoptosis, and frequent adenotonsillar hypertrophy. Other factors predisposing to OSA include obesity and generalized hypotonia with upper airway muscle malfunction. Central sleep apnea can be caused by dysfunction of the central respiratory control at the brainstem level. However, not all the sleep disturbances in Down syndrome patients can be explained by sleep apnea [4]. The patients have a reduced quantity of REM sleep and decreased REM sleep density. Sleep fragmentation and arousals independent of respiratory events and periodic limb movements, and even restless legs syndrome have also been reported. Therefore, daytime sleepiness is not a surprising consequence of poor nocturnal sleep quality.

Coincidence with imperative sleepiness and cataplexy is, however, extremely rare. Dominguez-Ortega et al. [5] described a unique case of Down syndrome without OSA and narcolepsy-like symptoms. The patient had almost continuous attacks of sudden loss of muscle tone when excited over her favorite TV program, being angry, laughing, and/or being very tired. She was also extremely drowsy during the day. HLA examination showed the DQB1*0602 haplotype. A borderline mean sleep latency on MSLT (8.8 min) with 4 SOREMs was found. The patient improved in response to imipramine treatment.

Sex chromosome abnormalities

Owing to "classic" sex chromosome abnormalities, the most common variant in phenotypic male patients is XXY (Klinefelter syndrome), and XXX or 45X0 (Turner syndrome) in female individuals. However, no sleep studies have yet appeared in the relevant literature. *Fragile X chromosome* belongs to the trinucleotid repeat disorders, but it is the most common cause of inherited mental retardation, with a rate of occurrence 1:4000 live births in males and 0.6 in females. The cause is an inherited X-linked mutation with amplification of a CGG repeat in the X mental retardation 1 (FMR1) gene (Xq27.3). Characteristic features are present at birth and include an elongated face, large ears and protruding jaw (Figure 30.1) and macroorchidism. Cognitive and language features comprise deficits consistent with the level of mental retardation, more pronounced deficits are in visual–spatial skills, attention and executive functioning. Behavioral features include increased social avoidance, anxiety and hyperactivity [6].

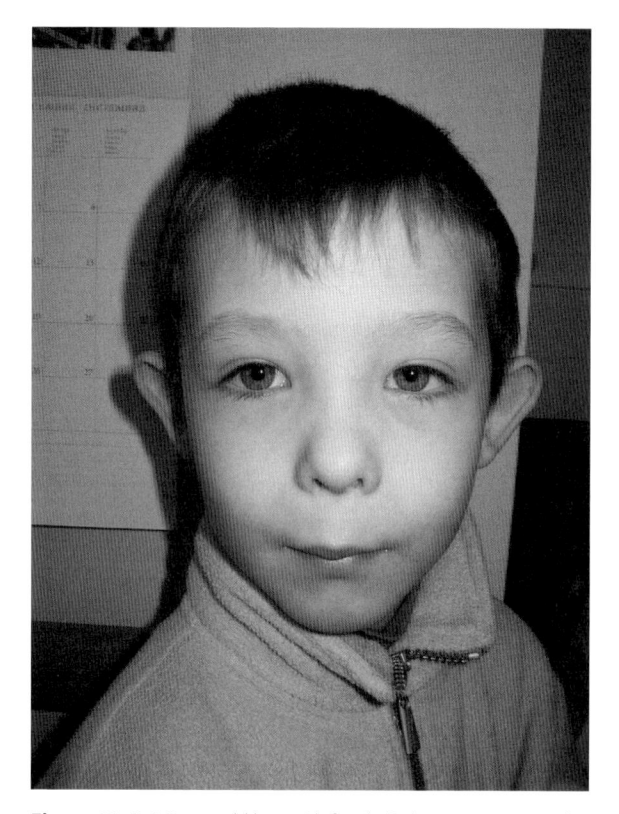

Figure 30.1 A 3-year-old boy with fragile X chromosome. Note his typical elongated face with large ears and protruding jaw. (See color plate section).

Sleep patterns have not been frequently studied. A correlation was found between REM sleep deficit and the level of mental retardation [6]. An increased risk of OSA, variable sleep duration, and sleep fragmentation are sporadically reported [4]. An interesting study [7] found increased levels of melatonin across the circadian cycle in young fragile X individuals, possibly explaining the difficulties in maintaining consistent sleep and increased number of night wake episodes. Hence, in some children, irritability can mask a higher level of sleepiness due to irregular melatonin secretion. Clonidine has been reported to have a beneficial effect on the hyperactivity and abnormal sleep patterns in the affected children [8]. Behavioral therapy has also been used with benefit [9].

Chromosomal anomalies in various dysmorphic syndromes

Conditions known as contiguous-gene syndromes do not result from a gross chromosomal deletion or duplication and they are not detectable with conventional cytogenetic technique. FISH analysis should be usually used for the detection of microdeletion syndromes. Patterns can be found of phenotypic expression resulting from inactivation or overexpression caused by the deletion, duplication, or other malformation of a set of adjacent genes in a specific chromosome region [2]. Typical examples include disorders showing genetic imprinting such as the Prader–Willi and Angelman syndromes. Genetic imprinting means differential expression of autosomal genes depending upon their parental origin. Thus, if the deletion involves the paternal chromosome 15(15q11–q13), the Prader–Willi syndrome results, if this gene is deleted in the maternal chromosome 15, the Angelman syndrome is present [10].

Prader–Willi syndrome is marked mainly by obesity, small stature, hyperphagia and mental retardation (Figure 30.2a. Hypogonadism also belongs to the characteristic features. The prevalence of this syndrome is estimated at 1 in 10 000 to 25 000 births. Approximately 70% of patients demonstrate a deletion of the proximal part of the long arm of chromosome 15 (15q11–q13), the rest having paternal derived 15th chromosome polymorphism or other abnormalities; the presence of point mutations is questionable.

EDS is the most common sleep-related symptom in the Prader–Willi syndrome. Although OSA may have a role to play in some patients, the primary cause of EDS is thought to lie in hypothalamic dysfunction. Camfferman et al. [11] reviewed a total of 110 cases (children and adults) with Prader–Willi syndrome as published in 13 studies designed to evaluate subjective and objective measurements of daytime sleepiness. In more than two-thirds of the cases (67.2%), caregivers or parents reported EDS. Eighty-nine patients underwent the MSLT and 37 subjects (41.6 %) showed a mean sleep latency of less than 5 mins, and in nearly one-third (32.7%) at least one SOREM was found. The authors concluded that EDS increases over childhood/puberty to reach stability and plateau in adulthood.

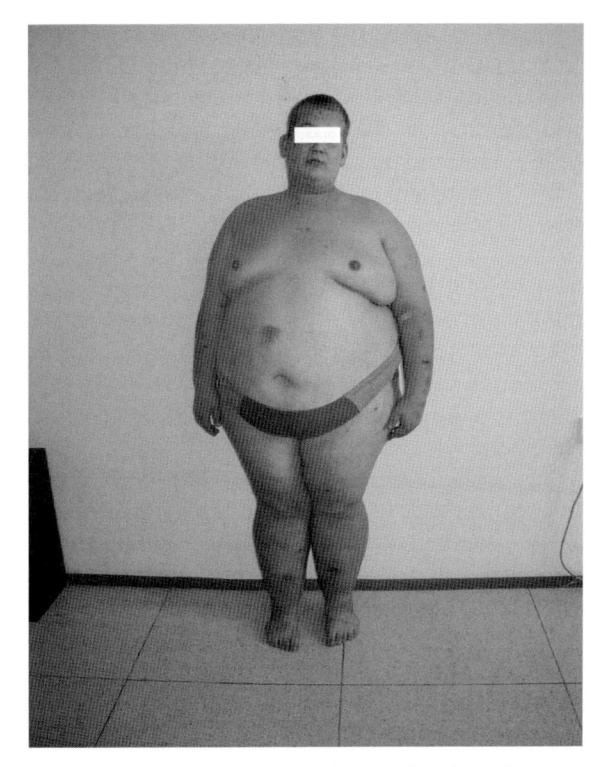

Figure 30.2a A 16-year-old boy with a typical Prader–Willi phenotype. (See color plate section).

Upper airway obstruction during sleep and sleep-related hypoventilation are broadly discussed as co-responsible for EDS. The risk factors for OSA include obesity and mass loading of the chest wall caused by the progression of restrictive lung disease (and resulting alveolar hypoventilation), obesity-related narrowing of the upper airway, facial dysmorphism, abnormalities of central respiratory control, reduced ventilatory response to hypoxia and hypercapnia, scoliosis and hypotonia [11]. However, no convincing correlation was found between OSA severity and EDS intensity. Some authors [12] speculate that hypoarousability and abnormal ventilation during sleep have hypothalamic dysregulation in common.

The hypothalamus is known to regulate NREM–REM cycles. REM abnormalities (narcolepsy-like symptoms) have a higher prevalence in patients with the Prader–Willi syndrome. Reviewing the relevant literature, Camfferman et al. [11] found cataplexy-like symptoms in 13 out of 63 patients (20.6%). Potential involvement of hypothalamic dysfunction can be supported by decreased CSF hypocretin-1 level [13]. In their study, Nevsimalova *et al.* [13] found that low hypocretin was also associated with shorter latencies to sleep onset on MSLT. However, no abnormalities in hypothalamic functioning, neuroimaging or post-mortem examinations [14] have been found, which is why the role of hypothalamic abnormalities and OSA in the etiology of EDS remains unclear.

CPAP (or BiPAP) is known to have been used for the control of OSA and produce EDS improvement [11]. Most patients benefit from modafinil, but no multicentric study has yet been done. Growth hormone therapy slightly decreases the risk of OSA, but again, there is no description of its effect on EDS. When epileptic seizures complicate the clinical picture, antiepileptic drugs should be used. Prednisolone has a beneficial effect in the management of continuous spike and waves during sleep (electrical status epilepticus during sleep) (Figure 30.2b).

Angelman syndrome is called the "happy puppet syndrome" because of the patients' characteristic jerky movements, happy disposition and frequent laughter. A deletion of the maternally derived 15q11–q13 is seen in some 75% of the affected children, some others have a defect in the imprinting center or in the gene involved in the ubiqutin-mediated protein degradation pathway. The incidence of this syndrome is less than 1 in 1000. The clinical picture is marked by severe mental retardation, microcephaly, and involuntary movements (jerks). Seizures are common and include almost every seizure type [2]. An open-mouth expression with tongue protrusion can resemble a face frequently found in early childhood cataplectic attacks.

A variety of sleep abnormalities are reported including prolonged sleep latency, frequent nocturnal awakenings, involuntary movements, bruxism, snoring, and an increased rate of parasomnias (enuresis, sleep terrors, sleepwalking). Nocturnal sleep time is reduced and some children have abnormal sleep–wake cycles, with short periods of diurnal and nocturnal sleep. Although an increase in total sleep time is reported [4], no detailed information on subjective and/or objective EDS tests are available.

Both behavioral and pharmacological methods are in use for the treatment of sleep disturbances. Melatonin (0.3 mg) before bedtime promotes less fragmented sleep and helps to regulate sleep–wake cycles [15].

Williams syndrome is a disorder marked by an unusual elfin-like facies, hyperacusis, infantile hypercalcemia, and significant physical and mental retardation. The condition is caused by a heterozygous deletion in chromosome 7q11.23 and its incidence is estimated at 1 in 10 000. The syndrome results from deletion of 25–30 genes, including the elastin gene; hence, vascular and connective tissue abnormalities are frequent, potentially leading to supravalvular aortic stenosis. Hypersociability with friendly behavior, talent for music and good language ability is a striking characteristic of young children, and contrasts with severe deficits of non-verbal tasks [2].

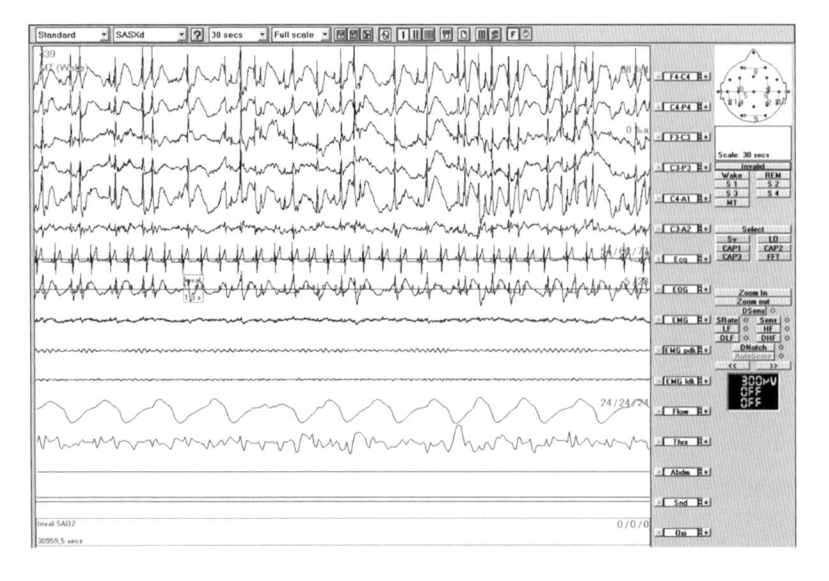

Figure 30.2b Polysomnographic record showing continuous discharges of spike and waves during sleep.

There are only a few studies dealing with sleep problems in these patients. While in children attention is focused on night sleep complaints, predominantly on periodic limb movements [16], Goldman *et al.* [17] used actigraphy to examine overnight sleep patterns in 23 adolescents and adults (mean age 25.5 ± 8.0 years) and completed their sleep data with a structured questionnaire. Although free to spend 9 h in bed, 95.2% of the subjects were tired and 77.3% were really sleepy during the day. The mean Epworth Sleepiness Scale (ESS) score was 8.7 ± 4.4, while over a third of the EDS patients (34.8%) exhibited an ESS score ≥ 10. As polysomnographic data are lacking, it is not known how disturbed nocturnal sleep can influence the daytime sleepiness.

Smith–Magenis syndrome is a severe neurodevelopmental disorder characterized by mental retardation with distinctive behavioral characteristics, dysmorphic features and an abnormal circadian pattern of melatonin ascribed to an intersticial deletion of chromosome 17 (17p11.2). The prevalence of this syndrome is estimated at 1 per 25 000 live births. All cases occur *de novo*, there is no parental imprinting [18]. Characteristic features include brachycephaly with a typical craniofacial appearance (midface hypoplasia, characteristic mouth with a "cupid's bow" shape, prognathism), ocular abnormalities (myopia, strabismus, iris anomalies), speech delay with hoarse and deep voice, short stature, brachydactyly, peripheral neuropathy and scoliosis (Figure 30.3a). Behavioral problems include aggression, self-injurious behaviors, repetitive behavior, impulsivity and hyperactivity with attention deficit [19].

Sleep disturbances (seen in 65–100% of cases) have a major impact on both the patients and other family members. All affected children display a phase shift in their circadian rhythm of melatonin secretion (Figure 30.3b) which parallels sleep disturbance and abnormal daytime behavior. Prominent sleep problems include early sleep onset, repeated and prolonged awakening during the night and early sleep offset. Most patients exhibit morning tiredness, temper tantrums when tired, and naps during the day. Almost consistently their sleep attacks come at the end of the day with sudden falling asleep during evening meals, even with a full mouth. The mechanism of the quantitatively normal but rhythmically abnormal melatonin secretion is, as yet, unknown. The best recommended treatment is a combination of evening melatonin administration and morning β1-adrenergic antagonist to reduce the daytime production of this hormone [18].

Coffin–Lowry Syndrome is a rare disorder characterized by moderate to severe mental retardation, facial dysmorphism, tapering digits, and skeletal deformity. The condition is transmitted by X-linked semidominant inheritance. The gene is located on the Xp22.2, with correlated mutation identified in the RSK-2 gene, a growth factor-regulated protein kinase [20].

Stimulus-induced drop episodes characterized by a sudden loss of muscle tone triggered by unexpected tactile or auditory stimuli occur in these patients. The events go under various names including cataplexy, non-epileptic collapses with atonia, exaggerated startle responses, hyperekplexia and drop episodes. Epileptic origin of the attacks can be excluded; no epileptiform activity was proved in any reported case. Drop attacks are never induced by laughter or anger, or on telling or hearing a joke, common triggers for

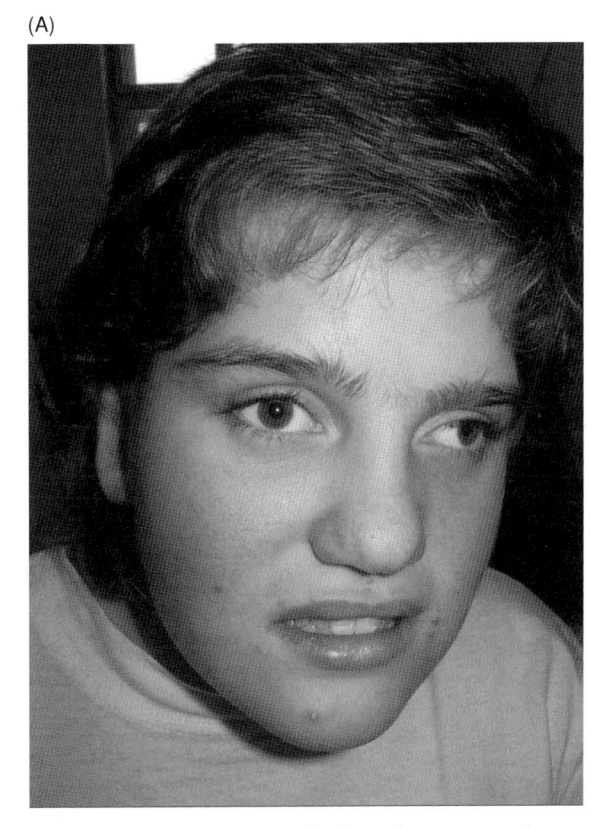

Figure 30.3 (A) A 13-year-old girl with Smith–Magenis syndrome. Note her craniofacial dysmorphic features with brachycephaly, midface hypoplasia and prognathism. (see color plate).

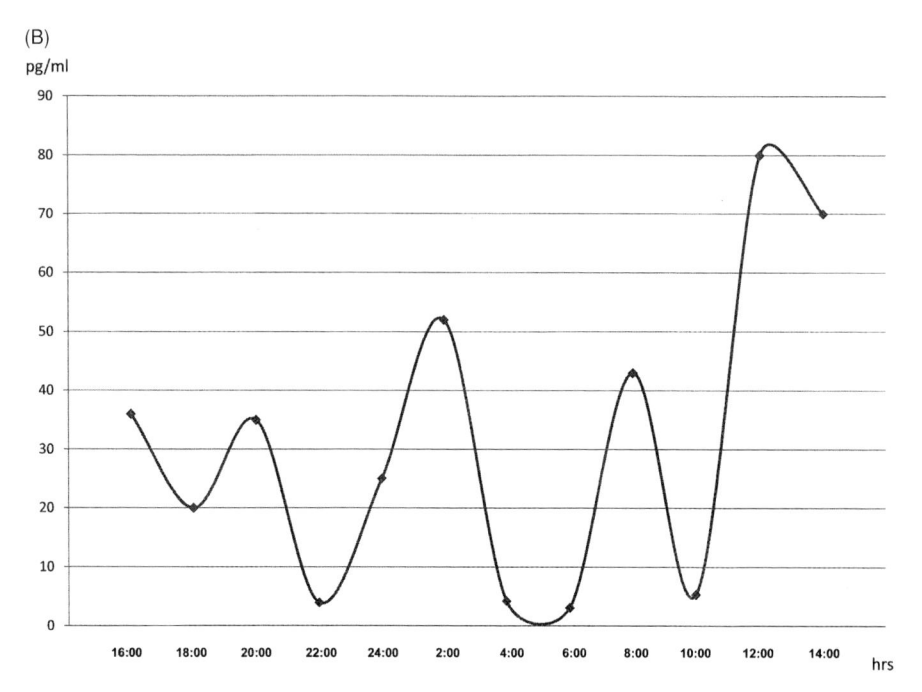

Figure 30.3 (B) An irregular 24-h profile of salvory melatonin with secretion peak in the midday and early afternoon hours in another 3-year-old boy with Smith–Magenis syndrome.

cataplexy. Recovery is immediate, the attacks last only a few seconds and always lead to a fall. This is also an unexpected feature for cataplexy. Sleepiness has not been described in any case. However, since neurophysiological studies do not point to hyperekplexia either, the pathophysiology of these cataplexy-like drop attacks remains unclear [21]. Treatment with conventional antiepileptic medication proved ineffective; in one case [22] clomipramine was effective, in two other cases [21] tiagabine – a potent GABA-uptake inhibitor – was used with a benefit.

Norrie disease is a rare X-linked disorder (microdeletion syndrome, Xp11.3–p11.4) characterized by infantile blindness, pseudotumorous retinal dysgenesis, and ocular atrophy. It is commonly associated with mental retardation, sensorineural deafness, dysmorphic features, and occasionally with atonic seizures. Vossler *et al.* [23] described three boys with this syndrome and found them to have cataplexy and abnormal REM sleep with no other signs of narcolepsy. During EEG-video-polysomnographic monitoring, attacks of cataplexy and inappropriate periods of REM sleep, during which the patients were unarousable, were detected. In all subjects, platelet monoamine oxidase (MAO)-B activity was absent, serum serotonin levels were markedly increased, and plasma catecholamine levels were normal. The authors suppose that the congenital absence of MAO in patients with Norrie disease is indirectly responsible for their cataplexy and REM sleep disturbance.

Some other congenital syndromes such as *Möbius, Pierre–Robin, Treacher–Collins, Goldenhar,* and/or centrofacial dysgenesia belong to neuroembryological and/or genetic programming malformations of the nervous system with difficulties primarily related to upper airway obstruction. A description of these syndromes would go beyond the scope of this chapter.

Inherited metabolic and neurodegenerative diseases of the nervous system

These diseases result from a single mutant gene coding for an enzymatic protein mostly involved in the catabolic pathway. The consequent homeostatic disturbances give rise to neurological or developmental abnormalities. Both groups of diseases arise from single-gene defects. However, in metabolic diseases the defective gene is normally expressed in one or more organs (not necessarily in the nervous system), and chemical analyses of tissues often have a diagnostic value. As a rule, neurodegenerative diseases result from a single defective gene, but that is mainly or exclusively expressed in the nervous system and chemical abnormalities of tissues or body fluids are lacking [24].

Inherited neurometabolic disorders

Sleepiness can be a sign of a number of progressive metabolic encephalopathies including disorders of amino acid metabolism, carbohydrate metabolism and/or organic acidurias. In these cases, however, it may well indicate a toxic accumulation of metabolites and subsequent episodes of altered consciousness.

An exception is *gamma-hydroxybutyric (GHB) aciduria*, caused by succinic semialdehyde dehydrogenase deficiency that causes neurological and cognitive disorders of varying severity. The non-specific nature and difficult detection of urinary GHB explain why this disorder is largely underdiagnosed. Out of 350 patients identified worldwide, only 8 adults with this aciduria have been reported in the literature [25]. Characteristic features include impaired psychomotor development with hypotonia and disturbances in motor coordination, impaired development of language, mainly due to poor auditory perception, and seizures and psychotic features in late adolescence and adulthood. Moreover, narcolepsy-like symptoms can be a relevant feature of the disease.

The most striking sleep disorders have been found in different lysosomal storage disorders, characterized by an accumulation of undergraded macromolecules within lysosomes. The most common representatives of lysosomal storage diseases are the glycogen storage diseases – glykogenoses (Pompe disease), mucopolysaccharidoses and mucolipidoses, glykoproteinoses together with sphingolipidoses, and neuronal ceroid lipofuscinoses. Almost all are autosomal recessive inherited diseases, and the combined prevalence of all lysosomal storage diseases is 1 in 6600 to 1 in 7700 live births [24].

Pompe disease results from acid α-glucosidase deficiency; its incidence is estimated at 1 in 40 000 individuals. The infantile form is usually fatal before the age of 2 years, the juvenile form progresses more slowly, but all patients develop involvement of respiratory muscles – predominantly of the diaphragm. Most die of respiratory failure in the second or third decade of life. However, recently introduced causal enzymatic treatment promises a better prognosis. Patients with the adult form may survive for decades following diagnosis. Respiratory insufficiency due to diaphragm weakness or sleep apnea may appear in any stage of the disease, and daytime sleepiness usually reflects the severity of impaired breathing [26].

Mucopolysaccharidoses are heterogeneous syndromes consisting of mental and physical retardation, multiple skeletal deformities, hepatosplenomegaly and clouding of the cornea in Hunter and Hurler syndromes. The large head, "inhuman" facies and deformed limbs are called gargoyle features. The syndrome comprises seven major entities, some subdivided into two or more subgroups that are distinguishable by their clinical picture, genetic transmission, enzyme defect, and urinary mucopolysaccharide pattern. Defective lysosomal catabolism of glycosaminoglycans leading to their specific accumulation is the common feature for all the types.

OSA is the most common sleep disorder in mucopolysaccharidoses. Upper airway obstruction has multiple causative factors, and progressive respiratory disease may severely affect morbidity and mortality. Leighton *et al*. [27] found OSA – ranging in severity from mild to severe – in 24 out of 26 examined patients. The most marked obstructive respiratory problems were found in Hurler syndrome followed by Hurler–Scheie syndrome and Hunter syndrome. OSA severity depends also on the patient's age. Surprisingly, children are more severely affected than adult patients [28]. Retropalatal and retroglossal spaces were found to be significantly smaller in children than in adults. Adenoid hypertrophy, too, had a significant role to play in all examined children. Daytime sleepiness could then be related to the severity of OSA and its response to treatment. However, insufficient data are available.

The most frequent and probably specific sleep disturbances have been found in the commonest mucopolysaccharidosis, Sanfilippo syndrome. These patients have extremely irregular sleep patterns, with several sleep episodes of variable duration with an irregular round-the clock distribution [29]. Guerrero *et al*. [30] examined urine melatonin excretion in 12 patients with Sanfilippo syndrome and found a significantly lower melatonin excretion at night and significantly higher concentration in the morning, with a slightly higher level also sustained during the day when compared with the controls. Analysis of the circadian rhythm alteration may explain the cause of sleep disorders found in these patients, and help establish melatonin as a beneficial treatment.

Niemann–Pick disease is a heterogeneous syndrome comprising different forms (A–D). However, its

Table 30.1 A cohort of 50 patients with Wilson disease – questionnaire data

Clinical forms	Asymptomatic $n = 5$	Hepatic $n = 20$	Neurologic $n = 25$	Significance
Mean age (years)	47.6 ± 13.5	33.6 ± 8.5*	45.3 ± 8.4	$P < 0.05$
Sleepiness:				
EDS	60% ($n = 3$)	40% ($n = 8$)	52% ($n = 13$)	NS
Daily attacks (n)	2.6 ± 2.1	1.2 ± 1.5*	2.6 ± 2.1	$P < 0.05$
ESS	10.2 ± 7.9	6.7 ± 2.6	9.2 ± 5.3	NS
Paroxysmal atonia ("cataplexy-like" attacks)	40% ($n = 2$)	25% ($n = 5$)	32% ($n = 8$)	NS
Sleep paralysis	40% ($n = 2$)	25% ($n = 5$)	32% ($n = 8$)	NS
Hypnagogic/hypnopompic hallucinations	40% ($n = 2$)	25% ($n = 5$)	28% ($n = 7$)	NS
RBD-SQ	3.6 ± 2.9	5.1 ± 3.6	5.1 ± 3.2	NS
RLS	40% ($n = 2$)	20% ($n = 4$)	28% ($n = 7$)	NS

RBD-SQ, REM Behavior Sleep Questionnaire.
RLS, Restless legs syndrome. EDS, Excessive Daytime Sleepiness. ESS, Epworth Sleepiness Scale.

significantly reduced total sleep time, sleep efficiency, percentages of REM sleep and NREM stage 2. The percentage of NREM stage 1 and the number of awakenings increase with age and clinical stage of the disease. Treatment with melatonin before bedtime may help to slightly improve the circadian rhythm in both NCL forms.

Inherited metabolic diseases also include disorders of metal metabolism. The most frequent disorder is copper metabolism – *Wilson disease (WD)*, also known as hepatolenticular degeneration. It is inherited as an autosomal recessive trait with a prevalence of around 1 in 30–50 000. More than 200 mutations have been identified in the responsible gene, ATP7B (chromosome 13q14.3). Mutations in the ATP7B gene result in reduced copper excretion into the bile and reduced incorporation into caeruloplasmin in the liver. Instead, the copper is accumulated in the liver, brain, cornea and other organs [24]. Four clinical subgroups have been verified – hepatic, neurological, mixed with hepatic and neurological symptoms, and asymptomatic, i.e. presymptomatic WD. Neuronal damage in the brain tissue of patients with WD affects predominantly basal ganglia and the brainstem, although copper can accumulate in any part of the CNS gray or white matter.

Sleep disturbances seem to be relatively frequent. In a questionnaire study [39], WD patients had a significantly higher number of nocturnal awakenings, failed to feel rested after sleep, during the day they felt tired and took frequent naps. Moreover, sleep paralysis and cataplexy occurred more often in the WD patients than in the reference group. Our cohort of 50 WD patients [40] who were asked to complete the standardized sleep questionnaire data were divided into three clinical forms (asymptomatic, hepatic, and subjects with predominantly neurological symptoms) (see Table 30.1). The group of 20 patients with hepatic involvement was younger and had fewer daily attacks of sleepiness than the other groups. However, we did not find any difference between the study groups in any other parameters. EDS was found in more than half of our patients with almost borderline values of ESS and with a relatively high frequency of other REM sleep phenomena (cataplexy-like attacks, sleep paralysis, hypnagogic/hypnopompic hallucinations). Also surprisingly high was the score of the REM Behavior Sleep Questionnaire (RBD-SQ) and an increased rate of restless legs syndrome. However, all data have yet to be verified by face-to-face interviews and polysomnography.

Neurodegenerative diseases of the nervous system

From the clinical point of view, heredodegenerative diseases can be categorized according to the anatomical structure involved. Heredodegenerative diseases of the basal ganglia were mentioned in the previous chapters, which is why attention will now be paid only to heredodegenerative diseases of cerebellum and brainstem and to some diffuse cerebral degenerative diseases in children. Degenerative diseases of the spinal cord are mentioned together with neuromuscular diseases in the next part of this chapter.

Spinocerebellar ataxias (SCA) include ataxias of childhood (with Friedreich's disease as the most common) and a large and heterogeneous group of adult ataxias. Sleepiness is only exceptionally a feature of the clinical picture. However, Valind *et al.* [41] described four patients with autosomal dominant cerebellar ataxia and deafness, in three of whom narcolepsy was diagnosed. EDS and REM sleep behavior disorder may well be a common component of Machado–Joseph disease (SCA-3). In a series of 22 affected patients, Friedman *et al.* [42] examined their ESS and found a mean a borderline value (9.1). More than 40 % of the patients had a score ≥ 10. The neurodegenerative process in this clinical entity involves substantia nigra, locus coeruleus and other brainstem and cerebellar structures. The cause of RBD and EDS can be similar to that of synucleinopathies.

However, the most exact literary data concerning sleep disorders are devoted to diffuse degenerative diseases in childhood, predominantly to the Rett syndrome.

Rett syndrome is a severe neurological disorder with an incidence 1 in 10 000 to 1 in 15 000 girls and belongs to one of the most frequent causes of mental retardation in female patients. It is generally caused by mutation in the MECP2 gene (Xq28), more than 200 mutations recorded. The condition is almost exclusively seen in girls because of the predominance of *de novo* mutations on the paternal X chromosome and also because of the early postnatal lethal effects of the disease-causing mutation in hemizygous boys [43]. The disorder is characterized by progressive intellectual and neurological impairment beginning after apparently normal psychomotor development for the first months of life. Early signs of Rett syndrome typically manifest at the age of 6–18 months. Characteristic features comprise: microcephaly, stereotyped hand movements (hand-wringing or washing), severely impaired language functioning, autistic behavior, regression of motor and intellectual functions, attacks of epilepsy and hyperventilation during wakefulness.

Several studies show that sleep patterns are changed from infancy. The affected girls sleep longer during the day and, on the other hand, wake and laugh in the middle of the night. Their sleep onset is very irregular and total daytime sleep remains prolonged instead of showing the normal age-related physiological decline. The immature sleep pattern seems to be a consequence of arrested brain development. Frequent daily napping has been reported in almost 80% of affected patients and found to increase with age [44]. Severity of sleep problems is also partly influenced by a specific mutation type. There are sporadic reports on the beneficial effect of L-carnitine on nocturnal sleep [4]. The sleep–wake rhythm can probably be better influenced by evening doses of melatonin, which synchronizes the nocturnal sleep and increases the arousal level in daytime [45].

Neurodevelopmental syndromes with genetic compound

This group represents a heterogeneous group of clinical entities including neurodevelopmental multistructure abnormalities (neurocutaneous syndromes, phakomatoses), developmental disorders of language and learning, and developmental disorders of behavior. The serious sleep disturbances were described in the spectrum of behavioral abnormalities, particularly in autism, attention deficit hyperactivity disorder (ADHD), and Tourette syndrome.

Autistic spectrum disorders

These are a behaviorally defined set of development disorders that affect up to 0.6% of the population and result from diverse biological, genetic and ecogenetic factors. Genetic etiology supports a higher concordance for autism in monozygotic twins, markedly increased prevalence in the siblings of affected children, and the existence of potential susceptibility genes (e.g. region 15q11–13). Case reports and series of patients with certain single-gene disorders and chromosomal abnormalities account for 5–14% of all children with autistic features [46].

Autism is characterized by impairment in the social interaction and communication. In addition, autistic patients have restricted, stereotyped, and repetitive patterns of activities, interests, and behaviors. The deficit is diagnosed, as a rule, in toddlers, if not already (in some of them) in infancy. Approximately half of the autistic population has an IQ above 50, and a quarter to a third above 70. About 20% have high-functioning autism with normal or even higher IQ levels.

Sleep difficulties have been reported in 49–89% of affected children [4]. The commonly reported sleep problems include difficulty falling asleep, restless sleep with frequent interruptions, sleep disordered breathing, bruxism and parasomnias. In their cohort of 108 autistic children, Liu et al. [47] found 45% of affected subjects having morning awakening problems and 31% suffering from daytime sleepiness. Increased risk of daytime sleepiness was connected with comorbid epilepsy, insomnia and parasomnias. The authors conclude that sleep problems in autistic children are caused by multiple biological, family and environmental factors, rather than by a single factor. Behavior therapy, together with parental sleep hygiene, education and behavioral intervention of the child's sleep, should be taken as important aspects of any treatment for autism.

Attention deficit hyperactivity disorder (ADHD)

ADHD refers to the covariation of inattention, hyperactivity and impulsivity. The second year of life is the earliest in which ADHD symptoms could be detected, and age of 3–5 years is the peak time of onset. Its prevalence ranges between 3 and 5% of school-age children. There is no single underlying cause of ADHD; however, it is highly heritable, probably based on multiple genes, each with a small effect size. Several linkage studies implicate a polymorphism of the dopamine receptor D4 (DRD4) gene, located on chromosome 11p15.5. Dopamine transporter (DAT) polymorphism has also been described. Increased concordance for ADHD in monozygotic compared to dizygotic twins, together with an increased incidence of ADHD in the first- and second-degree relatives also provide a clue to ADHD genetic etiology [46].

The hypothesis of sleep problems in close association with ADHD helped to define one of the diagnostic criteria for ADHD in DSM-III. Difficulties in initiating and maintaining sleep are estimated to affect 25–50% of children with this condition. There is also an increased rate of periodic limb movements (PLMs) and restless legs syndrome [48]. Sleep problems believed to mimic ADHD symptoms may be associated with or exacerbated by ADHD. Psychotropic medication (e.g. methylphenidate) used for ADHD control may also result in sleep problems [49]. However, a debate still continues over whether or not children with ADHD have significantly altered sleep patterns. As some studies suggest, increased variability from night to night or instability of sleep–wake patterns may help distinguish the sleep patterns of ADHD children from those of the controls. However, there are no consistent findings concerning stable differences in sleep quantity or in other variables [1]. Moreover, some previous studies may have been influenced by comorbidity with tics or even with Tourette syndrome.

Tourette syndrome (TS)

TS is characterized by multiple, uncontrollable muscular and vocal ticks, often associated with obsessive and compulsive behavior and ADHD. It is most common in boys (prevalence 1:2000 or more according to diagnostic criteria); a hypothesis of autosomal dominant transmission is currently proposed, though not yet clearly proved [43]. A variety of sleep disturbances have been documented including night terrors, somnambulism, PLMs, reduced sleep time with longer sleep latency and a number of awakenings, but clear EDS does not belong among the characteristic clinical features. The TS gene is believed to confer life-long susceptibility to disorders of ventilatory control during sleep, resulting in a higher incidence of such conditions as infantile apnea and sudden infant death syndrome early in life, and sleep apnea later on in older children and adults [50].

Neuromuscular diseases

Neuromuscular diseases include a wide spectrum of motor unit diseases starting with the affection of motor neuron in the brainstem and spinal cord – spinal muscular atrophies (SMA), continuing through myasthenic syndromes, muscle dystrophies and congenital myopathies, myotonic syndromes and ending with hereditary motor and sensory polyneuropathies (HMSN). The most frequent are SMA, Duchenne muscular dystrophy and HMSN. The sleep mechanisms leading to clinical manifestation of EDS are similar in all these clinical entities.

Patients suffering from neuromuscular diseases are at an increased risk of sleep-related breathing disorders (SRBD) such as obstructive sleep apnea syndrome (OSAS) and hypoventilation, as well as central sleep apnea. SRDB increases particularly due to diaphragmatic weakness, and can precede abnormalities during wakefulness by months to years. Hypoventilation becomes more severe as the disease progresses, but in some cases SRBD can still be present

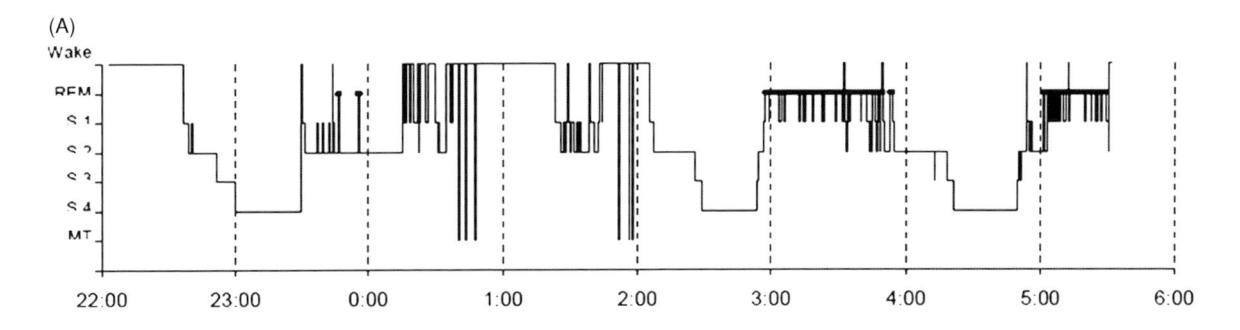

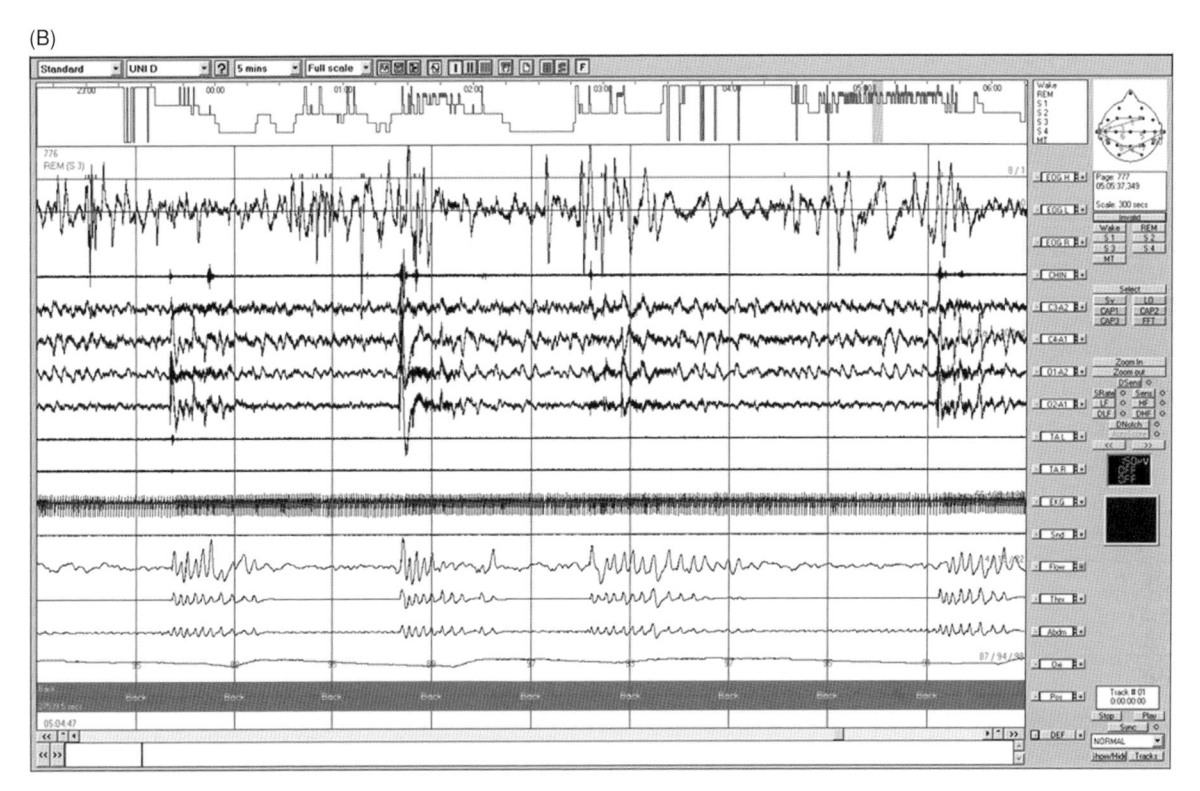

Figure 30.5 (A) Hypnogram of a 15-year-old boy with Duchenne muscular dystrophy with many awakenings disrupting predominantly REM sleep. (B) A compressed polysomnographic recording illustrating a number of central sleep apnea episodes during REM sleep accompanied by awakenings. (See color plate section).

in early stages of neuromuscular diseases. Sleep-related hypoxemia is predominantly seen in REM sleep (Figure 30.5), because of the loss of accessory muscle support to breathing in the development of diaphragmatic weakness. REM-related desaturations are also frequently associated with recurring apnea and hypopnea. These apneas are mostly of central origin, but obstructive apnea can develop if upper airway muscle contraction is impaired [51]. Later on, SRBD also appear during NREM sleep. A decrease in blood oxygen saturation can reach values of 60–80% in connection with increased compensatory breathing effort and nocturnal awakening reactions.

Nocturnal sleep-related ventilatory alterations lead to sleep inertia in the morning with headaches, daytime somnolence, fatigue and inappropriate napping. Daytime tests may show excessive somnolence proportional to the nocturnal alteration. Pediatric EDS can contribute to declining school grades or poor work performance at a later age. Noninvasive nocturnal breathing support is the adequate treatment for

SRBD in all the above-mentioned types of neuromuscular diseases [52].

Spinal muscular atrophy (SMA)

SMA is transmitted by an autosomal recessive gene and manifested by widespread muscular denervation and atrophy. The incidence is 1 in 10 000–25 000 as this is the most widespread hereditary neuromuscular disease, second only to Duchenne dystrophy. Four main clinical variants exist: infantile (SMA 1) with the most rapid course, intermediate (SMA 2) which constitutes approximately half of all cases, juvenile (SMA 3) with much slower progression, and the adult form (SMA 4). All three forms appearing in childhood are caused by mutations in a survival motor neuron gene 1 (SMN1) on the fifth chromosome [53].

SRBD are a classical feature mainly in SMA 1 and 2. In these two conditions, the intercostal muscles are more affected than the diaphragm, resulting in paradoxical breathing (inspiratory efforts cause the rib cage to move inward as the abdomen moves outward), and in the development of a characteristic bell-shaped chest deformity and pectus excavatum. Non-invasive mechanical ventilation can improve both the growth and development of the lung parenchyma and the chest wall, slow down or reverse the progression of the chest wall deformity, and increase the duration and quality of life. In the past 15 years, non-invasive ventilation has become a standard part of the healthcare system in all advanced countries. In each SMA-affected child suffering from a sleep disorder with hypercapnia, somnolence, morning headaches, and attention deficit during daytime, non-invasive intermittent positive pressure ventilation consolidates the nocturnal sleep architecture and improves his/her daytime functioning [51].

Duchenne muscular dystrophy (DMD)

DMD belongs to a group of dystrophinopathies, resulting from a mutation in the dystrophin gene, located on the short arm of the X chromosome (Xp21) and transmitted in a sex-linked recessive manner. The incidence of DMD, the most widespread neuromuscular disease, is approximately 1 in 3000 male births [53]. The clinical picture includes classic myopathic features (difficulty in climbing stairs, rising from the floor, progressive muscle wasting with increased lordosis and diminished tendon reflexes). In contrast to the general atrophy, there is striking pseudohypertrophy of the calves. Approximately at the age of 10–12 years, the children start being wheelchair-bound and developing cardiomyopathy.

Signs of early respiratory insufficiency are usually first detectable in sleep, so polysomnographic examination is most advisable. Annual monitoring is recommended if the vital capacity declines to <65%; the patients should undergo twice-yearly visits to pediatric specialists in pneumology and cardiology and to a somnologist after confinement to a wheelchair, after the vital capacity drops below 80%, and/or after the age of 10 years. Increased risk for SRBD includes hypopnea, central and obstructive apneas, and hypoxemia. The gradually increasing rate of nocturnal awakenings leads to daytime sleepiness and morning headaches. Treatment with non-invasive ventilatory support may improve quality of life and reduce the high morbidity and early mortality associated with DMD [51].

Hereditary motor and sensory neuropathy (HMSN, Charcot–Marie–Tooth disease, CMT)

This represents a widely heterogeneous group of diseases as regards the genetic background, mode of transmission, and clinical and neurophysiological manifestations. As the most common form, CMT1 is characterized by progressive peroneal muscular atrophy, and transmitted, as a rule, by an autosomal dominant type of inheritance. From the pathological point of view, extensive segmental demyelination and remyelination of peripheral nerves are characteristic features. Their prevalence is 3.8 in a population of 10 000, and most cases are caused by a submicroscopic duplication of the proximal portion of the short arm of chromosome 17 (17p11.2) [43]. The clinical picture varies from very mild up to the quite severe wheelchair-bound handicap phenotype.

Restrictive pulmonary impairment has been described in association with phrenic nerve dysfunction, diaphragm dysfunction, or thoracic cage abnormalities. Central sleep apnea may be associated with diaphragm dysfunction and hypercapnia, whereas OSA is reported as possibly caused by a pharyngeal neuropathy. Restless legs and PLMs during sleep are found in a large proportion of patients with prominent axonal nerve atrophy (CMT2). Vocal cord dysfunction, possibly due to laryngeal nerve involvement, is found in association with several CMT types and can often mimic asthma. EDS, if present, adds to the severity of SRDB. Bilevel positive airway pressure (BiPAP) is a more appropriate treatment than continuous positive airway pressure (CPAP). The prominence of peripheral neuropathy as a cause of the restless legs syndrome in CMT may justify treatment with neuropathic medication (e.g. gabapentin) which is better than dopaminergic agents [54].

References

1. **Dorris L**, **Scott N**, **Zuberi S**, et al. Sleep problems in children with neurological disorders. *Develop Neurorehab*, 2008; **11**:95–114.

2. **Menkes J H**, **Falk E**. Chromosomal anomalies and contiguous-gene syndromes. In: Menkes J H, Sarnat H B, Maria B L, Eds. *Child Neurology* (7th Ed.), Philadelphia Lippincott Williams and Wilkins, 2006: 227–257.

3. **Harvey MT**, **Kennedy CH**. Polysomnographic phenotypes in developmental disabilities. *Int J Devl Neuroscience*, 2002; **20**: 443–448.

4. **Rack MJ**. Sleep disorders associated with mental retardation. In: Culebras A, Ed. *Sleep Disorders and Neurologic Diseases* (2nd Ed.). New York, NY: Informa Healthcare, 2007: 27–37.

5. **Dominguez-Ortega L**, **Salin-Pascual R J**, **Diaz-Gallego E**. Narcolepsy-like symptoms in a patient with Down syndrome and without obstructive sleep apnea. *Sleep*, 2003; **26**:285–86.

6. **Harvey M T**, **Kennedy C H**. Polysomnographic phenotypes in developmental disabilities. *Int J Dev Neurosci*, 2002; **20**:443–48.

7. **Gould E L**, **Loesch D Z**, **Martin M J**, et al. Melatonin profiles and sleep characteristics in boys with fragile X syndrome: a preliminary study. *Am J Med Genet*, 2000; **95**:307–15.

8. **Hagerman R**. Fragile X: treatment of hyperactivity. *Pediatrics*, 1997; **99**:753.

9. **Weiskop S**, **Richdale A**, **Matthews J**. Behavioural treatment to reduce sleep problems in children with autism or fragile X syndrome. *Dev Med Child Neurol*, 2005; **47**:94–104.

10. **Pulst S M** (Ed). *Neurogenetics*. New York, NY: Oxford University Press, 2000.

11. **Camfferman D**, **McEvoy R D**, **O'Donoghue F**, et al. Prader Willi syndrome and excessive daytime sleepiness. *Sleep Med Rev*, 2008; **12**:65–75.

12. **Menendez A A**. Abnormal ventilatory responses in patients with Prader–Willi syndrome. *Eur J Pediatr*, 1999; **158**:941–42.

13. **Nevsimalova S**, **Vankova J**, **Stepanova I**, et al. Hypocretin deficiency in Prader–Willi syndrome. *Eur J Neurol*, 2005; **12**:70–72.

14. **Fronczek R**, **Lammers G J**, **Balesar R**, et al. The number of hypothalamic hypocretin (orexin) neurons is not affected in Prader–Willi syndrome. *J Clin Endocrinol Metab*, 2005; **90**:5466–70.

15. **Zhdanova I V**, **Wurtman R J**, **Wagstaff J**. Effect of a low dose of melatonin on sleep in children with Angelman syndrome. *J Pediatr Endocrinol Metab*, 1999; **12**:57–67.

16. **Arens R**, **Wright B**, **Elliot J**, et al. Periodic limb movement in sleep in children with Williams syndrome. *J Pediatr*, 1998; **133**:670–74.

17. **Goldman S E**, **Malow B A**, **Newman K D**, et al. Sleep patterns and daytime sleepiness in adolescents and young adults with Williams syndrome. *J Intel Dis Res*, 2009; **53**:182–88.

18. **De Leersnyder H**. Inverted rhythm of melatonin secretion in Smith–Magenis syndrome: from symptoms to treatment. *Trends Endocrin Metab*, 2006; **17**:291–98.

19. **Shelley B P**, **Robertson M M**. The neuropsychiatry and multisystem features of the Smith–Magenis syndrome. a review. *J Neuropsychiatry Clin Neurosci*, 2005; **17**:91–97.

20. **Trivier E**, **De Cesare D**, **Jacquot S**, et al. Mutation in the kinase Rsk-2 associated with Coffin–Lowry syndrome. *Nature*, 1996; **384**:567–70.

21. **Nelson G B**, **Hahn J S**. Stimulus-induced drop episodes in Coffin–Lowry syndrome. *Pediatrics*, 2003; **111**:e197–202.

22. **Caraballo R**, **Tesi Rocha A**, **Medina C**, et al. Drop episodes in Coffin–Lowry syndrome: an unusual type of startle response. *Epileptic Disord*, 2000; **2**: 173–76.

23. **Vossler D G**, **Wyler A R**, **Wilkus R J**, et al. Cataplexy and monoamine oxidase deficiency in Norrie disease. *Neurology*, 1996; **46**:1258–61.

24. **Menkes J H**, **Wilcox W R**. Inherited metabolic diseases of the nervous system. In: Menkes J H, Sarnat H B, Maria B L, Eds. *Child Neurology* (7th Ed.). Philadelphia, PA: Lippincott Williams and Wilkins, 2006: 29–141.

25. **Philippe A**, **Deron J**, **Genevieve, D**, et al. Neurodevelopmental pattern of succinic semialdehyde dehydrogenase deficiency (gamma-hydroxybutyric aciduria). *Develop Med Child Neurol*, 2004; **46**: 564–68.

26. **Mellies U**, **Stehling F**, **Dohna-Schwake C**, et al. Respiratory failure in Pompe disease: treatment with noninvasive ventilation. *Neurology*, 2005; **64**:1465–67.

27. **Leighton S E J**, **Papsin B**, **Vellodi A**, et al. Disordered breathing during sleep in patients with

mucopolysaccharidoses. *Int J Pediatr Otorhinolaryngol*, 2001; **58**:127–38.

28. **Santamaria F, Andreucci M V, Parenti G**, *et al*. Upper airway obstructive disease in mucopolysaccharidoses: polysomnography, computed tomography and nasal endoscopy findings. *J Inherit Metab Dis*, 2007; **30**:743–49.

29. **Fraser J, Wraith J E, Delatycki M B**. Sleep disturbance in mucopolysaccharidoses type III (Sanfilippo syndrome): a survey of managing clinicians. *Clin Genet*, 2002; **62**:418–21.

30. **Guerrero J M, Pozo D, Diaz-Rodrigues J L**, *et al*. Impairment of the melatonin rhythm in children with Sanfilippo syndrome. *J Pineal Res*, 2006; **40**:192–93.

31. **Vankova J, Stepanova I, Jech R**, *et al*. Sleep disturbances and hypocretin deficiency in Niemann–Pick disease type C. *Sleep*, 2003; **26**:427–30.

32. **Kanbayashi T, Abe M, Fujimoto S**, *et al*. Hypocretin deficiency in Niemann–Pick type C with cataplexy. *Neuropediatrics*, 2003; **34**:52–53.

33. **Nishino S, Kanbayashi T**. Symptomatic narcolepsy, cataplexy and hypersomnia, and their implications in the hypothalamic hypocretin/orexin system. *Sleep*, 2005; **9**:269–310.

34. **Oyama K, Takahashi T, Shoji Y**, *et al*. Niemann–Pick disease type C: cataplexy and hypocretin in cerebrospinal fluid. *Tokohu J Exp Med*, 2006; **209**:263–67.

35. **Vanier MT**. Biochemical studies in Niemann–Pick disease. I. Major sphingolipids of liver and spleen. *Biochim Biophys Acta*, 1983; **750**:178–84.

36. **Challamel M J, Mazzola M E, Nevsimalova S**, *et al*. Narcolepsy in children. *Sleep*, 1994; **17**:17–20.

37. **Kirveskari E, Partinen M, Santavuori P**. Sleep and its disturbance in a variant form of late infantile neuronal ceroid lipofuscinosis (CLN5). *J Child Neurol*, 2001; **16**:707–13.

38. **Kirveskari E, Partinen M, Salmi T**, *et al*. Sleep alteration in juvenile neuronal ceroid-lipofuscinosis. *Pediatr Neurol*, 2000; **22**:347–54.

39. **Portala K, Westermark K, Ekselius L**, *et al*. Sleep in patients with treated Wilson's disease. A questionnaire study. *Nord J Psychiatry*, 2002; **56**:291–97.

40. **Nevsimalova S, Buskova J, Skibova J**, *et al*. Sleep disorders in Wilson disease – a questionnaire study. The 50th anniversary of paradoxical sleep discovery, Lyon, 7–10 January 2009.

41. **Valind S, Nennesmo I, Lundberg P O**, *et al*. Neuroimaging study in autosomal dominant cerebellar ataxias, deafness, and narcolepsy. *Neurology*, 1999; **53**:2190–92.

42. **Friedman J H, Fernandez H H, Sudarsky L R**. REM behavior disorder and excessive daytime somnolence in Machado–Joseph disease (SCA-3). *Mov Disord*, 2003; **18**:1520–22.

43. **Menkes J H**. Heredodegenerative diseases. In: Menkes J H, Sarnat H B, Maria B L, Eds. *Child Neurology* (7th Ed.). Philadelphia, PA: Lippincott Williams and Wilkins, 2006: 163–226.

44. **Young D, Nagarajn L, de Klerk N**, *et al*. Sleep problems in Rett syndrome. *Brain Dev*, 2007; **29**:609–16.

45. **Nomura Y**. Neurophysiology of Rett syndrome. *Brain Dev*, 2001; **23**:S50–57.

46. **Kinsbourne M, Wood F B**. Disorders of mental development. In: Menkes J H, Sarnat H B, Maria B L, Eds. *Child Neurology* (7th Ed.). Philadelphia, PA: Lippincott Williams and Wilkins, 2006: 1097–156.

47. **Liu X, Hubbard J A, Fabes R A**, *et al*. Sleep disturbances and correlates of children with autism spectrum disorders. *Child Psychiatry Hum Dev*, 2006; **37**:179–91.

48. **Mann S C, Campbell E C, Caroff S N**, *et al*. Psychiatric aspects of movement disorders in sleep. In: Chokroverty S, Hening W A, Walkers A S, Eds. *Sleep and Movement Disorders*. Philadelphia, PA: Butterwoth Heinemann, 2003: 511–26.

49. **Owens J A**. The ADHD and sleep conundrum: a review. *J Dev Behav Ped*, 2005; **26**:312–22.

50. **Rodnitzky R L**. Sleep in Parkinson's disease. In: Culebras A, Ed. *Sleep Disorders and Neurologic Diseases* (2nd Ed.). New York, NY: Informa Healthcare, 2007: 205–28.

51. **Alves R S C, Resende M B D, Skomro R**, *et al*. Sleep and neuromuscular disorders in children. *Sleep Med Rev*, 2009; **13**:133–48.

52. **Culebras A**. Sleep disorders and neuromuscular disorders. In: Culebras A, Ed. *Sleep Disorders and Neurologic Diseases* (2nd Ed.). New York, NY: Informa Healthcare, 2007: 387–403.

53. **Sarnat H B, Menkes J H**. Diseases of the motor unit. In: Menkes J H, Sarnat H B, Maria B L, Eds. *Child Neurology* (7th Ed.). Philadelphia, PA: Lippincott Williams and Wilkins, 2006: 969–1024.

54. **Aboussouan L S, Lewis R A, Shy M E**. Disorders of pulmonary functions, sleep and the upper airway in Charcot–Marie–Tooth disease. *Lung*, 2007; **185**: 1–7.

Section 3 Chapter 31

Medical, Psychiatric and Neurological Causes of Sleepiness

Brain tumors, infections, and other CNS causes of sleepiness

Mari Viola-Saltzman and Nathaniel F. Watson

Introduction

Excessive daytime sleepiness (EDS) is a pervasive symptom with a wide variety of clinical descriptors including "somnolence", "hypersomnia", and "drowsiness". Other words and phrases such as "tiredness", "lethargy" or "decreased energy" are common synonyms used by the general public to convey their sleepiness to health care practitioners. Patients may be unaware of their own sleepiness and often confuse it with related symptoms such as fatigue, despite the fact that fatigue is a physical and psychological sense of exhaustion as opposed to a propensity to sleep. Sleepiness should not be confused with "stupor", "obtundation" or "coma"; terms often used to describe changes in alertness in patients with CNS masses. According to Plum and Posner, both sleep and coma are characterized by a reduced level of consciousness. However, sleep is a reversible, regulated state whereas obtundation or stupor requires repeated or continuous stimulation to generate wakefulness. A comatose patient may not be arousable [1].

In patients with focal or diffuse CNS insults the clinician should be aware that the CNS process itself can induce primary sleep disorders, such as sleep-disordered breathing (SDB), restless legs syndrome (RLS), or insomnia, which can precipitate sleepiness. Furthermore, comorbid medical or psychiatric issues, such as renal failure or depression, and numerous medications are notorious for being somnogenic. Therefore when considering sleepiness in the CNS injured patient, it is imperative to perform a thorough evaluation for sleep disorders, medication side-effects, or sleep-disrupting medical or psychiatric issues as the causative factor.

Clinical subjective and objective measures of sleepiness have been described in detail in other chapters and will not be discussed here. Similarly, this chapter primarily focuses on CNS pathology directly causing sleepiness, as opposed to pathology that causes sleep disorders that result in sleepiness. From a nosological perspective, the American Academy of Sleep Medicine, as published in the International Classification of Sleep Disorders-2 (ICSD-2), classifies sleepiness due to a neurologic cause as "narcolepsy due to medical condition" (also known as "secondary narcolepsy") or "hypersomnia due to medical condition." Both require that excessive daytime sleepiness be present almost daily for the past three months, a multiple sleep latency test (MSLT) with a mean sleep-onset latency of less than 8 min (if no definitive cataplexy), and a "significant" neurologic (or medical) disorder present to account for the sleepiness. Importantly, the sleepiness cannot be explained by another sleep disorder, psychiatric disorder, medication, or substance use [2]. All of the disorders covered in this chapter fall into these ICSD-2 categories, although not all have been objectively defined.

Neuroanatomical review of sleepiness

A salient discussion of the CNS causes of sleepiness requires a firm grasp of the neuroanatomy of sleep and wakefulness. The hypothalamic ventrolateral preoptic nucleus (VLPO) promotes sleep via projections to multiple wakefulness controlling regions in the CNS, including the tuberomammillary nuclei, raphe nuclei, locus coeruleus, lateral hypothalamus, and the pedunculopontine and laterodorsal tegmental nuclei. The basal forebrain, dorsal raphe nuclei, solitary tract nuclei, and thalamus drive non-rapid eye movement

---

Sleepiness: Causes, Consequences and Treatment, ed. Michael J. Thorpy and Michel Billiard. Published by Cambridge University Press. © Cambridge University Press 2011.

(NREM) sleep while rapid eye movement (REM) sleep is promoted by the pedunculopontine and laterodorsal tegmental regions of the brainstem and gigantocellular tegmental field of the pons. Wakefulness is generated by the diffusely projecting brainstem reticular activating system (RAS). The thalamus, hypothalamus, locus coeruleus, and cerebral cortices also support the wakeful state [3, 4].

Many hormones and peptides play key roles in regulating sleep and wakefulness. NREM sleep involves the activity of gamma-aminobutyric acid (GABA), galanin, serotonin, norepinephrine, and adenosine. GABA, acetylcholine, and dopamine are the main substances involved with REM sleep promotion. Wakefulness primarily involves the activity of acetylcholine, dopamine, serotonin, glutamate, histamine, hypocretin (orexin), and norepinephrine [3, 4]. Hypothalamic hypocretin-containing neurons are a key regulator of state stability in sleep and wakefulness with projections throughout the CNS and a readily measurable biomarker in the cerebrospinal fluid (CSF). Low or undetectable CSF hypocretin levels are highly sensitive and specific for idiopathic narcolepsy with cataplexy. Levels of this neuropeptide can also be reduced in symptomatic cases of EDS and secondary narcolepsy (e.g. CNS tumor/trauma/infection, leukemia, Guillain–Barré syndrome, and repeated generalized tonic–clonic seizures) and have been shown to rise with improvement or resolution of disease.

A cerebral insult leading to sleepiness may be either focal (such as a hypothalamic craniopharyngioma) or diffuse (such as a purulent meningitic infection lining the cerebral hemispheres). Focal lesions cause sleepiness by directly involving one (or more) of the neuroanatomic regions subserving sleep or wakefulness. Lesions may also cause sleepiness indirectly, such as a pineal tumor applying pressure on the hypothalamus causing narcoleptic symptoms, or a cerebral mass clogging the ventricular system leading to obstructive hydrocephalus and increased intracranial pressure. Space-occupying lesions or infarcts can produce cerebral parenchymal edema creating increased intracranial pressure, sleepiness, and in some cases, herniation. Diffuse cortical processes must be bihemispheric to induce sleepiness. In summary, sleepiness likely results from the coordinated activation of multiple sleep-promoting areas within the brain with possible coincident deactivation of wakefulness regions.

Neoplasms and paraneoplastic processes causing sleepiness

Cerebral tumors, especially those involving the sellar or suprasellar regions, typically induce sleepiness through direct neoplastic involvement or exertion of pressure on the hypothalamus, with reduced hypocretin production thought to be the causative factor. Sellar or suprasellar tumors can also induce endocrine dysfunction by disrupting thyroid function, or altering cortisol or growth hormone secretion. The resulting hormonal imbalance can indirectly induce sleepiness by causing obesity and subsequent obstructive sleep apnea (OSA).

Craniopharyngioma, a benign tumor arising from remnants of Rathke's pouch, is one of the most commonly studied sleepiness-inducing tumors. This diencephalic neoplasm typically originates from the pituitary stalk with extension to the hypothalamus. In a study of 79 patients with childhood craniopharyngioma, the average Epworth Sleepiness Scale score (ESS) in those with severe obesity (defined as a body mass index (BMI) ≥ 4 standard deviations (SD) above the mean) was 10, but only 4.5 in those with less significant obesity (BMI <4 SD above the mean). Reduced nocturnal salivary melatonin was noted in the sleepy group [5]. In another study of 21 craniopharyngioma patients, the mean ESS score was 8.1; not significantly different from healthy controls (5.7). However, approximately a third of these patients had an ESS score >10, and almost all of them were obese [6]. Another study of 115 childhood craniopharyngioma patients revealed 30% with an ESS score >10, but only 40% of them were obese. Ten of the 14 sleepy obese patients underwent polysomnography (PSG) and only 2 were found to have SDB [7]. Therefore, although obesity and subsequent OSA is a major cause of sleepiness in patients with craniopharyngioma, other factors contribute as well, likely due to hypothalamic compromise or effects on melatonin production. Another tumor with a predilection for hypothalamic involvement and effects on BMI and sleepiness is the pilocytic astrocytoma, which commonly occurs in the diencephalon, as well as the third and fourth ventricles. In 19 patients with childhood hypothalamic pilocytic astrocytoma, the average ESS was 11 among those with severe obesity (BMI ≥ 4 SD above the mean) but only 6 if the BMI was <4 SD above the mean [5].

Adenomas involving the pituitary gland, which lies in the sella turcica below the hypothalamus, may be non-functional (25–30%) or produce prolactin (25%), growth hormone (20%), or adrenocorticotropic hormone (10%). Among 76 patients with non-functioning pituitary macroadenomas treated by transsphenoidal surgery, the ESS score was increased compared to controls (7.6 vs. 4.8). Although this was within normal limits, the ESS significantly correlated with 15 of 21 quality-of-life parameters [8]. Other tumors of the sellar region have been associated with sleepiness. A 16-year-old girl complained of severe somnolence and atypical cataplexy after resection of a suprasellar germinoma. Despite an extremely elevated BMI of 52, her apnea–hypopnea index (AHI) was normal. Her secondary narcolepsy was confirmed by an MSLT mean sleep latency of 0.25 min with a mean REM latency of 2.1 min [9]. Similarly, a 28-year-old woman developed secondary narcolepsy after treatment (pinealectomy, chemotherapy, and radiation therapy) for a choroid plexus carcinoma of the pineal gland. Her ESS score was 15, MSLT showed 3 sleep onset REM periods (SOREMPs), and mean sleep latency was 7.5 min. Interestingly, her CSF hypocretin level was within the normal range [10]. Lastly, a gangliocytoma of the third ventricle caused hydrocephalus in a 55-year-old man. He had a shunt placed and received radiation therapy, but suffered from progressive sleepiness, hyperphagia, obesity, and memory impairment [11]. The secondary narcolepsy or sleepiness in all three cases was likely due to radiation, hydrocephalic pressure, and instrumentation of the third ventricle and diencephalic structures, most notably the hypothalamus. Importantly, sleepiness is not a given with diencephalic tumors. In a study of 27 patients with craniopharyngioma and 38 age-, gender-, and BMI-matched patients with non-functioning macroadenomas of the pituitary, the ESS score was within normal limits for both groups and did not differ significantly (mean score 7.7 vs. 7.5) [12].

Neoplastic involvement of the brainstem reticular activating system (RAS) has demonstrated effects on sleep and wakefulness as well. A subependymoma, a slow-growing tumor often found in the fourth ventricle, caused narcoleptic symptoms in a 50-year-old woman. The tumor was found to extend from the fourth ventricle to the midbrain tectum and rostral pons [13]. Brainstem gliomas have also been reported to induce sleepiness, with disruption of the RAS the likely cause [14, 15].

Hemispheric tumors have demonstrated somnogenic capabilities. A 30-year-old man with EDS and cataplexy was found to have a B-cell lymphoma occupying the left temporal lobe. MSLT showed a mean sleep latency of 40 s and 3 SOREMPs, consistent with secondary narcolepsy. He received treatment with radiation therapy, steroids, and methotrexate, and MSLT repeated at 3 months, 1, and 3 years showed resolution of the disorder. The authors proposed that tumor infiltration of the basal forebrain and hypothalamus induced sleepiness [16]. Another case of B-cell lymphoma and hypersomnia involved a 46-year-old man. Magnetic resonance imaging (MRI) revealed an infiltrative hyperintensity in the left basal ganglia, thalamus, cerebral pedunculus, splenium of the corpus callosum, and the right internal temporal lobe. Hypocretin was undetectable but normalized after treatment with steroids and chemotherapy, improving the ESS [17]. Lastly, an arachnoid cyst was found in the cerebellopontine angle of a 24-year-old woman with sleepiness and cataplexy since 14 years of age. Surgical correction resolved her symptoms, thought due to distortion of brainstem nuclei [18].

Paraneoplastic disorders such as anti-Ma2 encephalitis are also associated with sleepiness. Ma-2 is an onconeuronal protein linked with testicular and lung cancer. Antibodies to anti-Ma2 can be seen in patients presenting with limbic or brainstem encephalitis. Neurologic symptoms usually precede a cancer diagnosis. Among 38 patients with anti-Ma2 encephalitis, 32% complained of sleepiness, with 2 patients having cataplexy [19]. In a 69-year-old man with progressive hypersomnia and anti-Ma2 encephalitis, MRI showed T2 and fluid attenuation inversion recovery (FLAIR) hyperintense lesions in the dorsal midbrain, amygdala, and paramedian thalami. PSG revealed no evidence of OSA, but secondary narcolepsy was diagnosed based on 4 SOREMPs and mean sleep latency of 7 min on MSLT and low CSF hypocretin (49 pg/ml). REM sleep behavior disorder was also diagnosed based on dream enactment. Underlying carcinoma was not found while the patient's neurologic condition deteriorated [20]. A similar case involved progressive sleepiness in a 71-year-old man with anti-Ma2 encephalitis. MRI showed high signal intensity in the hypothalamus and hippocampi and hypocretin (orexin) was low. An underlying lung carcinoma was discovered and steroids improved his somnolence [21].

Treatment of cranial tumors can also induce sleepiness. Surgical manipulation and resection may damage nearby cortical tissue with somnogenic consequences. Radiation used to treat cerebral tumors usually has a field extending beyond tumor boundaries resulting in neuronal disruption in wakefulness-promoting regions. A 60-year-old man with acromegaly developed narcolepsy with cataplexy 2 weeks after completing radiation therapy for a pituitary adenoma [22]. Radiation therapy has been implicated in "somnolence syndrome", a poorly described hypersomnia in children receiving cranial irradiation for acute lymphocytic leukemia. Chemotherapeutics and immunomodulators used to treat cerebral tumors may also be somnogenic, although fatigue and insomnia are more frequently associated with these medications. In addition to direct neoplastic treatment improving sleepiness in these patients, alerting medications are often helpful. Methylphenidate, amphetamines, and modafinil are effective in the treatment of sleepiness in children with brain tumors [23].

Infectious causes of sleepiness

Infectious processes of the CNS, both diffuse and focal, can result in excessive sleepiness. Meningitis can cause alterations of consciousness or somnolence due to cerebral edema or obstructive hydrocephalus. Sleep disruption, which may lead to sleepiness, was found to be a frequent long-term consequence of both bacterial and viral meningitis, regardless of the severity of neurological symptoms [24].

Human immunodeficiency virus (HIV), a retrovirus, is transmitted by bodily fluids and can lead to immune system failure or acquired immunodeficiency syndrome (AIDS). One study of 128 HIV-infected individuals (median time with HIV 10 years) found an elevated mean ESS of 11 [25]. Even asymptomatic persons infected with HIV appear to suffer from multiple awakenings, although sleep difficulties increase with severity of disease [26–28]. Antiretroviral drugs, efavirenz and nevirapine have been linked to sleep disruption and vivid dreams, and zidovudine causes insomnia [29]. Infectious mononucleosis (IM), caused by the B-lymphocytic infection by Epstein–Barr virus (EBV), causes fever, sore throat, swollen lymph glands, and sleepiness. A study of 12 patients with suspected EBV revealed EDS both acutely and long term [30]. In some instances, EBV infection may be the cause of idiopathic hypersomnia.

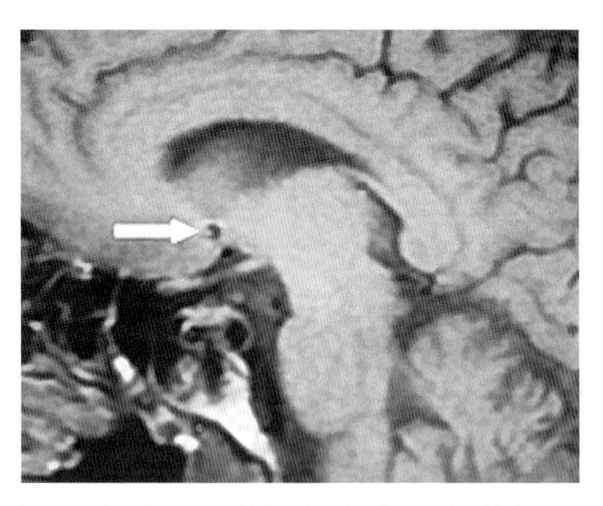

Figure 31.1 T1-weighted MRI lesion showing cysticerci lesion in the left lateral hypothalamus in a patient with sleepiness. Reprinted from [31] with permission from the American Academy of Sleep Medicine.

Neurocysticercosis, the most common parasitic infection to involve the CNS, is acquired by ingesting the eggs of a tapeworm (*Taenia solium*) found in water and foods contaminated with feces. A 54-year-old man developed neurocysticercosis and sleepiness following a trip to the Amazon River. He had an ESS of 22, mean sleep onset latency of 6.5 min, and 2 SOREMPs despite sleeping 22 h prior to the MSLT. He was found to have a cysticerci in his hypothalamus, and although his CSF hypocretin value was normal, he was diagnosed with secondary narcolepsy [31] (Figure 31.1). Lyme disease, caused by the tick-borne spirochete *Borrelia burgdorferi*, is associated with a wide variety of neurologic manifestations. Fatigue and sleep disturbances are common. In 11 patients with late Lyme disease, 8 (73%) complained of "unintentional sleep episodes when inactive", despite the MSLT mean sleep onset latency being within normal limits [32]. African trypanosomiasis, also known as "sleeping sickness", is a protozoal parasitic disease transmitted to the host by the tsetse fly through blood and lymph. The neurological phase of the disease is associated with confusion, fatigue, and mania that progresses to daytime sleepiness and nighttime insomnia, likely related to disruption of the anterior hypothalamus.

Sleepiness may also result from somnogenic aspects of the inflammatory response itself. Bacterial endotoxins induce interleukin-1 (IL-1) production resulting in sleepiness [33]. Tumor necrosis factor-alpha (TNF-α) and IL-1β also induce sleepiness in the

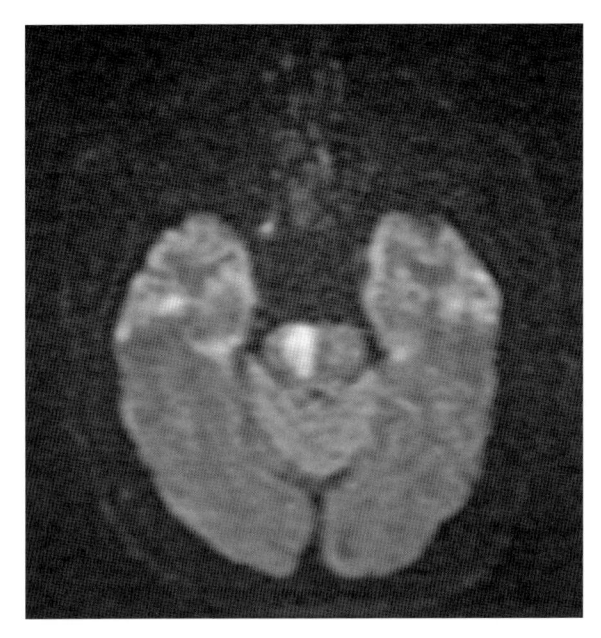

31. Brain tumors, infections, and other CNS causes

Figure 31.2 Diffusion-weighted MRI showing acute pontine infarct in a patient with sleepiness. Courtesy of the University of Washington.

early stages of the acute phase response to viral and bacterial infections [34].

Vascular causes of sleepiness

Sleepiness and sleep disturbances are common comorbidities in acute stroke and can evolve into chronic issues. Studies reveal that approximately two-thirds of stroke patients have SDB, a common cause of EDS [35, 36]. Absent this stroke comorbidity, stroke location can precipitate sleepiness with thalamic, subthalamic, mesencephalic, and pontine strokes often implicated due to ascending RAS disruption (Figure 31.2). Hypersomnia is most profound after bilateral, as opposed to unilateral, thalamic infarcts with symptom improvement over time [37]. In addition to thalamic involvement, hypothalamic strokes can cause hypersomnia due to disruption of the hypocretin system. This clinical scenario is exemplified by a 23-year-old man who developed secondary narcolepsy due to bilateral hypothalamic strokes following craniopharyngioma resection. His MSLT showed 4 SOREMPs and his CSF hypocretin was reduced. Sleepiness and cataplexy persisted for 5 years post-surgery [38].

Hemispheric strokes can reduce sleep efficiency, total sleep time, and in the acute setting, the amount of REM sleep. In a study of 27 first-ever hemispheric stroke patients (median National Institute of Health Stroke Scale (NIHSS) 7), 26% had an increased ESS score (>3 points) and 38% reported increased sleep duration (>2 h) following stroke. This phenomenon was predominantly observed in patients with large hemispheric strokes. Importantly, patients were excluded if they had an AHI >15 or >10 with complaints of sleepiness, ensuring the observed hypersomnia was not due to coincident SDB [39]. Sleepiness was likely caused by disruption of the arousal system through brainstem displacement by cerebral edema [40].

Sleepiness has been observed in CNS vascular diseases other than stroke. Hypersomnia was the presenting complaint in two cases of hypothalamic CNS angiitis [41, 42]. Hypersomnia and secondary narcolepsy have been described following hypoxic encephalopathy due to cardiopulmonary insufficiency [43]. In all of these cases, the hypersomnia was likely due to a complex interplay between location and extent of the CNS insult and somnogenic properties of the inflammatory response.

As previously mentioned, stroke can lead to sleep disorders that contribute to sleepiness, particularly SDB, present in 60–70% of patients following a stroke [44]. Stroke directly causes obstructive and central sleep apnea by compromising nerves subserving airway patency and respiratory control centers. Conversely, SDB can precipitate cerebrovascular disease and daytime somnolence is associated with increased stroke incidence (RR = 1.4, 95% CI = 1.1–1.8), with those reporting >8 h of sleep/night and sleepiness exhibiting the greatest stroke risk (RR = 1.9, 95% CI = 1.2–3.1) [45]. The tight link between stroke and SDB causes one to consider which came first. In most cases, sleep apnea is thought to precede stroke for a number of reasons. First, there is no relationship between SDB and stroke subtype, location or vascular territory. Second, there is no correlation between stroke severity and extent of SDB. Third, the presence of sleep apnea is not higher in stroke than transient ischemic attack (TIA) patients.

Other stroke-related sleep disrupters include insomnia, parasomnias, seizures, RLS, and depression. Insomnia can result from ischemic or hemorrhagic damage to the dorsal/tegmental brainstem, paramedian/lateral thalamus or select subcortical regions [40]. Parasomnias, such as REM sleep behavior disorder, can occur following cerebrovascular damage to the pontine tegmentum. Post-stroke epilepsy can disrupt normal sleep architecture, fragment sleep, and

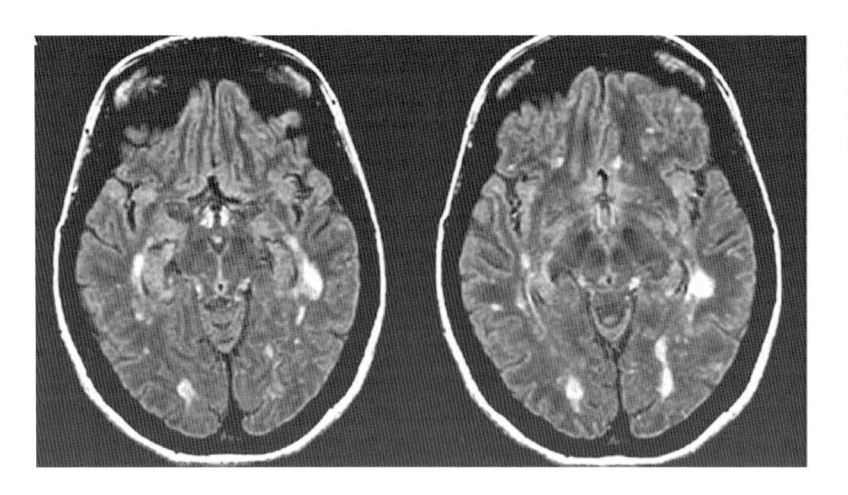

Figure 31.3 MRI T2 FLAIR lesions of the bilateral hypothalamus in a 37-year-old woman with relapsing-remitting MS and sleepiness. Reprinted from [50], with permission from Elsevier.

cause daytime somnolence. Infarction of the pyramidal tracts or basal ganglia can precipitate RLS resulting in sleep onset and maintenance insomnia, sleep fragmentation, and sleepiness. The astute clinician should consider all these potential stroke comorbidities when evaluating the patient with post-stroke hypersomnia.

Treatment of post-stroke somnolence involves the usual stimulant medications and is often challenging. Improvement has been reported with the use of amphetamines, modafinil, methylphenidate, levodopa, and dopamine agonists [40, 46]. Treating associated depression and primary sleep disorders may also improve the sleepiness.

Demyelinating causes of sleepiness

Multiple sclerosis (MS) is an immune-mediated inflammatory disease that attacks the myelin of CNS axons and typically occurs in adult, Caucasian females, living in northern latitudes. Neurologic symptoms can vary greatly between patients and may remit and relapse or progress unabated. Fatigue is common and often treated with modafinil. There are multiple case reports of MS patients presenting with acute hypersomnia, signifying disease recurrence [47–51]. Most of these involve neuroimaging that displays hypothalamic lesion(s) and low CSF hypocretin levels (<40 pg/ml), both of which improve, along with the hypersomnia, following steroid administration [47, 48, 50, 52, 53] (Figure 31.3). Some case reports include objective sleepiness testing and report findings consistent with severe sleepiness and/or secondary narcolepsy [49,51,53,54]. In one report, a 22-year-old woman with MS presented with acute-onset hypersomnia. The MSLT showed a mean sleep onset latency of 2.8 min and 5 SOREMPs. CSF hypocretin was undetectable. Two months following steroid therapy, her sleep onset latency was normal at 17.4 min with one SOREMP. Four months later, her sleep onset latency remained normal at 14.8 min, SOREMPs were absent, and CSF hypocretin normalized [49].

As with stroke, neoplastic, and infectious causes of sleepiness, lesion location in MS is critical to the presence or absence of sleepiness. In a case of new-onset MS, a 31-year-old woman presented with sleepiness and T2 MRI showed lesions in the bilateral basal ganglia, thalamus, and brainstem [52]. Although the causative lesion in this case could not be definitively established, the sleepiness was felt to be most likely due to compromise of the brainstem RAS.

Large studies of MS patients have examined the presence of sleepiness, fatigue, and other sleep-related issues. In a cross-sectional survey of 1063 people with MS, researchers mailed the Women's Health Initiative Insomnia Rating scale and Medical Outcomes Study Sleep measures to study participants. Results were compared to those from chronically ill patients and "healthy" individuals representing the general population in the United States. The authors concluded that MS patients have more sleep disturbances (and daytime somnolence) than either of the non-MS groups [55]. Conversely, multiple studies dispute sleepiness as an MS symptom. Two studies with a total of 122 MS patients revealed ESS scores at the high end of normal [56, 57]. Another study of 60 patients showed a median ESS score of only 7 with no correlation between the ESS and measures of sleep disturbance. In this particular study, the authors note their results may have been biased by the fact that 20 patients were on medications affecting sleep and wakefulness, including modafinil, amantadine, selective serotonin reuptake inhibitors (SSRI), tricyclic antidepressants (TCA), and hypnotics [58].

Using an alternate approach, researchers investigated 48 patients with relapsing-remitting MS or monosymptomatic optic neuritis for sleepiness and CSF hypocretin levels at two time points: during a disease attack, and when in remission. The ESS was "normal" (mean 5.4 during attack and 5.8 in remission) during both conditions and CSF hypocretin levels were unchanged, arguing against sleepiness as a part of the MS symptom complex [59]. Lastly, 61 MS patients and 42 age-matched healthy controls were examined with a pupillographic sleepiness test (PST), an unconventional test measuring daytime sleepiness based on spontaneous pupillary oscillations. MS patients had a mean ESS of 7.4 and a normal pupillary unrest index. Ironically, more controls (38%) than MS patients (26%) had ESS scores > 10 [60].

Due to the conflicting evidence regarding sleepiness in MS, researchers have focused their studies on the fatigued subset of MS patients. Fifteen MS patients with fatigue (Fatigue Severity Scale (FSS) ≥5) were compared to 15 MS patients without fatigue. The fatigued group had a mean ESS score of 10.5, significantly higher than those without fatigue (3.3) [61]. In another study of 60 patients, the ESS and FSS scores were significantly correlated [58]. Other investigations of sleepiness involving fatigued MS patients provide conflicting results, with studies of 27 and 6 patients revealing normal ESS scores (both <6) with the latter study demonstrating normal sleep latencies on MSLT [62, 63].

When present, sleepiness in MS is likely due to lesions that disrupt wakefulness pathways and comorbid illness. Insomnia is present in up to 40% of MS patients, and pain, nocturia, depression, and periodic limb movements (PLM) are common in MS and disruptive to sleep [64]. In addition, neuromodulators such as interferon commonly used in the management of MS may contribute to insomnia and feelings of sleepiness. Generally speaking, poor sleep in MS has been found to be an independent predictor of quality of life [65].

Acute disseminated encephalomyelitis (ADEM) is an immune-mediated, central demyelinating, monophasic illness closely related to MS from a pathophysiological perspective. Onset is acute, commonly following viral illness or vaccination, with a predilection for children. While disturbance of consciousness is common, seen in up to 70% of cases, sleepiness is less frequently reported [66, 67]. A handful of case reports, however, suggest an association between ADEM and somnolence. A 12-year-old girl diagnosed with ADEM presented with profound drowsiness and MRI showed high intensity signals in the hypothalamus, midbrain, caudate, putamen, and periventricular and subcortical white matter. MSLT showed a mean sleep onset latency of 4.5 min without SOREMPs. Her CSF hypocretin was decreased (102 pg/mLl and drowsiness improved with steroid treatment [68]. A 7-year-old Japanese girl diagnosed with ADEM presented with hypersomnia, seizures, and visual complaints. MRI showed bilateral white matter, basal ganglia, and hypothalamic lesions. CSF hypocretin was low (146 pg/mL) at presentation. After steroid therapy, EDS and CSF hypocretin levels improved [69]. A 5-year-old girl with hypersomnia due to ADEM was found to have lesions in the posterior hypothalamus, midbrain, lentiform nucleus, posterior limb of internal capsule, and thalamus. Her sleepiness improved rapidly with steroids [70]. Lastly, ADEM was diagnosed in a 38-year-old woman with hypersomnolence resulting in 16 h of sleep a day. MSLT was consistent with secondary narcolepsy, with 4 SOREMPs, an average sleep latency of 4.4 min, and CSF hypocretin was decreased (87 pg/ml). Six months following steroid treatment, subjective sleepiness was only mildly improved, MSLT findings were unchanged, and CSF hypocretin increased to 148 pg/ml [71].

Inflammatory causes of sleepiness

Inflammatory disorders are also implicated as a CNS cause of sleepiness. Sarcoidosis, a chronic, multisystem, non-caseating granulomatous disease most frequently affects the lungs in young African American women. CNS involvement is thought to occur in about 10% of those with systemic sarcoidosis, but is likely underdiagnosed. Neurosarcoidosis can affect any part of the nervous system; however, granulomas are most frequently discovered in the hypothalamus and pituitary gland [72]. Various case reports of patients with hypothalamic sarcoid granulomas revealed symptoms of sleepiness and/or narcoleptic features along with personality changes, hyperphagia, polydipsia, and variations in body temperature [73–76]. Some patients have improvement of symptoms with steroid treatment and/or whole-brain irradiation [75, 77].

Systemic lupus erythematosus (SLE) is another inflammatory disease associated with sleepiness, although the disorder is more commonly associated with fatigue. SLE is a chronic, multisystem disorder, typically affecting young women. A study of 35 SLE patients found 51% with MSLT- and ESS-confirmed sleepiness [78]. Sleep studies in these patients showed impaired sleep efficiency, elevated arousal index, increased stage 1 sleep, decreased slow-wave sleep, and alpha intrusion [78, 79]. Further evidence of sleep disruption in patients with SLE is provided by a study that found 62% of patients with poor sleep as indicated by a score ≥6 on the Pittsburgh Sleep Quality Index (PSQI) [80]. Sjogren's syndrome and Behcet's disease are other inflammatory diseases with neurologic involvement that have been associated with sleepiness, although the literature in support of this is sparse [81].

Epilepsy as a cause of sleepiness

The association of sleepiness and epilepsy has been extensively studied, with evidence both for and against an association. Positive studies demonstrate EDS in 17–28% of epilepsy patients [82, 83]. Seizure control appears to be a contributing factor, as one study of 270 patients found significantly more sleepiness in patients with uncontrolled epilepsy versus those seizure-free for at least one year [84]. Another study of 244 patients found that seizure frequency was significantly associated with increased ESS scores [85]. Studies demonstrating improvement in sleepiness with better seizure control are lacking. Conversely, some studies find no difference in ESS scores in those with epilepsy compared to controls [86–88]. Although the ESS score was not significantly different in a study of 486 partial epilepsy patients and 492 controls, there was a significant increase in sleepiness on the Sleep Diagnosis List, the Medical Outcomes Study Sleep Scale, and Groningen Sleep Questionnaire [86].

The nature of the ictal focus likely influences the expression of sleepiness in patients with epilepsy. Patients with nocturnal frontal lobe epilepsy have increased sleep fragmentation and EDS [89]. In a retrospective review of video electroencephalography (EEG), patients with frontal lobe epilepsy were found to have seizures occurring more often during sleep compared to patients with temporal lobe epilepsy, although the temporal lobe seizures were overall more common and generalized more frequently during sleep [90]. Sleepiness was similar in a study comparing 33 patients with nocturnal frontal lobe epilepsy and 27 controls; however, "tiredness after awakening" and "spontaneous mid-sleep awakenings" were more common in the patients with frontal lobe epilepsy [91].

Sleepiness in epilepsy patients no doubt extends beyond the effects of the disease itself. Direct medication effects are thought to play an important role with many antiepileptic drugs (AED) known to induce sleepiness. Because most studies on the topic do not involve treatment of naive subjects, it can be difficult to know whether to attribute the sleepiness to the epilepsy or the medications. The role of medication side-effects on sleepiness in patients with epilepsy is demonstrated by two studies showing a significant correlation between ESS and number of AEDs, with and without adjustment of seizure frequency [85, 92]. That said, many epilepsy patients complain of sleepiness before medications are started or even after they are discontinued.

AEDs can indirectly contribute to increased sleepiness in the epileptic patient. A number of AEDs contribute to weight gain, possibly causing or worsening SDB. Also, benzodiazepines and barbiturates may reduce responsiveness to hypercarbia and/or hypoxia and reduce airway muscle tone resulting in sleep apnea and sleepiness. Lastly, a number of AEDs are known to lead to restless legs symptoms and/or PLMs, which can cause sleep disruption and sleepiness. Certainly, clinicians should consider medication side-effects in an epileptic with a complaint of daytime somnolence.

Epileptics have an increased risk of OSA, seizures are more common in those with sleep apnea, and seizures increase the likelihood of sleep apnea. A study of 26 children with epilepsy (and age-matched controls) found that symptoms of SDB and parasomnias were independent predictors of sleepiness, leading the researchers to conclude that somnolence in these children is likely due to comorbid sleep disorders [93]. Lastly, treatment of OSA may reduce seizure frequency [85, 92, 94].

Insomnia is also frequently reported in epileptic patients, present in up to 28% of patients, and possibly contributes to sleepiness in these individuals [83]. A study of 100 epilepsy patients devoid of hypnotic therapy found that sleep-maintenance insomnia was more frequent in the patients with epilepsy compared to a control population [87].

Depression and sleepiness are also linked in patients with epilepsy. A study of 136 patients found depression to be the main predictor of sleepiness. Interestingly, depression did not correlate with seizure frequency or number of AEDs [95]. Another study of 332 children following first seizure (and 225 sibling controls) found that epileptics with sleep disturbances had worse neuropsychological functioning across all domains [96].

Few novel therapies have been proposed for the treatment of sleepiness in epileptics. In a unique study, 15 medically refractory epileptic patients had placement of a vagus nerve stimulator (VNS, set at low stimulus intensities) and showed significant improvement in MSLT mean sleep latencies and ESS scores. This despite the fact that VNS is known to precipitat SDB in some patients [97, 98]. Interestingly, there was no reduction in seizure frequency and AEDs remained constant [(99].

In conclusion, sleepiness is an important symptom in patients with epilepsy as the impact on quality of life is substantial. It may represent undertreatment of the seizure disorder, a medication side-effect, or a co-existing sleep disorder. Additionally, careful evaluation is required, since sleepiness can be mistaken for absence seizures, especially in children [100].

Structural causes of sleepiness

Lastly, structural brain malformations may also lead to sleepiness. Arnold–Chiari malformations, a downward herniation of the cerebellar tonsils and brainstem through the foramen magnum, may lead to an array of neurologic complaints. Somnolence may be an indirect result of associated obstructive or central sleep apnea [101]. Syringomyelia, a fluid-filled cavity within the spinal cord, has been associated with PLMs, which also may indirectly cause sleepiness [102].

Conclusion

The neuroanatomy of sleep and wakefulness is a complex interplay between numerous wake- and sleep-promoting centers and circadian factors. Correspondingly, when considering CNS causes of sleepiness, lesion location is more important than lesion etiology. Hypothalamic damage, whether from neoplasm, stroke, MS plaque or neurocysticercosis, can result in the same secondary narcolepsy phenotype. Indeed, even small lesions in the key location can have devastating consequences for an individual's ability to remain awake. Other important factors include somnogenic properties of any associated inflammatory response, sleep disruption due to symptoms of a CNS disorder (e.g. pain, primary sleep disorders), and medication side-effects. The clinical approach to sleepiness in CNS disease must address all these considerations to be successful.

The literature regarding CNS causes of sleepiness often lacks subjective and/or objective measures of sleepiness. The vast majority of publications are case reports. Many of the studies do not exclude patients taking sleep-altering medications, which can complicate findings of "sleepiness". Additionally, there is often no attempt to evaluate or exclude those with an underlying sleep disorder, which may be a major contributing factor. Therefore it appears that CNS causes of sleepiness are an understudied yet important topic requiring further research.

References

1. **Posner J B**, **Plum F**. *Plum and Posner's Diagnosis of Stupor and Coma* (4th Ed). Oxford, New York: Oxford University Press, 2007.

2. **American Academy of Sleep Medicine**. *The International Classification of Sleep Disorders: Diagnostic and Coding Manual*. 2nd Ed. Westchester, IL: American Academy of Sleep Medicine, 2005.

3. **Espana R A**, **Scammell T E**. Sleep neurobiology for the clinician. *Sleep*, 2004; **27**:811–20.

4. **Saper C B**, **Scammell T E**, **Lu J**. Hypothalamic regulation of sleep and circadian rhythms. *Nature*, 2005; **437**:1257–63.

5. **Muller H L**, **Handwerker G**, **Gebhardt U**, *et al*. Melatonin treatment in obese patients with childhood craniopharyngioma and increased daytime sleepiness. *Cancer Causes Control*, 2006; **17**:583–89.

6. **Poretti A**, **Grotzer M A**, **Ribi K**, *et al*. Outcome of craniopharyngioma in children: long-term complications and quality of life. *Dev Med Child Neurol*, 2004; **46**:220–29.

7. **Muller H L**, **Muller-Stover S**, **Gebhardt U**, *et al*. Secondary narcolepsy may be a causative factor of increased daytime sleepiness in obese childhood craniopharyngioma patients. *J Pediatr Endocrinol Metab*, 2006; **19**(Suppl 1):423–29.

8. **Van Der Klaauw A A**, **Dekkers O M**, **Pereira A M**, *et al*. Increased daytime somnolence despite normal sleep patterns in patients treated for nonfunctioning pituitary macroadenoma. *J Clin Endocrinol Metab*, 2007; **92**:3898–903.

9. **Marcus C L**, **Trescher W H**, **Halbower A C**, *et al*. Secondary narcolepsy in children with brain tumors. *Sleep*, 2002; **25**:435–39.

10. **Krahn L E**, **Boeve B F**, **Oliver L**, *et al*. Hypocretin (orexin) and melatonin values in a narcoleptic-like sleep disorder after pinealectomy. *Sleep Med*, 2002; **3**:521–23.

11. **Beal M F**, **Kleinman G M**, **Ojemann R G**, *et al*. Gangliocytoma of third ventricle: hyperphagia, somnolence, and dementia. *Neurology*, 1981; **31**:1224–28.

12. **Van Der Klaauw A A**, **Biermasz N R**, **Pereira A M**, *et al*. Patients cured from craniopharyngioma or nonfunctioning pituitary macroadenoma (NFMA) suffer similarly from increased daytime somnolence despite normal sleep patterns compared to healthy controls. *Clin Endocrinol (Oxf)*, 2008; **69**:769–74.

13. **Ma T K**, **Ang L C**, **Mamelak M**, *et al*. Narcolepsy secondary to fourth ventricular subependymoma. *Can J Neurol Sci*, 1996; **23**:59–62.

14. **Schoenhuber R**, **Angiari P**, **Peserico L**. Narcolepsy symptomatic of a pontine glioma. *Ital J Neurol Sci*, 1981; **2**:379–80.

15. **Stahl S M**, **Layzer R B**, **Aminoff M J**, *et al*. Continuous cataplexy in a patient with a midbrain tumor: the limp man syndrome. *Neurology*, 1980; **30**:1115–18.

16. **Onofrj M**, **Curatola L**, **Ferracci F**, *et al*. Narcolepsy associated with primary temporal lobe B-cells lymphoma in a HLA DR2 negative subject. *J Neurol Neurosurg Psychiatry*, 1992; **55**:852–53.

17. **Dauvilliers Y**, **Abril B**, **Charif M**, *et al*. Reversal of symptomatic tumoral narcolepsy, with normalization of CSF hypocretin level. *Neurology*, 2007; **69**:1300–01.

18. **Nakano H**, **Ogashiwa M**. Complete remission of narcolepsy after surgical treatment of an arachnoid cyst in the cerebellopontine angle. *J Neurol Neurosurg Psychiatry*, 1995; **58**:264.

19. **Dalmau J**, **Graus F**, **Villarejo A**, *et al*. Clinical analysis of anti-Ma2-associated encephalitis. *Brain*, 2004; **127**:1831–44.

20. **Compta Y**, **Iranzo A**, **Santamaria J**, *et al*. REM sleep behavior disorder and narcoleptic features in anti-Ma2-associated encephalitis. *Sleep*, 2007; **30**:767–69.

21. **Rojas-Marcos I**, **Graus F**, **Sanz G**, *et al*. Hypersomnia as presenting symptom of anti-Ma2-associated encephalitis: case study. *Neuro Oncol*, 2007; **9**:75–77.

22. **Dempsey O J**, **McGeoch P**, **de Silva R N**, *et al*. Acquired narcolepsy in an acromegalic patient who underwent pituitary irradiation. *Neurology*, 2003; **61**:537–40.

23. **Meeske K**, **Katz E R**, **Palmer S N**, *et al*. Parent proxy-reported health-related quality of life and fatigue in pediatric patients diagnosed with brain tumors and acute lymphoblastic leukemia. *Cancer*, 2004; **101**:2116–25.

24. **Schmidt H**, **Cohrs S**, **Heinemann T**, *et al*. Sleep disorders are long-term sequelae of both bacterial and viral meningitis. *J Neurol Neurosurg Psychiatry*, 2006; **77**:554–58.

25. **Salahuddin N**, **Barroso J**, **Leserman J**, *et al*. Daytime sleepiness, nighttime sleep quality, stressful life events, and HIV-related fatigue. *J Assoc Nurses AIDS Care*, 2009; **20**:6–13.

26. **Darko D F**, **McCutchan J A**, **Kripke D F**, *et al*. Fatigue, sleep disturbance, disability, and indices of progression of HIV infection. *Am J Psychiatry*, 1992; **149**:514–20.

27. **Moeller A A**, **Oechsner M**, **Backmund H C**, *et al*. Self-reported sleep quality in HIV infection: correlation to the stage of infection and zidovudine therapy. *J Acquir Immune Defic Syndr*, 1991; **4**:1000–03.

28. **Norman S E**, **Chediak A D**, **Kiel M**, *et al*. Sleep disturbances in HIV-infected homosexual men. *AIDS*, 1990; **4**:775–81.

29. **Morlese J F**, **Qazi N A**, **Gazzard B G**, *et al*. Nevirapine-induced neuropsychiatric complications, a class effect of non-nucleoside reverse transcriptase inhibitors? *AIDS*, 2002; **16**:1840–41.

30. **Guilleminault C**, **Mondini S**. Mononucleosis and chronic daytime sleepiness. A long-term follow-up study. *Arch Intern Med*, 1986; **146**:1333–35.

31. **Watson N F**, **Doherty M J**, **Zunt J R**. Secondary narcolepsy following neurocysticercosis infection. *J Clin Sleep Med*, 2005; **1**:41–42.

32. **Greenberg H E**, **Ney G**, **Scharf S M**, *et al*. Sleep quality in Lyme disease. *Sleep*, 1995; **18**:912–16.

33. **Dinarello C A**, **Cannon J G**, **Wolff S M**. New concepts on the pathogenesis of fever. *Rev Infect Dis*, 1988; **10**:168–89.

34. **Kelley K W**, **Bluthe R M**, **Dantzer R**, *et al*. Cytokine-induced sickness behavior. *Brain Behav Immun*, 2003; **17**(Suppl 1):S112–18.

35. **Parra O**, **Arboix A**, **Bechich S**, *et al*. Time course of sleep-related breathing disorders in first-ever stroke or transient ischemic attack. *Am J Respir Crit Care Med*, 2000; **161**:375–80.

36. **Turkington P M**, **Allgar V**, **Bamford J**, *et al*. Effect of upper airway obstruction in acute stroke on functional outcome at 6 months. *Thorax*, 2004; **59**:367–71.

37. **Hermann D M**, **Siccoli M**, **Brugger P**, *et al*. Evolution of neurological, neuropsychological and sleep wake

disturbances after paramedian thalamic stroke. *Stroke*, 2008; **39**:62–68.

38. **Scammell T E**, **Nishino S**, **Mignot E**, *et al*. Narcolepsy and low CSF orexin (hypocretin) concentration after a diencephalic stroke. *Neurology*, 2001; **56**:1751–53.

39. **Vock J**, **Achermann P**, **Bischof M**, *et al*. Evolution of sleep and sleep EEG after hemispheric stroke. *J Sleep Res*, 2002; **11**:331–38.

40. **Bassetti C L**. Sleep and stroke. *Semin Neurol*, 2005; **25**:19–32.

41. **Nakaji K**, **Ikeda A**, **Oka Y**, *et al*. Hypersomnia caused by isolated angiitis of the CNS. *Intern Med*, 2005; **44**:883–85.

42. **Tsutsumi S**, **Ito M**, **Yasumoto Y**, *et al*. Isolated angiitis in the hypothalamus mimicking brain tumor. *Neurol Med Chir (Tokyo)*, 2008; **48**:33–36.

43. **Rivera V M**, **Meyer J S**, **Hata T**, *et al*. Narcolepsy following cerebral hypoxic ischemia. *Ann Neurol*, 1986; **19**:505–08.

44. **Turkington P M**, **Bamford J**, **Wanklyn P**, *et al*. Prevalence and predictors of upper airway obstruction in the first 24 hours after acute stroke. *Stroke*, 2002; **33**:2037–42.

45. **Qureshi A I**, **Giles W H**, **Croft J B**, *et al*. Habitual sleep patterns and risk for stroke and coronary heart disease: a 10-year follow-up from NHANES I. *Neurology*, 1997; **48**:904–11.

46. **Autret A**, **Lucas B**, **Mondon K**, *et al*. Sleep and brain lesions: a critical review of the literature and additional new cases. *Neurophysiol Clin*, 2001; **31**:356–75.

47. **Iseki K**, **Mezaki T**, **Oka Y**, *et al*. Hypersomnia in MS. *Neurology*, 2002; **59**:2006–07.

48. **Kato T**, **Kanbayashi T**, **Yamamoto K**, *et al*. Hypersomnia and low CSF hypocretin-1 (orexin-A) concentration in a patient with multiple sclerosis showing bilateral hypothalamic lesions. *Intern Med*, 2003; **42**:743–45.

49. **Oka Y**, **Kanbayashi T**, **Mezaki T**, *et al*. Low CSF hypocretin-1/orexin-A associated with hypersomnia secondary to hypothalamic lesion in a case of multiple sclerosis. *J Neurol*, 2004; **251**:885–86.

50. **Vetrugno R**, **Stecchi S**, **Plazzi G**, *et al*. Narcolepsy-like syndrome in multiple sclerosis. *Sleep Med*, 2009; **10**:389–91.

51. **Wang C Y**, **Kawashima H**, **Takami T**, *et al*. [A case of multiple sclerosis with initial symptoms of narcolepsy]. *No To Hattatsu*, 1998; **30**:300–06.

52. **Hashiguchi S**, **Ogasawara N**, **Mine H**, *et al*. Multiple sclerosis with caudate lesions on MRI. *Intern Med*, 2001; **40**:358–62.

53. **Schluter B**, **Aguigah G**, **Andler W**. [Hypersomnia in multiple sclerosis]. *Klin Padiatr*, 1996; **208**:103–05.

54. **Schrader H**, **Gotlibsen O B**, **Skomedal G N**. Multiple sclerosis and narcolepsy/cataplexy in a monozygotic twin. *Neurology*, 1980; **30**:105–08.

55. **Bamer A M**, **Johnson K L**, **Amtmann D**, *et al*. Prevalence of sleep problems in individuals with multiple sclerosis. *Mult Scler*, 2008; **14**:1127–30.

56. **Rammohan K W**, **Rosenberg J H**, **Lynn D J**, *et al*. Efficacy and safety of modafinil (Provigil) for the treatment of fatigue in multiple sclerosis: a two centre phase 2 study. *J Neurol Neurosurg Psychiatry*, 2002; **72**:179–83.

57. **Zifko U A**, **Rupp M**, **Schwarz S**, *et al*. Modafinil in treatment of fatigue in multiple sclerosis. Results of an open-label study. *J Neurol*, 2002; **249**:983–87.

58. **Stanton B R**, **Barnes F**, **Silber E**. Sleep and fatigue in multiple sclerosis. *Mult Scler*, 2006;**12**:481–86.

59. **Knudsen S**, **Jennum P J**, **Korsholm K**, *et al*. Normal levels of cerebrospinal fluid hypocretin-1 and daytime sleepiness during attacks of relapsing-remitting multiple sclerosis and monosymptomatic optic neuritis. *Mult Scler*, 2008; **14**:734–38.

60. **Frauscher B**, **Egg R**, **Brandauer E**, *et al*. Daytime sleepiness is not increased in mild to moderate multiple sclerosis: a pupillographic study. *Sleep Med*, 2005; **6**:543–47.

61. **Heesen C**, **Nawrath L**, **Reich C**, *et al*. Fatigue in multiple sclerosis: an example of cytokine mediated sickness behaviour? *J Neurol Neurosurg Psychiatry*, 2006; **77**:34–39.

62. **Kaynak H**, **Altintas A**, **Kaynak D**, *et al*. Fatigue and sleep disturbance in multiple sclerosis. *Eur J Neurol*, 2006; **13**:1333–39.

63. **Vetrugno R**, **Stecchi S**, **Scandellari C**, *et al*. Sleep–wake and body core temperature rhythms in multiple sclerosis with fatigue. *Clin Neurophysiol*, 2007; **118**:228–34.

64. **Tachibana N**, **Howard R S**, **Hirsch N P**, *et al*. Sleep problems in multiple sclerosis. *Eur Neurol*, 1994; **34**:320–23.

65. **Merlino G**, **Fratticci L**, **Lenchig C**, *et al*. Prevalence of 'poor sleep' among patients with multiple sclerosis: an independent predictor of mental and physical status. *Sleep Med*, 2009; **10**:26–34.

66. **Dale R C**, **de Sousa C**, **Chong W K**, *et al*. Acute disseminated encephalomyelitis, multiphasic disseminated encephalomyelitis and multiple sclerosis in children. *Brain*, 2000; **123**:2407–22.

67. **Hynson J L**, **Kornberg A J**, **Coleman L T**, *et al*. Clinical and neuroradiologic features of acute

disseminated encephalomyelitis in children. *Neurology*, 2001; **56**:1308–12.

68. **Kubota H**, **Kanbayashi T**, **Tanabe Y**, *et al.* A case of acute disseminated encephalomyelitis presenting hypersomnia with decreased hypocretin level in cerebrospinal fluid. *J Child Neurol*, 2002; **17**:537–39.

69. **Yoshikawa S**, **Suzuki S**, **Kanbayashi T**, *et al.* Hypersomnia and low cerebrospinal fluid hypocretin levels in acute disseminated encephalomyelitis. *Pediatr Neurol*, 2004; **31**:367–70.

70. **Kanbayashi T**, **Goto A**, **Hishikawa Y**, *et al.* Hypersomnia due to acute disseminated encephalomyelitis in a 5-year-old girl. *Sleep Med*, 2001; **2**:347–50.

71. **Gledhill R F**, **Bartel P R**, **Yoshida Y**, *et al.* Narcolepsy caused by acute disseminated encephalomyelitis. *Arch Neurol*, 2004; **61**:758–60.

72. **Stern B J**, **Krumholz A**, **Johns C**, *et al.* Sarcoidosis and its neurological manifestations. *Arch Neurol*, 1985; **42**:909–17.

73. **Martin J B**, **Riskind P N**. Neurologic manifestations of hypothalamic disease. *Prog Brain Res*, 1992; **93**:31–40; discussion 40–42.

74. **Mathe J F**, **Mussini J M**, **Nomballais F**, *et al.* [Unusual involvement of the CNS in a case of neuro-sarcoidosis (author's transl)]. *Rev Neurol (Paris)*, 1980; **136**:33–41.

75. **Rubinstein I**, **Gray T A**, **Moldofsky H**, *et al.* Neurosarcoidosis associated with hypersomnolence treated with corticosteroids and brain irradiation. *Chest*, 1988; **94**:205–06.

76. **Servan J**, **Marchand F**, **Garma L**, *et al.* [Narcolepsy disclosing neurosarcoidosis]. *Rev Neurol (Paris)*, 1995; **151**:281–83.

77. **Bejar J M**, **Kerby G R**, **Ziegler D K**, *et al.* Treatment of central nervous system sarcoidosis with radiotherapy. *Ann Neurol*, 1985; **18**:258–60.

78. **Iaboni A**, **Ibanez D**, **Gladman D D**, *et al.* Fatigue in systemic lupus erythematosus: contributions of disordered sleep, sleepiness, and depression. *J Rheumatol*, 2006; **33**:2453–57.

79. **Valencia-Flores M**, **Resendiz M**, **Castano V A**, *et al.* Objective and subjective sleep disturbances in patients with systemic lupus erythematosus. *Arthritis Rheum*, 1999; **42**:2189–93.

80. **Chandrasekhara P K**, **Jayachandran N V**, **Rajasekhar L**, *et al.* The prevalence and associations of sleep disturbances in patients with systemic lupus erythematosus. *Mod Rheumatol*, 2009; **19**:407–15.

81. **Abad V C**, **Sarinas P S**, **Guilleminault C**. Sleep and rheumatologic disorders. *Sleep Med Rev*, 2008; **12**:211–28.

82. **Malow B A**, **Bowes R J**, **Lin X**. Predictors of sleepiness in epilepsy patients. *Sleep*, 1997; **20**:1105–10.

83. **Piperidou C**, **Karlovasitou A**, **Triantafyllou N**, *et al.* Influence of sleep disturbance on quality of life of patients with epilepsy. *Seizure*, 2008; **17**:588–94.

84. **Manni R**, **Tartara A**. Evaluation of sleepiness in epilepsy. *Clin Neurophysiol*, 2000; **111**(Suppl 2):S111–14.

85. **Manni R**, **Ratti M T**, **Sartori I**, *et al.* Sleepiness and its associated factors in epilepsy patients. *Sleep* [abstract], 1998; **21**:175.

86. **de Weerd A**, **de Haas S**, **Otte A**, *et al.* Subjective sleep disturbance in patients with partial epilepsy: a questionnaire-based study on prevalence and impact on quality of life. *Epilepsia*, 2004; **45**:1397–404.

87. **Khatami R**, **Zutter D**, **Siegel A**, *et al.* Sleep–wake habits and disorders in a series of 100 adult epilepsy patients – a prospective study. *Seizure*, 2006; **15**:299–306.

88. **Manni R**, **Politini L**, **Sartori I**, *et al.* Daytime sleepiness in epilepsy patients: evaluation by means of the Epworth sleepiness scale. *J Neurol*, 2000; **247**:716–17.

89. **Zucconi M**, **Oldani A**, **Smirne S**, *et al.* The macrostructure and microstructure of sleep in patients with autosomal dominant nocturnal frontal lobe epilepsy. *J Clin Neurophysiol*, 2000; **17**:77–86.

90. **Bazil C W**, **Walczak T S**. Effects of sleep and sleep stage on epileptic and nonepileptic seizures. *Epilepsia*, 1997; **38**:56–62.

91. **Vignatelli L**, **Bisulli F**, **Naldi I**, *et al.* Excessive daytime sleepiness and subjective sleep quality in patients with nocturnal frontal lobe epilepsy: a case-control study. *Epilepsia*, 2006; **47**(Suppl 5):73–77.

92. **Sanchez de Leon I F N**, **Marsilio D**, **Dinner D S**. Effect of seizure frequency and antiepileptic drugs on daytime alertness as measured by the Epworth Sleepiness Scale in patients with epilepsy. *Epilepsia* [abstract], 1997; **38**:56.

93. **Maganti R**, **Hausman N**, **Koehn M**, *et al.* Excessive daytime sleepiness and sleep complaints among children with epilepsy. *Epilepsy Behav*, 2006; **8**:272–77.

94. **Chihorek A M**, **Abou-Khalil B**, **Malow B A**. Obstructive sleep apnea is associated with seizure occurrence in older adults with epilepsy. *Neurology*, 2007; **69**:1823–27.

95. **Jenssen S**, **Gracely E**, **Mahmood T**, *et al.* Subjective somnolence relates mainly to depression among patients in a tertiary care epilepsy center. *Epilepsy Behav*, 2006; **9**:632–35.

96. **Byars A W**, **Byars K C**, **Johnson C S**, *et al.* The relationship between sleep problems and neuropsychological functioning in children with first recognized seizures. *Epilepsy Behav*, 2008; **13**:607–13.

97. **Ebben M R**, **Sethi N K**, **Conte M**, *et al.* Vagus nerve stimulation, sleep apnea, and CPAP titration. *J Clin Sleep Med*, 2008; **4**:471–73.

98. **Gschliesser V**, **Hogl B**, **Frauscher B**, *et al.* Mode of vagus nerve stimulation differentially affects sleep related breathing in patients with epilepsy. *Seizure*, 2009; **18**:339–42.

99. **Malow B A**, **Edwards J**, **Marzec M**, *et al.* Vagus nerve stimulation reduces daytime sleepiness in epilepsy patients. *Neurology*, 2001; **57**:879–84.

100. **Macleod S**, **Ferrie C**, **Zuberi S M**. Symptoms of narcolepsy in children misinterpreted as epilepsy. *Epileptic Disord*, 2005; **7**:13–17.

101. **Dauvilliers Y**, **Stal V**, **Abril B**, *et al.* Chiari malformation and sleep related breathing disorders. *J Neurol Neurosurg Psychiatry*, 2007; **78**:1344–48.

102. **Nogues M**, **Cammarota A**, **Leiguarda R**, *et al.* Periodic limb movements in syringomyelia and syringobulbia. *Mov Disord*, 2000; **15**:113–19.

Section 3 Medical, Psychiatric and Neurological Causes of Sleepiness

Chapter 32

Hypothyroidism and other endocrine causes of sleepiness

Hideto Shinno

Introduction

The relationship of the endocrine system to sleep has been documented by many studies. Insomnia has been associated with hyperthyroidism, Cushing's syndrome, menopause and other female hormonal conditions. Excessive sleepiness has been associated with hypothyroidism, acromegaly, poorly controlled type 2 diabetes, androgen excess, Cushing's syndrome, female hormonal changes and obesity, in part due to the co-occurrence of obstructive sleep apnea syndrome.

Sleep is known to have important modulatory effects on various components of the endocrine system. Marked increases in the secretion of growth hormone (GH) and prolactin (PRL) are observed during sleep, while the release of cortisol and thyrotropin (TSH) is inhibited [1]. Awakenings that interrupt sleep cause the inhibition of nocturnal GH and PRL secretions, and increases in cortisol and TSH. Sleep exerts modulatory effects on hormones of the hypothalamic–pituitary axis. Furthermore, these effects are associated with hormones controlling carbohydrate metabolism, appetite, and electrolyte balance. Sleep disturbance is considered to affect these hormone secretions and metabolism, which may have clinical relevance [1]. In this chapter, I will describe the influence of alterations in various endocrinological systems on sleep architecture, especially alterations that are associated with prolonged nocturnal sleep and/or daytime somnolence.

Physiology of the thyroid axis during sleep and while awake

Previous studies on the diurnal TSH rhythm demonstrated that daytime levels of plasma TSH are low, and then begin to elevate rapidly in the early evening. In the later part of the sleep period, TSH levels decline progressively, and then daytime values resume shortly after morning awakening [2]. Sleep during daytime hours does not induce a significant suppression of TSH secretion below normal daytime levels. When prior sleep deprivation causes an increase in the depth of sleep, the nocturnal TSH rise is more markedly inhibited. Slow-wave sleep (SWS) may be the primary determinant of the sleep-associated fall of TSH levels [2]. Consistent associations between descending slopes of TSH concentrations and slow-wave stages have been demonstrated, and TSH fluctuations are negatively cross-correlated to relative spectral power in the delta range [3]. Awakenings that interrupt nocturnal sleep are considered to relieve the inhibition of TSH, and to be consistently associated with short-term TSH elevation.

Thyroid hormones are bound to serum proteins and their peripheral concentrations are affected by diurnal variations in hemodilution. In contrast to those of TSH, the circadian and sleep-related variations of thyroid hormone are difficult to demonstrate. The increased amplitude of the TSH rhythm may result in a detectable increase in plasma triiodothyronine (T3) under particular conditions such as sleep deprivation [4]. Prolonged sleep loss has been suggested to be associated with an upregulation of the thyroid axis.

CSF homovanillic acid, a major metabolite of dopamine, has shown a negative correlation with plasma TSH and T3 in healthy humans [5], indicating the physiological significance of the interaction between dopamine and thyroid hormone in the central nervous system of the normal, euthyroid human. As clinical and experimental data have suggested, thyroid hormone influences central neurochemical systems, and may also affect wake-promoting systems. The

---

Sleepiness: Causes, Consequences and Treatment, ed. Michael J. Thorpy and Michel Billiard. Published by Cambridge University Press. © Cambridge University Press 2011.

pathogenesis of idiopathic hypersomnia is unknown, but the involvement of alterations in the hypothalamo-pituitary–thyroid (HPT) axis remains to be elucidated, although neuroendocrinological investigations have been performed in narcolepsy [6].

Hypothyroidism

History

Apneic breathing in myxedema has been documented since the 1960s. As described below, several mechanisms explain the association between sleep apnea and hypothyroidism.

Pathology

Hypothyroidism and sleep-disordered breathing

Myxedema is associated with sleep apnea, and several mechanisms have been proposed to explain the association with hypothyroidism. Patients with hypothyroidism commonly present with disordered breathing. However, hypothyroidism is uncommon in patients with obstructive sleep apnea syndrome (OSAS) [7]. The development of hypothyroidism appears to be related to OSAS, although the precise mechanism is not quite clear. The pathophysiology seems to involve myxedematous infiltration of tissues, and impaired function and reduced central drive of the upper airway muscles [7].

Alterations in neuronal signaling and hypothyroidism

The histaminergic tuberomammillary nucleus of the hypothalamus [8] and the noradrenergic locus coeruleus of the pons [9] are major wakefulness-promoting nuclei, and also play a role in autonomic regulation. However, thyroid hormones have been reported to serve as co-transmitters with some neurotransmitters such as histamine and noradrenaline [10]. Levothyroxine administration raises the histamine level of the hypothalamus and cerebral cortex [11]. Previous reports have suggested that T3 is localized in brain nuclei receiving strong noradrenergic innervation [12], and concentrated in both noradrenergic centers and noradrenergic projection sites [10]. It is possible that the altered thyroid function or the serum TSH level may affect the arousal-promoting system.

Clinical findings

Sleep apnea in hypothyroidism

Obstructive sleep apnea (OSA) often causes difficulty in maintaining sleep continuity. Patients usually complain of excessive daytime sleepiness, fatigue, snoring, decreased libido, and impaired concentration. Several studies have demonstrated that OSA is more prevalent among patients with hypothyroidism than among control subjects [13–16], and other studies have focused on how strongly hypothyroidism correlates with OSA. Lin et al. also compared hypothyroidism in patients with OSA, with hypothyroid patients without OSA, and suggested that age and body weight were related to the development of OSA [13]. Table 32.1 shows the results obtained by previous studies that investigated OSA in patients with hypothyroidism.

Sleep architecture in hypothyroidism

It is well known that patients with hypothyroidism usually exhibit daytime sleepiness. As described previously, sleep apnea and its related arousal at night may reduce the quality of nocturnal sleep and promote daytime somnolence. While sleep apnea may cause sleepiness, a primary central effect of hypothyroidism on sleep is also possible in some patients. There are few studies that have investigated sleep architecture in patients with hypothyroidism, but some articles have reported alterations in polysomnographic variables. Ruíz-Primo et al. examined nine myxedematous patients with overnight polysomnography [17]. In that study, polysomnography was carried out under three conditions: (1) baseline or myxedematous state; (2) with acute replacement hormone therapy; and (3) with chronic replacement therapy. Either a complete absence or very low level of slow-wave sleep (SWS) was found in the myxedematous state. After replacement hormone therapy, a restoration of the normal sleep pattern was demonstrated in three of the four patients that were followed. The latency for REM sleep was reported to increase during acute replacement therapy, and to become normal when euthyroidism was achieved. These findings may support the proposal that thyroid hormones exert central effects on the adult central nerve system.

Latent hypothyroidism

Latent hypothyroidism is a subclinical state, and is characterized by normal thyroid hormones (normal free T3 and free thyroxine (T4) levels) and

3. Medical, Psychiatric and Neurological Causes

Table 32.1 Summary of studies investigating the prevalence of sleep apnea in hypothyroidism (including latent hypothyroidism)

Authors	Year	Subjects	Results
Hypothyroidism			
Lin et al. [13]	1992	20 hypothyroid patients	all patients: snoring, 2 patients: moderate to severe OSA, 3 patients: mild OSA
Pelttari et al. [14]	1994	26 hypothyroid patients vs. 188 euthyroid controls	(1) some episodes of partial or complete upper airway obstruction were observed in 50% of hypothyroid patients and 29.3% of control subjects (2) severe OSAs were observed in 7.7% of hypothyroid patients and 1.5% of control subjects
Jha et al. [15]	2006	50 hypothyroid patients	30% of patients have sleep-disorder breathing. In 10 of 12 patients, sleep-disordered breathing recovered after levothyroxine replacement.
Misiolek et al. [16]	2007	15 hypothyroid patients	After the thyroid hormone stabilization, snoring severity was significantly decreased. ESS score showed significant improvement, while the desaturation index was at the same level.
Latent hypothyroidism			
Resta et al. [20]	2005	(Group A) subjects with normal TSH and thyroid function (Group B) subclinical hypothyroidism treated with levothyroxine (Group C) subclinical hypothyroidism never treated with levothyroxine	The percentage of OSA, BMI, RDI and AHI were not different among the 3 groups. When compared between Group B and C, the prevalence and severity of OSA were not different. ESS score was significantly increased in Group C.

AHI, apnea–hypopnea index; BMI, body mass index; ESS, Epworth Sleepiness Scale; OSA, obstructive sleep apnea; RDI, respiratory disturbance index.

increased TSH. Patients with latent hypothyroidism do not yet exhibit significant physical findings such as myxedema, tachycardia, or bradycardia that may be induced by altered thyroid function. The characteristics of sleep in latent hypothyroidism have not been documented, probably due to a subclinical and quiescent state. There is a report describing two cases of excessive daytime somnolence in latent hypothyroidism [18]. Both subjects had complained of excessive daytime sleepiness and prolonged nocturnal sleep. They had not felt refreshed after naps, and it was difficult for them to wake up in the morning. Excessive daytime sleepiness and prolonged nocturnal sleep started when they were 16–18 years of age, and continued for more than a year. Their respective polysomnography findings demonstrated short sleep latency, prolonged sleep time, a normal apnea/hypopnea index, and normal REM sleep latency. Both patients were considered to meet the ICSD-2 diagnostic criteria for idiopathic hypersomnia with long sleep time [19]. Their laboratory examinations demonstrated normal levels of free T3 and free T4, and elevated TSH (6–8 micro-unit/ml). There were no physical symptoms associated with altered thyroid function or obesity. The prolonged nocturnal sleep and excessive daytime sleepiness were successfully treated with levothyroxine.

There have not been sufficient data on the association between latent hypothyroidism and sleep-disordered breathing. Resta et al. investigated and compared the prevalence of sleep apnea, body mass index, and respiratory disturbance index among three groups [20]. Subjects with normal TSH and thyroid function comprised the first group. The second group included patients with subclinical hypothyroidism treated with levothyroxine. The third group consisted of patients with subclinical hypothyroidism never treated with levothyroxine. The percentage of OSA, neck circumference, and body mass index did not significantly differ amongst the three groups. The respiratory disturbance index as well as the percentage of the total number of apnea–hypopneas by total sleep time did not differ amongst the groups. The only significant difference between patients with and without treatment was the mean scores on the Epworth Sleepiness Scale (Table 32.1). In patients with latent hypothyroidism, levothyroxine treatment did not influence the prevalence or severity of OSA, while daytime sleepiness was worse in untreated latent hypothyroidism.

Congenital hypothyroidism

As reviewed by Hughes [21], spindles develop in humans at 6 weeks gestational age. Spindles initially demonstrate a low amplitude, with a gradual increase in amplitude, and especially in duration, achieving the maximum at 13 weeks. The duration then rapidly decreases with age to 23 weeks and thereafter slowly decreases to the end of the first year. The pause between spindles is usually inversely related to the spindle duration and stabilizes after 23 weeks. The complex of spindle and pause is longest at 10 weeks, then decreases with age and stabilizes at 17 weeks. Synchronous spindles develop from a low value of 10% to around 30% value by the end of the year, while asynchronous spindles maintain the same value for most of the year. The reticular nucleus of the thalamus has been suggested as the generator of spindles.

Thyroid hormone is known to play a major role in the process of brain development. Deficiencies in the interactions between the brain and thyroid hormones in humans may cause irreversible damage to the brain [22]. Recently, a study investigated the influence of congenital hypothyroidism on the features of polysomnographic sleep recordings in 40 children [23]. First, the study examined the percentage of children with respiratory alterations detected at different ages, and demonstrated that a high proportion of infants (43%) displayed central apnea as well as hypopnea (83%). The proportion of infants displaying central apnea decreased as the age increased. Comparison of sleep architecture between patients with congenital hypothyroidism and controls demonstrated a significant increase in non-REM sleep stage I and II and a decrease in SWS, regardless of age and treatment. There were no significant differences in the percentage of REM sleep or REM sleep latency. However, the percentage of REM sleep was shown to be positively correlated with the age of the child at the beginning of treatment, and negatively correlated with their age at the time of the study. Correlation analysis also showed a strong negative correlation between respiratory alterations and gestational age, age at the time of the study, and the duration of hormonal treatment [23].

Natural history

Myxedema often causes OSA in patients with hypothyroidism. Some reports have suggested improvement of sleep apnea in hypothyroid patients when the patients became euthyroid [15, 16], while other reports have suggested that there was no significant reduction in the apnea index, irrespective of the body mass index [24].

In congenital hypothyroidism, deficiency in interaction between the brain and thyroid hormones results in irreversible damage to the brain, presenting clinically as cretinism. Congenital hypothyroidism is readily detected in newborn babies by mass screening procedures, and hormonal replacement readily prevents many of the consequences. However, the effects of hormone replacement on brain development have not been sufficiently understood.

Management

Hypothyroidism and sleep apnea

To treat hypothyroidism, thyroid hormone replacement, such as with levothyroxine administration, is generally prescribed in clinical practice, but clinicians would like to know whether successful thyroid hormone replacement improves the OSA. Despite several studies, the results obtained in studies investigating the effects of thyroid hormone replacement on sleep apnea in patients with hypothyroidism have been inconsistent.

Some reports have suggested that sleep apnea in hypothyroid patients improved when the patients became euthyroid [15, 16], while other reports suggested that there was no significant reduction in the apnea index irrespective of body mass index [24].

Myxedema often causes OSA in patients with hypothyroidism. Studies reporting improvement of OSA after thyroid hormone replacement have concluded that myxedema may be a reversible cause of OSA. However, there are several studies reporting the failure to resolve OSA after thyroxine treatment. Hypothyroidism may induce long-term changes in upper airway mechanics [24] or breathing control, which do not resolve immediately after a euthyroid state is achieved.

Congenital hypothyroidism

Congenital hypothyroidism is known to cause irreversible damage to the brain. Optimal management of congenital hypothyroidism, therefore, requires early diagnosis by mass screening procedures in newborn babies, and prompt treatment to avoid an abnormal neuro-developmental outcome. As described previously, central sleep apnea is common in children with congenital hypothyroidism [23]. A significant correlation has been reported between respiratory alterations and the duration of hormone replacement [23]. The question whether high-dose thyroid hormone replacement is more beneficial than low-dose of initial thyroid hormone replacement for intellectual development and sleep-disordered breathing, however, remains to be elucidated.

Hypothalamo-pituitary–thyroid axis and alertness

Thyrotropin releasing hormone (TRH) is now known to be distributed widely in the CNS, and its receptors are reported to exist in structures such as the pituitary, cortex, brainstem, thalamus, hippocampus, amygdala, and spinal cord [25]. Besides its role in stimulating the release of thyroid-stimulating hormone (TSH) and prolactin, TRH has been shown to exhibit various neuromodulating effects that are separate from its hormonal effects [26]. These actions include CNS stimulant and antidepressant effects as well as neurotrophic effects. The clinical application of exogenous TRH, however, appears to be greatly limited because of a short biological half-life and limited access to the CNS. Therefore, biologically stable TRH analogues have been developed for possible clinical application.

Several reports have demonstrated the association between TRH and alertness in narcolepsy, while the association remains unclear in other disorders such as idiopathic hypersomnia and sleep apnea syndrome. Reports of the effect of TRH analogues in dogs with narcolepsy, such as acute and chronic oral administration of CG-3703, a TRH analogue, have demonstrated significantly reduced daytime sleep as well as cataplexy [6]. TRH and TRH analogues are also known to enhance dopaminergic transmission in the nucleus accumbens, which is important for locomotor activation and arousals [27]. It is possible that the effect of TRH on sleep and wakefulness may be mediated by enhancement of dopamine turnover, which is a common mechanism for most CNS stimulants [28].

TRH analogues could be beneficial for excessive daytime sleepiness, but evidence has not yet been accumulated in other types of hypersomnia. Further investigations are necessary in idiopathic hypersomnia, and symptomatic hypersomnia caused by endocrinological disorders such as hypothyroidism.

Acromegaly

History

In 1886, Roxburgh and Collis described daytime somnolence, and Chappell and Booth reported upper airway obstruction. The association between sleep apnea and acromegaly was, however, insufficiently understood in the nineteenth century, and sleep-disordered breathing in acromegaly has only been investigated since the 1970s.

Pathology

Sleep apnea in acromegaly is believed to be secondary to macroglossia causing narrowing of the hypopharynx. Although there are several endoscopic and cephalometric studies, the precise cause is unknown. However, studies have shown that some patients with acromegaly have a high rate of central apnea [29]. Grunstein *et al.* suggested that the central sleep apnea may be associated with increased ventilatory response to carbon dioxide, and that growth hormone (GH) hypersecretion may be related to the high prevalence of central apnea [30].

Clinical findings

Acromegaly is a disorder of dysregulated GH excess in adults, and is usually secondary to a GH-secreting pituitary adenoma. Patients with acromegaly exhibit the insidious development of coarsening of facial features, bony proliferation, soft tissue swelling [31]. Several studies have demonstrated the association between acromegaly and sleep apnea, whereas there have been no reports of the influence of increased GH secretion on the sleep architecture. The sleep apnea associated with increased GH usually induces poor sleep continuity and excessive daytime somnolence.

Sleep-disordered breathing is common in acromegaly. Studies on the prevalence and severity of sleep apnea in acromegaly have shown that at least 60% of patients have sleep apnea [29], and that heavy snoring occurs in most patients. Obesity has less influence on the prevalence of sleep apnea, while sleep-related breathing disorders become more prevalent with increasing age in keeping with typical sleep apnea [29]. Increases in body mass index in acromegaly may be due to increases in muscle weight but not due to body fat [31].

Management

High levels of insulin-like growth factor-1 (IGF-1) and high levels of GH reflect increased GH secretion, which reflect disease activity. Surgical treatment is usually required to resect a pituitary adenoma, and cure of the disease is associated with a physiologic 24-h GH secretion pattern, normal IGF-1 levels, and normal GH responses to glucose.

Sleep apnea in acromegaly may persist after surgical treatment of a pituitary adenoma. Reports have shown that there was no correlation between disease activity and sleep apnea, and that there were no significant differences in mean GH and IGF-1 levels in acromegaly patients with and without sleep apnea [29]. A study of a somatostatin analogue, octreotide, revealed a marked reduction in GH levels with a decrease in apnea severity [29]. The study, however, also reported that the decrease in apnea was not related to that in GH levels.

The reason sleep apnea occurs in patients cured of acromegaly is not sufficiently understood. It remains necessary to investigate: (i) how long the effects of acromegaly persist after the GH secretion is corrected, and (ii) whether there are permanent effects on upper airway function, or sleep breathing regulation.

Alteration in testosterone

History and pathology

Since the 1980s, there have been many reports describing the effects of testosterone on the development of sleep apnea [31]. Several studies examined the effects of exogenous testosterone on sleep-disordered breathing, and exogenous testosterone has been reported to increase sleep apnea in hypogonadal patients [32]. These reports suggest that alteration in the testosterone level may affect the regulation of breathing during sleep and the pathogenesis of sleep apnea, which may subsequently induce daytime sleepiness.

On the other hand, reduced levels of testosterone are reported in men with sleep apnea [33]. Androgen abnormalities in sleep apnea have distinct features from those reported in obesity. Decreases in sex hormone-binding globulin (SHBG) and free and total testosterone have been reported in men with sleep apnea, whereas men with obesity demonstrated decreased SHBG and total testosterone, but normal free testosterone. In sleep apnea, there were no significant increases in basal plasma luteinizing hormone and follicle-stimulating hormone levels, although plasma free and total testosterone levels were reduced. These findings suggest a hypothalamic abnormality.

Clinical findings

Due to increased sleep apnea and alteration in sleep architecture, patients with testosterone excess complain of sleep discontinuation and daytime sleepiness.

Sleep-disordered breathing in the hypogonadal state

As reported previously, administration of testosterone causes the development of sleep apnea. Furthermore, a placebo-controlled, double-blind trial of testosterone in healthy elderly men demonstrated that testosterone reduced total sleep time, increased the duration of hypoxemia, and disrupted breathing during sleep [34]. In this study using short-term, high-dose testosterone [34], the alterations did not appear to be due to upper airway narrowing, because changes in upper airway dimension were not significant despite the expected effects on body composition.

The influence of the hypogonadal state on sleep architecture

Some studies have investigated the influence of testosterone on sleep architecture. Leibenluft et al. examined the role of testosterone in the regulation of sleep and melatonin, prolactin, and TSH in men with pharmacologically induced hypogonadism, with and without gonadal steroid replacement [35]. Patients revealed significant decreases in 24-h prolactin levels and in the percentage and time of stage 4 non-REM sleep in the hypogonadal state compared with testosterone replacement. On the other hand, there were no differences in melatonin or TSH secretion or in the timing or duration of sleep between the two hormonal conditions. It appears that testosterone may have relatively specific and discrete effects on sleep and hormonal rhythms in men [35]. In patients with gonadotropin-releasing hormone deficiency, melatonin secretion was reported to be increased [36]. Taking these findings into consideration, the hypogonadal state may be associated with excessive daytime sleepiness.

Testosterone levels in sleep apnea

Although several studies have demonstrated decreased libido and low testosterone levels in men with sleep apnea, it may be argued whether the reduction of testosterone in sleep apnea is caused by sleep disturbance, (nocturnal or daytime) hypoxemia, or obesity. Grunstein et al. reported the reduced hormone level induced by sleep apnea was independent of age, degree of obesity, and the presence of awake hypoxemia and hypercapnia [33]. Testosterone levels are significantly reduced by sleep deprivation and fragmentation.

Management

After treatment of sleep apnea with nasal CPAP or uvulopalatopharyngoplasty, testosterone levels increase [33]. The alteration in testosterone observed in patients with sleep apnea appears not to be associated with age or obesity. Another study reported that mean and area under the curve (AUC) values of testosterone and LH increased during CPAP [37]. Sleep apnea in men is considered to be associated with dysfunction of the pituitary–gonadal axis. The central suppression of nocturnal testosterone in patients with sleep apnea is partially corrected during chronic CPAP treatment.

As several data have indicated, alteration in androgen levels is associated with sleep-disordered breathing. When androgen replacement is carried out, clinicians should closely assess for the development of sleep apnea symptomatology, and monitor the patient's therapy for the development of sleep-disordered breathing and daytime somnolence.

Menopause and altered female hormone status

Pathology

Many studies on the 24-h physiological variations in female hormones have demonstrated that plasma luteinizing hormone (LH) is markedly modulated by the menstrual cycle. In the early follicular phase, LH pulses are large and infrequent, and a marked slowing of the frequency of secretory pulses occurs during sleep. In the mid-follicular phase, pulse amplitude is decreased, pulse frequency is increased, and the frequency modulation of LH pulsatility by sleep is less apparent. Pulse amplitude increases again by the late follicular phase. In the early luteal phase, the pulse amplitude is markedly increased, pulse frequency is decreased, and nocturnal slowing of pulsatility is again evident. In the mid and late luteal phase, pulse amplitude and frequency are decreased and there is no modulation by sleep [1].

In post-menopausal women, on the other hand, gonadotropin levels are elevated, but these levels do not show any consistent circadian pattern. Studies have shown that sleep-disordered breathing is more prevalent in post-menopausal women [38], and hormone replacement therapy has been associated with a lower risk of sleep apnea [39]. The influence of the alteration in estrogen levels on sleep has not been sufficiently investigated. Estrogen deficiency after menopause may cause central obesity [40], which is likely to be the main factor for the increased prevalence of sleep apnea in the post-menopausal period. While progesterone levels fall after menopause, there have been no data on the therapeutic effect of progesterone in sleep apnea.

Clinical findings

While the effects of the menstrual cycle and the administration of oral contraceptives on sleep architecture have not been adequately studied, the prevalence of obstructive sleep apnea in women shows a significant increase with menopause [38], and may lead to daytime sleepiness. Body composition seems to be associated in complex ways with midlife aging, with menopause, and with sleep apnea, making it difficult to control for confounding factors due to increased weight and fat deposition. A study evaluated the differences in sleep between women of early (less than 5 years after menopause) and late (more than 5 years after menopause) post-menopause [41]. Polysomnography variables, subjective sleepiness (measured by the Epworth Sleepiness Scale), and other subjective complaints (body pain, bruxism, anxiety, depression, and lack of concentration) were compared between patients in the early and late stages of menopause. Subjective complaints were more frequent in the late postmenopause group, although polysomnographic findings did not detect significant differences.

Management

A high prevalence of sleep-disordered breathing poses a public health burden, because it might lead to cerebrovascular and cardiovascular complications such as stroke, heart failure, myocardial infarction, arrhythmias, and hypertension. Sleep apnea results in excessive daytime somnolence and disturbed activities of daily living (ADL). The question of whether hormone replacement therapy reduces cardiovascular risk in menopausal women has long been investigated, but the results are inconclusive. With regard to the effect of hormone replacement on obstructive sleep apnea, there have been several polysomnographic studies. The prevalence of obstructive sleep apnea (apnea/hypopnea index over 15) among hormone-treated patients was demonstrated to be approximately half the prevalence among non-treated patients [39].

Hyperprolactinemia

Pathology

Sleep apnea is also associated with reduced prolactin secretory pulse frequency [42]. Although there has not been a sufficient volume of studies investigating the association between sleep and alteration in prolactin secretion, some experimental studies demonstrated interesting findings. In rats rendered hyperprolactinemic with anterior pituitary grafts, short- and long-term administrations of prolactin markedly increased REM sleep, while the pituitary grafts affected neither growth hormone plasma concentration nor pituitary mRNA levels [43]. Both the duration and the frequency of the REM sleep episodes increased and persisted during weeks 4–7 post-implantation, which indicated that the enhancements in REM sleep persist during hyperprolactinemia.

Clinical findings in prolactinoma

A report demonstrated that patients with prolactinoma have enhanced SWS compared with control subjects [44]. This may result in the excessive daytime somnolence in humans. The patients in that report exhibited secondary hypogonadism, but there were no other endocrine abnormalities. There were no differences in REM sleep variables between patients with prolactinoma and control subjects. As indicated in the previous section on pathology, rats with experimentally elevated levels of prolactin demonstrated enhanced REM sleep. However, the chronic excessive elevation of prolactin levels appear to exert different influences on sleep architecture in humans compared with those in rats. These findings may account for the good sleep quality in patients with prolactinoma.

Corticosteroid and sleep

Cushing's syndrome refers to the clinical manifestations induced by chronic exposure to excess glucocorticoids. Three pathological conditions are known to result in the chronic oversecretion of endogenous cortisol. The most frequent is Cushing's disease, where adrenocorticotropic hormone (ACTH) is overproduced by a pituitary corticotroph adenoma. Rarely, ACTH can be overproduced by a non-pituitary tumor. Finally, cortisol can be directly oversecreted in an adrenal cortex due to either a benign or a malignant tumor. Patients with Cushing's syndrome are characterized by truncal obesity, hypertension, and depression.

There is little information on the alteration of sleep in patients exhibiting disordered corticosteroid secretion. Shipley et al. reported that 32% of patients with Cushing's syndrome had at least mild sleep apnea, and 18% had moderate to severe sleep apnea [45]. These patients demonstrated a tendency toward greater complaints of excessive daytime sleepiness compared to control subjects. When polysomnography variables were compared between non-apneic patients and control subjects, there were striking differences in sleep structure. Patients revealed lighter and more fragmented sleep, significantly shorter REM latency and increased REM density, which were similar to those in patients with major depression. There are similarities in the pathophysiology of altered sleep structure between Cushing's syndrome and depression, and a number of studies have suggested that major depression, as well as Cushing's syndrome, is involved with a dysfunction of the HPA axis. These findings may account for poor sleep continuity and excessive daytime sleepiness.

Diabetes

Clinical findings

There have not been any specific alterations in sleep architecture reported in patients with diabetes. A report on sleep disturbances in young patients with insulin-dependent diabetes mellitus demonstrated that sleep architecture was not disturbed by nocturnal hypoglycemia and there were no changes in sleep stages, fragmentation, or arousals [46].

Sleep apnea is common in diabetes, which often causes daytime sleepiness and tiredness. Central obesity is a more crucial determinant of morbidity and mortality than total adiposity. Obesity is, indeed, common in both diabetes and sleep apnea, but OSA has been demonstrated to be associated with the increased insulin resistance independent of obesity [47].

Alternatively, there are fewer studies investigating whether sleep apnea promotes or contributes to the development of obesity. It remains controversial whether OSA plays an independent role in the development of glucose intolerance or diabetes mellitus. The prevalence of diabetes mellitus in obstructive sleep apnea was demonstrated to be higher than that in control subjects (25.9% vs. 8.2%) [48]. The study also demonstrated that 62% of patients received a diagnosis of impaired glucose tolerance or diabetes mellitus, and that insulin resistance was associated with body mass index but not with apnea/hypopnea index [48].

There have been several studies that have reported altered serotonergic sensitivity in the hypothalamus. Because of the effect of the serotonin precursor, L-5-hydroxytryptophan, or reuptake inhibitors on OSA, OSA may involve an altered serotonergic system. Hudgel *et al.* examined the cortisol response to the ingestion of L-5-hydroxytryptophan that is decarboxylated in the brain, and reported that patients with obstructive sleep apnea showed significantly higher cortisol production after L-5-hydroxytryptophan administration compared with control non-apneic subjects, which was not readily explained by changes in body weight [49]. These findings suggested the cortisol response to L-5-hydroxytryptophan was elevated in apneic patients most likely as a result of increased hypophyseal serotonin activity. A serotonergic-deficient state was indicated to cause the supersensitivity of post-synaptic serotonergic receptors in the hypothalamus. Short periods of sleep deprivation may produce evidence of increased serotonin turnover. The speculation that chronic sleep fragmentation and hypoxemia due to sleep apnea produce serotonin depletion in the hypothalamus and other regions, however, remains to be elucidated.

Management

Obstructive sleep apnea is associated with increased insulin resistance independent of body mass index [47]. It may be argued whether treatment of sleep apnea can increase insulin sensitivity and improve glycemic control. Although there have not been consistent data on the effect of treating sleep apnea on insulin sensitivity in diabetic and non-diabetic subjects, some studies demonstrated the effects. Babu *et al.* examined changes in interstitial glucose levels and measured hemoglobin (Hb)A1C levels in patients with type 2 diabetes mellitus before and after continuous positive airway pressure (CPAP) treatment for sleep-disordered breathing using a 72-h continuous glucose monitoring system [50]. The mean 1-h postprandial glucose values were significantly reduced for every meal with about 12-weeks' CPAP treatment. Only in patients who were treated for more than 4 h/day, the reduction in HbA1C level was significantly correlated with days of CPAP treatment. It may be possible that sleep-disordered breathing is pathophysiologically related to impaired glucose homeostasis. CPAP may be an important therapeutic approach for diabetic patients with sleep-disordered breathing, although further investigations are mandatory.

Conclusions

In any patient with an endocrine disorder, alterations in sleep architecture and/or increased sleep apnea are usually present, which can cause daytime somnolence. It is also important to consider the potential development of sleep apnea and daytime sleepiness in patients who are receiving certain hormonal replacements.

Further investigations into the possible roles of hormones in regulating sleep, alertness and circadian rhythms in humans are necessary.

References

1. **Van Cauter E**. Endocrine physiology. In: Kryger M, Roth T, Dement W, Eds. *Principles and Practice of Sleep Medicine*. 4th Ed. Philadelphia, PA: Elsevier Saunders, 2005: 266–82.

2. **Brabant G**, **Prank K**, **Rant U**, *et al.* Physiological regulation of circadian and pulsatile thyrotropin secretion in normal man and woman. *J Clin Endocrinol Metab*, 1990; **70**:403–09.

3. **Goichot B**, **Brandenberger G**, **Saini J**, *et al.* Nocturnal plasma thyrotropin variations are related to slow-wave sleep. *J Sleep Res*, 1992; **1**:186–90.

4. **Allan J S**, **Czeisler C A**. Persistence of the circadian thyrotropin rhythm under constant conditions and after light-induced shifts of circadian phase. *J Clin Encocrinol Metab*, 1994; **79**:508–12.

5. **Strawn J R**, **Ekhator N N**, **D'Souza B B**, *et al*. Pituitary–thyroid state correlates with central dopaminergic and serotonergic activity in healthy humans. *Neuropsychobiology*, 2004; **49**:84–87.

6. **Riehl J**, **Honda K**, **Kwan M**, *et al*. Chronic oral administration of CG-3703, a thyrotropin releasing hormone analog, increases wake and decreases cataplexy in canine narcolepsy. *Neuropsychopharmacology*, 2000; **23**:34–45.

7. **Grunstein R R**, **Sullivan C E**. Hypothyroidism and sleep apnea. Mechanisms and management. *Am J Med*, 1988; **85**:775–79.

8. **Steininger T L**, **Alam M N**, **Gong H**, *et al*. Sleep–waking discharge of neurons in the posterior lateral hypothalamus of the albino rat. *Brain Res*, 1999; **840**:138–47.

9. **Wu M F**, **Gulyani S A**, **Yau E**, *et al*. Locus coeruleus neurons: cessation of acting during cataplexy. *Neuroscience*, 1999; **91**:1389–99.

10. **Dratman M B**, **Gordon J T**. Thyroid hormones as neurotransmitters. *Thyroid*, 1996; **6**:639–47.

11. **Upadhyaya L**, **Agrawal J K**. Effect of l-thyroxine and carbimazole on brain biogenic amines and amino acids in rats. *Endocr Res*, 1993; **19**:87–99.

12. **Dratman M B**, **Futaesaku Y**, **Crutschfield F L**, *et al*. Iodine-125-labeled triiodothyronine in rat brain: evidence for localization in discrete neural systems. *Science*, 1982; **215**:309–12.

13. **Lin C C**, **Tsan K W**, **Chen P J**. The relationship between sleep apnea syndrome and hypothyroidism. *Chest*, 1992; **102**:1663–67.

14. **Pelttari L**, **Rauhala E**, **Polo O**, *et al*. Upper airway obstruction in hypothyroidism. *J Intern Med*, 1994; **236**:177–81.

15. **Jha A**, **Sharma S K**, **Tandon N**, *et al*. Thyroxine replacement therapy reverses sleep-disordered breathing in patients with primary hypothyroidism. *Sleep Med*, 2006; **7**:55–61.

16. **Misiolek M**, **Marek B**, **Namyslowski G**, *et al*. Sleep apnea syndrome and snoring in patients with hypothyroidism with relation to overweight. *J Physiol Pharmacol*, 2007; **58**(Suppl 1):77–85.

17. **Ruíz-Primo E**, **Jurado J L**, **Solís H**, *et al*. Polysomnographic effects of thyroid hormones in primary myxoedema. *Electroencephalogr Clin Neurophysiol*, 1982; **53**:559–64.

18. **Shinno H**, **Inami Y**, **Inagaki T**, *et al*. Successful treatment with levothyroxine for idiopathic hypersomnia patients with subclinical hypothyroidism. *Gen Hosp Psychiatry*, 2009; **31**:190–93.

19. **American Academy of Sleep Medicine**. *The International Classification of Sleep Disorders: Diagnostic and Coding Manual* (2nd Ed.). Westchester, IL: American Academy of Sleep Medicine, 2005.

20. **Resta O**, **Carratù P**, **Carpagnano G E**, *et al*. Influence of subclinical hypothyroidism and T4 treatment on the prevalence and severity of obstructive sleep apnoea syndrome (OSAS). *J Endocrinol Invest*, 2005; **28**:893–98.

21. **Hughes J R**. Development of sleep spindles in the first year of life. *Clin Electroencephalogr*, 1996; **27**:107–15.

22. **Buyukgebiz A**. Newborn screening for congenital hypothyroidism. *J Pediatr Endocrinol Metab*, 2006; **19**:1291–98.

23. **Terán-Pérez G**, **Arana-Lechuga Y**, **González-Robles R O**, *et al*. Polysomnographic features in infants with early diagnosis of congenital hypothyroidism. *Brain Dev*, 2010; **32**:332–37.

24. **Petrof B J**, **Kelly A M**, **Rubinstein N A**, *et al*. Effect of hypothyroidism on myosin heavy chain expression in rat pharyngeal dilator muscles. *J Appl Physiol*, 1992; **73**:179–87.

25. **Winokur A**, **Manaker S**, **Kreider M**. TRH and TRH receptors in the spinal cord. *Ann N Y Acad Sci*, 1989; **553**:314–24.

26. **Kolesnick R N**, **Gershengorn M C**. Thyrotropin-releasing hormone and the pituitary: new insights into the mechanisms of stimulated secretion and clinical usage. *Am J Med*, 1985; **79**:729–39.

27. **Momiyama T**, **Ishihara K**, **Kimura K**, *et al*. Long-term antiepileptic effects of chronic intake of CNK-602A, a thyrotropin-releasing hormone analogue on spontaneously-epileptic rats. *Epilepsia*, 1996; **37**:328–31.

28. **Wisor J P**, **Nishino S**, **Sora I**, *et al*. Dopaminergic role in stimulant-induced wakefulness. *J Neurosci*, 2001; **21**:1787–94.

29. **Grunstein R R**, **Ho K Y**, **Sullivan C E**. Acromegaly and sleep apnea. *Ann Intern Med*, 1991; **115**:527–32.

30. **Melmed D**. Acromegaly. *N Engl J Med*, 1990; **322**:966–77.

31. **Sandblom R E**, **Matsumoto A M**, **Schoene R B**, *et al*. Obstructive sleep apnea induced by testosterone administration. *N Engl J Med*, 1983; **308**:506–10.

32. **Schneider B K**, **Pickett C K**, **Zwillich C W**, *et al*. Influence of testosterone on breathing during sleep. *J Appl Physiol*, 1986; **61**:618–24.

33. **Grunstein R R**, **Handelsman D J**, **Lawrence S**, *et al.* Neuroendocrine dysfunction in sleep apnea: reversal by nasal continuous positive airway pressure. *J Clin Endocrinol Metab*, 1989; **68**:352–58.

34. **Liu P Y**, **Yee B**, **Wishart S M**, *et al.* The short-term effects of high-dose testosterone on sleep, breathing, and function in older men. *J Clin Endocrinol Metab*, 2003; **88**:3605–13.

35. **Leibenluft E**, **Schmidt P J**, **Turner E H**, *et al.* Effects of leuprolide-induced hypogonadism and testosterone replacement on sleep, melatonin, and prolactin secretion in man. *J Clin Endocrinol Metab*, 1997; **82**:3203–07.

36. **Luboshitzky R**, **Wagner O**, **Lavi S**, *et al.* Abnormal melatonin secretion in male patients with hypogonadism. *J Mol Neurosci*, 1996; **7**:91–98.

37. **Luboshitz R**, **Lavie L**, **Shen-Orr Z**, *et al.* Pituitary–gonadal function in men with obstructive sleep apnea. The effect of continuous positive airways pressure treatment. *Neuro Endocrinol Lett*, 2003; **24**:463–67.

38. **Young T**, **Finn L**, **Austin D**, *et al.* Menopausal status and sleep-disordered breathing in the Wisconsin Sleep Cohort Study. *Am J Respir Crit Care Med*, 2003; **167**:1181–85.

39. **Shahar E**, **Redline S**, **Young T**, *et al.* Hormone replacement therapy and sleep-disordered breathing. *Am J Respir Crit Care Med*, 2003; **167**:1186–92.

40. **Carr M C**. The emergence of the metabolic syndrome with menopause. *J Clin Endocrinol Metab*, 2003; **88**:2404–11.

41. **Hachul H**, **Bittencourt L R**, **Soares J M** Jr, *et al.* Sleep in post-menopausal women: differences between early and late post-menopause. *Eur J Obstet Gynecol Reprod Biol*, 2009; **145**:81–84.

42. **Spiegel K**, **Follenius M**, **Krieger J**, *et al.* Prolactin secretion during sleep in obstructive sleep apnoea patients. *J Sleep Res*, 1995; **4**:56–62.

43. **Obál F Jr**, **Kacsóh B**, **Bredow S**, *et al.* Sleep in rats rendered chronically hyperprolactinemic with anterior pituitary grafts. *Brain Res*, 1997; **25**:130–36.

44. **Frieboes R M**, **Murck H**, **Stalla G K**, *et al.* Enhanced slow wave sleep in patients with prolactinoma. *J Clin Endocrinol Metab*, 1998; **83**:2706–10.

45. **Shipley J E**, **Schteingart D E**, **Tandon R**, *et al.* Sleep architecture and sleep apnea in patients with Cushing's disease. *Sleep*, 1992; **15**:514–18.

46. **Porter P A**, **Byrne G**, **Stick S**, *et al.* Nocturnal hypoglycaemia and sleep disturbances in young teenagers with insulin dependent diabetes mellitus. *Arch Dis Child*, 1996; **75**:120–23.

47. **Punjabi N M**, **Ahmed M M**, **Polotsky V Y**, *et al.* Sleep-disordered breathing, glucose intolerance, and insulin resistance. *Respir Physiol Neurobiol*, 2003; **136**:167–78.

48. **Otake K**, **Sasanabe R**, **Hasegawa R**, *et al.* Glucose intolerance in Japanese patients with obstructive sleep apnea. *Inter Med*, 2009; **48**:1863–68.

49. **Hudgel D W**, **Gorden E A**, **Meltzer H Y**. Abnormal serotonergic stimulation of cortisol production in obstructive sleep apnea. *Am J Respir Crit Care Med*, 1995; **152**:186–92.

50. **Babu A R**, **Herdegen J**, **Fogelfeld L**, *et al.* Type 2 diabetes, glycemic control, and continuous positive airway pressure in obstructive sleep apnea. *Arch Intern Med*, 2005; **165**:447–52.

Section 3 Chapter 33

Medical, Psychiatric and Neurological Causes of Sleepiness

Toxic and metabolic causes of sleepiness

Fabio Cirignotta and Fabio Pizza

Introduction

According to the International Classification of Sleep Disorders (ICSD), excessive daytime sleepiness (EDS) due to toxic and metabolic factors is a hypersomnia that can be diagnosed when the subjective EDS complaint coexists with a "medical or neurological disorder", and can be evaluated with nocturnal polysomnography possibly coupled with a multiple sleep latency test (MSLT) to exclude other sleep disturbances. Nevertheless, the ICSD states that most of the features of this nosographic category are "not applicable or not known" and that this area is "understudied" [1].

We reviewed the current evidence available on EDS, looking for similarities and differences between different metabolic disturbances and for potential confounders such as daytime fatigue and sleep-disordered breathing (SDB).

Infections and inflammatory response

Clinical findings

It is empirically known since antiquity that during sickness (particularly, infectious) otherwise normal subjects experience increased sleep pressure and daytime sleepiness, along with body temperature elevation and symptoms of malaise in the context of the immune-mediated host defense [2]. EDS is therefore one of the prominent features of the so-called "sickness behavior", a physiological adaptive response to infection documented in all animal species, that seems to change an individual's priorities to promote recovery following infection [3].

Laboratory investigations and pathophysiological hypotheses

EDS during inflammation and infection has been closely linked to the central role of cytokines, the humoral links between the immune and central nervous systems signaling the brain in health and disease [4]. Experimental studies on humans and animals showed that endotoxin administration induces an increase of proinflammatory cytokines such as IL-1, IL-6, and TNF-α associated with increased sleepiness perception and altered sleep [3, 5]. Moreover, experimental data suggest that significant exogenous stimuli can evoke a combined immune (cytokines) and neuroendocrine (hypothalamic–pituitary–adrenal (HPA) axis) activation associated with fever disrupting sleep continuity [2, 4].

Obesity, insulin resistance, and metabolic syndrome

Clinical findings

After the discovery of obstructive sleep apnea (OSA) and its intrinsic link to obesity, little attention has been paid to the presence of EDS in obesity out of the context of SDB. Recently, obesity has again been associated with EDS even in the absence of sleep apnea, with the additional evidence that the increased sleep propensity during daytime is not merely the expression of altered nocturnal sleep, as obese patients that had higher sleep efficiency at night were the ones with prominent EDS. Moreover, nocturnal sleep of obese subjects showed a circadian shift of REM sleep towards early morning hours, suggesting a circadian rhythm abnormality [6].

Sleepiness: Causes, Consequences and Treatment, ed. Michael J. Thorpy and Michel Billiard. Published by Cambridge University Press. © Cambridge University Press 2011.

Accordingly, a large epidemiological study confirmed that in the general population EDS is more strongly associated with metabolic factors and depression than with SDB or sleep disruption. The most significant risk factors for EDS were body mass index, age, sleep duration, diabetes, smoking and, lastly, sleep apnea [7]. Therefore, EDS is a morbid characteristic of obesity and not, or not always, the consequence of sleep disturbances.

The independent association of EDS and diabetes in the general population points to the causal role of glucose metabolism in the pathogenesis of EDS [7]. Similarly, 80% of 50 women with polycystic ovary syndrome (PCOS), a premenopausal endocrine disorder characterized by insulin resistance, complained of EDS, whereas SDB was diagnosed only in 17% of them, and 70% of non-obese PCOS women compared to 22.5% of non-obese controls showed EDS, reflecting an association between EDS and insulin resistance independent from SDB or obesity [8]. Accordingly, it has been proposed to subtype obesity into two phenotypes: the first associated with normothymia, high sleep efficiency and EDS; the second associated with depression, low sleep efficiency, and fatigue [9]. These evidences suggested a top-down interpretation of the relation between obesity, SDB, and EDS: sleep apnea itself could be regarded as a consequence of obesity, with inflammation, insulin resistance, visceral adiposity and central neural mechanisms playing a major role in the pathogenesis of SDB, EDS and cardiovascular comorbidities [10]. SDB and sleepiness may be manifestations of a severe dysmetabolism, the so-called metabolic syndrome. It includes EDS in obese patients without sleep apnea as well as EDS associated with insulin resistance and PCOS, and promotes a feed-forward pernicious cycle between obesity, EDS, SDB, inflammation and insulin resistance [11].

Laboratory investigations and pathophysiological hypotheses

The link between EDS and obesity has been explored by laboratory investigations on plasma factors. A study on morning plasma concentrations of IL-1, IL-6, and TNF-α in sleep disorders characterized by EDS such as narcolepsy, idiopathic hypersomnia, and sleep apnea, disclosed an association between TNF-α, IL-6 and EDS, with the additional evidence of a strong positive correlation between IL-6 and BMI [12]. Normal subjects have a biphasic circadian pattern of IL-6, that changes its profile, but not the overall secretion amount, during a sleep deprivation challenge with nighttime undersecretion and daytime oversecretion, the latter probably contributing to day-long somnolence and fatigue [13]. In the complex interplay between sleep apnea and obesity, the amount of visceral fat, rather than BMI per se, appeared as a predisposing factor associated with SDB. Moreover, both visceral fat and SDB contributed in a dose–response fashion to hypercytokinemia, hyperleptinemia and fasting hyperinsulinemia in patients with SDB compared to controls [14]. A study on women with PCOS, obese subjects, and normal controls disclosed higher levels of IL-6 in women with PCOS and intermediate levels in obese patients compared to non-obese controls. Additionally, in the obese group IL-6 was correlated with BMI, whereas in PCOS patients IL-6 levels were correlated with indices of insulin resistance such as fasting plasma glucose, but not with BMI, suggesting a pathophysiological link between glucose dysregulation and hypercytokinemia [15].

Renal insufficiency – end stage kidney disease

Clinical findings

Daytime sleepiness and sleep disturbances are common complaints in patients with chronic renal failure and end stage kidney disease (ESKD) undergoing dialysis treatment [16]. Epidemiological studies with questionnaire-based assessment of EDS showed prevalences in ESKD patients undergoing dialysis, that ranged from 12 to 77%, partially attributable to the different criteria applied [17–20]. Although most studies concordantly showed a high prevalence of EDS and of other disabling sleep disorders, such as poor sleep quality, insomnia, SDB, and restless legs syndrome, only a few support the hypothesis that SDB could explain the EDS in ESKD patients as compared to the general population [19]. Therefore, it seems that the metabolic condition of ESKD requiring dialysis treatment intrinsically leads to EDS. Many ESKD patients undergoing long-term hemodialysis (HD) also complain of daytime fatigue, a subjective sense of weakness, lack of energy and tiredness. Fatigue semantically overlaps with daytime sleepiness and depression, also sharing with EDS the difficulty of being adequately recognized with validated tools in this patient population [21]. To our knowledge, studies evaluating EDS and fatigue in light of coexistent sleep disturbances in ESKD are lacking.

Few studies have attempted to characterize the EDS of renal patients in light of circadian factors. Hsu and co-workers showed that one-third of HD patients complained of impaired vigilance, fatigue, and unrefreshing sleep, with patients on the evening HD shift having better sleep quality and less daytime sleepiness, albeit not in a pathological range [22]. Merlino and co-workers found an association between sleep complaints, but not EDS by itself, and morning HD shift [18], whereas Bastos and collaborators did not replicate any of these findings [20]. Barmar and colleagues showed a similar level of EDS in patients with chronic renal failure and those with ESKD undergoing HD. Objectively, by studying sleep–wake behavior by means of wrist actigraphy, they showed that HD patients frequently displayed an unstable sleep–wake pattern, with different sleep schedules between days with or without HD, that was strongly associated with EDS and influenced by low HD efficiency and the morning shift [23].

Only a few studies have characterized nocturnal sleep using polysomnography and daytime sleepiness with the MSLT or the maintenance of wakefulness test (MWT). Stepanski and collaborators studied 81 peritoneal dialysis patients, and showed that half of them reported unintentional daytime napping, confirmed by a short sleep latency on MSLT (mean of 6±3 min, with only 2 out of 18 subjects above 10 min), and only partially explained by the presence of a significant SDB (11 out of 18 patients) or periodic leg movements during sleep (six patients) [24]. Parker and co-workers evaluated a well-controlled sample of 46 HD patients, excluding potential confounders, such as other chronic medical conditions or use of medications with central nervous system effects, as well as patients with symptoms of sleep disturbances obviously leading to EDS, such as restless legs and snoring. They found that one-third (15) of patients had mean MSLT sleep latencies ≤8 min, consistent with EDS, with 6 patients under the sleep latency threshold of 5 min, suggesting severe EDS, and that 8 subjects also had at least 2 sleep onset REM sleep periods. Another third of patients (14) complained of subjective EDS at the Epworth Sleepiness Scale (ESS), but subjective and objective sleepiness seemed unrelated. Finally, mild SDB and periodic leg movements during sleep characterized the group, and SDB was related to objective, but not subjective, EDS [25]. Hanly et al. studied 24 HD patients not selected on the basis of sleep disturbance and re-evaluated nocturnal sleep and daytime sleepiness of 15 subjects after a switch from diurnal to nocturnal HD. Baseline polysomnography showed sleep fragmentation associated with a high prevalence of SDB and periodic leg movements, regardless of whether the recordings were performed on the HD day or two days later. Daytime sleepiness was highly prevalent; 46% of patients had a pathological ESS score, with increased subjective sleepiness closer to HD day, and 42% and 54% of patients had a mean MSLT sleep latency <5 min on the HD day or two days after HD, respectively. The major determinants of objective EDS were nocturnal periodic leg movements, but not SDB, and blood urea nitrogen, the latter being significantly correlated with sleep latencies on MSLT. The shift to nocturnal HD was associated with an amelioration of blood urea nitrogen and of SDB, and a correlation analysis between relative changes of nocturnal sleep parameters, blood urea nitrogen and MSLT sleep latencies showed that periodic leg movements play an independent role in the pathogenesis of EDS in these patients [26]. A single study evaluated the impact of erythropoietin therapy on nocturnal sleep and daytime sleepiness, assessed by means of the MWT in 10 HD patients that had sleep complaints such as poor sleep quality, nocturnal awakenings, daytime fatigue, but not restless legs syndrome or "significant" sleep apnea. Erythropoietin significantly improved hematocrit, periodic leg movements, and EDS with the mean MWT sleep latency increasing from 9.7 to 17.7 min [27]. Therefore, an intrinsic link between periodic leg movements during sleep and EDS in ESKD patients undergoing HD could exist.

Laboratory investigations and pathophysiological hypotheses

Despite many epidemiological studies showing an increased prevalence of EDS in ESKD patients undergoing long-term dialysis treatment, only a few reported an association of EDS with clinical or laboratory parameters assessing the uremic condition severity. Chen and co-workers found that patients with EDS (18% of 600 subjects, according to the ESS) were older, had higher levels of hemoglobin, lower HD duration, and lower albumin concentration, with additional clinical evidence supporting coexistent SDB [19]. Bastos et al. disclosed that subjects with EDS (28% out of 100 patients, according to the

ESS) showed lower HD efficacy [20]. Nevertheless, a study evaluating EDS in patients with chronic renal failure and in patients undergoing long-term HD showed comparable EDS prevalence in both clinical conditions [23], whereas a single study prospectively evaluating patients with chronic renal failure for three years disclosed a progressive decline of sleep quality, assessed by means of the Pittsburg Sleep Quality Index (PSQI), in parallel with decreasing renal function, assessed by serum creatinine concentration, even if highly influenced by age [28]. These studies could support the hypothesis that the decline of renal function, with its intrinsic metabolic alterations due to reduced kidney clearance, negatively impacts on sleep and, probably, on daytime functioning.

Several pathogenetic considerations could explain EDS in renal patients, especially those with ESKD undergoing long-term HD.

First, subclinical uremic encephalopathy is common in dialysis patients and could be reflected by EDS. The commonest electroencephalographic finding supporting this hypothesis is the presence of mild slow-wave frontal abnormalities during wakefulness, highly correlated to changes in biochemical indexes of uremia such as blood urea nitrogen and creatinine [29]. Similarly, hyperparathyroidism is frequent in renal insufficiency, namely secondary hyperparathyroidism, and elevation of the parathyroid hormone has neurotoxic effects associated with slow electroencephalographic activities in both uremic animals and patients undergoing long-term HD [30].

Second, many lines of evidence prove that HD clearly influences circadian rhythms, therefore a negative impact on the quality of nocturnal sleep and on daytime alertness is highly expected. A simple study evaluating the effect of HD on body temperature and sleepiness disclosed that HD induces chronic, episodic elevations of body temperature that persist for at least two hours, and that the HD timing plays a role on temperature rhythm disruption and on enhanced daytime sleepiness [31]. Chronic renal insufficiency also affects melatonin concentration, further supporting the hypothesis of a detrimental effect on the circadian regulation of human activities [32].

Third, chronic uremia is associated with low plasma levels of tyrosine, an amino acid precursor of norepinephrine and dopamine, two neurotransmitters involved in neurologic arousal [33]. Moreover, metabolites of creatinine, i.e. guanidine compounds that have been found increased in the cerebrospinal fluid and brain of uremic patients, inhibit responses to the inhibitory neurotransmitters gamma-aminobutyric acid and glycine in cultured rodents' neurons, and might interfere with sleep neurotransmission [34]. Therefore, uremia is associated with complex neurotransmission imbalances that could lead to reduced daytime alertness (hypoaminergic condition) as well as to altered nocturnal sleep (inhibited gamma-aminobutyric acid response).

Fourth, dialysis treatment induces significant elevations of proinflammatory cytokines that share hypnogenic properties. Peritoneal dialysis could trigger a persistent overproduction of IL-1, IL-6, TGF-β, and fibroblast growth factor acting via bacterial peritonitis [35], whereas HD performed with complement activating membranes increases leucocyte expression of IL-1, TNF-α, and IL-8 [36]. Cytokine overproduction may play a role in different aspects of uremia, such as anemia, that has a negative effect on nocturnal sleep of these patients [27], as well as directly affecting circadian rhythms including body temperature and sleep–wake cycles [37]. Consistently, ESKD patients undergoing HD treatment have high levels of systemic inflammation that were associated with poor subjective sleep quality [38].

Liver failure

Clinical findings

Little attention has been paid to EDS in patients with liver failure. Compared to other chronic medical conditions, daytime sleepiness frequently overlaps with fatigue, and tools to clearly distinguish these symptoms have not been validated in hepatic patients.

Newton *et al.* evaluated nocturnal sleep quality and sleep–wake patterns by using wrist actigraphy, subjective daytime sleepiness, and measures of fatigue in 48 women with primary biliary cirrhosis (PBC) compared with normal controls. They showed that patients with PBC complained of poorer sleep quality and higher subjective EDS than controls, with the EDS highly correlated with fatigue. Patients with PBC objectively slept more during the daytime than controls, and this difference could be mainly ascribed to the subgroup of PBC subjects with high fatigue levels, further corroborating the subjective complaints. A subsample of 9 patients with PBC and severe EDS was also investigated by polysomnography that showed coexistent SDB in only a single subject, suggesting that hepatic insufficiency by itself has a pathogenetic role for EDS and fatigue occurrence [39]. The same group evaluated patients with histologically proven non-alcoholic fatty liver disease (NAFLD) in comparison with normal controls using subjective EDS and fatigue assessments coupled with activity monitoring by means of pedometer actigraphy. When compared to controls, patients with NAFLD showed higher levels of fatigue, comparable to patients with PBC, that was associated with subjective EDS at the ESS. Fatigue severity was inversely correlated with activity (i.e. higher fatigue associated with lower activity) and directly with depression (i.e. higher fatigue associated with higher depression level). Conversely, fatigue severity was not related with laboratory and histological parameters measuring underlying liver disease or insulin resistance [40]. Mostacci and collaborators compared 178 patients with non-alcohol-related liver cirrhosis to a control group using a semi-structured interview coupled with the Basic Nordic Sleep Questionnaire and the ESS for sleep complaints and daytime sleepiness. Cirrhotic patients frequently complained of bad sleep (26% vs. 8%), that was significantly associated with daytime sleepiness and frequent napping according to the Basic Nordic Sleep Questionnaire. Overall, 16% of patients with cirrhosis had EDS according to the ESS (vs. 13% of controls) and frequently complained of insomnia. Patients with minimal hepatic encephalopathy were more frequently insomniac and sleepy, without any other significant clinical or laboratory correlate [41]. Another study evaluated sleep complaints in cirrhotic patients without overt hepatic encephalopathy in comparison with patients with chronic renal failure and healthy controls. Both patient groups showed a higher prevalence of sleep disturbances than the controls, with the additional evidence that patients with unsatisfactory subjective sleep quality reported worse nocturnal sleep and daytime functioning with frequent and prolonged napping. Cirrhotic patients did not show any association between sleep disturbances and clinical or laboratory parameters, whereas cirrhotic patients with sleep disturbances frequently had a delayed bedtime, delayed wake-up time, and evening chronotypology according to Horne and Ostberg's questionnaire, and both renal and hepatic patients with unsatisfactory sleep had higher anxiety and depression scores. Wrist actigraphy disclosed reduced motor activity in cirrhotics, with increased nocturnal activity and altered circadian rhythm, as measured by the ratio between daytime and nighttime activity. The altered distribution of motor activity was more pronounced in patients with unsatisfactory sleep, in which a shift toward later hours of the day confirmed the subjective evening circadian preference [42].

Laboratory investigations and pathophysiological hypotheses

As outlined above, none of the clinical studies on patients with hepatic insufficiency showed a significant relationship between sleepiness or sleep disturbances and laboratory, including serum ammonia, or clinical parameters characterizing liver disease [39, 40], apart from an association with minimal hepatic encephalopathy [41]. Within the clinical spectrum of hepatic encephalopathy, a decline of consciousness is a typical symptom that should be promptly identified in order to remove potential precipitating factors and avoid the progression to a comatosed state. Hepatic encephalopathy has been linked to raised brain concentration of ammonia and to increased gamma-aminobutyric acid neurotransmission [43]. In hepatic failure, several neurotransmitters other than gamma-aminobutyric acid, such as glutamate, dopamine, serotonin, opioids, and histamine have shown abnormalities, that could play a role in the pathogenesis of sleep disturbances and EDS, as long as they are involved in the regulation of the sleep–wake cycle [43, 44].

Second, Córdoba *et al.* disclosed an association between unsatisfactory sleep and evening chronotype, corroborated by a shift in the circadian profile of motor activity towards the later hours of the day, and associated with increased daytime napping [42]. Accordingly, a study on the 24-h plasma melatonin profile in cirrhotic patients with subclinical hepatic encephalopathy and healthy controls showed a delay in the time of onset and the peak of circadian neurohormone secretion together with markedly elevated concentrations during daytime hours. The analysis of sleep–wake patterns on sleep diaries showed an increased number of daytime naps and nocturnal awakenings in cirrhotic patients, with the additional evidence that the hepatic patients lacking diurnal rhythmicity of the melatonin profile, and with higher levels, were the ones with the highest number of naps and awakenings [45].

Third, several studies suggest a potential role of proinflammatory cytokines in the pathogenesis of sleep disturbances, EDS, and fatigue in hepatic patients. Studies on PBC have shown complex abnormalities of cytokine expression in liver tissue, suggesting that cytokines produced by T-helper lymphocytes have a pathogenetic role in PBC [46, 47]. Moreover, B lymphocytes of patients with PBC displayed an increased IL-6 response to bacterial stimuli, further connecting the pathogenesis of PBC to similar findings in EDS disorders [12, 48]. Similarly, patients with non-alcoholic steatohepatitis have increased plasma levels of IL-6 and TNF-α [49], whereas obesity itself could play a role in the pathogenesis of cirrhosis acting through complex inflammatory mechanisms triggered by exposure to lipopolysaccharide [50].

Fourthly, EDS in cirrhotics could be also partially explained by the coexistence of SDB, the prevalence of which increases in parallel to the severity of the liver disease [51], and when ascites complicates the clinical condition [52].

Chronic pulmonary diseases

Clinical findings

Few studies have evaluated nocturnal sleep together with daytime sleepiness in patients with pulmonary diseases that lead to severe metabolic alterations such as hypoxia and hypercapnia.

Dancey *et al*. evaluated 19 adults with cystic fibrosis (CF) and 10 controls with polysomnography and MSLT. CF patients reported more nocturnal awakenings, with the objective evidence of longer sleep latency, reduced total sleep time, and reduced sleep efficiency, the last significantly associated, and correlated, with hypoxemia during wakefulness and, more significantly, during sleep. Despite the above findings, CF patients showed subjective (ESS) and objective (MSLT) levels of daytime sleepiness within the normal range and comparable to that of healthy controls. Conversely, daytime fatigue was higher in patients with CF than in controls [53].

Orr and collaborators evaluated 14 patients with chronic obstructive pulmonary disease (COPD) and severe hypoxemia. Despite the presence of severe hypoxemia during sleep, associated with short and fragmented nocturnal sleep, none of the COPD patients had EDS either subjective, or objective on the MSLT [54]. The Sleep Heart Health Study, evaluated the potential association between obstructive airway disease (OAD) and SDB, without a significant overlap in the general population. In the absence of SDB, patients with OAD had slightly shorter total sleep time, but did not differ in sleep latency, sleep efficiency, and subjective sleepiness (ESS) compared to community-dwelling adults [55].

Few data are available on bronchial asthma (BA). A sleep questionnaire survey comparing 267 BA patients with 2394 controls disclosed that BA is associated with poor sleep quality, nocturnal symptoms of SDB, and daytime sleepiness and tiredness. After adjusting for possible confounders, a potential association between BA and EDS was confirmed. In asthmatic patients EDS, together with tiredness, was associated with allergic rhinitis and with bronchial hyperresponsiveness [56]. Teodorescu and collaborators evaluated EDS and its correlates in a population of 115 BA patients, finding that 55% of patients complained of daytime sleepiness, with 47% having a pathological ESS score, and with 86% or 38% reporting snoring or habitual snoring. The ESS score was independently associated with SDB symptoms and male gender, but not with BA severity. EDS seemed a frequent complaint in patients with BA, with its severity correlating to underlying symptoms of SDB that would require further diagnostic and therapeutic approaches [57]. Krishnan and co-workers explored subjective sleep quality, daytime sleepiness, and quality of life in 41 patients with idiopathic pulmonary fibrosis (IPF), an inflammatory disease of the lower respiratory tract characterized by extreme fatigue and poor prognosis. The authors reported a lower sleep quality associated, and correlated, with higher levels of subjective EDS compared to a non-age-matched control group. Neither the ESS nor the PSQI were correlated with any demographic or clinical patient characteristic, including pulmonary function tests. Moreover, quality-of-life domains were variably correlated with subjective sleep quality, but not with EDS [58].

Laboratory investigations and pathophysiological hypotheses

As outlined above, chronic pulmonary diseases are clearly associated with poor sleep quality, but can be dichotomized into disorders without EDS, such as CF, COPD, OAD, and those with EDS, such as BA and IPF. The last are clearly characterized by underlying pathogenetic inflammatory processes. Concerning the metabolic alterations intrinsic to pulmonary insufficiency, none of the studies provide any correlation between pulmonary function, hypoxia and EDS, suggesting that even extreme hypoxia does not cause EDS, whereas it could contribute to poor sleep quality and fatigue. Conversely, experimental data proved that intermittent hypoxia activates an inflammatory response with expression of IL-6, without altering the clock genes profile [59]. These experimental data could explain the vicious cycle of intermittent hypoxia, inflammation, and EDS in SDB, and could conversely clarify why constant, albeit severe, hypoxia is not associated with EDS in chronic pulmonary diseases without prominent inflammation.

Chronic heart failure

Clinical findings

Even if heart failure (HF) is not characterized by intrinsic dysmetabolism, it induces severe consequences on the perfusion of other organs, such as the kidney with secondary insufficiency, as well as on the plasma concentration of several circulatory factors, such as the atrial natriuretic peptide, that have important metabolic functions. Recently, patients with HF have been investigated to characterize their sleep disturbances and EDS. Redeker and Stein, using wrist actigraphy and questionnaires, compared 59 patients with HF to controls. HF patients showed poorer objective indexes of sleep continuity on wrist actigraphy, of subjective sleepiness on the ESS, and of subjective sleep quality on the PSQI [60]. Nevertheless, studies applying polysomnography in HF patients frequently disclosed SDB. Ferrier and colleagues found 68% of SDB in 87 stable HF patients: 53% were of obstructive type, and 15% of central type, the latter significantly associated with lower left ventricular ejection fraction. HF patients with SDB did not have subjective EDS [61]. A large epidemiological study compared nocturnal indexes and subjective daytime sleepiness of 155 HF patients and of 1139 random community subjects with SDB of variable severity, confirming that subjects with HF had significantly less subjective sleepiness for any severity of SDB, despite lower objective sleep quality. In patients with HF, the association between obesity and sleep apnea was significantly weaker, without the expected increase of body mass index with increasing SDB severity [62]. Hastings and co-workers evaluated 39 patients with HF using objective measures of daytime sleepiness, namely wrist actigraphy and a single behavioral daytime wakefulness test, together with polysomnography. They found that 22 patients had SDB, 12 of central and 10 of obstructive type, with a negative impact on sleep continuity on polysomnographic and actigraphic assessments. Strikingly, HF patients with SDB were significantly sleepier than HF patients with normal nocturnal breathing when sleepiness was evaluated with objective measures during daytime, but did not show any difference in terms of subjective sleepiness on the ESS. Therefore a "dissociation" between objective and subjective measures of daytime sleepiness characterized HF patients with SDB, with the potential limitation that the ESS could be an unreliable tool in this patient population [63]. Hanly and Zuberi-Khokar evaluated 7 patients with HF and Cheyne–Stokes respiration in comparison with 7 patients with HF and 9 controls using polysomnography coupled with sleepiness assessment using the ESS and the MSLT. SDB was associated with sleep fragmentation, i.e. arousals occurring in the hyperpneic phase of Cheyne–Stokes breathing, and objective sleepiness, i.e. low sleep latencies on MSLT, again without significant differences in terms of subjective sleepiness. Moreover, as long as nocturnal oxygen saturation did not differ between HF patients with or without SDB, the authors suggested that objective daytime sleepiness could reflect sleep fragmentation more than hypoxia itself [64].

Laboratory investigations and pathophysiological hypotheses

The current literature clearly suggests that daytime sleepiness in patients with HF is generally associated with underlying SDB, with the specificity that EDS could be objectively evaluated, but not subjectively perceived [61–64]. Therefore, it seems that the HF condition itself is not characterized by prominent EDS. Moreover, when considering the potential contribution of cytokines or obesity to EDS disclosed in other metabolic disturbances, HF patients did not show the usual association between SDB severity and body mass index, further suggesting that HF is an atypical condition with regard to EDS [62].

Nevertheless, even if EDS in patients with HF is due to SDB, Zilberman and collaborators found another distinguishing feature when evaluating 38 HF patients with anemia before and after treatment with erythropoietin and intravenous iron. Thirty-seven had SDB at baseline, and after treatment the authors found a significant amelioration of SDB, including obstructive and central events, and Cheyne–Stokes breathing, that was associated with a significant improvement of the ESS and of cardiologic functional status, without changing periodic leg movements during sleep. Therefore, a contribution of anemia to SDB could be intrinsic to HF, probably due to several factors, such as reduced cardiac function, impaired systemic oxygenation, and tissue swelling of the upper airways predisposing to obstruction [65].

Exposure to toxins

Clinical findings

Despite widespread knowledge that exposure to toxins could result in various neurological disorders, there is no scientific literature of studies evaluating sleep disturbances and daytime sleepiness either with instrumental methods or with questionnaires commonly used in sleep medicine. Viaene et al. recently reviewed the evidence available on solvent exposure, showing that acute exposure could cause a prenarcotic syndrome, whereas long-lasting exposure could induce an irreversible toxic encephalopathy [66]. Several studies have shown a decrease of sleep quality, with difficulty falling asleep and early awakenings that could be within the symptoms related to an acute or chronic encephalopathy, but without detailing the type of sleep disturbances and without excluding the coexistence of SDB in exposed subjects. Moreover, similar to alcohol, toxin exposure can also augment SDB of both obstructive and central type, but studies objectively evaluating this possible effect using polysomnographic methods are lacking [66].

Conclusions

Reviewing the literature, we found convincing data to affirm that EDS can be a feature characterizing infectious or inflammatory diseases, obesity, insulin resistance, renal and hepatic failure, and pulmonary diseases such as bronchial asthma and idiopathic pulmonary fibrosis, even in the absence of other common sleep disturbances such as SDB. Conversely, neither other chronic pulmonary diseases, such as CF, COPD, OAD, nor chronic cardiac insufficiency seemed significantly associated with EDS, suggesting that EDS is not the mere expression of a chronic and disabling medical condition.

Several lines of evidence could support common pathophysiological mechanisms underlying the association between EDS and the above-mentioned diseases: first, an inflammatory condition with high concentrations of proinflammatory cytokines resulting in enhanced daytime somnolence is proved in infections, obesity, insulin resistance, renal and hepatic failure, BA and IPF; second, a metabolic encephalopathy is associated with renal and hepatic failure, as well as with toxin exposure, intrinsically related to altered central nervous system neurotransmission, and possibly resulting in a decreased level of daytime vigilance; third, an alteration of circadian rhythms has been demonstrated in infectious and inflammatory diseases, obesity, renal and hepatic failure, contributing to disturbed sleep and EDS. We suggest the need to verify these potential mechanistic associations in further studies with objective measures of EDS and advanced polysomnographic techniques commonly used in the sleep medicine field.

The paucity and heterogeneity of the literature on EDS in metabolic conditions intrinsically limits the strength of the association. Further studies are highly warranted to validate sleep questionnaires in chronic medical conditions assuring their reliability, and to evaluate the relations between EDS and fatigue, a subjective symptom frequently experienced in patients with chronic medical diseases. We emphasize the need to investigate these categories of patients with advanced polysomnographic techniques that could rule out SDB as a misleading cause of EDS, and search for potential characteristics of sleep alterations, including SDB. Therapeutic studies on sleep disorders and EDS occurring in the context of metabolic alterations are needed to assess whether specific treatments, other than those generally recommended for the sleep disorders or for the coexistent medical condition per se, could achieve better results.

To summarize, EDS is frequently associated with chronic metabolic diseases that have high prevalence and heavy socio-economical impact. Given the well-known negative impact of EDS on quality of life and, possibly, on long-term prognosis, it is important to investigate EDS in this context to determine the potential contribution to a poor, and possibly reversible, medical outcome.

References

1. **American Academy of Sleep Medicine**. *The International Classification of Sleep Disorders: Diagnostic and Coding Manual* (2nd Ed.). Westchester, IL: American Academy of Sleep Medicine, 2005.

2. **Schuld A, Haack M, Hinze-Selch D**, *et al.* Experimental studies on the interaction between sleep and the immune system in humans. *Psychother Psychosom Med Psychol*, 2005; **55**:29–35.

3. **Kelley K W, Bluthé R M, Dantzer R**, *et al.* Cytokine-induced sickness behavior. *Brain Behav Immun*, 2003; **17**(Suppl 1):S112–18.

4. **Kapsimalis F, Basta M, Varouchakis G**, *et al.* Cytokines and pathological sleep. *Sleep Med*, 2008; **9**:603–14.

5. **Hermann D M, Mullington J, Hinze-Selch D**, *et al.* Endotoxin-induced changes in sleep and sleepiness during the day. *Psychoneuroendocrinology*, 1998; **23**:427–37.

6. **Vgontzas A N, Bixler E O, Tan T L**, *et al.* Obesity without sleep apnea is associated with daytime sleepiness. *Arch Intern Med*, 1998; **158**:1333–37.

7. **Bixler E O, Vgontzas A N, Lin H M**, *et al.* Excessive daytime sleepiness in a general population sample: the role of sleep apnea, age, obesity, diabetes, and depression. *J Clin Endocrinol Metab*, 2005; **90**:4510–15.

8. **Vgontzas A N, Legro R S, Bixler E O**, *et al.* Polycystic ovary syndrome is associated with obstructive sleep apnea and daytime sleepiness: role of insulin resistance. *J Clin Endocrinol Metab*, 2001; **86**:517–20.

9. **Vgontzas A N, Bixler E O, Chrousos G P**. Obesity-related sleepiness and fatigue: the role of the stress system and cytokines. *Ann N Y Acad Sci*, 2006; **1083**:329–44.

10. **Vgontzas A N**. Does obesity play a major role in the pathogenesis of sleep apnoea and its associated manifestations via inflammation, visceral adiposity, and insulin resistance? *Arch Physiol Biochem*, 2008; **114**:211–23.

11. **Vgontzas A N, Bixler E O, Chrousos G P**. Metabolic disturbances in obesity versus sleep apnoea: the importance of visceral obesity and insulin resistance. *J Intern Med*, 2003; **254**:32–44.

12. **Vgontzas A N, Papanicolaou D A, Bixler E O**, *et al.* Elevation of plasma cytokines in disorders of excessive daytime sleepiness: role of sleep disturbance and obesity. *J Clin Endocrinol Metab*, 1997; **82**:1313–16.

13. **Vgontzas A N, Papanicolaou D A, Bixler E O**, *et al.* Circadian interleukin-6 secretion and quantity and depth of sleep. *J Clin Endocrinol Metab*, 1999; **84**:2603–07.

14. **Vgontzas A N, Papanicolaou D A, Bixler E O**, *et al.* Sleep apnea and daytime sleepiness and fatigue: relation to visceral obesity, insulin resistance, and hypercytokinemia. *J Clin Endocrinol Metab*, 2000; **85**:1151–58.

15. **Vgontzas A N, Trakada G, Bixler E O**, *et al.* Plasma interleukin 6 levels are elevated in polycystic ovary syndrome independently of obesity or sleep apnea. *Metabolism*, 2006; **55**:1076–82.

16. **Parker K P**. Sleep disturbances in dialysis patients. *Sleep Med Rev*, 2003; **7**:131–43.

17. **Hui D S, Wong T Y, Ko F W**, *et al.* Prevalence of sleep disturbances in Chinese patients with end-stage renal failure on continuous ambulatory peritoneal dialysis. *Am J Kidney Dis*, 2000; **36**:783–88.

18. **Merlino G, Piani A, Dolso P**, *et al.* Sleep disorders in patients with end-stage renal disease undergoing dialysis therapy. *Nephrol Dial Transplant*, 2006; **21**:184–90.

19. **Chen W C, Lim P S, Wu W C**, *et al.* Sleep behavior disorders in a large cohort of Chinese (Taiwanese) patients maintained by long-term hemodialysis. *Am J Kidney Dis*, 2006; **48**:277–84.

20. **Bastos J P, Sousa R B, Nepomuceno L A**, *et al.* Sleep disturbances in patients on maintenance hemodialysis: role of dialysis shift. *Rev Assoc Med Bras*, 2007; **53**:492–96.

21. **Jhamb M, Weisbord S D, Steel J L**, *et al.* Fatigue in patients receiving maintenance dialysis: a review of definitions, measures, and contributing factors. *Am J Kidney Dis*, 2008; **52**:353–65.

22. **Hsu C Y, Lee C T, Lee Y J**, *et al.* Better sleep quality and less daytime symptoms in patients on evening hemodialysis: a questionnaire-based study. *Artif Organs*, 2008; **32**:711–16.

23. **Barmar B, Dang Q, Isquith D**, *et al.* Comparison of sleep/wake behavior in CKD stages 4 to 5 and hemodialysis populations using wrist actigraphy. *Am J Kidney Dis*, 2009; **53**:665–72.

24. **Stepanski E, Faber M, Zorick F**, *et al.* Sleep disorders in patients on continuous ambulatory peritoneal dialysis. *J Am Soc Nephrol*, 1995; **6**:192–97.

25. **Parker K P, Bliwise D L, Bailey J L**, *et al.* Daytime sleepiness in stable hemodialysis patients. *Am J Kidney Dis*, 2003; **41**:394–402.

26. **Hanly P J, Gabor J Y, Chan C**, *et al.* Daytime sleepiness in patients with CRF: impact of nocturnal hemodialysis. *Am J Kidney Dis*, 2003; **41**:403–10.

27. **Benz R L, Pressman M R, Hovick E T**, *et al.* A preliminary study of the effects of correction of anemia with recombinant human erythropoietin therapy on sleep, sleep disorders, and daytime sleepiness in hemodialysis patients (The SLEEPO study). *Am J Kidney Dis*, 1999; **34**:1089–95.

28. **Sabbatini M, Pisani A, Crispo A**, *et al.* Sleep quality in patients with chronic renal failure: a 3-year longitudinal study. *Sleep Med*, 2008; **9**:240–46.

29. **Hughes J R**. Correlations between EEG and chemical changes in uremia. *Electroencephalogr Clin Neurophysiol*, 1980; **48**:583–94.

30. **Goldstein D A, Feinstein E I, Chui L A**, et al. The relationship between the abnormalities in electroencephalogram and blood levels of parathyroid hormone in dialysis patients. *J Clin Endocrinol Metab*, 1980; **51**:130–34.

31. **Parker K P, Bliwise D L, Rye D B**. Hemodialysis disrupts basic sleep regulatory mechanisms: building hypotheses. *Nurs Res*, 2000; **49**:327–32.

32. **Vaziri N D, Oveisi F, Reyes G A**, et al. Dysregulation of melatonin metabolism in chronic renal insufficiency: role of erythropoietin-deficiency anemia. *Kidney Int*, 1996; **50**:653–56.

33. **Fürst P**. Amino acid metabolism in uremia. *J Am Coll Nutr*, 1989; **8**:310–23.

34. **De Deyn P P, Macdonald R L**. Guanidino compounds that are increased in cerebrospinal fluid and brain of uremic patients inhibit GABA and glycine responses on mouse neurons in cell culture. *Ann Neurol*, 1990; **28**:627–33.

35. **Lai K N, Lai K B, Lam C W**, et al. Changes of cytokine profiles during peritonitis in patients on continuous ambulatory peritoneal dialysis. *Am J Kidney Dis*, 2000; **35**:644–52.

36. **Rousseau Y, Haeffner-Cavaillon N, Poignet J L**, et al. In vivo intracellular cytokine production by leukocytes during haemodialysis. *Cytokine*, 2000; **12**:506–17.

37. **Pertosa G, Grandaliano G, Gesualdo L**, et al. Clinical relevance of cytokine production in hemodialysis. *Kidney Int Suppl*, 2000; **76**:S104–11.

38. **Chiu Y L, Chuang Y F, Fang K C**, et al. Higher systemic inflammation is associated with poorer sleep quality in stable haemodialysis patients. *Nephrol Dial Transplant*, 2009; **24**:247–51.

39. **Newton J L, Gibson G J, Tomlinson M**, et al. Fatigue in primary biliary cirrhosis is associated with excessive daytime somnolence. *Hepatology*, 2006; **44**:91–98.

40. **Newton J L, Jones D E, Henderson E**, et al. Fatigue in non-alcoholic fatty liver disease (NAFLD) is significant and associates with inactivity and excessive daytime sleepiness but not with liver disease severity or insulin resistance. *Gut*, 2008; **57**:807–13.

41. **Mostacci B, Ferlisi M, Baldi Antognini A**, et al. Sleep disturbance and daytime sleepiness in patients with cirrhosis: a case control study. *Neurol Sci*, 2008; **29**:237–40.

42. **Córdoba J, Cabrera J, Lataif L**, et al. High prevalence of sleep disturbance in cirrhosis. *Hepatology*, 1998; **27**:339–45.

43. **Jones E A, Weissenborn K**. Neurology and the liver. *J Neurol Neurosurg Psychiatry*, 1997; **63**:279–93.

44. **Lozeva V, Tuomisto L, Tarhanen J**, et al. Increased concentrations of histamine and its metabolite, tele-methylhistamine and down-regulation of histamine H3 receptor sites in autopsied brain tissue from cirrhotic patients who died in hepatic coma. *J Hepatol*, 2003; **39**:522–27.

45. **Steindl P E, Finn B, Bendok B**, et al. Disruption of the diurnal rhythm of plasma melatonin in cirrhosis. *Ann Intern Med*, 1995; **123**:274–77.

46. **Martinez O M, Villanueva J C, Gershwin M E**, et al. Cytokine patterns and cytotoxic mediators in primary biliary cirrhosis. *Hepatology*, 1995; **21**:113–19.

47. **Nagano T, Yamamoto K, Matsumoto S**, et al. Cytokine profile in the liver of primary biliary cirrhosis. *J Clin Immunol*, 1999; **19**:422–27.

48. **Kakumu S, Shinagawa T, Ishikawa T**, et al. Interleukin 6 production by peripheral blood mononuclear cells in patients with chronic hepatitis B virus infection and primary biliary cirrhosis. *Gastroenterol Jpn*, 1993; **28**:18–24.

49. **Abiru S, Migita K, Maeda Y**, et al. Serum cytokine and soluble cytokine receptor levels in patients with non-alcoholic steatohepatitis. *Liver Int*, 2006; **26**:39–45.

50. **Yang S Q, Lin H Z, Lane M D**, et al. Obesity increases sensitivity to endotoxin liver injury: implications for the pathogenesis of steatohepatitis. *Proc Natl Acad Sci USA*, 1997; **94**:2557–62.

51. **Ogata T, Nomura M, Nakaya Y**, et al. Evaluation of episodes of sleep apnea in patients with liver cirrhosis. *J Med Invest*, 2006; **53**:159–66.

52. **Crespo J, Cifrián J, Pinto J A**, et al. Sleep apnea obstructive syndrome: a new complication previously undescribed in cirrhotic patients with ascites. *Am J Gastroenterol*, 2003; **98**:2815–16.

53. **Dancey D R, Tullis E D, Heslegrave R**, et al. Sleep quality and daytime function in adults with cystic fibrosis and severe lung disease. *Eur Respir J*, 2002; **19**:504–10.

54. **Orr W C, Shamma-Othman Z, Levin D**, et al. Persistent hypoxemia and excessive daytime sleepiness in chronic obstructive pulmonary disease (COPD). *Chest*, 1990; **97**:583–85.

55. **Sanders M H, Newman A B, Haggerty C L**, et al. Sleep and sleep-disordered breathing in adults with predominantly mild obstructive airway disease. *Am J Respir Crit Care Med*, 2003; **167**:7–14.

56. **Janson C, De Backer W, Gislason T**, et al. Increased prevalence of sleep disturbances and daytime sleepiness in subjects with bronchial asthma: a

population study of young adults in three European countries. *Eur Respir J*, 1996; **9**:2132–38.

57. Teodorescu M, Consens F B, Bria W F, et al. Correlates of daytime sleepiness in patients with asthma. *Sleep Med*, 2006; **7**:607–13.

58. Krishnan V, McCormack M C, Mathai S C, et al. Sleep quality and health-related quality of life in idiopathic pulmonary fibrosis. *Chest*, 2008; **134**:693–98.

59. Burioka N, Koyanagi S, Fukuoka Y, et al. Influence of intermittent hypoxia on the signal transduction pathways to inflammatory response and circadian clock regulation. *Life Sci*, 2009; **85**:372–78.

60. Redeker N S, Stein S. Characteristics of sleep in patients with stable heart failure versus a comparison group. *Heart Lung*, 2006; **35**:252–61.

61. Ferrier K, Campbell A, Yee B, et al. Sleep-disordered breathing occurs frequently in stable outpatients with congestive heart failure. *Chest*, 2005; **128**:2116–22.

62. Arzt M, Young T, Finn L, et al. Sleepiness and sleep in patients with both systolic heart failure and obstructive sleep apnea. *Arch Intern Med*, 2006; **166**:1716–22.

63. Hastings P C, Vazir A, O'Driscoll D M, et al. Symptom burden of sleep-disordered breathing in mild-to-moderate congestive heart failure patients. *Eur Respir J*, 2006; **27**:748–55.

64. Hanly P, Zuberi-Khokhar N. Daytime sleepiness in patients with congestive heart failure and Cheyne–Stokes respiration. *Chest*, 1995; **107**:952–58.

65. Zilberman M, Silverberg D S, Bits I, et al. Improvement of anemia with erythropoietin and intravenous iron reduces sleep-related breathing disorders and improves daytime sleepiness in anemic patients with congestive heart failure. *Am Heart J*, 2007; **154**:870–76.

66. Viaene M, Vermeir G, Godderis L. Sleep disturbances and occupational exposure to solvents. *Sleep Med Rev*, 2009; **13**:235–43.

Section 3 Medical, Psychiatric and Neurological Causes of Sleepiness

Chapter 34

Excessive sleepiness due to medications and drugs

Paula K. Schweitzer

Introduction

Sleepiness is a common side-effect of drugs which affect the central nervous system. Sleep–wake state is controlled by a complex interaction between sleep-promoting and wake-promoting systems involving nuclei in the hypothalamus and brainstem [1–3]. Drugs can cause sedation by multiple mechanisms which affect the balance between these systems. Most hypnotics and many antiepileptic medications cause sedation by gamma-aminobutryic acid (GABA) agonism which directly affects the sleep-promoting system. The sedating side-effect of many drugs involves inhibition of the wake-promoting system, in particular via antagonism of histamine type 1 (H_1), alpha adrenergic type 1 (α_1), and serotonin type 2 ($5HT_2$) receptors. In fact, H_1 antagonism is a principal mechanism for the sedating activity of numerous drugs including the "classic" antihistamines such as diphenhydramine, a number of antidepressants including amitriptyline, doxepin, mirtazepine, and trazodone, as well as antipsychotic medications such as clozapine and quetiapine. Drugs such as melatonin receptor agonists and melatonin may produce sedation via effects on the circadian timing system. Sedation may also be caused by effects on other neurotransmitters and neuropeptides involved in sleep-wake regulation including acetylcholine, adenosine, dopamine, glutamate, and orexin/hypocretin. In addition to receptor binding profile, factors which determine the degree of sedation produced by a drug include dose, half-life, lipid solubility (which determines the degree of central nervous system penetration), presence or absence of active metabolites, interactions with other drugs, and time of administration.

This chapter reviews drugs for which sleepiness is considered a side-effect. Evaluation of data is complicated by imprecise terminology (e.g. sleepiness, sedation, somnolence, fatigue, drowsiness are used interchangeably) and variable methodology ranging from spontaneous reports to objective measurement. Most data describing sleepiness are obtained through subjective reports. Subjective measurement scales and objective tests such as polysomnography (PSG) and the multiple sleep latency test (MSLT) are less commonly used. While PSG measurements are typically employed to evaluate desirable sedation (e.g. as treatment for insomnia), these findings may be used cautiously to infer undesirable sedation if the same drug is taken during the daytime. While the consequences of sleepiness (impaired function) may be a critical issue, care must be taken in attributing deficits in cognitive and neurobehavioral performance to sleepiness, as underlying disease or other drug effects may be involved.

Hypnotics

Drugs approved for the treatment of insomnia in the USA include specific benzodiazepine receptor agonists (Table 34.1) a melatonin receptor agonist, and an H_1 antagonist. Other drugs used as hypnotics include anxiolytic benzodiazepines, sedating antidepressants, antiepileptics, antihistamines (present in most over-the-counter hypnotics), antipsychotics, barbiturates, sodium oxybate, and valerian. The mechanism for sedation for benzodiazepine receptor agonists and barbiturates is GABA agonism, but varies for other drugs. While the sedating properties of these drugs are useful for the treatment of insomnia, residual sedation may occur as a result of the desired drug action continuing into the wake period. The magnitude of residual sedation is related to duration of action, which depends on pharmacokinetic properties and drug dose. Both

---

Sleepiness: Causes, Consequences and Treatment, ed. Michael J. Thorpy and Michel Billiard. Published by Cambridge University Press. © Cambridge University Press 2011.

Table 34.1 Benzodiazepine receptor agonists listed in order of decreasing half-life, grouped by indication

Drug	Half-life (h)	FDA Indication for drugs available in USA	Indication for drugs not available in USA
Flunitrazepam	36–200[1]		Insomnia
Flurazepam	48–120[1]	Insomnia	
Quazepam	15–120[1]	Insomnia	
Nitrazepam	20–50		Insomnia
Estazolam	10–24[1]	Insomnia	
Lormetazepam	10–12		Insomnia
Temazepam	8–20	Insomnia	
Loprazolam	6–12		Insomnia
Eszopiclone	5–6	Insomnia	
Zopiclone	4–6		Insomnia
Midazolam	1.8–6.4	Pre-operative sedation	Insomnia
Zolpidem extended release	1.6–4.5	Insomnia	
Zolpidem	1.5–2.4	Insomnia	
Triazolam	1.5–5	Insomnia	
Zaleplon	1.0	Insomnia	
Nordazepam	50–120[1]		Anxiety
Chlordiazepoxide	36–120[1]	Anxiety	
Clorazepate	36–100[1]		Anxiety
Halazapam	30–100[1]		Anxiety
Diazepam	36–100[1]	Anxiety, panic disorder	
Prazepam	30–100[1]		Anxiety
Clonazepam	24–56	Seizures, panic disorder	
Lorazepam	12–16[1]	Anxiety	
Bromazepam	10–20		Anxiety
Alprazolam	10–15	Anxiety, panic disorder	
Clobazam	8–60		Anxiety, seizures
Oxazepam	6–11	Anxiety	

[1] Range includes elimination half-life of active metabolite.

epidemiological and experimental studies of benzodiazepine receptor agonists indicate that drugs with long half-lives or active metabolites and drugs used in higher doses are more likely to cause next-day sleepiness or impair next-day function [4–6]. Time of administration and amount of time allotted for sleep are also important factors. Most short- to intermediate-acting benzodiazepine receptor agonists do not impair next-day performance when used in typical pre-sleep doses [6]. Zopiclone, however, despite its shorter half-life, has been linked to residual impairment in driving performance 10–11 h after bedtime administration [7]. When given only 4–5 h prior to driving, zolpidem but not zaleplon impaired driving [8].

Psychotherapeutic drugs

Anti-anxiety drugs

Drugs most commonly used in the treatment of anxiety disorders include benzodiazepine receptor agonists, antidepressants, and buspirone. Beta antagonists, antiepileptics, and atypical antipsychotics are sometimes used. Pharmacological profiles of anxiolytic benzodiazepines (e.g. alprazolam, clonazepam, diazepam, lorazepam) are similar to those of benzodiazepines used for insomnia. However, half-lives of the anxiolytic drugs are intermediate to long (Table 34.1), and these drugs are administered during the daytime. Thus, sedation may be more problematic. Sleepiness has been confirmed objectively by a study of non-anxious subjects who showed decreased MSLT latencies (increased sleep tendency) with alprazolam and diazepam on both day 1 and 7 of treatment [9]. Performance impairment, including driving, has been noted in studies of both normal subjects and patient groups for treatment periods of up to three weeks, particularly at higher doses [10]. Risk for traffic accidents appears to be higher for anxiolytic benzodiazepines than for hypnotic benzodiazepines, likely because of their longer half-lives [11]. The risk decreases with duration of use, suggesting development of tolerance. Men were more likely than women to have accidents as were those under 60 years of age [12]. As with benzodiazepine hypnotics, risk for accidents was higher for drugs with longer half-lives [11, 13].

Buspirone is not sedating, as it has no affinity for the benzodiazepine receptors and does not affect GABA binding. It appears to act primarily as a $5HT_{1A}$ partial agonist, but also has effects on dopamine D_2 receptors [14].

Antidepressants

Antidepressant drugs have effects at multiple receptors (Table 34.2), affecting mood likely through 5HT and norepinephrine (NE) receptors. Sedation may result from antagonism at H_1, α_1, and $5HT_2$ receptors. The most sedating antidepressants include the tricyclic antidepressants (TCAs) amitriptyline, doxepin, and trimipramine, as well as trazodone and mirtazapine. These drugs are frequently used off-label in lower doses for treatment of insomnia [15, 16]. Information on sedation comes from subjective reports, studies on the effects of these drugs on nocturnal sleep, and evaluations of cognitive and psychomotor performance. There are no studies objectively evaluating sleepiness during the daytime.

TCAs differ from one another in their relative effects in blocking 5HT or NE reuptake as well as in the degree of antagonism of muscarinic cholinergic receptors and H_1 receptors [17, 18]. The more sedating TCAs tend to be more anticholinergic (amitriptyline) and more antihistaminergic (doxepin, trimipramine) but also exhibit proportionately greater inhibition of 5HT reuptake than NE reuptake. Doxepin is a potent antihistamine at antidepressant doses. In addition, at very low doses (1–6 mg), it is relatively selective for H_1 receptors, which has led to its evaluation as a hypnotic [19]. The secondary amines (desipramine, nortriptylline, protriptyline) which are more potent in blocking NE reuptake than 5HT reuptake and also have lower affinity for H_1 receptors are much less likely to be sedating. TCAs have half-lives of approximately 15–30 h, with active metabolites having slightly longer half-lives [20]. Thus residual sedation is a potential problem when these drugs are used as hypnotics, even at lower doses. When used at antidepressant doses, sedation is very likely, particularly with initial use. These drugs are subjectively sedating and objectively decrease sleep latency and increase total sleep time when studied polysomnographically [21, 22]. Cognitive and psychomotor performance including driving are likely to be impaired at least initially [23]. There is conflicting evidence on the development of tolerance to sedation and performance impairment [24, 25].

Trazodone has complex effects on the 5HT system [26, 27]. It is a relatively weak but specific 5HT uptake inhibitor with minimal effects on NE. It also antagonizes $5HT_{1A}$, $5HT_{1C}$, and $5HT_2$ receptors while its active metabolite is a potent 5HT agonist. The sedating effects of trazodone are likely the result of moderate α_1 and H_1 antagonism. While half-life is approximately 5–9 h, its active metabolite has a half-life of 4–14 h. Drowsiness is its most frequently reported side-effect [28]. Trazodone is commonly used off-label to treat insomnia at doses of 25–150 mg. Well-controlled studies evaluating efficacy in insomnia are limited and there are no published studies on primary insomnia [29]. PSG studies indicate trazodone decreases sleep latency and increases slow-wave sleep, but effects on sleep continuity are inconsistent. Trazodone impairs performance in healthy individuals [30], but data on depressed individuals are inconclusive.

Nefazodone is structurally similar to trazodone, but its affinity for α_1 receptors is less and it has no affinity for H_1 receptors [26]. Thus it is less consistently sedating than trazodone. None the less, somnolence is a frequently reported side-effect. Objective data are limited.

Table 34.2 Half-life and receptor pharmacology of sedating antidepressant drugs[1,2,3]

Drug	Drug Class	Half-life (hours)	5HT reuptake	NE reuptake	α_1 antagonism	M antagonism	H_1 antagonism	$5HT_2$ receptor antagonism	Other effects
Amitriptyline	Tricyclic, tertiary	5–45	++	+	+++	+++	++	+	
Clomipramine	Tricyclic, tertiary	15–60	+++	+	+++	+++	+	+	
Doxepin	Tricyclic, tertiary	10–25	0/+	+	+++	++	+++	+	
Imipramine	Tricyclic, tertiary	5–30	+++	+	++	++	+	0/+	
Trimipramine	Tricyclic, tertiary	15–40	0	0	+++	++	+++	+	
Nortriptyline	Tricyclic, secondary	15–35	+	++	++	+	++	+	
Amoxapine	Tetracyclic	6–30	0/+	+	++	0	+	+	
Trazodone	Phenylpiperazine	3–14	+	0	++	0	+	++	$5\text{-}HT_{1A}$, $5\text{-}HT_{1C}$, α_2 antagonism
Nefazodone	Phenylpiperazine	2–18	++	0/+	+	0	0	++	
Mirtazapine	Noradrenergic and specific serotonergic antidepressant	20–40	0	0/+	+	+	+++	++	$5\text{-}HT_1$, α_2 antagonism

[1] References: [18, 26, 32].
[2] Strength of effect is indicated relative to other drugs in table; "0" indicates no significant effect.
[3] Abbreviations: NE, Norepinephrine; 5HT, Serotonin; α, Alpha adrenergic; M, Muscarinic cholinergic; H, Histamine.

Table 34.3 Half-life and receptor pharmacology of antispychotic drugs[1,2,3]

Drug	Half-life (h)	D1	D2	5HT$_2$	M	α1	H$_1$	5HT$_{1A}$
Typical								
Chlorpromazine	18–40	+	++	+++	++	+++	+	0
Haloperidol	18–40	+++	+++	+	0	++	0	0
Thioridazine	18–40	+	+	++	++	+++	+	0
Atypical								
Aripiprazole	75–94	+	+++	++	0	++	++	+++
Clozapine	12	++	+	+++	+++	+++	+++	+
Olanzapine	36	+++	++	+++	+++	++	+++	0
Quetiapine	6	+	+	+	0	+++	++	+
Risperidone	3	++	++	+++	0	+++	+	+
Ziprasidone	7	+	++	+++	0	++	++	+++

[1] References [37, 38, 39].
[2] Receptor binding strength is given relative to other drugs in table; "0" indicates no significant effect.
[3] Abbreviations: D, dopamine; 5HT, serotonin; M, muscarinic anticholinergic.

Mirtazapine disinhibits both 5HT and NE via blockade of $α_2$ receptors [31]. It is a potent antagonist of H$_1$ and 5HT$_2$ receptors, which likely accounts for its highly sedating activity [32]. Limited PSG studies indicate improvements in sleep latency and sleep continuity [33, 34]. Mirtazapine impairs driving performance and attention acutely in normals [35].

While selective serotonin reuptake inhibitors (SSRIs) and selective norepinephrine reuptake inhibitors (SNRIs) are more likely to be associated with subjective reports of insomnia, sedation is sometimes reported. PSG studies generally show sleep disruption and REM suppression [36]. Daytime impairment is not commonly reported.

Antipsychotics

Antipsychotic drugs have complex pharmacological profiles (Table 34.3) [37–39]. Sedation is more likely in drugs with relatively more potent antagonism of H$_1$, $α_1$, or 5HT$_2$ receptors.

Among the older drugs, chlorpromazine and thioridazine appear to be more sedating than haloperidol, probably because of H$_1$ antagonism. Clozapine, which is a strong antagonist of H$_1$, $α_1$, and 5HT$_{2a}$, is even more sedating [40], while aripiprazole is the least sedating among the second-generation drugs.

While ziprasidone and quetiapine would be expected to be sedating given their pharmacological profiles, they appear less sedating than other drugs, possibly because of their short half-lives. Olanzapine and quetiapine have been used as hypnotics in non-psychotic patients. Small-sample studies indicate that olanzapine, quetiapine, and ziprasidone decrease nocturnal sleep latency and improve sleep continuity [37, 41, 42]. Uncontrolled studies suggest that clozapine, haloperidol, and risperidone also improve sleep [43]. There are no studies that objectively evaluate daytime sleepiness. Although antipsychotics cause cognitive impairment in healthy subjects [44], some of these drugs may improve cognitive function in patients despite significant sedation, presumably because of treatment of the underlying disorder [45].

Antiepileptic drugs

Sedation is one of the most common adverse effects of antiepileptic drugs [46]. For many of these drugs the mechanism for sedation involves effects on GABA (agonism, reuptake inhibition, GABA transaminase inhibition) [47]. Sedation is most common with the older drug phenobarbital, but is also quite frequent with carbamazapine and phenytoin, and slightly less common with newer drugs [48]. Some of the newer drugs have multiple mechanisms of action which has led to their use in other disorders such as neuropathic pain, fibromyalgia, migraine, restless legs syndrome, anxiety, schizophrenia, bipolar disorder, and insomnia [49]. Lamotrigine, which has an unknown mechanism of action, has been approved for treatment of bipolar disorder. Topiramate, while approved for seizures, has been evaluated for depression, psychotic disorders, eating disorders, and substance use disorders, in addition to neuropathic pain. Topiramate has multiple pharmacological properties including increasing GABA possibly by activating a site on the GABAa receptor and enhancement of GABA-activated chloride channels. Tiagabine, which inhibits GABA uptake and binds to H_1, $5HT_{1B}$, benzodiazepine, and chloride channel receptors, has been evaluated for insomnia. Gabapentin and pregabalin are used frequently to treat neuropathic pain and fibromyalgia, but have also been used for insomnia, bipolar disorder, migraine, and periodic limb movement disorder. Gabapentin and pregabalin are structural analogue of GABA but do not bind to either $GABA_A$ or $GABA_B$ receptors, are not converted into GABA or GABA agonists, and do not inhibit GABA reuptake [50]. Both drugs bind to the α_2-δ subunit of presynaptic voltage-gated calcium channels resulting in decreased excitatory neurotransmitter release. Sedation is reported to occur in 15–25% of patients using these drugs to treat neuropathic pain [51, 52].

PSG studies show that the older antiepileptic drugs generally decrease sleep latency and improve sleep continuity [53], while the newer drugs show variable effects, with some increasing slow-wave sleep [54]. Studies of tiagabine in primary insomnia show dose-dependent increases in slow-wave sleep but inconsistent effects on total sleep time and sleep efficiency [55, 56]. Gabapentin and pregabalin improve subjective sleep quality in patients treated for pain [57].

Compared to healthy controls or patients with untreated epilepsy, patients on phenobarbital, carbamazepine, phenytoin, or valproate have shown increased sleepiness on MSLT or decreased alertness on a wake maintenance test [58–60]. Similar studies with the newer drugs levetiracetam [61], gabapentin, and topiramate [58] showed no change in daytime assessments of sleepiness or alertness. Impairment in short-term memory, concentration, and attention appear to be more common with the older drugs, particularly phenobarbital and phenytoin, while the newer drugs appear to have few negative effects with the exception of topiramate [62, 63]. Placebo-controlled studies are needed to confirm these findings, however.

Antihistamines

Drugs currently classified as antihistamines are not truly histamine antagonists but inverse agonists, as they stabilize the receptor in its inactive state [64]. Among the classic antihistamines, drugs have been divided into two groups by their sedative potential. First-generation H_1 antihistamines (chlorpheniramine, cyproheptadine, diphenhydramine, doxylamine, hydroxyzine, meclizine, and promethazine) are lipophilic molecules which easily cross the blood–brain barrier, demonstrating H_1 receptor occupancy of up to 60% or more [65, 66]. In addition to H_1 antagonism, they show muscarinic cholinergic and α-adrenergic antagonism and also affect 5HT transmission which may also influence sedation. Elimination half-lives range from 4–8 h for diphenhydramine to 20–27 h for hydroxyzine and chlorpheniramine; doxylamine has a half-life of 10 h. Second-generation antihistamines (cetirizine, desloratadine, fexofenadine, levocetirizine, loratadine) are hydrophilic molecules which do not easily penetrate the central nervous system. Although they are much more selective than the first-generation antihistamines, H_1 receptor occupancy varies from almost negligible (e.g. fexofenadine) to 30% (cetirizine) [67].

Most over-the-counter drugs marketed as hypnotics or combination analgesic–hypnotics contain diphenhydramine; some contain doxylamine. Studies evaluating efficacy of diphenhydramine in treating insomnia show mixed results [68, 69]. However, typical daytime dosing used for treatment of seasonal or environmental allergy symptoms, results in increased physiological sleep tendency as measured by MSLT and decreased performance [70, 71]. While these studies suggest that tolerance may develop within three to four days, there is evidence that driving performance may continue to be impaired [72]. Other first-generation antihistamines are less well studied.

The second-generation antihistamines are generally non-sedating and less likely to impair performance when used in recommended doses [73, 74]. However, consistent with its higher degree of H_1 receptor occupancy, cetirizine appears to produce more subjective sedation and performance impairment than fexofenadine [67].

While histamine-2 (H_2) antagonists have limited central nervous system activity, sedation may emerge with increase in dose [75] or interaction with other drugs. For example, cimetidine slows the clearance of some benzodiazepine receptor agonists which may make carry-over effects of hypnotics more of a problem. Benzodiazepine-produced impairment of psychomotor and cognitive function was prolonged with concomitant administration of cimetidine and ranitidine in healthy volunteers [76].

Antihypertensive drugs

Both sedation and insomnia have been reported with some antihypertensive drugs and may be caused by effects on adrenergic receptors involved in sleep–wake regulation. Sedation is the most common side-effect of the α_2 agonists clonidine and methyldopa, occurring in 30–75% of patients, but tolerance may develop over time [77]. Increased nocturnal sleep time has been shown in healthy subjects given clonidine acutely [78], but there are no studies which quantify daytime sedation objectively. However, microsleeps were reported in one study of a single morning dose of clonidine in young healthy subjects [79]. While both disturbed sleep and sedation have been reported with beta antagonists, central nervous system effects are relatively infrequent and appear to be more likely with non-selective beta-antagonists [80] (e.g. propranolol) which also have higher affinity for 5HT receptors [81]. Fatigue or sedation have been reported, at least transiently, in beta antagonists with vasodilating properties which also block α_1 receptors (e.g. carvedilol, labetolol) [82] and with α_1 antagonists (e.g. prazosin, terazosin).

Dopamine agonists

Daytime sleepiness is a common complaint in patients with Parkinson's disease and likely has multiple causes, including abnormalities in sleep–wake regulation caused by the disease, comorbid sleep and medical disorders, or medications. The principal drugs used to treat Parkinson's disease are levodopa/carbidopa and dopamine agonists. Dopamine agonists differ somewhat in their selectivity for dopamine receptor classes and subtypes [83]. The ergot agonists pergolide and apomorphine have both D_1 and D_2 agonist activity while the non-ergot agonists pramipexole, ropinirole, and rotigotine are selective for D_2 and have higher specificity for the D_3 subtype than the D_2 subtype.

Both ergot and non-ergot drugs have been associated with increases in daytime sleepiness, including sudden "sleep attacks" [84, 85]. While increased sleepiness with higher drug doses [86, 87] suggests a drug effect, higher doses are associated with more advanced disease. MSLT studies in patients indicate no differences in sleepiness among various dopamine agonists including pramipexole, ropinirole, bromocriptine, or pergolide [88–90]. However, somnolence and fatigue have been reported by healthy individuals [91] and non-Parkinson patients treated for restless legs symptoms with pramipexole or ropinirole [92]. In addition, two small studies in normals showed decreased mean MSLT latency with both pramipexole [93] and ropinirole [94] but not bromocriptine [93]. The mechanism for sedation is unclear, as enhanced dopaminergic transmission is generally associated with wakefulness. However, molecular genetic and pharmacologic studies in animals suggest that stimulation of post-synaptic D_1 and D_2 receptors facilitate arousal while activation of D_3 receptors induces sedation [95]. Relative receptor activation may also play a role as animal studies indicate that low doses of D_2 agonists appear more likely to induce sedation while higher doses increase wake.

Pain medications

The neurobiology of pain is complex and involves both peripheral and central mechanisms. Multiple neurotransmitters modulate pain processing, including substance P, endorphins (via mu opioid receptors), norepinephrine (α_2 adrenoceptors), and serotonin ($5HT_{1b/d}$ and $5HT_3$ receptors) [96]. Drugs used in the treatment of pain include analgesics (non-steroidal anti-inflammatory drugs and opiates), antidepressants (particularly TCAs and SNRIs), antiepileptics, and skeletal muscle relaxants [97, 98]. The antidepressant duloxetine is approved for treatment of diabetic neuropathy and the antiepileptic drugs gabapentin and pregabalin (discussed further in the section on antiepileptic drugs) are approved for treatment of post-herpetic neuralgia. Pregabalin is also approved for treatment of peripheral neuropathy and fibromyalgia.

Opioids act at multiple central nervous system receptors, including mu, kappa, delta, and nociceptin/orphanin FQ [99]. While all of these receptor subtypes appear to be involved in the analgesic effect of opioids, the mechanism for sedation involves mu and kappa receptors [100]. The mu subtype is also involved in respiratory control. The most common clinically used opioids are relatively selective for mu receptors. Opioid peptides (enkephalins, endorphins, dynorphins) are involved in the regulation of blood pressure, respiration, mood, pain perception, and possibly sleep [101]. Somnolence is a common side-effect of opioid medication [102], and varies with drug dose, duration of use, age, and severity of underlying disease [103, 104]. Morphine, oxycodone, codeine, and fentanyl have half-lives of 2–5 h, levorphanol 12–16 h, and methadone 24 h. Tramadol, meperidine and propoxyphene have active metabolites which extend their half-lives to 6–9, 14–21, and 30–40 h, respectively. Limited PSG data indicate that opioids used acutely in young healthy individuals have no effect on total sleep time or wake after sleep onset but markedly decrease slow-wave sleep [105], and may decrease REM in higher doses [106]. In current or former addicts opioids decrease total sleep time and increase wake after sleep onset [107]. Data evaluating sleepiness objectively are limited. Epidemiologic studies suggest an increased risk for vehicle accidents in patients using prescription opiate medications [108–110].

The most serious adverse effect of opioids is respiratory depression, especially during sleep or following surgery. Limited data suggest that clinically significant respiratory depression is rare in healthy individuals using standard doses acutely [111]. However, central sleep apnea is common with chronic opioid use [112] and sustained hypoxemia during sleep is more likely in patients with pulmonary disease or obstructive sleep apnea [113, 114].

Skeletal muscle relaxants have diverse pharmacological profiles [115], but most have central nervous system effects and cause sedation [116]. These drugs have similar onset of action (generally 30–60 min) but elimination half-life ranges from 1 h (methocarbamol) to over 18 h (cyclobenzaprine). Antispastic agents include baclofen, a $GABA_B$ receptor agonist, and tizanadine, a centrally acting α_2 agonist. Antispasmodic drugs include cyclobenzaprine, which is structurally similar to amitriptyline and exhibits anticholinergic, noradrenergic, and $5HT_2$ antagonist activity; orphenadrine which is structurally similar to diphenhydramine and binds to both H_1 receptors and NMDA receptors; and a number of drugs with unknown mechanisms of action but which depress the central nervous system. These include metaxolone, methocarbamol, and carisoprodol which is metabolized to meprobamate. While sedation is a frequently cited adverse event, there are no studies objectively evaluating sleep, sleepiness, or cognitive function.

Triptans, which are selective $5HT_{1B/D}$ agonists, are the primary treatment for acute migraine. Sedation is a common side-effect and more likely with lipophilic drugs with active metabolites (e.g. eletriptan, zolmitriptan, rizatriptan) [117].

Alcohol

Alcohol is initially stimulating at low to moderate doses while plasma concentration is rising to peak levels, but is sedating at higher doses and following peak concentration [118]. Degree of sedation depends on dose and time of ingestion and is potentiated by prior sleep loss and concomitant use of sedating drugs [119]. The principal mechanism for sedation is via $GABA_A$ receptor binding.

Alcohol is commonly used as a sleep aid. When ingested acutely by non-alcoholics within an hour of bedtime, low to moderate doses of alcohol decrease sleep latency and increase total sleep time during the first part of the night. However, sleep is disrupted during the latter part of the night, likely the result of withdrawal as alcohol is rapidly metabolized. Alcohol-induced sleep disruption may decrease next-day alertness and performance [120]. Tolerance to the initial sedation may develop within a few nights. In alcoholics, sleep onset during periods of drinking may be rapid but sleep duration is short and fragmented. Disrupted sleep may persist for long periods during abstinence [121].

MSLT studies indicate increased sleep latency at peak breath concentration but decreased latencies (increased sleepiness) as alcohol concentration falls [118], accompanied by impaired performance which persists at least 2 h following complete alcohol metabolism [122]. Increased basal sleepiness as a result of sleep restriction/deprivation or circadian time interacts with alcohol to worsen sleepiness and performance impairment [119]. Alcohol increases risk for motor vehicle accidents [109, 110].

Conclusions

Sleepiness is a common side-effect of drugs which act on the central nervous system. Drugs cause sedation via effects on the neural systems involved in sleep–wake regulation, primarily by increasing GABA or inhibiting histamine, norepinephrine, or serotonin. Important factors affecting degree of sedation include receptor binding profile, dose, half-life, and time of administration. The consequences of daytime sleepiness which include impaired performance and increased risk of accidents must be considered when prescribing these medications.

References

1. **Saper C B**, **Scammell T**, **Lu J**. Hypothalamic regulation of sleep and circadian rhythms. *Nature*, 2005; **437**:1257–63.
2. **Monti J**, **Jantos H**. The roles of dopamine and serotonin, and of their receptors, in regulating sleep and waking. *Prog Brain Res*, 2008; **172**:625–46.
3. **Szabadi E**. Drugs for sleep disorders: mechanisms and therapeutic prospects. *Br J Clin Pharmacol*, 2006; **61**:761–66.
4. **Vermeeren A**. Residual effects of hypnotics: epidemiology and clinical implications. *CNS Drugs*, 2004; **18**:297–328.
5. **Roehrs T**, **Kribbs N**, **Zorick F**, *et al*. Hypnotic residual effects of benzodiazepines with repeated administration. *Sleep*, 1986; **9**:309–17.
6. **Verster J C**, **Veldhuijzen D S**, **Volkerts E R**. Residual effects of sleep medication on driving ability. *Sleep Med Rev*, 2004; **8**:309–25.
7. **Vermeeren A**, **Danjou P E**, **O'Hanlon J F**. Residual effects of evening and middle-of-the-night administration of zaleplon 10 and 20 mg on memory and actual driving performance. *Hum Psychopharmacol*, 1998; **13**(Suppl 2):S98–107.
8. **Zammit G**, **Corser B**, **Dohramji K**, *et al*. Sleep and residual sedation after administration of zaleplon, zolpidem, and placebo during experimental middle-of-the-night awakening. *J Clin Sleep Med*, 2006; **2**:417–23.
9. **Seidel W F**, **Cohen S A**, **Wilson L**, *et al*. Effects of alprazolam and diazepam on the daytime sleepiness of non-anxious subjects. *Psychopharmacology*, 1985; **87**:194–97.
10. **O'Hanlon J F**, **Vermeeren A**, **Uiterwijk M M C**, *et al*. Anxiolytics' effects on the actual driving performance of patients and healthy volunteers in a standardized test. *Neuropsychobiology*, 1995; **31**:81–88.
11. **Neutel C I**. Risk of traffic accident injury after a prescription for a benzodiazepine. *Ann Epidemiol*, 1995; **5**:239–44.
12. **Neutel C I**. Benzodiazepine-related traffic accidents in young and elderly drivers. *Hum Psychopharmacol*, 1998; **13**(Suppl 2):S115–23.
13. **Barbone F**, **McMahon A D**, **Davey P G** *et al*. Association of road-traffic accidents with benzodiazepine use. *Lancet*, 1998; **352**:1331–36.
14. **Eison A S**, **Temple D L**. Buspirone: review of its pharmacology and current perspectives on its mechanism of action. *Am J Med*, 1986; **80**(Suppl 3):61–68.
15. **Walsh J K**, **Schweitzer P K**. Ten-year trends in the pharmacological treatment of insomnia. *Sleep*, 1999; **22**:371–75.
16. **Walsh J K**. Drugs used to treat insomnia in 2002: regulatory-based rather than evidence-based medicine. *Sleep*, 2004; **27**:1441–42.
17. **Maurer I**, **Volz H**. Cell-mediated side effects of psychopharmacological treatment. *Arzneimittelforschung*, 2001; **51**:785–92.
18. **Nelson J C**. Tricyclic and tetracyclic drugs. In: Schatzberg A, Nemeroff C, Eds. *The American Psychiatric Publishing Textbook of Psychopharmacology*. Washington, DC: American Psychiatric Publishing, 2009: 263–87.
19. **Roth T**, **Rogowski R**, **Hull S**, *et al*. Efficacy and safety of doxepin 1 mg, 3 mg, and 6 mg in adults with primary insomnia. *Sleep*, 2007; **30**:1555–61.
20. **Rudorfer M V**, **Potter W Z**. Metabolism of tricyclic antidepressants. *Cell Mol Neurobiol*, 1999; **19**:373–409.
21. **Mayers A G**, **Baldwin D S**. Antidepressants and their effect on sleep. *Hum Psychopharmacol*, 2005; **20**:533–59.
22. **Wilson S**, **Argyropoulos S**. Antidepressants and sleep. A qualitative review of the literature. *Drugs*, 2006; **65**:927–47.
23. **Brunnauer A**, **Laux G**, **Geiger E**, *et al*. Antidepressants and driving ability: results from a clinical study. *J Clin Psychiatry*, 2006; **67**:1776–81.
24. **Volz H-P**, **Sturm Y**. Antidepressant drugs and psychomotor performance. *Neuropsychobiology*, 1995; **31**:146–55.
25. **Sakulsripong M**, **Curran H V**, **Lader M**. Does tolerance develop to the sedative and amnesic effects of antidepressants? A comparison of amitriptyline, trazodone and placebo. *Eur J Clin Pharmacol*, 1991; **40**:43–48.
26. **Golden R N**, **Dawkins K**, **Nicholas L**. Trazadone and Nefazodone. In: Schatzberg A, Nemeroff C, Eds. *The American Psychiatric Publishing Textbook of Psychopharmacology*. Washington, DC: American Psychiatric Publishing, 2009: 403–14.
27. **Caccia S**. Metabolism of the newer antidepressants. An overview of the pharmacological and pharmacokinetic implications. *Clin Pharmacokinet*, 1998; **34**:281–302.

28. **Cunningham L A**, **Borison R L**, **Carman J S**, et al. A comparison of venlafaxine, trazodone, and placebo in major depression. *J Clin Psychopharmacol*, 1994; **14**:99–106.

29. **Mendelson W B**. A review of the evidence for the efficacy and safety of trazodone in insomnia. *J Clin Psychiatry*, 2005; **66**:469–76.

30. **Hindmarch I**, **Kerr J**. Behavioural toxicity of antidepressants with particular reference to moclobemide. *Psychopharmacology*, 1992; **106**:S49–55.

31. **De Boer T**. The pharmacologic profile of mirtazapine. *J Clin Psychiatry*, 1996; **57**(Suppl 4):19–25.

32. **Schatzberg A F**. Mirtazapine. In: Schatzberg A, Nemeroff C, Eds. *The American Psychiatric Publishing Textbook of Psychopharmacology*. Washington, DC: American Psychiatric Publishing, 2009: 429–37.

33. **Ruigt G S**, **Kemp B**, **Groenhout C M**, et al. Effect of the antidepressant Org 3770 on human sleep. *Eur J Clin Pharmacol*, 1990; **38**:551–54.

34. **Winokur A**, **DeMartinis NA** 3rd, **McNally D P**, et al. Comparative effects of mirtazapine and fluoxetine on sleep physiology measures in patients with major depression and insomnia. *J Clin Psychiatry*, 2003; **64**:1224–29.

35. **Wingen M**, **Bothmer J**, **Langer S**, et al. Actual driving performance and psychomotor function in healthy subjects after acute and subchronic treatment with escitalopram, mirtazapine, and placebo: a crossover trial. *J Clin Psychiatry*, 2005; **66**:436–43.

36. **DeMartinis N A**, **Winokur A**. Effects of psychiatric medications on sleep and sleep disorders. *CNS Neuroll Dis Drug Targets*, 2007; **6**:17–29.

37. **Krystal A**, **Goforth H**, **Roth T**. Effects of antipsychotic medications on sleep in schizophrenia. *Int Clin Psychopharmacol*, 2008; **23**:150–60.

38. **Nasrallah H A**, **Tandon R**. Classic antipsychotic medications. In: Schatzberg A, Nemeroff C, Eds. *The American Psychiatric Publishing Textbook of Psychopharmacology*. Washington, DC: American Psychiatric Publishing, 2009: 533–54.

39. **Buckley P F**, **Foster A E**. Quetiapine. In: Schatzberg A, Nemeroff C, Eds. *The American Psychiatric Publishing Textbook of Psychopharmacology*. Washington, DC: American Psychiatric Publishing, 2009: 599–612.

40. **Fitton A**, **Heel R C**. Clozapine: a review of its pharmacological properties and therapeutic use in schizophrenia. *Drugs*, 1990; **40**:722–47.

41. **Sharpley A L**, **Vassallo C M**, **Cowen P J**. Olanzapine increases slow-wave sleep: evidence for blockade of central 5-HT(2C) receptors in vivo. *Biol Psychiatry*, 2000; **47**:468–70.

42. **Cohrs S**. Sleep disturbance in patients with schizophrenia: impact and effect of antipsychotics. *CNS Drugs*, 2008; **22**:939–62.

43. **Wetter T C**, **Lauer C J**, **Gillich G**, et al. The electroencephalographic sleep pattern in schizophrenic patients treated with clozapine or classical antipsychotic drugs. *J Psychiatr Res*, 1996; **30**:411–19.

44. **Vitiello B**, **Martin A**, **Hill J**, et al. Cognitive and behavioral effects of cholinergic, dopaminergic, and serotonergic blockade in humans. *Neuropsychopharmacology*, 1997; **16**:15–24.

45. **Meltzer H**, **McGurk S**. The effects of clozapine, risperidone, and olanzapine on cognitive function in schizophrenia. *Schizophrenia Bull*, 1999; **25**:233–55.

46. **Kennedy G M**, **Lhatoo S D**. CNS adverse events associated with antiepileptic drugs. *CNS Drugs*, 2008; **22**:739–60.

47. **Sammaritano M**, **Sherwin A**. Effect of anticonvulsants on sleep. *Neurology*, 2000; **54**:S16–24.

48. **Malow B A**, **Bowes R J**, **Lix X**. Predictors of sleepiness in epilepsy patients. *Sleep*, 1997; **20**:1105–10.

49. **Johannessen Landmark C**. Antiepileptic drugs in non-epilepsy disorders. *CNS Drugs*, 2008; **22**:27–47.

50. **Frye M A**, **Moore K M**. Gabapentin and pregabalin. In: Schatzberg A, Nemeroff C, Eds. *The American Psychiatric Publishing Textbook of Psychopharmacology*. Washington, DC: American Psychiatric Publishing, 2009: 767–79.

51. **Guay D R**. Pregabalin in neuropathic pain: a more "pharmaceutically elegant" gabapentin? *Am J Geriatr Pharmacother*, 2005; **3**:274–87.

52. **Arnold L M**, **Goldenberg D L**, **Stanford S B**, et al. Gabapentin in the treatment of fibromyalgia: a randomized, double-blind, placebo-controlled, multicenter trial. *Arthritis Rheum*, 2007; **56**:1336–44.

53. **Bazil C W**. Effects of antiepileptic drugs on sleep structure. Are all drugs equal? *CNS Drugs*, 2003; **17**:719–28.

54. **Sammaritano M**, **Sherwin A**. Effect of anticonvulsants on sleep. *Neurology*, 2000; **54**:S16–24.

55. **Walsh J K**, **Zammit G**, **Schweitzer P K**, et al. Tiagabine enhances slow wave sleep and sleep maintenance in primary insomnia. *Sleep Med*, 2006; **7**:155–61.

56. **Walsh J K**, **Perlis M**, **Rosenthal M**, et al. Tiagabine increases slow-wave sleep in a dose-dependent fashion without affecting traditional efficacy measures in adults with primary insomnia. *J Clin Sleep Med*, 2006; **2**:35–41.

57. **Gilron I**. Gabapentin and pregabalin for chronic neuropathic and early postsurgical pain: current

evidence and future directions. *Curr Opin Anaesthesiol*, 2007; **20**:456–72.

58. **Salinsky M**, **Storzbach D**, **Oken B**, *et al*. Topiramate effects on the EEG and alertness in healthy volunteers: a different profile of antiepileptic drug neurotoxicity. *Epilepsy Behav*, 2007; **10**:463–69.

59. **Roeder-Wanner U U**, **Noachter S**, **Wolf P**. Response of polygraphic sleep to phenytoin treatment for epilepsy: a longitudinal study of immediate, short- and long-term effects. *Acta Neurol Scand*, 1987; **76**:157–67.

60. **Palm L**, **Anderson H**, **Elmqvist D**, *et al*. Daytime sleep tendency before and after discontinuation of antiepileptic drugs in preadolescent children with epilepsy. *Epilepsia*, 1992; **33**:687–91.

61. **Cicolin A**, **Magliola U**, **Giordano**, *et al*. Effects of levetiracetam on nocturnal sleep and daytime vigilance in healthy volunteers. *Epilepsia*, 2006; **47**:82–85.

62. **Manni R**, **Ratti M T**, **Perucca E**, *et al*. A multiparametric investigation of daytime sleepiness and psychomotor function in epileptic patients treated with phenobarbital and sodium valproate: a comparative controlled study. *Electroencephalogr Clin Neurophysiol*, 1993; **86**:322–28.

63. **Martin R**, **Kuzniecky R**, **Ho S**, *et al*. Cognitive effects of topiramate, gabapentin, and lamotrigine in healthy young adults. *Neurology*, 1999; **52**:321–27.

64. **Timmerman H**, **Leurs R**, **Brann M R**, *et al*. In vitro pharmacology of clinically used central nervous system-active drugs as inverse H1 receptor agonists. *J Pharmacol Exp Ther*, 2007; **322**:172–79.

65. **Okamura N**, **Yanai K**, **Higuchi M**, *et al*. Functional neuroimaging of cognition impaired by a classical antihistamine, d-chlorpheniramine. *Br J Pharmacol*, 2000; **129**:115–23.

66. **Tashiro M**, **Mochizuki H**, **Iwabuchi K**, *et al*. Roles of histamine in regulation of arousal and cognition: functional neuroimaging of histamine H1 receptors in human brain. *Life Sci*, 2002; **72**:409–14.

67. **Tashiro M**, **Sakurada Y**, **Iwabuchi K**, *et al*. Central effects of fexofenadine and cetirizine: measurement of psychomotor performance, subjective sleepiness, and brain histamine H1-receptor occupancy using 11C-doxepin positron emission tomography. *J Clin Pharmacol*, 2004; **44**:890–900.

68. **Morin C M**, **Koetter U**, **Bastien C**, *et al*. Valerian-hops combination and diphenhydramine for treating insomnia: a randomized placebo-controlled clinical trial. *Sleep*, 2005; **28**:1465–71.

69. **Glass J R**, **Sproule B A**, **Herrmann N**, *et al*. Effects of 2-week treatment with temazepam and diphenhydramine in elderly insomniacs: a randomized, placebo-controlled trial. *J Clin Psychopharmacol*, 2008; **28**:182–88.

70. **Schweitzer P K**, **Muehlbach M J**, **Walsh J K**. Sleepiness and performance during three-day administration of cetirizine or diphenhydramine. *J Allergy Clin Immunol*, 1994; **94**:716–24.

71. **Richardson G S**, **Roehrs R A**, **Rosenthal L**, *et al*. Tolerance to daytime sedative effects of H1 antihistamines. *J Clin Psychopharmacol*, 2002; **22**:511–15.

72. **Verster J C**, **Volkerts E R**. Antihistamines and driving ability: evidence from on-the-road driving studies during normal traffic. *Ann Allergy Asthma Immunol*, 2004; **92**:294–303.

73. **Shamsi Z**, **Hindmarch I**. Sedation and antihistamines: a review of inter-drug differences using proportional impairment ratios. *Hum Psychopharmaclogy Clin Exp*, 2000; **15**:S3–30.

74. **Bender B**, **Berning S**, **Dudden R**, *et al*. Sedation and performance impairment of diphenhydramine and second-generation antihistamines: a meta-analysis. *J Allergy Clin Immunol*, 2003; **111**:770–76.

75. **Raemaekers J**, **Vermeeren A**. All antihistamines cross blood–brain barrier. *BMJ*, 2000; **321**:572.

76. **Sanders L D**, **Whitehead C**, **Gildersleve C D**, *et al*. Interaction of H2-receptor antagonists and benzodiazepine sedation. A double-blind placebo-controlled investigation of the effects of cimetidine and ranitidine on recovery after intravenous midazolam. *Anaesthesia*, 1993; **48**: 286–92.

77. **Paykel E S**, **Fleminger R**, **Watson J P**. Psychiatric side effects of antihypertensive drugs other than reserpine. *J Clin Psychopharmacol*, 1982; **2**:14–39.

78. **Kanno O**, **Clarenbach P**. Effects of clonidine and yohimbine on sleep in man: Polygraphic study and EEG analysis by normalized slope descriptors. *Electroencephalogr Clin Neurophysiol*, 1985; **60**:478–84.

79. **Carskadon M A**, **Cavallo A**, **Rosekind M R**. Sleepiness and nap sleep following a morning dose of clonidine. *Sleep*, 1989; **12**:338–44.

80. **Dahlöf C**, **Dimenäs E**. Side effects of beta-blocker treatments as related to the central nervous system. *Am J Med Sci*, 1990; **299**:236–44.

81. **Yamada Y**, **Shibuya F**, **Hamada J**, *et al*. Prediction of sleep disorders induced by adrenergic receptor blocking agents based on receptor occupancy. *J Pharmacokinet Biopharm*, 1995; **23**:131–45.

82. **Pearce C J**, **Wallin J D**. Labetalol and other agents that block both alpha- and beta-adrenergic receptors. *Cleve Clin J Med*, 1994; **61**:59–69.

83. **Kvernmo T**, **Houben J**, **Syite I**. Receptor-binding and pharmacokinetic properties of dopaminergic agonists. *Curr Top Med Chem*, 2008; **8**:1049–67.

84. Etminan M, Samii A, Takkouche B, et al. Increased risk of somnolence with the new dopamine agonists in patients with Parkinson's disease: a meta-analysis of randomised controlled trials. *Drug Saf*, 2001; **24**:863–68.

85. Happe S, Berger K. The association of dopamine agonists with daytime sleepiness, sleep problems and quality of life in patients with Parkinson's disease – a prospective study. *J Neurol*, 2001; **248**:1062–67.

86. Suzuki K, Miyamoto T, Miyamoto M, et al. Excessive daytime sleepiness and sleep episodes in Japanese patients with Parkinson's disease. *J Neurol Sci*, 2008; **271**:47–52.

87. Kaynak D, Kiziltan G, Kaynak H, et al. Sleep and sleepiness in patients with Parkinson's disease before and after dopaminergic treatment. *Eur J Neurol*, 2005; **12**:199–207.

88. Razmy A, Lang A E, Chapiro C M. Predictors of impaired daytime sleep and wakefulness in patients with Parkinson disease treated with older (ergot) vs newer (nonergot) dopamine agonists. *Arch Neurol*, 2004; **61**:97–102.

89. Roth T, Rye D B, Borchert L D, et al. Assessment of sleepiness and unintended sleep in Parkinson's disease patients taking dopamine agonists. *Sleep Med*, 2003; **4**:275–80.

90. Shpirer I, Miniovitz A, Klein C, et al. Excessive daytime sleepiness in patients with Parkinson's disease: a polysomnography study. *Mov Disord*, 2006; **21**:1432–38.

91. Hamidovic A, Kang U J, de Wit H. Effects of low to moderate acute doses of pramipexole on impulsivity and cognition in healthy volunteers. *J Clin Psychopharmacol*, 2008; **28**:45–51.

92. Baker W L, White C M, Coleman C I. Effect of nonergot dopamine agonists on symptoms of restless legs syndrome. *Ann Fam Med*, 2008; **6**:253–62.

93. Micallef J, Rey M, Eusebio A, et al. Antiparkinsonian drug-induced sleepiness: a double-blind placebo-controlled study of L-dopa, bromocriptine and pramipexole in healthy subjects. *Br J Clin Pharmacol*, 2009; **67**:333–40.

94. Ferreira J J, Galitzky M, Thalamas C, et al. Effect of ropinirole on sleep onset: a randomized, placebo-controlled study in healthy volunteers. *Neurology*, 2002; **58**:460–62.

95. Monti J M, Monti D. The involvement of dopamine in the modulation of sleep and waking. *Sleep Med Rev*, 2007; **11**:113–33.

96. Schug S, Garrett W, Gillespie G. Opioid and non-opioid analgesics. *Best Pract Res Clin Anaesthesiol*, 2003; **17**:91–110.

97. Roehrs T, Roth T. Sleep and pain: interaction of two vital functions. *Semin Neurol*, 2005; **25**:106–16.

98. Zin C, Nissen L, Smith M, et al. An update on the pharmacological management of post-herpetic neuralgia and painful diabetic neuropathy. *CNS Drugs*, 2008; **22**:417–22.

99. Gutstein H, Akil H. Opioid analgesics. In: Hardman J, Limbird L, Gilman A, Eds. *Goodman and Gilman's the Pharmacological Basis of Therapeutics* (11th Ed.). New York, NY: McGraw-Hill, 2005.

100. Schug S, Garrett W, Gillespie G. Opioid and non-opioid analgesics. *Best Pract Res Clin Anaesthesiol*, 2003; **17**:91–110.

101. Wilson L, Dorosz L. Possible role of the opioid peptides in sleep. *Med Hypotheses*, 1984; **14**:269–80.

102. Inturrisi C. Clinical pharmacology of opioids for pain. *Clin J Pain*, 2002; **18**:S3–13.

103. Clemons M, Regnard C, Appleton T. Alertness, cognition and morphine in patients with advanced cancer. *Cancer Treat Rev*, 1996; **122**:451–68.

104. Nikolaus T, Zeyfang A. Pharmacological treatments for persistent non-malignant pain in older persons. *Drugs Aging*, 2004; **21**:19–41.

105. Dimsdale J, Norman D, DeJardin D, et al. The effects of opioids on sleep architecture. *J Clin Sleep Med*, 2007; **3**:33–36.

106. Walder B, Tramer M, Blois R. The effects of two single doses of tramadol on sleep: a randomized, cross-over trial in healthy volunteers. *Eur J Anaesthesiol*, 2001; **18**:36–42.

107. Cronin A, Keifer J, Davies M, et al. Postoperative sleep disturbance: influences of opioids and pain in humans. *Sleep*, 2001; **24**:39–44.

108. Engeland A, Skurtveit S, Mørland J. Risk of road traffic accidents associated with the prescription of drugs: a registry-based cohort study. *Ann Epidemiol*, 2007; **17**:597–602.

109. Drummer O H, Gerostamoulos J, Batziris H, et al. The incidence of drugs in drivers killed in Australian road traffic crashes. *Forensic Sci Int*, 2003; **134**:154–62.

110. Mura P, Kintz P, Ludes B, et al. Comparison of the prevalence of alcohol, cannabis and other drugs between 900 injured drivers and 900 control subjects: results of a French collaborative study. *Forensic Sci Int*, 2003; **133**:79–85.

111. Wang D, Teichtahl H. Opioids, sleep architecture and sleep-disordered breathing. *Sleep Med Rev*, 2007; **11**:35–46.

112. Wang D, Teichtahl H, Drummer O, et al. Central sleep apnea in stable methadone maintenance treatment patients. *Chest*, 2005; **128**:1348–56.

113. **Farney R**, **Walker J**, **Cloward T**, *et al.* Sleep-disordered breathing associated with long-term opioid therapy. *Chest*, 2003; **123**:632–39.

114. **Catley D**, **Thornton C**, **Jordan C**, *et al.* Pronounced, episodic oxygen desaturation in the postoperative period: its association with ventilatory pattern and analgesic regimen. *Anesthesiology*, 1985; **63**:20–28.

115. **Wishart D S**, **Knox C**, **Guo A C**, *et al.* DrugBank: a knowledgebase for drugs, drug actions and drug targets. *Nucl Acids Res*, 2008; **36**(Database issue):D901–06.

116. **See S**, **Ginzburg R**. Skeletal muscle relaxants. *Pharmacotherapy*, 2008; **28**:207–13.

117. **Dodick D**, **Martin V**. Triptans and CNS side-effects: pharmacokinetic and metabolic mechanisms. *Cephalalgia*, 2004; **24**:417–24.

118. **Papineau K L**, **Roehrs T A**, **Petrucelli N**, *et al.* Electrophysiological assessment (The Multiple Sleep Latency Test) of the biphasic effects of ethanol in humans. *Alcohol Clin Exp Res*, 1998; **22**:231–35.

119. **Roehrs T**, **Roth T**. Sleep, sleepiness, sleep disorders and alcohol use and abuse. *Sleep Med Rev*, 2001; **5**:287–97.

120. **Roehrs T**, **Yoon J**, **Roth T**. Nocturnal and next-day effects of ethanol and basal level of sleepiness. *Hum Psychopharmacol*, 1991; **6**:307–11.

121. **Colrain I**, **Turlington S**, **Baker F**. Impact of alcoholism on sleep architecture and EEH power spectra in men and women. *Sleep*, 2009; **32**:1341–52.

122. **Roehrs T**, **Claiborue D**, **Knox M**, *et al.* Residual sedating effects of ethanol. *Alcohol Clin Exp Res*, 1994; **18**:831–34.

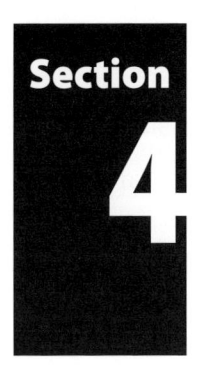

Section 4: Therapy of Excessive Sleepiness

Section 4 Chapter 35

Therapy of Excessive Sleepiness

Amphetamines, methylphenidate and excessive sleepiness

Una D. McCann

History

Amphetamine is a synthetic sympathomimetic stimulant that bears close structural similarity to the endogenous compounds, epinephrine and norepinephrine (Figure 35.1a–c). The word "amphetamine" is an acronym for **a**lpha-**m**ethyl**phe**nethyl**amine** [1]. It was first synthesized in 1887, by the Romanian chemist Lazăr Edeleanu, who named the compound phenylisopropylamine [2]. Amphetamine is the basic structural element in a number of centrally active compounds that are collectively known as "amphetamines" and that range in activity from central stimulants to hallucinogens [3]. Amphetamines that are approved for use for the treatment of narcolepsy include dextroamphetamine (the more active D-isomer of racemic amphetamine), racemic amphetamine, and various combinations of D-amphetamine and racemic amphetamine. The American Academy of Sleep Medicine's Practice Parameters for the Treatment of Narcolepsy and Other Hypersomnias of Central Origin [4] indicate that methamphetamine (Figure 35.1d) is also an effective treatment. However, use of methamphetamine for this purpose is off-label. Brand names of the drugs in the United States that contain, or metabolize into, amphetamine include Adderall, Vyvanse, and Dexedrine. The brand name for methamphetamine is Desoxyn.

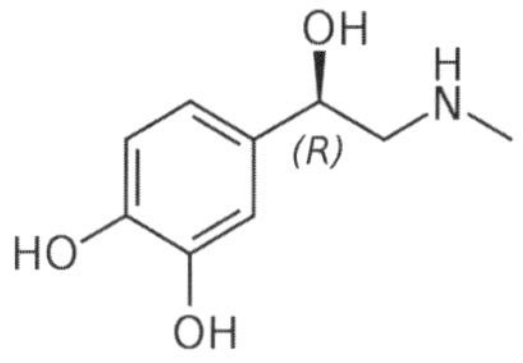

Although initially synthesized in 1887, no clinical use was found for amphetamine until 1927, when the chemist and psychopharmacologist Gordon Alles, while working with the allergist George Piness, re-synthesized it in search of an artificial replacement for ephedrine. The bronchodilator and hypertensive properties of amphetamines, as well as their ability to reverse barbiturate anesthesia, were recognized shortly

Figure 35.1a

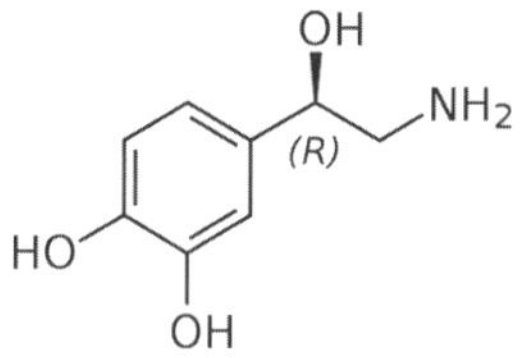

Figure 35.1b

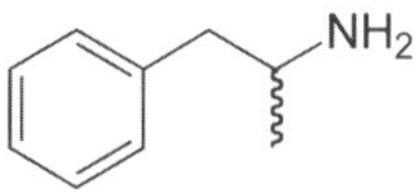

Figure 35.1c

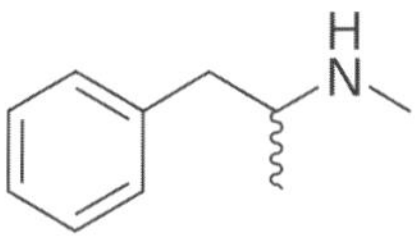

Figure 35.1d

thereafter, and amphetamines were marketed as nasal inhalers to relieve nasal congestion [5].

Between 1932 and 1946, the pharmaceutical industry developed a list of more than three dozen accepted clinical uses for amphetamines, including the treatment of schizophrenia, morphine and codeine addiction, tobacco smoking, heart block, head injuries, infantile cerebral palsy, radiation sickness, low blood pressure, and seasickness [5, 6]. Many of the purported benefits of amphetamines were false or exaggerated, a problem that was compounded by the fact that amphetamines were promoted as lacking a risk for addiction. It took several decades for the abuse

Sleepiness: Causes, Consequences and Treatment, ed. Michael J. Thorpy and Michel Billiard. Published by Cambridge University Press. © Cambridge University Press 2011.

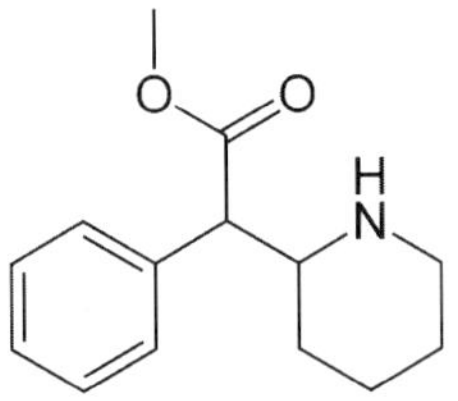

Figure 35.2

liability, addictive properties, and psychiatric side-effects of the amphetamines to be fully recognized [7]. Amphetamine and methamphetamine are both Schedule II compounds.

Interest in the utility of amphetamines for various ailments by both the medical and lay communities in the 1930s to the 1950s, and the availability of various amphetamines in both oral and intravenous preparations set the stage for a series of epidemics of amphetamine abuse and addiction in the United States and abroad. Methamphetamine abuse and addiction continues to be a major public health threat worldwide [8].

Methylphenidate is another central psychostimulant that is approved for the treatment of narcolepsy, and that is also used for other causes of excessive daytime sleepiness (Figure 35.2). Methylphenidate bears some structural similarities to the amphetamines, but is a member of the piperidine class of compounds.

Methylphenidate was first synthesized in 1944 and its stimulant effects were identified a decade later. It is currently the most commonly prescribed psychostimulant, principally for the treatment of attention deficit hyperactivity disorder. It is also approved for the treatment of narcolepsy, and is used off-label for the treatment of other types of centrally based excessive daytime sleepiness [4]. Many patients prefer methylphenidate to other psychostimulants because of its short half-life. Methylphenidate is available in both oral and patch formulations. Brand names for methylphenidate include Ritalin, Attenta, Focalin, Methylin, Metadate, Equasym, Rubifen, Motiron, Stimdate, Concerta, Biphentin and Daytrana.

Like the amphetamines, methylphenidate has abuse potential. A recent systematic review of the literature provided consistent evidence that methylphenidate is misused, largely in older adolescents and college students [9]. Less difficult to discern is the underlying motivation for methylphenidate misuse. In particular, in addition to euphorigenic effects, reasons that have been cited for methylphenidate misuse include studying, staying awake and improved alertness, in addition to "getting high/partying" and experimenting [9].

Despite the abuse liability of amphetamine, dextroamphetamine and methamphetamine, all three agents are effective for the treatment of excessive daytime sleepiness of central origin. As stated in a recent American Academy of Sleep Medicine report [4], these compounds have a long history of effective use in clinical practice but have limited information available on benefit-to-risk ratio. The lack of these data was hypothesized to reflect the limited sources of research funding for medications available in generic form rather than clinical utility of these medications.

Mechanisms of action

Amphetamines act primarily as indirect monoaminergic agonists, by increasing intrasynaptic concentrations of central dopamine and norepinephrine through release from presynaptic terminals. In particular, amphetamines enter neurons via monoaminergic transporters (at neuronal terminals) or by diffusion. From there, they displace biogenic amines from storage vesicles, ultimately causing release of dopamine, norepinephrine and/or serotonin release into the synaptic cleft. At higher dosages, monoamine oxidase inhibition and reuptake blockade occur, with the strength of these effects differing among the various amphetamine derivatives. Amphetamines have no direct actions at monoaminergic receptors [10, 11].

In contrast to the amphetamines, methylphenidate's primary mechanism of action is related to catecholamine reuptake inhibition, rather than presynaptic release. Therefore, in a fashion similar to cocaine, methylphenidate increases synaptic catecholamines by impeding reuptake inactivation of impulse-released dopamine and norepinephrine from the synaptic cleft [12, 13].

Pharmacokinetics

Amphetamine and methamphetamine are well absorbed from the gastrointestinal tract and are primarily metabolized through hepatic enzymatic pathways. In brief, six different chemical processes are important in the pathway of amphetamines: aromatic hydroxylation, aliphatic hydroxylation, *N*-dealkylation, oxidative deamination, *N*-oxidation, and conjugation of the nitrogen [14]. Significant amounts of methamphetamine and amphetamine are excreted unchanged, but the amount and distribution of the metabolites are dramatically influenced by urinary pH [14–17]. Under normal physiological conditions, the mean excretion of intact amphetamine and methamphetamine is approximately 30 and 43%, respectively [14, 15]. However, acidification of the urine can dramatically reduce reabsorbtion of drug, so that excretion of intact drug can range from as little as 1–2% in highly alkaline urine to as much as 74–76% in strongly acidic urine [14, 15]. Reabsorbtion of amphetamine leads to further metabolic breakdown (and increased drug half-life) leading to further variability in pharmacokinetic parameters. There are slight differences in the pharmacokinetics of the different enantiomers of amphetamine. Therefore, the formulation (as well as preparation) of the particular amphetamine compound can influence amphetamine pharmacokinetics.

Methylphenidate is nearly completely absorbed from the gastrointestinal tract in humans [18] and is very rapidly hydrolyzed at its methyl ester linkage to ritalinic acid, an inactive metabolite [19]. Methylphenidate's metabolites are primarily excreted in the urine (approximately 70%) within 48–96 h [20].

Use for the treatment of sleepiness

As reviewed elsewhere in this volume, before considering use of amphetamines or methylphenidate to treat sleepiness, it is imperative that an accurate diagnosis of a specific hypersomnia of central origin be identified. Other disorders, including sleep-disordered breathing syndromes, periodic limb movements, insufficient sleep, psychiatric disorders, medications, and circadian rhythm disorders can all mimic hypersomnia of central origin, and the underlying medical or behavioral source of sleepiness should be the target of treatment.

If it is determined that the basis for excessive daytime sleepiness is related to one of the 12 disorders that fall under the category of hypersomnia of central origin in the International Classification of Sleep Disorders, Second Edition (ICSD-2) [21], then use of psychostimulants, including the amphetamines and methylphenidate are primary modes of therapy. However, since the approval of modafinil for the treatment of narcolepsy, many clinicians consider amphetamines and methylphenidate second-line treatments because modafinil has a preferable abuse profile.

Table 35.1 Typical dosing range of amphetamines and methylphenidate for the treatment of sleepiness of central origin[1]

Stimulant compound	Usual daily doses[2]	Half-life (h)
d-amphetamine sulfate	5–60 mg (15–100 mg)	10–12
Methamphetamine HCl	5–60 mg (15–80 mg)	4–5
Methylphenidate HCl	10–60 mg (30–100 mg)	3–4

[1] Adapted from [23].
[2] Doses recommended by the American Sleep Disorders Association are listed in parentheses (usual starting dose and maximal dose recommended).

Typically, when treating a patient with amphetamines or methylphenidate for excessive daytime sleepiness, a patient is started at a low dose, with a gradual increase in dose over weeks to months until a satisfactory benefit is achieved. Interestingly, although patients will often report that stimulants lead to improved daytime alertness, objective sleep measures are never normalized [22]. Typical ranges of amphetamine, methamphetamine and methylphenidate used to treat hypersomnia of central origin are provided in Table 35.1. The final dose of stimulant varies substantially from patient to patient, and is often related to the emergence of unacceptable side-effects. The dose, formulation, and treatment should be tailored to the individual patient's needs. For example, a patient who has an occupation that requires continuous and sustained high levels of alertness may prefer continuous-release formulations of drug, whereas other patients may prefer amphetamines with short half-lives that permit naps and are free of unwanted side-effects in between dosages. Even at therapeutic dosages, symptoms such as jitteriness, headache, anxiety, irritability, excessive sweating, gastrointestinal disturbance, anorexia and increased heart rate can occur. The ultimate dosing regimen should not only take into account levels of alertness, but an individual patient's ability to tolerate side-effects. Ultimately, the regimen selected should be the optimal balance between desired and undesired effects, leading to optimal daytime functioning.

Toxicity/adverse effects

Acute toxicity

The toxic effects of amphetamines and methylphenidate are, in large part, an exaggeration of their clinically desired effects. At therapeutic dosages, amphetamines and methylphenidate lead to increased energy and alertness, increased confidence, improved mood, elevated heart rate and blood pressure, vasoconstiction, bronchodilation and mildly elevated body temperature. The extent and duration of these effects depend upon the formulation of the psychostimulant (e.g. immediate versus extended release), the dosage, and to a certain extent an individual patient's tolerance. At excessive dosages, amphetamines and methylphenidate can lead to irritability, paranoia, aggressive behavior, hyperpyrexia, arrhythmias, malignant hypertension, stroke, seizures, rhabdomyalysis, renal failure, coronary and cerebral vasospasm, cardiovascular collapse, and death [11].

Neurotoxicity

More than 25 years ago, evidence emerged indicating that methamphetamine has neurotoxic potential toward brain dopamine and/or serotonin neurons [24–27]. In particular, animals treated with repeated (or sufficiently high) doses of methamphetamine develop long-lasting depletions of dopamine and 5-HT, reductions in tyrosine hydroxylase (TH) and tryptophan hydroxylase (TPH) activity, reduced concentrations of dopamine and serotonin metabolites, reduced dopamine and serotonin transporter density, and reductions in the vesicular monoamine transporter (serotonin VMAT) (for reviews, see [28–30]). Lasting neurotoxic effects of methamphetamine have been subsequently documented in numerous rodent and primate species [31–35], with partial recovery over time [32]. Morphological studies indicate that the reductions in presynaptic dopamine and serotonin axonal markers are related to destruction of DA and serotonin axons and axon terminals [36–38], typically with sparing of nerve cell bodies [34–39] (but see [40, 41]). Silver staining studies have documented degeneration of axon terminals in the striatum of methamphetamine treated animals [39, 42–44]. Collectively, these data strongly suggest that methamphetamine has the potential to produce a distal axotomy of brain dopamine and serotonin neurons.

Several studies have been conducted in an effort to evaluate the potential for methamphetamine to produce dopamine neurotoxicity in humans, by measuring the dopamine transporter (DAT), a structural component of the dopamine terminal using molecular neuroimaging methods [45–51]. There is a general consensus among studies that methamphetamine can lead to a loss of brain dopamine transporters, but there is less agreement regarding the extent and duration of the loss, with some studies suggesting that damage lasts months to years [46, 49–51], but one study showing no significant dopamine transporter reductions in methamphetamine subjects who reported having abstained from methylphenidate use for 15 ($\pm$7) months [50]. Only one study has evaluated the status of brain serotonin transporters in the brains of living human methamphetamine abusers [52]. This study reported global reductions in serotonin transporter density, and that transporter density and aggressive behavior were inversely related.

Ellison and colleagues [36] were the first to report the dopaminergic neurotoxic potential of amphetamine toward dopamine neurons in rats that received constant infusions of amphetamine. Shortly thereafter, it was demonstrated that single or repeated systemic dosages of amphetamine also damaged brain dopamine, but not brain serotonin neurons [53, 54]. Since that time, there have been numerous additional studies that have demonstrated the dopaminergic neurotoxic effects of amphetamine, including studies in monkeys and baboons that were treated with oral dosages of amphetamine similar to those used for the treatment of attention deficit hyperactivity disorder [55]. It is not known whether amphetamine-induced dopamine neurotoxicity occurs in humans.

Three studies have assessed the potential for methylphenidate to damage brain monoaminergic neurons [53, 56, 57]. All three showed no lasting effect of methylphenidate, even when given repeatedly, systemically and at high dosages. The finding that methamphetamine lacks neurotoxic potential toward brain DA or 5-HT neurons may be an important consideration for patients who will require chronic treatment with psychostimulants.

Conclusions/future directions

Although the utility of amphetamines and methylphenidate for improving daytime alertness is widely accepted, there is a paucity of controlled data demonstrating this effect. Further, there are no head-to-head comparisons of the older stimulants with more recently developed drugs, such as modafinil and pemoline, making comparisons difficult. Importantly, the traditional stimulants (amphetamine, methamphetamine, dextroamphetamine, and methylphenidate) are available in less-expensive generic forms, and therefore might be preferable to some patients. There is a need for large-scale randomized controlled studies comparing older and newer agents, both with regard to efficacy and safety.

A major drawback of the amphetamines, and of methylphenidate to a lesser degree, is their abuse potential. The United Nations Office on Drugs and Crime has identified abuse of amphetamine-type stimulants to be secondary only to abuse of marijuana globally [58], and in the United States, methamphetamine abuse and dependence poses major public health and law enforcement problems [8]. Given concerns about abuse liability, use of amphetamines and, to a lesser extent, methylphenidate for the treatment of sleepiness of central origin should be judicious, particularly in patients with a personal or family history of substance use or dependence. Given the availability of other agents without documented abuse potential, amphetamines (and, possibly methylphenidate) should not be the first line of pharmacologic treatment.

In addition to the problem of abuse liability, the amphetamines (but not methylphenidate) have the potential to produce brain dopamine neurotoxicity. Clear evidence of dopaminergic injury has been shown in methamphetamine abusers using modern molecular neuroimaging methods. Although similar studies have not been conducted in amphetamine abusers, a study in baboons treated with a drug regimen modeled after dosing regimens used for the treatment of attention deficit hyperactivity disorder demonstrated loss of dopaminergic axons and axon terminals. Whether similar dopaminergic injury occurs in humans who use amphetamine or methamphetamine for excessive daytime sleepiness is not known, nor is it known whether there is recovery of normal dopaminergic innervation or function over time.

Future research should include head-to-head comparisons of recently developed psychostimulants with amphetamines, so that meaningful comparisons regarding safety and efficacy can be made. Molecular imaging studies similar to those that have been conducted in methamphetamine abusers should be conducted in patients who are prescribed amphetamines for sleepiness. These studies should aim to determine whether dopaminergic neurotoxicity occurs following dosages of methamphetamine and amphetamine that are used clinically, whether toxicity, if it occurs is associated with functional consequences, and whether recovery of dopamine neuronal integrity and function occurs over time.

References

1. **Nichols D E**. Medicinal chemistry and structure–activity relationships. In: Cho L A K, Segal D S, Eds. *Amphetamine and its Analogs: Psychopharmacology, Toxicology and Abuse*. San Diego, CA: Academic Press, 1994: 3–41.
2. **Edeleanu L**. Uber einige Derivate der Phenylmethacrylsaure und der Phenylisobuttersaure. *Ber Deutsch Chem Ges* 1887; **20**:616.
3. **Cho A K, Segal D S**. Preface. In: Cho A K, Segal D S, Eds. *Amphetamine and its Analogs: Psychopharmacology, Toxicology and Abuse*. New York, NY: Academic Press, 1994: xix–xxi.
4. **Morgenthaler T I, Kapur V K, Brown T**, *et al*. Practice parameters for the treatment of narcolepsy and other hypersomnias of central origin. Standards of Practice Committee of the American Academy of Sleep Medicine. *Sleep*, 2007; **30**:1705–11.
5. **Miller M A, Hughes A L**. Epidemiology of amphetamine use in the United States. In: Cho A K, Segal D S, Eds. *Amphetamine and its Analogs: Psychopharmacology, Toxicology, and Abuse*. New York, NY: Academic Press, 1994: 439–57.
6. **Grinspoon L, Hedblom P**. *The Speed Culture: Amphetamine Use and Abuse in America*. Cambridge, MA: Harvard University Press, 1975: 11–39.
7. **Lemere F**. The danger of amphetamine dependency. *Am J Psychiatry*, 1966; **123**:569–72.
8. **Rawson R A, Condon T P**. Why do we need an *Addiction* supplement focused on methamphetamine? *Addiction*, 2007; **102**(Suppl 1):1–4.
9. **Wilens T E, Adler L A, Adams J**, *et al*. Misuse and diversion of stimulants prescribed for ADHD: a systematic review of the literature. *J Am Acad Child Adolesc Psychiatry*, 2008; **47**:21–31.
10. **Snyder S H, Taylor K M, Coyle J T**, *et al*. The role of brain dopamine in behavioral regulation and the actions of psychotropic drugs. *Am J Psychiatry*, 1970; **127**:199–207.
11. **White S R**. Amphetamine toxicity. *Semin Respir Crit Care Med*, 2002; **23**:27–36.
12. **Froimowitz M, Patrick K, Cody V**. Conformational analysis of methylphenidate and its structural relationship to other dopamine reuptake blockers such as CFT. *Pharm Res*, 1995; **12**:1430–34.
13. **Patrick K S, Straughn A B, Perkins J S**, *et al*. Evolution of stimulants to treat ADHD: transdermal

methylphenidate. *Hum Psychopharmacol*, 2009; **24**:1–17.

14. Musshoff F. Illegal or legitimate use? Precursor compounds to amphetamine and methamphetamine. *Drug Metab Rev*, 2000; **32**:15–44.

15. Beckett H, Rowland M. Urinary excretion of methylamphetamine in man. *Nature*, 1965; **206**:1260–61.

16. Beckett A H, Salmon J A, Mitchard M. The relation between blood levels and urinary excretion of amphetamine under controlled acidic and under fluctuating urinary pH values using [14C] amphetamine. *J Pharm Pharmacol*, 1969; **21**: 251–58.

17. Davis J M, Kopin I J, Lemberger L. Effects of urinary pH on amphetamine metabolism. *Ann N Y Acad Sci*, 1971; **179**:493–501.

18. Faraj B A, Israili Z H, Perel J M, *et al*. Metabolism and disposition of methylphenidate-14C: studies in man and animals. *J Pharmacol Exp Ther*, 1974; **191**: 535–47.

19. Lin S N, Andrenyak D M, Moody D E, *et al*. Enantioselective gas chromatography-negative ion chemical ionization mass spectrometry for methylphenidate in human plasma. *J Anal Toxicol*, 1999; **23**:524–30.

20. Eichhorst J, Etter M, Lepage J, *et al*. Urinary screening for methylphenidate (Ritalin) abuse: a comparison of liquid chromatography–tandem mass spectrometry, gas chromatography–mass spectrometry, and immunoassay methods. *Clin Biochem*, 2004; **37**:175–83.

21. American Academy of Sleep Medicine. *The International Classification of Sleep Disorders: Diagnostic & Coding Manual* (2nd Ed.). Westchester, IL: American Academy of Sleep Medicine, 2005.

22. Mitler M M, Hajdukovic R. Relative efficacy of drugs for the treatment of sleepiness in narcolepsy. *Sleep*, 1991; **14**:218–20.

23. Mignot E, Nishino S. Pathophysiological and pharmacologic aspects of the sleep disorder narcolepsy. In: Davis K L, Charney D, Cole J T, Nemeroff C, Eds. *Neuropsychopharmacology: The Fifth Generation of Progress*. Philadelphia, PA: Lippincott, Williams and Wilkins, 2002: 1907–22.

24. Seiden L S, Fischman M W, Schuster C R. Long-term methamphetamine induced changes in brain catecholamines in tolerant rhesus monkeys. *Drug Alcohol Depend*, 1976; **1**:215–19.

25. Kogan F J, Nichols W K, Gibb J W. Influence of methamphetamine on nigral and striatal tyrosine hydroxylase activity and on striatal dopamine levels. *Eur J Pharmacol*, 1976; **36**:363–71.

26. Ricaurte G A, Schuster C R, Seiden L S. Long-term effects of repeated methylamphetamine administration on dopamine and serotonin neurons in the rat brain: a regional study. *Brain Res*, 1980; **193**:153–63.

27. Hotchkiss A J, Gibb J W. Long-term effects of multiple doses of methamphetamine on tryptophan hydroxylase and tyrosine hydroxylase activity in rat brain. *J Pharmacol Exp Ther*, 1980; **214**:257–62.

28. Gibb J W, Hanson G R, Johnson M. Neurochemical mechanisms of toxicity. In: Cho A K, Segal D S, Eds. *Amphetamine and its Analogs: Neuropsychopharmacology, Toxicology and Abuse*. New York, NY: Academic Press, 1994: 269–89.

29. Seiden L S, Ricaurte G A. Neurotoxicity of methamphetamine and related drugs. In: Meltzer H Y, Ed. *Psychopharmacology – A Generation of Progress*. New York, NY: Raven Press, 1987: 359–66.

30. Lew R, Malberg J E, Ricaurte G A, *et al*. Evidence for and mechanism of action of neurotoxicity of amphetamine related compounds. In: Kostrzewa R M, Ed. *Highly Selective Neurotoxins: Basic and Clinical Applications*. Totowa, NJ: Humana Press, 1997: 235–68.

31. Harvey D C, Lacan G, Tanious S P, *et al*. Recovery from methamphetamine induced long-term nigrostriatal dopaminergic deficits without substantia nigra cell loss. *Brain Res*, 2000; **871**:259–70.

32. Melega W P, Raleigh M J, Stout D B, *et al*. Recovery of striatal dopamine function after acute amphetamine- and methamphetamine-induced neurotoxicity in the vervet monkey. *Brain Res*, 1997; **766**:113–20.

33. Melega W P, Lacan G, Harvey D C, *et al*. Dizocilpine and reduced body temperature do not prevent methamphetamine-induced neurotoxicity in the vervet monkey: [11C]WIN 35,428-positron emission tomography studies. *Neurosci Lett*, 1998; **258**:17–20.

34. Woolverton W L, Ricaurte G A, Forno L S, *et al*. Long-term effects of chronic methamphetamine administration in rhesus monkeys. *Brain Res*, 1989; **486**:73–78.

35. Villemagne V, Yuan J, Wong D F, *et al*. Brain dopamine neurotoxicity in baboons treated with doses of methamphetamine comparable to those recreationally abused by humans: evidence from [11C]WIN-35,428 positron emission tomography studies and direct in vitro determinations. *J Neurosci*, 1998; **18**:419–27.

36. Ellison G, Eison M S, Huberman H S, *et al*. Long-term changes in dopaminergic innervation of caudate nucleus after continuous amphetamine administration. *Science*, 1978; **201**:276–78.

37. Molliver M E, Berger U V, Mamounas L A, *et al*. Neurotoxicity of MDMA and related compounds:

anatomic studies. *Ann N Y Acad Sci*, 1990; **600**:640–64.

38. **Axt K J, Molliver M E**. Immunocytochemical evidence for methamphetamine-induced serotonergic axon loss in the rat brain. *Synapse*, 1991; **9**:302–13.

39. **Ricaurte G A, Guillery R W, Seiden L S**, *et al.* Dopamine nerve terminal degeneration produced by high doses of methylamphetamine in the rat brain. *Brain Res*, 1982; **235**:93–103.

40. **Sonsalla P K, Jochnowitz N D, Zeevalk G D**, *et al.* Treatment of mice with methamphetamine produces cell loss in the substantia nigra. *Brain Res*, 1996; **38**:172–75.

41. **Hirata H, Cadet J L**. Methamphetamine-induced serotonin neurotoxicity is attenuated in p53-knockout mice. *Brain Res*, 1997; **768**:345–48.

42. **Ricaurte G A, Seiden L S, Schuster C R**. Further evidence that amphetamines produce long-lasting dopamine neurochemical deficits by destroying dopamine nerve fibers. *Brain Res*, 1984; **303**:359–64.

43. **Ryan L J, Linder J C, Martone M E**, *et al.* Histological and ultrastructural evidence that D-amphetamine causes degeneration in neostriatum and frontal cortex of rats. *Brain Res*, 1990; **518**:67–77.

44. **O'Callaghan J P, Miller D**. Neurotoxicity profiles of substituted amphetamines in the C57BL/6J mouse. *J Pharmacol Exp Ther*, 1994; **270**:741–51.

45. **McCann U D, Wong D F, Yokoi F**, *et al.* Reduced striatal dopamine transporter density in abstinent methamphetamine and methcathinone users: evidence from positron emission tomography studies with [11C]WIN-35,428. *J Neurosci*, 1998; **18**:8417–22.

46. **McCann U D, Kuwabara H, Kumar A**, *et al.* Persistent cognitive and dopamine transporter deficits in abstinent methamphetamine users. *Synapse*, 2008; **62**:91–100.

47. **Sekine Y, Iyo M, Ouchi Y**, *et al.* Methamphetamine-related psychiatric symptoms and reduced brain dopamine transporters studied with PET. *Am J Psychiatry*, 2001; **158**:1206–14.

48. **Sekine Y, Minabe Y, Ouchi Y**, *et al.* Association of dopamine transporter loss in the orbitofrontal and dorsolateral prefrontal cortices with methamphetamine-related psychiatric symptoms. *Am J Psychiatry*, 2003; **160**:1699–701.

49. **Volkow N D, Chang L, Wang G J**, *et al.* Association of dopamine transporter reduction with psychomotor impairment in methamphetamine abusers. *Am J Psychiatry*, 2001a; **158**:377–82.

50. **Volkow N D, Chang L, Wang G J**, *et al.* Loss of dopamine transporters in methamphetamine abusers recovers with protracted abstinence. *J Neurosci*, 2001b; **21**:9414–18.

51. **Johanson C E, Lundahl L H, Lockhart N**, *et al.* Intravenous cocaine discrimination in humans. *Exp Clin Psychopharmacol*, 2006; **14**:99–108.

52. **Sekine Y, Ouchi Y, Takei N**, *et al.* Brain serotonin transporter density and aggression in abstinent methamphetamine abusers. *Arch Gen Psychiatry*, 2006; **63**:90–100.

53. **Wagner G C, Ricaurte G A, Johanson C E**, *et al.* Amphetamine induces depletion of dopamine and loss of dopamine uptake sites in caudate. *Neurology*, 1980; **30**:547–50.

54. **Fuller R W, Hemrick-Luecke S**. Long-lasting depletion of striatal dopamine by a single injection of amphetamine in iprindole-treated rats. *Science*, 1980; **209**:305–07.

55. **Ricaurte G A, Mechan A O, Yuan J**, *et al.* Amphetamine treatment similar to that used in the treatment of adult attention-deficit/hyperactivity disorder damages dopaminergic nerve endings in the striatum of adult nonhuman primates. *J Pharmacol Exp Ther*, 2005; **315**:91–98.

56. **Zaczek R, Battaglia G, Contrera J F**, *et al.* Methylphenidate and pemoline do not cause depletion of rat brain monoamine markers similar to that observed with methamphetamine. *Toxicol Appl Pharmacol*, 1989; **100**:227–33.

57. **Yuan J, McCann U, Ricaurte G**. Methylphenidate and brain dopamine neurotoxicity. *Brain Res*, 1997; **767**:172–75.

58. **United Nations Office On Drugs and Crime**. World Drug Report. Available online at: http://www.unodc.org/pdf/research/wdr07/WDR_2007.pdf

Section 4 Chapter 36

Therapy of Excessive Sleepiness

Modafinil/armodafinil in the treatment of excessive daytime sleepiness

Renee Monderer and Michael J. Thorpy

Introduction

Excessive daytime sleepiness (EDS), a common problem that affects a substantial portion of the general population, is often the cardinal presenting feature of sleep disorders such as narcolepsy, shift work disorder (SWD), and obstructive sleep apnea (OSA). Modafinil, an effective wake-promoting agent with good safety and tolerability measures in addition to having low abuse potential, has been studied extensively in the treatment of daytime sleepiness associated with these sleep disorders, as well as other medical conditions such as Parkinson's disease, multiple sclerosis, depression, and chronic fatigue syndrome. More recently, a longer form of modafinil, armodafinil, the R-enantiomer, has been approved for the treatment of narcolepsy, SWD, and EDS associated with OSA. The following is a review of the therapeutic efficacy, tolerability and mode of action of modafinil and armodafinil for approved and off-label treatment of excessive sleepiness.

Modafinil for the treatment of excessive sleepiness associated with OSA

The treatment of choice for obstructive sleep apnea is continuous positive airway pressure (CPAP), which when used effectively, can alleviate respiratory disturbances, oxygen desaturations, and daytime sleepiness. However, a significant number of patients with treated obstructive sleep apnea continue to experience residual excessive sleepiness [1, 2]. Modafinil has been studied as a wake-promoting agent to alleviate symptoms of daytime sleepiness in patients with OSA treated by CPAP.

A 4-week randomized, double-blind, placebo-controlled, parallel study evaluated the efficacy of modafinil (200 mg/d, week 1; 400 mg/d, weeks 2–4) in 157 patients with obstructive sleep apnea (Respiratory Disturbance Index (RDI) $\geq$ 15) and residual daytime sleepiness while compliant with CPAP therapy [3]. As defined in previous literature, CPAP compliance required that patients use the machine for $\geq$ 4 h per night on 70% of nights [4]. The Epworth Sleepiness Scale (ESS) was used to assess subjective daytime sleepiness, while the Multiple Sleep Latency Test (MSLT) was used to evaluate objective sleepiness. Additionally, the Clinical Global Impression Scale of Change (CGI-C) looked at illness severity.

The mean changes from baseline in ESS scores at weeks 1 and 4 showed a significantly greater improvement in daytime sleepiness in patients using CPAP plus modafinil as compared to CPAP plus placebo ($p < 0.001$) [3]. Additionally, at week 4, 51% of patients in the modafinil group had an ESS less than 10 (i.e. within the normal range), as compared to 27% in the placebo group ($p < 0.01$). Furthermore, at week 4, the mean sleep latency on MSLT improved from a baseline of 7.4 to 8.6 min in patients receiving CPAP plus modafinil, as compared to a decrease in sleep latency from 7.5 min at baseline to 7.2 min at week 4 in the CPAP plus placebo group. CGI-C ratings were significantly more improved in the modafinil group as compared with the placebo group ($p = 0.035$).

There was a small but significant increase in the arousal index in the patients receiving modafinil compared to controls (14.3 vs. 11.8, $p = 0.018$), but no significant change in either group in the number of hours of CPAP use [3]. The most common side-effects reported were headaches (modafinil 23%; placebo 11%) and nervousness (modafinil 12%; placebo 3%). Sitting systolic blood pressure was slightly but

---

Sleepiness: Causes, Consequences and Treatment, ed. Michael J. Thorpy and Michel Billiard. Published by Cambridge University Press. © Cambridge University Press 2011.

significantly increased in the modafinil group compared to placebo (modafinil 1.0 mmHg; placebo −2.6 mmHg; $p = 0.035$).

A follow-up 12-week open-label study of 125 patients previously randomized to the above 4-week study was done to evaluate the longer-term effects of modafinil on residual sleepiness (ESS ≥ 10) in patients with obstructive sleep apnea (RDI ≥ 15) on CPAP [5]. The patients received a dose that the investigator determined was the most desirable for each individual patient (200, 300, or 400 mg). During the entire 12-week study, the significant improvement seen on the ESS during the 4-week trial was maintained with CPAP plus modafinil. More than 93% of patients were clinically improved on the CGI-C from weeks 2 to 12 of the open-label study. However, unlike the 4-week trial, in this open-label study there was a small but significant drop in the mean nightly CPAP use with modafinil compared to baseline at the start of the study (modafinil 5.9 h/night; double-blind baseline 6.3 h/night; $p = 0.004$). Once again, headache and nervousness were the most common adverse effects. In the modafinil group increases in heart rate at week 1 (2.1 beats/min) and standing diastolic blood pressure at weeks 6 and 12 (1.9 mmHg) were not deemed clinically significant; however, 8 patients (6%) reported cardiovascular adverse events (hypertension, $n = 4$; palpitations, $n = 2$; tachycardia, $n = 2$).

A smaller randomized, double-blind, placebo-controlled cross-over study with 32 patients was designed to evaluate the efficacy of modafinil in obstructive sleep apnea patients using CPAP [6]. Participants received either 400 mg of modafinil or placebo for 2 weeks followed by a washout period for 1 week and then either 400 mg of modafinil or placebo for the last 2 weeks. The study only found a significant improvement in mean sleep latency on the Maintenance of Wakefulness Test (MWT, modafinil 18.3 ± 3.9 min; placebo 16.6 ± 5.0 min; $p < 0.02$). However, no significant effect on sleepiness was found on the MSLT or ESS. Additionally, quality of life, the Short Form 36 (SF-36) and Functional Outcomes of Sleep Questionnaire (FOSQ), which measure the effects of sleepiness on multiple domains of everyday living and quality of life, and cognitive performance by the Surrogate Reference Task (SURT) and Paced Auditory Serial Addition Task (PASAT), and global evaluations were also unchanged in the modafinil group. There was a small but significant reduction in CPAP use with modafinil (modafinil 6.3 ± 1 h/night; placebo 6.5 ± 1 h/night; $p = 0.03$). Modafinil was associated with more side-effects, but there were no statistically significant differences for any individual adverse effect. Arousal indices, blood pressure measurements, and EKG findings were not statistically different between the two groups. The authors of the paper speculated that they did not find a significant improvement with modafinil on multiple efficacy measures because of the short duration of the study and the small number of patients who were included in it [6].

A more recent, large 12-week double-blind, placebo-controlled parallel study, was conducted with 309 sleep apnea patients compliant with CPAP who were randomized to receive either 400 mg of modafinil, 200 mg of modafinil, or placebo [7]. Wakefulness was significantly improved on the MSLT with both the 400 and 200 mg of modafinil as compared to control on weeks 4, 8, and 12. At week 12, mean sleep latency on MSLT increased by 1.6 min (200 mg modafinil) and 1.5 min (400 mg modafinil) as compared to 1.1 min for those receiving placebo ($p < 0.0001$). The ESS scores decreased by 4.5 points in both modafinil groups in contrast to the placebo group, which had a 1.8-point decrease ($p < 0.0001$). Additionally, overall clinical condition improved, as seen on the CGI-C, by 61 and 68% of patients in the 200 and 400 mg modafinil groups, respectively, as compared with 37% of patients receiving placebo ($p < 0.001$). Vigilance, general productivity, and activity level subscale scores on FOSQ improved with modafinil.

In this 12-week study, the most frequent adverse effects with modafinil were headache, nausea, and anxiety [7]. Modafinil did not significantly change sleep parameters on PSG, hours of nightly CPAP use, or blood pressure measurements. Fifty-five percent of patients entered the study with a history of hypertension and a relatively small percentage of patients reported hypertension as a side-effect (200 mg group, 4.6%; 400 mg group, 7.6%; placebo, 1.9%). Seven of the 13 patients in the modafinil group who developed new-onset hypertension were considered to have hypertension related to the study drug.

Based on the above studies (Table 36.1), the American Academy of Sleep Medicine (AASM) recommended modafinil as standard treatment for residual excessive sleepiness in treated obstructive sleep apnea patients [8]. Other causes of sleepiness must be addressed prior to starting modafinil such as CPAP non-compliance, insufficient sleep, poor sleep

4. Therapy of Excessive Sleepiness

Table 36.1 Outcomes for modafinil

Disorder	Measures	Modafinil 200 mg Baseline	Modafinil 200 mg Change from baseline	Modafinil 400 mg Baseline	Modafinil 400 mg Change from baseline
OSA I study [3]	ESS	–	–	14.2	−4.6
	MSLT	–	–	7.4	+1.2
OSA II study [7]	ESS		−4.5		−4.5
	MWT	13.1	+1.6	13.6	+1.5
SWD [18]	KSS	7.3	−1.5	–	–
	MSLT	2.1	+1.7	–	–
	PVT	12.5	−2.6	–	–
Narcolepsy I [22]	ESS	17.9	−3.5	17.1	−4.1
	MSLT	2.9	+1.8	3.3	+1.9
	MWT	5.8	+2.3	6.6	+2.3
Narcolepsy II [23]	ESS	17.4	−4.4	18.0	−5.7
	MSLT	3.0	+1.9	2.7	+2.4
	MWT	6.1	+2.1	5.9	+1.9

* MSLT and MWT values represent mean sleep latency in minutes.
* PVT values represent number of lapses.
Abbreviations: OSA, obstructive sleep apnea; SWD, shift work disorder; MSLT, Multiple Sleep Latency Test; MWT, Maintenance of Wakefulness Test; PVT, Psychomotor Vigilance Test; ESS, Epworth Sleepiness Scale; KSS, Karolinska Sleepiness Scale.

hygiene, mask leaks, depression, and other sleep disorders.

Armodafinil for the treatment of excessive sleepiness associated with OSA

Two large 12-week randomized, double-blind, placebo-controlled studies were done to evaluate the efficacy of armodafinil for the treatment of residual daytime sleepiness in patients with OSA on CPAP therapy [9, 10]. Patients included had excessive sleepiness defined as an ESS $\geq$ 10, despite effective (apnea–hypopnea index $\leq$ 10 on polysomnogram) and regular ($\geq$ 4 h/night on 70% of nights) CPAP use for $\geq$ 4 weeks. The results from these two studies of armodafinil were pooled in a third paper to analyze the effects of wakefulness, cognition, fatigue, safety and tolerability [11]. Of the 651 patients in the study, 41% had a history of hypertension at baseline.

Armodafinil significantly improved wakefulness as measured by mean sleep latency on MWT at 4 weeks, 8 weeks and 12 weeks. The mean change from baseline in mean sleep latency at week 12 was a 2-min increase for armodafinil 150 and 250 mg/day, compared with a 1.5-min decrease for placebo ($p < 0.0001$). Armodafinil also improved late day wakefulness (mean sleep latency on the MWTs last three naps) compared to placebo at the final visit ($p < 0.05$). Wakefulness on the ESS was significantly improved at all visits in the armodafinil group compared to controls ($p < 0.0001$). At 12 weeks, 49% of patients in the armodafinil group had an ESS$\leq$10 compared to 26% in the placebo group [11].

Episodic secondary memory, a measure of long-term memory that measures the ability to recall verbal and visual information, was significantly improved in quality with armodafinil compared to placebo ($p < 0.05$). This improvement in episodic secondary memory was not consistently found in the individual studies [9, 10], but the pooled analysis showed improvement. However, the speed of memory, power of attention, and continuity of attention between treatment groups did not reach statistical significance [11]. Global fatigue scores (measured by the Brief Fatigue Inventory) were significantly improved in both armodafinil groups as compared to placebo ($p < 0.01$).

Armodafinil was generally well tolerated, with headache being the most commonly reported adverse effect (armodafinil 17%; placebo 8%). The most frequently encountered adverse effects that led to discontinuation of armodafinil were headache ($n = 5$) and nausea ($n = 4$). No serious adverse effects were attributed to the study drug. No meaningful changes in systolic or diastolic blood pressures and heart rates

Table 36.2 Outcomes for armodafinil

Disorder	Measures	Armodafinil 150 mg Baseline	Armodafinil 150 mg Change from Baseline	Armodafinil 250 mg Baseline	Armodafinil 250 mg Change from baseline
OSA I [9]	MWT	21.5	+1.7	23.3	+2.2
OSA II [10]	MWT	23.7	+2.3	–	–
SWD [20]	MSLT	2.3	+3.0	–	–
Narcolepsy [32]	MWT	12.1	+1.3	9.5	+2.6

* MSLT and MWT values represent mean sleep latency in minutes.
Abbreviations: OSA, obstructive sleep apnea; SWD, shift work disorder; MSLT, Multiple Sleep Latency Test; MWT, Maintenance of Wakefulness Test.

were found [11]. Clinically meaningful changes in blood pressure were defined a priori as greater than or equal to 140 mmHg with at least a 10% increase for systolic blood pressure, and greater than or equal to 90 mmHg with at least a 10% increase for diastolic blood pressure. The incidence of newly diagnosed hypertension was less than 1% in both the armodafinil and placebo groups. Worsening hypertension was found in 3% of patients in the armodafinil group and 2% of patients in the placebo group [11] (Table 36.2).

There was a significant reduction in hours of nightly CPAP use in the armodafinil group compared to the placebo group [armodafinil, −0.3 (0.7) h; placebo, −0.1 (0.6) h; $p<0.0001$] [11]. Nocturnal polysomnogram variables, including apnea–hypopnea indices, remained unchanged throughout the studies in both the armodafinil and placebo groups.

In summary, both modafinil and armodafinil appear to be effective treatments for residual sleepiness in patients with OSA despite CPAP treatment. No comparison studies have been done between modafinil and armodafinil in this patient population. In the above studies, both medications improved levels of wakefulness and overall clinical condition. The most common side-effect reported was headache. A small but significant increase in blood pressure was reported in this patient population, highlighting the need to monitor blood pressure when using modafinil or armodafinil in sleep apnea patients.

Modafinil in shift work disorder

Almost 17% of the workforce is made up of shift workers working either a steady night shift or rotating night shifts [12]. Research has shown that night shift workers have a significantly higher prevalence of excessive sleepiness compared to day workers, with up to 32% of shift workers meeting criteria for shift work disorder [13]. This often leads to more frequent absenteeism, depression, sleep-related accidents, and other physical, social, and personal consequences [13–16]. Modafinil has been assessed for the treatment of the excessive sleepiness seen in shift work disorder.

Thirty-two healthy volunteers participated in a randomized, double-blind, placebo-controlled study to evaluate the effect of modafinil 200 mg on simulated night shifts [17]. For 4 days and 4 nights, subjects participated in multiple tests to determine alertness and vigilance between the hours of 2300 and 0700 and monitored by polysomnography each day beginning at approximately 0815. The mean sleep latency on MWT was significantly improved on the four nights in the modafinil group compared to the placebo group. Almost 94% of participants in the modafinil group had a mean sleep latency >15 min compared to only 62.5% on the placebo group ($p = 0.33$). Additionally, vigilance and reaction times, as measured by the reaction time of the Psychomotor Vigilance Test (PVT), were between 40 and 200% higher in the placebo group than in the modafinil group. No significant differences were found on the Digit Symbol Substitution Test (DSST), the Stanford Sleepiness Scale (SSS), or the Karolinska Sleepiness Scale (KSS). On executive function testing, the modafinil group scored better than the placebo group in areas of verbal flexibility and verbal originality. On polysomnography, the placebo group seemed to fall asleep slightly faster than the modafinil group (placebo, 6.0 ± 4.8 min; modafinil 8.9 ± 4.8 min). No other significant side-effects were seen in this study.

In a 12-week, double-blind, placebo-controlled study, 209 patients with shift work sleep disorder were randomly assigned to receive either 200 mg of modafinil or placebo prior to starting their nighttime shift [18]. Mean sleep latencies were significantly improved in the modafinil group from 2.1 min at baseline to 3.8 min at 12 weeks ($p < 0.001$), but not in the placebo group (baseline 2.04 min, final visit 2.37 min; $p = 0.24$). This improvement in sleep latency was seen at the 2am and 4am naps, but not at the 6am and 8am naps. Significantly more patients had clinical improvement on the CGI-C test with modafinil than with placebo (74 vs. 36%, $p < 0.001$). Additionally, modafinil was associated with a significant reduction in frequency and duration of performance lapses on the PVT.

Additionally in this study, subjective levels of sleepiness as rated by the KSS were also significantly reduced in the modafinil group ($p < 0.001$) [18]. Patient diaries reported that modafinil reduced the level of sleepiness both during the night shift and on the commute home. In the modafinil group, fewer patients reported having had accidents or near-accidents during the commute home (modafinil 29%, placebo 54%, $p < 0.001$). Despite these effects, there were no statistically significant effects on intentional or unintentional naps, caffeine intake, and accidents or near-accidents. Insomnia was more commonly reported by patients in the modafinil group than in the placebo group (6 vs. 0%, $p = 0.01$); however, there were no significant differences on any polysomnographic parameters. It is noteworthy that despite the benefits seen with modafinil, most patients continued to have high levels of sleepiness (sleep latencies < 5 min) and impaired performance on testing at night.

Given the physical, social, and personal consequences of shift work disorder [13–16], a second 12-week, randomized, double-blind, placebo-controlled study sought to evaluate the effects of modafinil on patient functioning and quality of life [19]. Two hundred and seventy-eight patients with shift work disorder were randomized to receive either modafinil 200 mg, 300 mg, or placebo prior to starting their shift each night. Modafinil 300 mg significantly improved total scores on the FOSQ (modafinil, 2.3; placebo, 1.6; $p < 0.05$). FOSQ scores for vigilance, activity, and productivity were significantly improved in the modafinil 300 mg group at the final visit. Significant improvements with both doses of modafinil were shown on the SF-36 mental component score from baseline to the final visit (mean change from baseline: modafinil 300 mg, 3.2; modafinil 200 mg, 3.7; placebo, 0.7 points). Modafinil 300 and 200 mg significantly increased the SF-36 domains for vitality, but only modafinil 300 mg increased the role–emotional domain. Daily diaries were not significantly different in terms of sleep parameters or caffeine intake.

In this second 12-week study, the most common adverse effects reported were headache (21.5%), nausea (12.4%), and nervousness (6.8%), which had higher rates of occurrence in the modafinil 300 mg group [19]. Other adverse events reported included insomnia, tachycardia, palpitations, and elevated liver enzymes. A higher number of patients withdrew from the study due to adverse events from the modafinil 300 mg group compared to the placebo and modafinil 200 mg groups (placebo, $n = 4$; modafinil 200 mg, $n = 5$; modafinil 300 mg, $n = 19$). Overall, modafinil 300 mg exhibited stronger effects on health-related quality of life and patient functioning, but more adverse effects and lower tolerability were also seen.

Armodafinil in shift work disorder

The efficacy of armodafinil was evaluated in a 12-week, randomized, placebo-controlled study with 254 permanent or rotating shift workers with SWD [20]. Armodafinil has a significantly longer half-life than modafinil; therefore, the aim of the study was to examine the effects of armodafinil on the latter part of the night and the commute home, times during which shift workers are most severely impaired. This was done by focusing on the mean sleep latencies for the later naps on MSLT.

Armodafinil significantly improved mean sleep latency on MSLT by 3.1 min compared to an increase of 0.4 min with placebo ($p < 0.001$). This greater increase in mean sleep latency was seen at all 5 time points for the armodafinil group as compared to placebo ($p < 0.001$ at 12am, 2am, 4am; $p = 0.007$ at 6am; $p = 0.02$ at 8am) [20]. Seventy-nine percent of patients receiving armodafinil were improved on the CGI-C ratings as compared to 59% of those receiving placebo ($p < 0.001$). At all visits, the KSS scores were significantly improved with armodafinil, and on electronic diaries, the armodafinil group was significantly improved in areas of maximum levels of sleepiness during the night shift and commute home, and in the mean number of mistakes, accidents, or near misses compared to placebo. Armodafinil also significantly improved speed of memory, episodic secondary memory, and power of attention.

The most common side-effects of armodafinil included headache (12%), nausea (7%), nasopharyngitis (6%), and anxiety (5%) [20]. The only serious adverse effect reported with armodafinil was suicidal ideations in a patient with a history of depression ($n = 1$), which the investigator thought might be related to the medication. Armodafinil did not significantly alter any sleep variable on polysomnography. Overall, armodafinil caused a sustained reduction in sleepiness throughout the night and improved memory and attention.

In summary, modafinil has been shown to be effective in improving symptoms of sleepiness in shift workers with shift work disorder; however, significant sleepiness persists in this population. The American Academy of Sleep Medicine has stated that modafinil is indicated to enhance alertness during the night shift for SWD [21], although there is still the need for the development of more effective therapies. Armodafinil shows a slight advantage of longer duration of effect in shift workers although there are no direct comparative studies with modafinil (see Tables 36.1 and 36.2).

Modafinil in narcolepsy

Narcolepsy is a central nervous system disorder that is characterized by severe daytime sleepiness, cataplexy, hypnagogic hallucinations, sleep paralysis, and disturbed nighttime sleep. For most patients, the inability to maintain daytime alertness is the most disabling feature of the disorder. In the past, amphetamines and other CNS stimulants were used to treat daytime sleepiness; however, these medications can have serious side-effects. Currently, modafinil and armodafinil are widely used for sleepiness associated with narcolepsy.

Two double-blind, placebo-controlled studies were done by the US Modafinil in Narcolepsy Multicenter Study Group to assess the efficacy of modafinil for sleepiness in narcolepsy [22, 23]. In both studies, objective measures of sleepiness were determined based on the MSLT and MWT. Subjective measures included the ESS and the CGI-C. Each study was 9 weeks in duration. A combined total of 558 narcolepsy patients (81% with cataplexy) were randomized to receive placebo, modafinil 200 mg, or modafinil 400 mg. Those patients unable or unwilling to stop anticataplectic medications during the trial period were excluded. At baseline, patients were noted to be severely sleepy, with a mean ESS between 17.1 and 18.3 and a maximum mean MSLT sleep latency of 3.3 min.

Both studies demonstrated a significant improvement in sleep latency on MSLT and MWT for 200 and 400 mg of modafinil [22, 23]. The combined results demonstrated a mean sleep latency on the MWT that increased by more than 2 min in both treatment groups, compared with a decrease of 0.7 min in the placebo group ($p < 0.001$). Additionally, mean ESS scores were significantly decreased for both modafinil 200 and 400 mg compared to placebo ($p < 0.001$). A significantly larger percentage of patients in both modafinil groups showed improvement in overall clinical condition on the CGI-C (61–66% modafinil vs. 37% for placebo; $p < 0.001$). No dose–response effect was seen for the 400 mg dose compared with the 200 mg dose in either study. There were no significant changes in sleep parameters seen on polysomnographic studies.

The second study included a 2-week treatment discontinuation phase to determine the effects of withdrawal on patients who had been taking modafinil [23]. During the discontinuation period, subjects in the modafinil groups experienced a loss of improvements in wakefulness that had been seen over the course of the study. No symptoms consistent with tolerance or abrupt withdrawal were seen. These discontinuation results were also supported by similar results from a Canadian study that ended with a 2-week double-blind discontinuation period [24].

It is noteworthy that the first study done used only a 1-day titration period for the 400 mg group, as compared to the second study in which both the 200 and 400 mg groups had a gradual titration over 8–9 days. In the first study, 12% of patients in the 400 mg group withdrew due to adverse events compared to only 1% of patients in the 400 mg group in the second study. This difference is likely due to the longer titration schedule [22, 23].

Modafinil was well tolerated in both studies. The most frequent adverse event was headache. There was no significant difference in the incidence of cataplexy between the treatment and placebo groups. However, it is likely that patients with severe cataplexy were underrepresented because those patients who could not discontinue anticataplectic medications were excluded.

Two smaller studies of 50 and 75 patients, using a cross-over design, showed similar improvements in daytime sleepiness [25, 26]. In the first study, subjects received 300 mg/day in two divided doses, whereas subjects in the second study were given modafinil 200 and 400 mg twice daily, at morning and noon. Significant improvements were seen on the MWT and in daily sleep logs in both studies. In these two smaller studies, the CGI-C did not significantly improve.

Based on many of these studies, the American Academy of Sleep Medicine recommended modafinil as standard of care for sleepiness in patients with narcolepsy in 2000 and 2007 [27, 28]. Modafinil is considered the "first-line" treatment for excessive daytime sleepiness in most patients diagnosed with narcolepsy.

Further studies were done to determine the optimal dosing protocols for modafinil in narcolepsy patients including the use of a single 200 mg dose, higher doses, and divided doses to achieve improvements in late afternoon and evening wakefulness. While the original placebo-controlled studies showed no dose–response effect for 400 compared to 200 mg, a later study, using a modified version of the MWT that included an evening test session, demonstrated significantly improved evening wakefulness with the 400 mg dose (whether in a single dose or divided dose) compared to the 200 mg dose. The greatest improvements in evening wakefulness were seen with the 400 mg split-dose regimen, as compared to the 200 and 400 mg once daily regimen [29].

A second study looking at dosing effects found a 600 mg split-dose regimen (400 mg in the morning and 200 mg in the early afternoon) was found to achieve more sustained wakefulness throughout the day compared to 400 mg once daily [30]. A third study showed that split-dose regimens of either 400 mg in the morning and 200 mg at noon or 200 mg in the morning and at noon were superior to a single dose of 200 mg in the morning [31]. Based on the above data, in narcolepsy patients with residual late afternoon or evening sleepiness, a split-dose regimen of modafinil may enhance wakefulness throughout the day.

Armodafinil in narcolepsy

A large, randomized, placebo-controlled, study of 196 patients with narcolepsy compared 150 and 250 mg of armodafinil with placebo [32]. For this study, the MWT was extended later in the day (9am to 3pm) to assess the longer duration of effect of armodafinil. Patients receiving armodafinil 150 and 250 mg/day experienced significantly increased MWT mean sleep latency compared to placebo. The mean sleep latencies increase over baseline at final visit were 1.3, 2.6, and 1.9 min in the 150 mg, 250 mg and combined groups, respectively, compared with a decrease of 1.9 min in the placebo group ($p < 0.01$). These significant changes were seen at all time points for the 150 mg dose, but statistical significance was not reached at weeks 8 and 12 for the 250 mg group.

The Clinical Global Impression Scale showed significant improvement at the final visit with proportions of 69, 73, and 71% for the 150 mg, 250 mg, and combined armodafinil groups, respectively, compared with 33% for placebo. Memory, attention, and fatigue showed statistically significant improvement with both doses of armodafinil ($p < 0.05$). Subjective sleepiness as measured by the ESS also showed significant improvements with both doses of armodafinil compared to placebo (150 mg, −4.1; 250 mg, −3.8; placebo, −1.9).

In summary, armodafinil at both doses enhanced wakefulness throughout the day and improved clinical condition, memory, and attention as compared to placebo. Comparisons with modafinil were not made.

Off-label uses of modafinil

Many off-label uses of modafinil have been investigated. Modafinil has been used for sleepiness or fatigue in Parkinson's disease, multiple sclerosis, depression, and chronic fatigue syndrome, as well as other neurological and psychiatric disorders (Table 36.3).

Parkinson's disease

Excessive daytime sleepiness is very common in Parkinson's disease, affecting up to 50% of patients [33]. Two studies have shown modafinil to be effective in the treatment of EDS in PD. Two double-blind studies of modafinil in PD, at doses of 100–200 mg/day, showed significant improvements in the ESS and the CGI-C, without any major side-effects or adverse effects on the motor features of PD [34, 35]. A third larger study found no significant improvement in ESS or MSLT with modafinil (200–400 mg/day) in PD [33]. No consistent evidence has shown that modafinil is effective for EDS associated with Parkinson's disease, but further studies are needed.

Multiple sclerosis

Fatigue is a common and disabling feature of multiple sclerosis [36]. One single-blind study with 72 patients

Table 36.3 Indications for modafinil

Diagnosis	Symptoms	FDA approval	Modafinil Doses studied	Armodafinil Doses studied
Obstructive sleep apnea	EDS	Yes	200–400 mg	150–250 mg
Shift work disorder	EDS	Yes	200–400 mg	150 mg
Narcolepsy	EDS	Yes	200–400 mg	150–250 mg
Depression	Fatigue	No	100–400 mg	N/A
Multiple sclerosis	Fatigue	No	200–400 mg	N/A
Parkinson's disease	EDS	No	100–400 mg	N/A
Chronic fatigue syndrome	Fatigue	No	200–400 mg	N/A
Traumatic brain injury	Fatigue EDS	No	100–400 mg	N/A

N/A = not applicable; EDS = Excessive Daytime Sleepiness.

found significant improvement on fatigue measures with modafinil 200 mg compared to placebo, but not with 400 mg of modafinil [37]. Additionally, mean ESS scores were significantly reduced with 200 and 400 mg of modafinil, but baseline ESS scores were already in the normal range. In contrast, two double-blind, placebo-controlled studies found no improvement in fatigue measures with either dose of modafinil [38, 39]. A recent retrospective study found that modafinil was most effective for patients with fatigue who also suffered from EDS [40]. Further studies need to be conducted in order to clarify the role of modafinil in patients with multiple sclerosis.

Depression

Sleep disturbances and fatigue are common symptoms of depression which may persist despite treatment with antidepressant medication [41]. Two large, randomized, double-blind, placebo-controlled studies evaluated the use of modafinil in the treatment of residual fatigue and sleepiness in partially treated patients with major depressive disorder [42, 43]. Both studies found a significant reduction in the Fatigue Severity Scale (FSS) and ESS in the first 1–2 weeks of the trial with modafinil compared to placebo; however, these differences were no longer significant at any other time point in either study. Interestingly, both studies showed a large placebo effect on reducing both the ESS and FSS scores. No differences in depression scales were found at any point. A third study that was open-label examined the use of modafinil in combination with paroxetine as initial therapy for major depression disorder [44]. This study found significant improvements on the FSS, ESS, and the Hamilton Rating Scale (depression scale); however, this study had no placebo group. Based on these studies, modafinil does not appear to be effective for treating major depressive disorder. However, modafinil is commonly used clinically to augment the effects of antidepressant therapy.

Chronic fatigue syndrome

One randomized, double-blind, placebo-controlled, cross-over study of 14 patients with chronic fatigue syndrome evaluated the use of modafinil 200 and 400 mg compared to placebo [45]. No consistent differences were found in self-ratings of fatigue, quality of life, mood, or cognition. Additional large studies are needed to further elucidate the role of modafinil in chronic fatigue syndrome.

Mode of action of modafinil

The exact mode of action of modafinil is not fully understood. There is no single receptor to which modafinil binds or that it inhibits [46]. In animal studies, modafinil has been shown to interact with dopaminergic, noradrenergic, glutamatergic, GABAergic, serotoninergic, hypocretinergic, and histaminergic pathways (Table 36.4).

Initial literature suggested that modafinil only weakly binds to dopamine receptors. Modafinil-induced hyperactivity in mice or modafinil-induced arousal in cats was not blocked by a dopamine-receptor antagonist [47, 48]. However, more recent evidence suggests that modafinil in vitro binds to the dopamine transporter (DAT) and inhibits dopamine transport leading to increased extracellular levels

4. Therapy of Excessive Sleepiness

Table 36.4 Mode of action of modafinil/armodafinil

Neurotransmitter	Method of action	Site of action
Dopamine	Inhibition of dopamine reuptake transporter	Multiple arousal systems
Norepinephrine (NE)	Inhibition of the NE reuptake transporter	VLPO
Hypocretin	Stimulation	Lateral hypothalamus
Histamine	Stimulation	Tuberomamillary nucleus

Table 36.5 Most common adverse effects

Adverse effects	Modafinil	Armodafinil
Headache	34%	17%
Nausea	11%	7%
Dizziness	5%	5%
Nervousness	7%	1%
Anxiety	5%	4%
Insomnia	5%	5%
Rhinitis	7%	Not reported
Back pain	6%	6%
Flu syndrome	4%	1%
Hypertension	3%	Not reported
Diarrhea	6%	4%

Based on data from prescribing information for modafinil and armodafinil [59, 62].

of dopamine [46]. The wake-promoting effects of modafinil are lost in DAT knockout mice [46].

Some studies have suggested that modafinil interacts with adrenergic alpha-1 systems. Various alpha-adrenoreceptor antagonists attenuate the modafinil response in animal studies [48, 49]. However, studies in canine narcolepsy and hypertension suggest otherwise. Adrenergic alpha-1 stimulation inhibits cataplexy and worsens hypertension, neither of which is found with modafinil [50].

Modafinil appears to reduce GABA levels and increase glutamate and serotonin levels in the cortex, indirectly. These activities do not appear to be involved in the clinical effects of modafinil [51].

C-fos activity is increased in the wake-promoting hypothalamic brain regions including the hypocretin neurons, tuberomamillary nucleus, and suprachiasmatic nucleus, and at higher doses in the striatum and cingulate cortex with administration of modafinil [52–54].

Modafinil increases the inhibitory effects of norepinephrine on the ventrolateral preoptic nucleus (VLPO), thereby promoting wakefulness [55]. Modafinil was also shown to increase levels of norepinephrine in the rat prefrontal cortex and medial hypothalamus [56].

In summary, modafinil action appears to be modulated through various neurotransmitters including dopamine, norepinephrine, histamine, glutamate, hypocretin and serotonin.

Mode of action of armodafinil

Modafinil is a racemic compound, with an R-enantiomer and an S-enantiomer. The R-enantiomer has a half-life of 10–14 h, whereas the S-enantiomer has a half-life of 3–4 h [57, 58]. Modafinil has equal amounts of the S-enantiomer and the R-enantiomer, but the S-enantiomer is eliminated three times faster than the R-enantiomer. Armodafinil is the R-enantiomer of modafinil. It is well absorbed and peak levels are obtained at 2 h [59]. Both modafinil and armodafinil are metabolized in the liver. The main pathway of metabolism of armodafinil is by amidehydrolysis, which is a non-CYP pathway [57, 58]. The mode of action appears to be similar to that of modafinil as discussed above.

Even though modafinil and armodafinil have similar half-lives, plasma concentrations are higher late in the day with armodafinil compared to modafinil. It is this difference in the monophasic decline of armodafinil compared to the biphasic decline of modafinil which results in higher plasma drug concentration at a later time [60].

Safety and tolerability of modafinil and armodafinil

Safety data have been reported from clinical trials, preclinical studies on drug interactions, post-marketing adverse event reporting, post-marketing surveillance programs, and studies on abuse and dependence potential. Modafinil and armodafinil are generally very well tolerated, with mostly mild to moderate side-effects reported (Table 36.5) [9, 11, 22, 23].

Headache is the most common side-effect reported for both modafinil and armodafinil. In most cases, headaches were reported as mild to moderate in severity and appeared to be dose related. Headache appears to be the most common reason reported for discontinuation of armodafinil [59].

Other side-effects commonly reported with modafinil and armodafinil were nausea, dizziness, and insomnia. Some slight increases in hepatic enzymes were reported with modafinil and armodafinil [19, 59]. Some studies on the use of modafinil for OSA have shown a slight rise in mean systolic and diastolic blood pressure, but this was not thought to be significant. However, more patients taking modafinil have required an increase in dose or an additional prescription for antihypertensive agents [5, 61]. Likewise, small but consistent increases in systolic and diastolic blood pressure have been seen with armodafinil [59].

Most studies have not reported any EKG changes with modafinil or armodafinil. Cases of chest pain, palpitations, dyspnea, and transient ischemic T-wave changes on EKG were reported with modafinil in patients with mitral valve prolapse and left ventricular hypertrophy [62]. It is recommended that modafinil and armodafinil not be used in patients with a history of left ventricular hypertrophy or in patients with mitral valve prolapse who have experienced the mitral valve prolapse syndrome when previously receiving CNS stimulants. Overall, the cardiovascular profile of modafinil and armodafinil is more favorable than with other stimulants.

Psychiatric symptoms, including mania, delusions, hallucinations, and suicidal ideation have been experienced in association with modafinil use. Controlled trials with modafinil and armodafinil have reported nervousness, confusion, agitation, and depression. Caution should be taken when modafinil or armodafinil is given to patients with a history of psychosis, depression, or mania.

In clinical trials of modafinil and armodafinil, no serious cases of skin rash were reported. Rare cases of serious or life-threatening rash such as Stevens–Johnson Syndrome (SJS), Toxic Epidermal Necrolysis (TEN), and Drug Rash with Eosinophilia and Systemic Symptoms (DRESS) have been reported in children and adults while taking modafinil [62]. Since it is not possible to predict whether a rash will become serious, modafinil/armodafinil should be discontinued on first sign of rash if it is not clear that the rash is not drug related. Rare cases of angioedema and multi-organ hypersensitivity reactions have been reported.

Modafinil has been tested with medications such as warfarin and oral contraceptives that induce the hepatic cytochrome P450 enzyme system [63, 64]. Modafinil was found to decrease the peak plasma concentration of ethinylestradiol. Women should be cautioned to use additional or alternative methods of contraceptive while taking modafinil and for one month after discontinuation. Blood levels of fluoxetine may be slightly increased by modafinil. Armodafinil is a moderate inhibitor of CYP2C19 and a moderate inducer of CYP3A4 and therefore adjustments in dosage should be made when administered with medications such as triazolam, diazepam, cyclosporine, and phenytoin.

Modafinil and armodafinil are Category C for pregnancy. It is recommended that pregnant women avoid taking either modafinil or armodafinil unless the risks of stopping the drug outweigh the benefits. The amount of modafinil/armodafinil excreted in breast milk in unknown.

Modafinil and armodafinil are both schedule IV medications. Studies have shown that modafinil/armodafinil have low potential for abuse, even at doses as high as 800 mg/day [65, 66]. There is no known modafinil withdrawal syndrome.

Conclusion

Modafinil has now been recommended by the AASM as standard therapy for treatment of excessive sleepiness associated with OSA with continued sleepiness despite treatment, SWD, and narcolepsy. Most controlled studies have shown that modafinil is efficacious in improving daytime sleepiness in these disorders, with improvements in measures of quality of life and some aspects of cognition. However, many of these patients continue to experience daytime sleepiness despite treatment, highlighting the need for further research in this area. Modafinil has not been shown to be consistently effective for the treatment of fatigue and sleepiness associated with Parkinson's disease, depression, multiple sclerosis, and chronic fatigue syndrome, although it is commonly used in these disorders.

Armodafinil has recently been approved for the treatment of daytime sleepiness in patients with narcolepsy, SWD, and sleepiness associated with treated OSA. Armodafinil appears to have a longer duration of effect with a similar efficacy profile to modafinil, which may benefit patients who experience late afternoon and early evening symptoms of sleepiness. Both modafinil and armodafinil are generally well tolerated. Headache and nausea are the most common side-effects reported, although they are generally mild to moderate in severity. Both medications have a low likelihood of tolerance and a limited abuse potential.

Further research is needed to study the effectiveness and appropriate dosing and timing of both modafinil and armodafinil in the treatment of sleepiness and fatigue in these sleep disorders, as well as in other neurological and psychiatric disorders.

References

1. **Sforza E**, **Kreiger J**. Daytime sleepiness after long-term continuous positive airway pressure (CPAP) treatment in obstructive sleep apnea syndrome. *J Neurol Sci*, 1992; **110**:21–26.
2. **Bedard M-A**, **Montplaisir J**, **Malo J**, et al. Persistent neuropsychological deficits and vigilance impairment in sleep apnea syndrome after treatment with continuous positive airways pressure (CPAP). *J Clin Exp Neuropsychol*, 1993; **15**:330–41.
3. **Pack A**, **Black J**, **Schwartz J**, et al. Modafinil as the adjunct therapy for daytime sleepiness in obstructive sleep apnea. *Am J Respir Crit Care Med*, 2001; **164**:1675–81.
4. **Kribbs N B**, **Pack A I**, **Kline L R**, et al. Objective measurement of patterns of nasal CPAP use by patients with obstructive sleep apnea. *Am Rev Respir Dis*, 1993; **147**:887–95.
5. **Schwartz J**, **Hirshkowitz M**, **Erman M**, et al. Modafinil as adjunct therapy for daytime sleepiness in obstructive sleep apnea. *Chest*, 2003; **124**:2192–99.
6. **Kingshott R**, **Vennelle M**, **Coleman E**, et al. Randomized, double-blind, placebo-controlled crossover trial of modafinil in the treatment of residual excessive daytime sleepiness in the sleep apnea/hypopnea syndrome. *Am J Respir Crit Care Med*, 2001; **163**:918–23.
7. **Black J**, **Hirshkowitz M**. Modafinil for treatment of residual excessive sleepiness in nasal continuous positive airway pressure-treated obstructive sleep apnea/hypopnea syndrome. *Sleep*, 2005; **28**:464–71.
8. **Morgenthaler T**, **Kapen S**, **Lee-Chiong T**, et al. Practice parameters for the medical therapy of obstructive sleep apnea. *Sleep*, 2006; **29**:1031–35.
9. **Roth T**, **White D**, **Schmidt-Nowara W**, et al. Effects of armodafinil in the treatment of residual excessive sleepiness associated with obstructive sleep apnea/hypopnea syndrome: a 12-week, multicenter, double-blind, randomized, placebo-controlled study in nCPAP-adherent adults. *Clin Ther*, 2006; **28**:689–706.
10. **Hirshkowitz M**, **Black J E**, **Wesner K**, et al. Adjunct armodafinil improves wakefulness and memory in obstructive sleep apnea/hypopnea syndrome. *Resp Med*, 2007; **101**:616–27.
11. **Roth T**, **Rippon G**, **Arora S**. Armodafinil improves wakefulness and long term episodic memory in n-CPAP adherent patient with excessive sleepiness associated with obstructive sleep apnea. *Sleep Breath*, 2008; **12**:53–62.
12. **Beers T**. Flexible schedules and shift work: replacing the '9-to5' workday? *Monthly Labor Rev*, 2000; **123**:33–40.
13. **Drake C**, **Roehrs T**, **Richardson G**, et al. Shift work sleep disorder: prevalence and consequences beyond that of symptomatic day workers. *Sleep*, 2004; **27**:1453–62.
14. **Jaffe M**, **Smolensky M**, **Wunn C**. Sleep quality and physical and social well-being in North American petrochemical shift workers. *South Med J*, 1996; **89**:305–12.
15. **Munakata M**, **Ichi S**, **Nunokawa T.**, et al. Influence of night shift work on psychologic state and cardiovascular and neuroendocrine responses in healthy nurses. *Hypertens Res*, 2001; **24**:25–31.
16. **Morikawa Y**, **Miura K**, **Ishizaki M**, et al. Sickness absence and shift work among Japanese factory workers. *J Hum Ergol*, 2001; **30**:393–98.
17. **Walsh J**, **Randazzo A**, **Stone K**, et al. Modafinil improves alertness, vigilance and executive function during simulated night shifts. *Sleep*, 2004; **27**: 434–39.
18. **Czeisler C**, **Walsh J**, **Roth T**, et al. Modafinil for excessive sleepiness associated with shift-work sleep disorder. *N Engl J Med*, 2005; **353**:476–86.
19. **Erman M**, **Rosenberg R**, For the US Modafinil Shift Work Sleep Disorder Study Group. Modafinil for excessive sleepiness associated with chronic shift work sleep disorder: effects on patient functioning and health-related quality of life. *Primary Care Companion. J Clin Psychiatry*, 2007; **9**:188–94.
20. **Czeisler C**, **Walsh J**, **Wesnes K**, et al. Armodafinil for treatment of excessive sleepiness associated with shift work disorder: a randomized controlled study. *Mayo Clin Proc*, 2009; **11**:958–72.
21. **Morgenthaler T**, **Lee-Chiong T**, **Alessi C**, et al. Practice parameters for the clinical evaluation and treatment of circadian rhythm sleep disorders. *Sleep*, 2007; **30**:1445–59.
22. **US Modafinil in Narcolepsy Multicenter Study Group**. Randomized trial of modafinil for the treatment of pathological somnolence in narcolepsy. *Ann Neurol*, 1998; **43**:88–97.
23. **US Modafinil in Narcolepsy Multicenter Study Group**. Randomized trial of modafinil as a treatment for the excessive daytime somnolence of narcolepsy. *Neurology*, 2000; **54**:1166–75.

24. **Moldofsky H, Broughton R, Hill J.** A randomized trial of long term, continued efficacy and safety of modafinil in narcolepsy. *Sleep Med*, 2000; **1**: 109–16.

25. **Billiard M, Besset A, Montplaisir J,** et al. Modafinil: a double blind multicenter study. *Sleep*, 1994; **17**(8 Suppl.):S107–12.

26. **Broughton R, Fleming J, George C,** et al. Randomized, double blind, placebo controlled, crossover trial of modafinil in the treatment of excessive daytime sleepiness in narcolepsy. *Neurology*, 1997; **49**:444–51.

27. **Littner M, Johnson S, McCall W,** et al. for the American Academy of Sleep Medicine Standard of Practice Committee. Practice parameters for the treatment of narcolepsy: an update for 2000. *Sleep*, 2001; **24**:451–66.

28. **Morgenthaler T, Kapur V, Brown T,** et al. Standards of Practice Committee of the American Academy of Sleep Medicine. Practice parameters for the treatment of narcolepsy and other hypersomnias of central origin. *Sleep*, 2007; **30**:1705–11.

29. **Schwartz J, Feldman N, Bogan R,** et al. Dosing regimen effects of modafinil for improving daytime wakefulness in patients with narcolepsy. *Clin Neuropharm*, 2003; **26**:252–57.

30. **Schwartz J, Nelson M, Schwarys E,** et al. Effects of modafinil on wakefulness and executive function in patients with narcolepsy experiencing late-day sleepiness. *Clin Neuropharmacol*, 2004; **27**:74–79.

31. **Schwartz J, Feldman N, Bogan R.** Dose effects of modafinil in sustaining wakefulness in narcolepsy patients with residual evening sleepiness. *J Neuropsychiatry Clin Neuosci*, 2005; **17**:405–12.

32. **Harsh J, Hayduk R, Rosenberg R,** et al. The efficacy and safety of armodafinil as treatment for adults with excessive sleepiness associated with narcolepsy. *Curr Med Res Opin*, 2006; **22**:761–74.

33. **Ondo W G, Fayle R, Atassi F,** et al. Modafinil for daytime somnolence in Parkinson's disease: double blind, placebo controlled parallel trial. *J Neurol Neurosurg Psych*, 2005; **76**:1636–39.

34. **Hogl B, Saletu M, Brandauer E,** et al. Modafinil for the treatment of daytime sleepiness in Parkinson's disease: a double-blind, randomized, crossover, placebo-controlled polygraphic trial. *Sleep*, 2002; **25**:905–09.

35. **Adler C H, Caviness J N, Hentz J G,** et al. Randomized trial of Modafinil for treating subjective daytime sleepiness in patients with Parkinson's disease. *Mov Disord*, 2003; **18**:287–93.

36. **Krupp L, Alvarez L, LaRocca N,** et al. Fatigue in multiple sclerosis. *Arch Neurol*, 1988; **45**:435–37.

37. **Rommohan K, Rosenberg J, Lynn D,** et al. Efficacy and safety of modafinil for the treatment of fatigue in multiple sclerosis: a two centre phase 2 study. *J Neurol Neurosurg Psychiatry*, 2002; **72**:179–83.

38. **Dowson A, Kliminster S, Salt R.** Provigil: a pilot, single-centre, double-blind, placebo-controlled crossover study in the treatment of fatigue in multiple sclerosis (abstract). Presented at the 12th meeting of the European Neurological Society, 22–26 June 2002, Berlin, Germany.

39. **Stankoff B, Aubant E, Confavreux C,** et al. Efficacy and safety of modafinil for the treatment of fatigue in multiple sclerosis: a randomized, placebo-controlled, double-blind multicenter study (abstract). Presented at the 13th meeting of the European Neurological Society, 14–18 June 2003, Istanbul, Turkey.

40. **Littleton E, Hobart J, Palace J.** Modafinil for multiple sclerosis fatigue: does it work? *Clin Neurol Neurosurg*, 2010; **112**:29–31.

41. **Nierenberg A, Keefe B, Leslie V,** et al. Residual symptoms in depressed patients who respond acutely to fluoxetine. *J Clin Psychiatry*, 1999; **60**:221–25.

42. **DeBattista C, Dogramji M, Menza M,** et al. Adjunct modafinil for short-term treatment of fatigue and sleepiness in patients with major depressive disorder: a preliminary double-blind, placebo-controlled study. *J Clin Psychiatry*, 2003; **64**:1057–64.

43. **Fava M, Thase M, DeBattista C.** A multicenter, placebo-controlled study of modafinil augmentation in partial responders to selective serotonin reuptake inhibitors with persistent fatigue and sleepiness. *J Clin Psychiatry*, 2005; **66**:85–93.

44. **Ninan P, Hassman H, Glass S,** et al. Adjunctive modafinil at initiation of treatment with selective serotonin reuptake inhibitors enhances the degree and onset of therapeutic effects in patients with major depressive disorder and fatigue. *J Clin Psychiatry*, 2004; **65**:414–20.

45. **Randall D, Cafferty F, Shneerson J,** et al. Chronic treatment with modafinil may not be beneficial in patients with chronic fatigue syndrome. *J Psychopharmacol*, 2005; **19**:647–60.

46. **Mignot E, Nishino S, Guilleminault C,** et al. Modafinil binds to the dopamine uptake carrier site with low affinity. *Sleep*, 1994; **17**:436–37.

47. **Simon P, Hemet C, Ramassamy C,** et al. Non-amphetaminic mechanism of stimulant locomotor effect of modafinil in mice. *Eur Neuropychopharmacol*, 1995; **5**:509–14.

48. **Lin J, Roussel B, Akaoka H,** et al. Role of catecholamines in the modafinil and amphetamine induced wakefulness, a comparative pharmacological study in the cat. *Brain Res*, 1992; **591**:319–26.

49. **Duteil J**, **Rambert F**, **Pessonnier J**, et al. Central alpha 1-adrenergic stimulation in relation to the behavior stimulating effect of modafinil: studies with experimental animals. *Eur J Pharmacol*, 1990; **180**:49–58.

50. **Mignot E**, **Renaud A**, **Nishino S**, et al. Canine cataplexy is preferentially controlled by adrenergic mechanisms: evidence using monoamine selective uptake inhibitors and release enhancers. *Psychopharmacology (Berl)*, 1993; **113**:76–82.

51. **Tanganelli S**, **Fuxe K**, **Ferraro L**, et al. Inhibitory effects of the psychoactive drug modafinil on gamma-aminobutyric acid outflow from the cerebral cortex of the awake freely moving guinea pig. *Arch Pharmacol*, 1992; **345**:461–65.

52. **Lin J**, **Hou Y**, **Jouvet M**. Potential brain neuronal targets for amphetamine-, methylphenidate-, modafinil-induced wakefulness, evidenced by c-fos immunocytochemistry in the cats. *Proc Natl Acad Sci USA*, 1996; **93**:14 128–33.

53. **Chemelli R**, **Williw J**, **Sinton C**, et al. Narcolepsy in orexin knockout mice: molecular genetics of sleep regulation. *Cell*, 1999; **98**:437–51.

54. **Scammell T**, **Estabrooke I**, **McCarthy M**, et al. Hypothalamic arousal regions are activated during modafinil-induced wakefulness. *J Neurosci*, 2000; **20**:8620–28.

55. **Gallopin T**, **Luppi P**, **Rambert F**, et al. Effects of the wake promoting agent modafinil on sleep-promoting neurons from the ventrolateral preoptic nucleus: an in vitro pharmacologic study. *Sleep*, 2004; **27**:19–25.

56. **de Saint Hilaire Z**, **Orosco M**, **Rouch C**, et al. Variations in extracellular monoamines in the prefrontal cortex and medial hypothalamus after modafinil administration: a microdialysis study in rats. *Neuroreport*, 2001; **12**:3533–37.

57. **Robertson P Jr**, **Hellriegel E**. Clinical pharmacokinetics profile of modafinil. *Clin Pharmacokinet*, 2003; **42**:123–37.

58. **Darwish M**, **Kirby M**, **Robertson P** Jr, et al. Interaction profile of armodafinil with medications metabolized by cytochrome P450 enzymes 1A2, 3A4 and 2C19 in healthy subjects. *Clin Pharmacokinet*, 2008; **47**:61–74.

59. **Nuvigil (armodafinil) tablets prescribing information**. (Tablets prescribing information, 2009.) http://www.nuvigil.com/media/full_prescribing_information.pdf

60. **Darwish M**, **Kirby M**, **Hellriegel E**, et al. Armodafinil and modafinil have substantially different pharmacokinetic profiles despite having the same terminal half-lives: analysis of data from three randomized, single-dose, pharmacokinetic studies. *Clin Drug Invest*, 2009; **29**:613–23.

61. **Roth T**, **Schwartz J**, **Hirshkowitz M**, et al. Evaluation of the safety of modafinil for treatment of excessive sleepiness. *J Clin Sleep Med*, 2007; **3**:595–602.

62. **FDA**. Provigil (modafinil) tablets prescribing information 2007. Available from http://www.accessdata.fda.gov/drugsatfda_docs/label/2007/020717s020s013s018lbl.pdf.

63. **Robertson P Jr**, **Hellriegel E**, **Arora S**, et al. Effect of modafinil on pharmacokinetics of ethinyl estradiol and triazolam in healthy volunteers. *Clin Pharmacol Ther*, 2002; **71**:46–56.

64. **Robertson P Jr**, **Hellriegel E**, **Arora S**, et al. Effect of modafinil at steady state on the single-dose pharmacokinetic profile of warfarin in healthy volunteers. *J Clin Pharmacol*, 2002; **42**:205–14.

65. **Myrick H**, **Malcolm R**, **Taylor B**, et al. Modafinil: preclinical, clinical, and post-marketing surveillance: a review of abuse liability issues. *Ann Clin Psychiatry*, 2004; **16**:101–09.

66. **Rush C**, **Kelly T**, **Hays L**, et al. Acute behavioral and psychological effects of modafinil in drug abusers. *Behav Pharmacol*, 2002; **13**:105–15.

Section 4 Chapter 37

Therapy of Excessive Sleepiness

Sodium oxybate for the treatment of excessive sleepiness

Neil T. Feldman

History

The development of sodium oxybate (SXB) as a therapeutic agent began about 50 years ago when the compound was first synthesized as an analogue of the inhibitory neurotransmitter γ-aminobutyric acid (GABA). Known at that time as 4-hydroxybutyrate or γ-hydroxybutyrate (GHB), it was hypothesized that it would possess the central activity of GABA but cross the blood–brain barrier permitting peripheral administration [1], and the general anesthetic properties of GHB were soon demonstrated in animals [2] and humans [3–5]. Although GHB proved to be an unsatisfactory anesthetic because it lacked analgesic properties and caused myoclonic jerking during induction and emergence [6, 7], it continues to be used in the field of anesthesia in Europe (Somsanit® Injection, Franz Köhler Chemie, Germany; Gamma-OH® Injection, CERNEP-Synthélabo, France), where it is generally administered in combination with an analgesic or other anesthetic agent. During this time, it became apparent that GHB possessed unique properties with respect to sleep. When administered to human subjects, GHB was found to induce slow, synchronized EEG patterns similar to the slow waves observed during normal sleep [8].

As described below, GHB was subsequently studied by several independent investigators in the United States and Europe for the treatment of narcolepsy beginning in the 1970s and continuing into the 1990s. Based on the promising results of this work, the National Organization of Rare Disorders (NORD) and the Office of Orphan Products Development at the Food and Drug Administration (FDA) encouraged a small pharmaceutical company which specialized in the development of orphan drugs (Orphan Medical, Inc., Minnetonka, MN) to develop SXB for the treatment of narcolepsy. Following the completion of several clinical trials which established the safety and efficacy of SXB, it received market approval in 2002 for the treatment of cataplexy in patients with narcolepsy (Xyrem® [sodium oxybate] oral solution). In 2005, SXB was also approved for the treatment of excessive sleepiness in patients with narcolepsy.

While the therapeutic uses of GHB were being explored, it was also being marketed in the USA during the 1980s as an unregulated dietary supplement. GHB was believed to stimulate the release of growth hormone and was being used by body builders for its alleged anabolic effects, but the sale of GHB was banned by the FDA in 1990 following reports of fatal overdose [9]. GHB was also being abused because of alcohol-like euphoria, and subsequent restrictions on the sale of GHB led to an increase in illicit GHB trafficking including the GHB analogues gamma-butyrolactone and 1,4-butanediol. By the mid 1990s, illicit GHB had become popular as a "club drug" and was being implicated in growing numbers of overdose [10] and drug-facilitated sexual assault [11]. Eventually, dependence and withdrawal following chronic use of high-dose GHB was reported [12]. Efforts to control GHB abuse and drug-facilitated sexual assault eventually led to the passage of the Hillory J. Farias and Samantha Reid Date-Rape Drug Prohibition Act of 2000 (Public Law [PL] 106–172) [13]. This law amended the Controlled Substances Act by listing GHB as a Schedule I agent, but created an exception which placed FDA-approved formulations of GHB in Schedule III, permitting the development of SXB as a treatment for narcolepsy to continue.

Neurobiology of γ-hydroxybutyrate

Soon after the effects of GHB were discovered, it was shown to be an endogenous compound in the

---

Sleepiness: Causes, Consequences and Treatment, ed. Michael J. Thorpy and Michel Billiard. Published by Cambridge University Press. © Cambridge University Press 2011.

mammalian brain [14, 15], where it appears to function as a neuromodulator or neurotransmitter; however, its exact function in the central nervous system remains unknown despite decades of research (for comprehensive reviews on the neurobiology of GHB, see [16, 17]). Evidence supporting the role of GHB as a neurotransmitter includes a synthesis pathway, vesicular storage, calcium-dependent release and subsequent re-uptake mechanisms. GHB is derived from the precursor molecule GABA and is known to bind with high specificity to high- and low-affinity GHB receptors [18]. These G-protein-coupled receptors [19] are widely distributed throughout the cortex and subcortical areas, including dopaminergic areas such as the hippocampus, amygdala, septum, basal ganglia and substantia nigra [20]. As GHB receptors are known to be colocalized with dopaminergic terminals, much work has been done to assess the effects of GHB on dopamine-rich areas of the brain. Current evidence suggests GHB may regulate dopaminergic transmission in nigrostriatal and mesocorticolimbic pathways [21, 22]. When present in pharmacological concentrations, GHB also binds to GABA-B receptors, which appear to mediate most of the hypnotic effects of the drug; however, GHB can also be metabolized to GABA, and it is unclear whether the GABA-B receptor-mediated effects are caused by GHB itself or by GABA which is derived from GHB [23].

The effects of GHB at the GHB receptors are excitatory while those at the GABA-B receptors are inhibitory. Consequently, the drug acts as a hypnotic when administered in therapeutic doses until it reaches low concentrations and the excitatory GHB receptor-mediated effects occur. When administered therapeutically at bedtime, this may cause patients to suddenly awaken during the night. Similar to other GABA-B agonists such as baclofen, GHB increases total sleep time and delta waves during sleep; however, the GABA-B agonist baclofen has no beneficial effect on either cataplexy or EDS [24], suggesting GHB improves the symptoms of narcolepsy via non-GABA-B mechanisms.

Pharmacokinetics of γ-hydroxybutyrate

Endogenous GHB is synthesized via transamination of GABA to succinic semialdehyde which is then reduced to GHB. When administered exogenously, GHB is known to be rapidly metabolized to succinic semialdehyde, and then oxidized to succinic acid, which enters the Krebs' cycle where it is metabolized to carbon dioxide. Minor routes of GHB metabolism include β-oxidation and conversion to GABA [25]. Urinary excretion is minimal [26].

GHB is rapidly but incompletely absorbed after oral administration, and increasing the oral dose of GHB results in disproportionately large increases in peak plasma concentrations. For example, doubling the dose from 4.5 to 9.0 g increases the area under the curve of a concentration vs. time plot by 3.7-fold. In some studies, the drug displayed non-linear pharmacokinetic properties following twice-nightly administration. For example, the oral administration of 3 g taken at bedtime and again after 4 h resulted in peak plasma concentrations of 62.8 and 91.2 µg/ml, respectively [27]; however, when 12 healthy subjects were randomized to receive SXB 2.25 g following a 10-h fast and a repeat dose of 2.25 g after an additional 4 h of fasting, the mean (±SD) C_{max} were 84.2 (15.4) and 93.0 (28.2) µg/ml, respectively, indicating an effect of residual food in the stomach (personal communication, Jazz Pharmaceuticals, Inc.). Clinically non-significant increases in peak plasma concentration have been shown to occur following chronic administration although the elimination half-life remained unchanged [28].

The elimination half-life is also dose dependent and has been reported to range from 20 to 42 min [28–30]. As the oral bioavailability of the drug is decreased by a high-fat meal [28], it is suggested that the nightly dose of SXB should be administered at the same time with respect to the evening meal.

Early clinical use of γ-hydroxybutyrate for narcolepsy

Mamelak and co-workers were the first clinical investigators to suggest GHB may be beneficial for the treatment of sleep disorders. In their first report, GHB was administered at bedtime to several patients with insomnia. This resulted in sleep induction characterized by normal sleep stages; however, they observed several other significant changes, including decreased sleep latency, increased total sleep time and slow-wave sleep, and a greater proportion of REM sleep during the first half of the night [31, 32]. Eventually, the unusual properties of GHB were studied in patients with narcolepsy where the administration of

GHB at bedtime resulted in improved sleep quality with decreased nocturnal awakenings. A dose of 1.5–2.25 g was given at bedtime with additional doses of 1–1.5 g repeated 1–2 times as needed to maintain sleep throughout the night. The observed increase in nocturnal sleep consolidation [33] was associated with decreased symptoms of narcolepsy, including a significant decrease in the duration of daytime naps although the number of naps remained unchanged [34].

The effects of GHB were also evaluated in 30 patients with narcolepsy for up to 30 weeks. GHB was administered in two nightly doses taken at bedtime and again 4 h later. The total nightly dose ranged from 5 to 7 g. Stimulant medications were administered as needed for the treatment of EDS. These changes corresponded with substantial reductions in daytime sleepiness, sleep attacks and other daytime symptoms of narcolepsy. Daytime naps decreased by an average of 48% after 3 weeks while sleep attacks decreased by 65%. Although daytime sleepiness was not completely eliminated, it was controlled with lower doses of stimulant medication than patients were taking before the study [35]. The early use of GHB for the treatment of narcolepsy was also reported by Montplaisir and Godbout. GHB was administered to 36 patients of whom 14 (39%) reported subjective improvements in EDS. In a subsequent 30-day trial, 4 of 10 patients (40%) reported improvements in EDS [36].

The first randomized, placebo-controlled study with GHB for the treatment of narcolepsy was conducted by Scrima and co-workers. Using a double-blind cross-over design, they administered placebo or GHB at a nightly dose of 25 mg/kg at bedtime followed by a repeat dose of 25 mg/kg 3 h later to 20 patients with narcolepsy for 29 days. Following a 6-day washout period, the alternate treatment was administered. Patients were maintained on methylphenidate ≤300 mg daily as needed. Subjective sleepiness and the number of sleep attacks were not significantly different for placebo-treated patients, although multiple sleep latency tests suggested marginally increased sleep latency mean during GHB treatment [37, 38]. While these results were not very robust, Lammers *et al.* treated 24 narcolepsy patients with GHB for 4 weeks at a nightly dose of 60 mg/kg in a randomized double-blind placebo-controlled cross-over trial. Compared to placebo, daytime sleep attacks and the severity of subjective daytime sleepiness were significantly reduced [39].

Clinical development of sodium oxybate

GHB acquired the official generic name of sodium oxybate (SXB) during the formal development as a treatment for narcolepsy. The clinical trials which included EDS as an outcome measure are described below. The effects of SXB on other outcome measures are not discussed in detail. These studies enrolled adult patients with narcolepsy based on a valid polysomnogram and diagnostic criteria established by the American Sleep Disorders Association. Subjects working in occupations requiring variable shifts or routine night shifts were excluded from enrollment. In all studies, the study drug was administered in two equally divided nightly doses at bedtime and 4 h later. For convenience, the doses of SXB used are expressed as total nightly doses. In each study, subjects were permitted to use stimulants for the treatment of EDS but were not allowed to change the dosage. Changes in subjective sleepiness were measured with the Epworth Sleepiness Scale (ESS) and objectively with the 40-min Maintenance of Wakefulness Test (MWT).

OMI-GHB-2 & 3 (Trial 1 in the Prescribing Information [PI])

Among the 136 patients enrolled in this randomized, double-blind, placebo-controlled trial study, 113 (83.1%) were maintained on a stable dose of stimulant throughout the trial. Subjects were randomized to receive placebo or 3, 6, or 9 g of SXB without titration. After 4 weeks, the SXB-treated patients demonstrated significant dose-related improvements in ESS scores, becoming significant at the 9 g dose. For some patients dosed at 9 g, their level of sleepiness as indicated by the ESS fell into the normal range. This improvement in wakefulness occurred while most patients remained on stable doses of stimulant medications. These patients also demonstrated a significant decrease in the number of sleep attacks at the 6 and 9 g doses [40].

Patients who completed the above study were permitted to enroll in a 12-month open-label SXB extension trial. Patients began SXB treatment at a dose of 6 g nightly. Based on clinical efficacy and tolerability, the dose was adjusted in 1.5 g increments at 2-week intervals but staying within the range of 3–9 g nightly. Of the 118 patients enrolled in the study, 104 (88.1%) were taking one or more concomitant

4. Therapy of Excessive Sleepiness

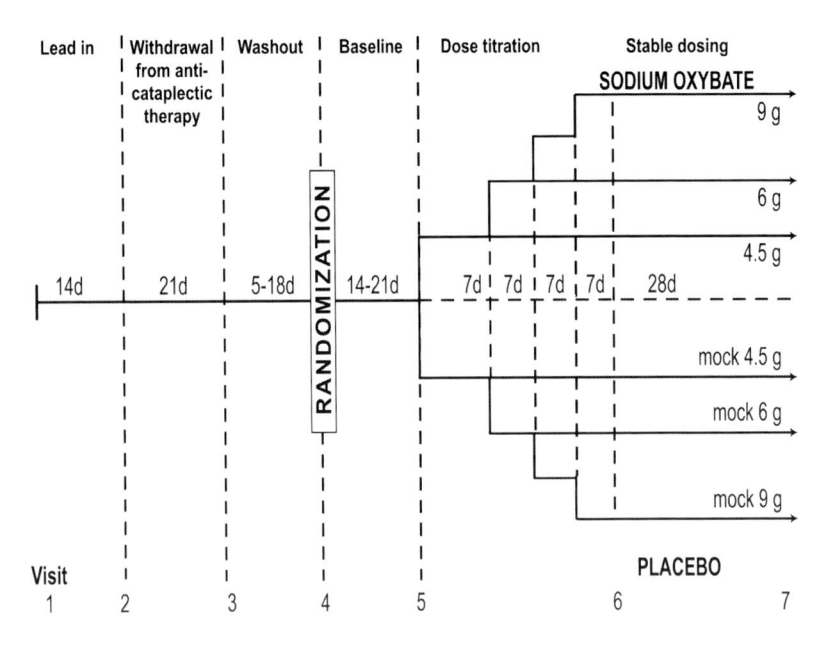

Figure 37.1 Following a 2-week baseline phase, anticataplectic medications were withdrawn over a 21-day period. The washout period was 5 days or 5 times the half-life of the withdrawn medication, whichever was longer. An additional 2 weeks were required for patients withdrawn from fluoxetine. To minimize the placebo effect, all patients were started on placebo during a single-blind fashion and recorded baseline cataplexy occurrences over a 2–3-week period. Patients were then titrated to their final dose of sodium oxybate or placebo as shown. Efficacy assessments were obtained at visits 2, 5, 6 and 7. Adapted from Xyrem® International Study Group, 2005 with permission [42].

stimulant medications. Significant improvements in baseline ESS scores occurred at every dosage used except 4.5 g (probably due to insufficient number of patients in this group) after 4 weeks, becoming maximal after 8 weeks. Across all doses used, the mean baseline ESS score decreased by approximately 30%. Other significant improvements reported by patients included nocturnal sleep quality, level of alertness, ability to concentrate, and a substantial decrease in the number and duration of sleep attacks [41].

OMI-SXB-15 (Trial 3 in the PI)

This study assessed the effects of nightly SXB administration on subjective and objective measures of EDS in 228 patients with narcolepsy [42]. It also characterized the effects of SXB on nocturnal sleep parameters. Stimulants were used by 178 (78%) patients for the treatment of EDS. Baseline MWT and ESS assessments were made during an initial 14-day baseline period while patients were treated with placebo drug in single-blind fashion. During a 4-week double-blind dose–titration phase, patients remained on placebo or were started on a dose of 3 g nightly (Figure 37.1). Some of these patients remained at 3 g nightly while an equal number of patients were titrated to receive 6 or 9 g nightly. Placebo-treated patients followed a similar mock titration protocol. All patients then continued at their assigned dose for the remaining 4 weeks of the study.

At the end of the trial, the median baseline ESS score of 19 had decreased to 15 and 12 among patients taking SXB at nightly doses of 6 and 9 g, respectively. The nightly use of SXB also resulted in significant, dose-related improvements in median MWT scores. Patients receiving 4.5 g of SXB displayed an increase of 1.75 min while patients treated with 9 g dose showed a median increase of more than 10 min. The dose-related decrease in the median baseline frequency of weekly sleep attacks was significant across all doses and significant among the 6 and 9 g dose groups when compared to placebo.

OMI-SXB-22 (Trial 4 in the PI)

The following double-blind, placebo-controlled trial recruited 231 patients maintained on stable doses of modafinil (200–600 mg/day) to characterize the efficacy of SXB alone and together with modafinil for the treatment of EDS in patients with narcolepsy [43]. Baseline MWT and ESS assessments were made during an initial 14-day baseline period while patients were treated with their usual dose of modafinil in single-blind fashion (Figure 37.2). Subsequently, patients were randomized to receive treatment with (1) SXB 6 g nightly, (2) modafinil, (3) SXB 6 g nightly and modafinil, or (4) placebo. After 4 weeks, the dose of SXB was increased to 9 g for an additional 4 weeks.

At the end of the trial, the mean average MWT sleep latency in the placebo group was 6.87 min,

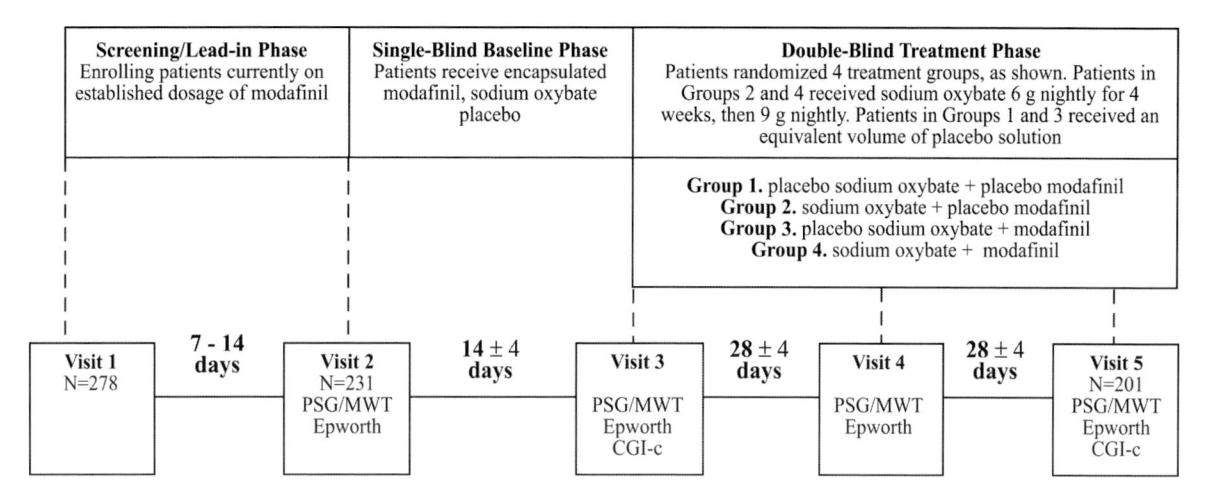

Figure 37.2 Following a 1–2 baseline phase, patients underwent a PSG and MWT while remaining on stable doses of modafinil. During a subsequent 2-week, single-blind, baseline phase, patients received placebo while remaining on modafinil. At Visit 3, patients were randomized into the four treatment groups as shown. The dose of sodium oxybate was increased from 6 g nightly to 9 g nightly after 4 weeks. The efficacy and safety measures were performed as indicated. Adapted from Black and Houghton, 2006 with permission [43].

which was significantly lower than the modafinil group (10.13 min), the SXB group (12.24 min) or the SXB/modafinil group (12.91 min). The greatest improvements occurred during the initial 4 weeks of the trial. The SXB/modafinil group demonstrated a significant mean increase in baseline mean sleep latency of 2.72 min. This represents the incremental improvement in EDS produced by the addition of SXB over the use of modafinil alone. The SXB and SXB/modafinil groups demonstrated significant reductions in ESS scores compared to patients treated with placebo at the end of the trial while the scores for the modafinil-treated patients did not significantly change and were not different from the placebo group.

The patients treated with SXB alone and SXB plus modafinil also demonstrated significantly fewer weekly sleep attacks at the end of the trial compared to modafinil and placebo groups. The mean number of weekly sleep attacks decreased from 10.05 at baseline to 7.10 in the SXB-treated patients and from 11.82 to 5.55 in the SXB/modafinil-treated group. There were no differences in sleep attacks in the modafinil- and placebo-treated groups.

Pivotal trials 3 and 4 established SXB as an effective treatment for EDS, and based on the evidence provided in those clinical trials, SXB has become recognized by the American Academy of Sleep Medicine as a standard treatment for daytime sleepiness in narcolepsy [44]. Interestingly, the nightly use of SXB is also associated with significant improvements in the quality and duration of nocturnal sleep; however, the improvements in sleep alone cannot explain the improvements observed in EDS.

The administration of triazolam to patients with narcolepsy improved nocturnal sleep efficiency and overall sleep quality without benefiting EDS [45]. The effects of SXB on EDS appear to be unique and unrelated to GABA-B activity. Similar to SXB, baclofen is also an agonist at the GABA-B receptor. In a recent study by Huang and Guilleminault, baclofen and SXB were administered at bedtime for 3 months to recently diagnosed patients with narcolepsy. Although both medications increased total sleep time and delta wave sleep, improvements in EDS and cataplexy occurred only in SXB-treated patients [24]. The mechanism by which SXB improves cataplexy and sleepiness does not appear to be mediated by GABA-B receptors.

The beneficial effects of SXB for the treatment of EDS do not appear to be limited to narcolepsy. Patients with Parkinson's disease also experience disrupted nocturnal sleep and EDS [46]. The nightly administration of SXB to patients with Parkinson's disease at doses generally used for narcolepsy (3–9 g) has been shown to significantly increase slow-wave sleep time and improve ESS and Fatigue Severity Scale scores in an open-label polysomnographic study [47].

In fact, SXB may improve both sleepiness and vigilance in normal volunteers with sleep deprivation

[48]. This was recently demonstrated in a study in which subjects underwent two consecutive nights of sleep deprivation followed each morning by a 3-h sleep opportunity. Prior to sleep, some subjects received SXB while others received placebo. Total sleep time was not significantly different between these groups; however, the mean duration of slow-wave sleep was approximately 88 min among the SXB-treated subjects and 57 min among the placebo-treated subjects ($p < 0.001$), while the amount of REM sleep in these two groups was approximately 12 and 35 min, respectively ($p < 0.001$). As a group, the subjects treated with SXB had significantly longer mean Multiple Sleep Latency Test (MSLT) on both days compared with the subjects treated with placebo. The SXB subjects rated themselves significantly less sleepy on the Karolinska Sleepiness Scale and displayed significantly faster reaction times on the Psychomotor Vigilance Task on the second day. These investigators suggest that SXB reduces the negative impact of sleep deprivation by increasing slow-wave sleep.

Safety

During clinical trials, the most common adverse events (>5%) occurring more frequently than placebo-treated patients were nausea (19%), dizziness (18%), headache (18%), vomiting (8%), somnolence (6%), urinary incontinence (6%), and nasopharyngitis (6%). Less common but more serious adverse events associated with SXB include confusion, depression and other neuropsychiatric events [49]. Since the launch of the product in the United States, Canada and the European Union through March 2008, an estimated 26 000 patients have received treatment with SXB. Adverse events reported with a frequency of ≥1% include nausea (2.2%), insomnia (1.4%), headache (1.4%), dizziness (1.3%), and vomiting (1.0%) [50]. It should be emphasized that these data represent the findings of a passive surveillance collection method and therefore almost certainly represent an underestimate of the actual frequency of adverse events. In addition, the duration of treatment of this population was not provided.

Early, unapproved forms of GHB were labeled as club drugs and associated with sexual assault [51], and despite early concerns that the commercial availability of SXB would lead to widespread abuse, such events have rarely been reported [52]. This is likely due to the restricted distribution program which has decreased the likelihood of product diversion for illicit uses. Since the launch of the product through March 2008, 14 cases of possible SXB abuse have been reported worldwide after market introduction [50].

The SXB prescribing information includes a black box warning which emphasizes the potential for respiratory depressant effects [49] and a case report describes the worsening sleep apnea symptoms in two patients [53]. One clinical trial examined the effects of SXB on sleep-disordered breathing and sleep architecture in patients with mild to moderate obstructive sleep apnea (OSA). This randomized, cross-over study enrolled 60 patients each with an apnea–hypopnea index (AHI) between 10/h and 40/h and nadir oxygen saturation (SpO_2) of >75%. Treatments included SXB 9 g nightly, SXB 9 g nightly + modafinil 200 mg daily, zolpidem 10 mg nightly, or placebo nightly. Patients were treated for four consecutive nights followed by overnight polysomnography. Among the 42 patients completing the study, the mean change in baseline AHI and mean SpO_2 values were not significantly different among the four treatment groups. Among the SXB-treated patients, central apneas increased and clinically significant decreases in oxygen saturation occurred in three patients [54]. Among narcolepsy patients with evidence of sleep-disordered breathing during baseline polysomnography, SXB should be prescribed only to those patients who fully comply with nasal continuous positive airway pressure therapy. During long-term treatment, the respiratory status of SXB-treated patients should be periodically evaluated with nocturnal oximetry and prescribers should remain vigilant for the possible development of sleep-disordered breathing [55]. Of special concern are recent reports of deaths in SXB-treated patients [56]. SXB is a CNS and respiratory depressant and the concomitant administration of drugs with additional respiratory depressant effects is contraindicated. Suggestions for the use of SXB in patients with sleep-disordered breathing have recently been published [55].

Conclusion

SXB can play a significant role in the treatment of excessive sleepiness associated with narcolepsy, although it does not normalize alertness in most patients. Optimal treatment usually requires the use of SXB in combination with modafinil or other stimulants. Patients taking SXB may display widely divergent therapeutic benefit, with some patients achieving a very robust therapeutic benefit while others receive no response. No demographic parameter or symptom complex predicts the success or failure of treatment in an individual patient.

The acceptance of SXB as a first-line therapy has been reduced by its adverse event profile, inconvenient nighttime dosing, a restricted distribution system and its association with illicit forms of GHB; however, the range of therapeutic options for this patient population is limited and the effectiveness of current treatments are also limited by adverse events and tolerance. Therefore, SXB should probably be utilized in narcolepsy more often than the current frequency. Hopefully, a formulation will soon be developed that will eliminate the need for a second dose of SXB during the night. Future clinical trials should be conducted that will assess the effects of SXB for the treatment of excessive sleepiness associated with other disorders.

References

1. **Laborit H, Buchard F, Laborit G**, et al. Use of sodium 4-hydroxybutyrate in anesthesia and resuscitation. *Agressologie*, 1960; **1**:549–60.
2. **Drakontides A, Schneider J, Funderburk W**. Some effects of sodium gamma-hydroxybutyrate on the central nervous system. *J Pharmacol, Exp Ther* 1962; **135**:275–84.
3. **Helrich M, McAslan T, Skolnik S**, et al. Correlation of blood levels of 4-hydroxybutyrate with state of consciousness. *Anesthesiology*, 1964; **25**:771–75.
4. **Solway J, Sadove M**. 4-Hydroxybutyrate: a clinical study. *Anesth Analg*, 1965; **44**:532–39.
5. **Yamada Y, Yamamoto J, Fujiki A**, et al. Effect of butyrolactone and gamma-hydroxybutyrate on the EEG and sleep cycle in man. *Electroencephalogr Clin Neurophysiol*, 1967; **22**:558–62.
6. **Vickers M**. Gamma-hydroxybutyric acid. *Proc R Soc Med*, 1968; **61**:821–24.
7. **Vickers M**. Gamma-hydroxybutyric acid. *Int Anesthesiol Clin*, 1969; **7**:75–89.
8. **Metcalf D, Emde R, Stripe J**. An EEG-behavioral study of sodium hydroxybutyrate in humans. *Electroencephalogr Clin Neurophysiol*, 1966; **20**:506–12.
9. **Centers for Disease Control**. Multistate outbreak of poisonings associated with illicit use of gamma-hydroxybutyrate. *JAMA*, 1991; **256**:447–48.
10. **Li J, Stokes S, Woeckener A**. A tale of novel intoxication: seven cases of γ-hydroxybutyric acid overdose. *Ann Emerg Med*, 1998; **31**:723–28.
11. **Schwartz R, Milteer R, LeBeau M**. Drug-facilitated sexual assault ('date rape'). *South Med J*, 2000; **93**:558–61.
12. **Craig K, Gomez H, McManus J**, et al. Severe gamma-hydroxybutyrate withdrawal: a case report and literature review. *J Emerg Med*, 2000; **18**:76–80.
13. Food and Drug Administration. *Fed Regist*, 2000; **65**:13 235–38.
14. **Bessman S, Fishbein W**. Gamma-hydroxybutyrate. A new metabolite in brain. *FASEB J*, 1963; **22**:334–35.
15. **Roth R**. Formation and regional distribution of gamma-hydroxybutyric acid in mammalian brain. *Biochem Pharmacol*, 1970; **19**:3013–19.
16. **Wong C, Chan K, Gibson K**, et al. Gamma-hydroxybutyric acid: neurobiology and toxicology of a recreational drug. *Toxicol Rev*, 2004; **23**:3–20.
17. **Pardi D, Black J**. Gamma-hydroxybutyrate/sodium oxybate: neurobiology, and impact on sleep and wakefulness. *CNS Drugs*, 2006; **20**:993–1018.
18. **Castelli M, Ferraro L, Mocci I**, et al. Selective gamma-hydroxybutyric acid receptor ligands increase extracellular glutamate in the hippocampus, but fail to activate G protein and to produce the sedative/hypnotic effect of gamma-hydroxybutyric acid. *J Neurochem*, 2003; **87**:722–32.
19. **Andriamampandry C, Taleb O, Viry S**, et al. Cloning and characterization of a rat brain receptor that binds the endogenous neuromodulator gamma hydroxybutyrate (GHB). *FASEB J*, 2003; **17**:1691–93.
20. **Hechler V, Gobaille S, Bourguignon J**, et al. Extracellular events induced by gamma-hydroxybutyrate in striatum: a microdialysis study. *J Neurochem*, 1991; **56**:938–44.
21. **Roth R, Doherty J, Walters J**. Gamma-hydroxybutyrate: a role in the regulation of central dopaminergic neurons? *Brain Res*, 1980; **189**:556–60.
22. **Nissbrandt H, Elverfors A, Engberg G**. Pharmacologically induced cessation of burst activity in nigral dopamine neurons: significance for the terminal dopamine efflux. *Synapse*, 1994; **17**:217–24.
23. **Crunelli V, Emri Z, Leresche N**. Unravelling the brain targets of gamma-hydroxybutyric acid. *Curr Opin Pharmacol*, 2006; **6**:44–52.
24. **Huang Y, Guilleminault C**. Narcolepsy: action of two gamma-aminobutyric acid type B agonists, baclofen and sodium oxybate. *Pediatr Neurol*, 2009; **41**:9–16.
25. **Maitre M**. The gamma-hydroxybutyrate signalling system in brain: organization and functional implications. *Prog Neurobiol*, 1997; **51**:337–61.

26. **Abanades S**, **Farré M**, **Segura M**, et al. Disposition of gamma-hydroxybutyric acid in conventional and nonconventional biologic fluids after single drug administration: issues in methodology and drug monitoring. *Ther Drug Monit*, 2007; **29**:64–70.

27. **Scharf M**, **Lai A**, **Branigan B**, et al. Pharmacokinetics of gamma-hydroxybutyrate (GHB) in narcoleptic patients. *Sleep*, 1998; **21**:507–14.

28. **Borgen L**, **Okerholm R**, **Lai A**, et al. The pharmacokinetics of sodium oxybate oral solution following acute and chronic administration to narcoleptic patients. *J Clin Pharmacol*, 2004; **44**:253–57.

29. **Ferrara S**, **Zotti S**, **Tedeschi L**, et al. Pharmacokinetics of gamma-hydroxybutyric acid in alcohol dependent patients after single and repeated oral doses. *Br J Clin Pharmacol*, 1992; **34**:231–35.

30. **Palatini P**, **Tedeschi L**, **Frison G**, et al. Dose-dependent absorption and elimination of gamma-hydroxybutyric acid in healthy volunteers. *Eur J Clin Pharmacol*, 1993; **45**:353–56.

31. **Mamelak M**, **Escriu J**, **Stokan O**. Sleep-inducing effects of gamma-hydroxybutyrate. *Lancet*, 1973; **2**:328–29.

32. **Mamelak M**, **Escriu J**, **Stokan O**. The effects of gamma-hydroxybutyrate on sleep. *Biol Psychiatry*, 1977; **12**:273–88.

33. **Broughton R**, **Mamelak M**. The treatment of narcolepsy–cataplexy with nocturnal gamma-hydroxybutyrate. *Can J Neurol Sci*, 1979; **6**:1–6.

34. **Broughton R**, **Mamelak M**. Effects of nocturnal gamma-hydroxybutyrate on sleep/wake patterns in narcolepsy–cataplexy. *Can J Neurol Sci*, 1980; **7**:23–31.

35. **Scharf M**, **Brown D**, **Woods M**, et al. The effects and effectiveness of γ-hydroxybutyrate in patients with narcolepsy. *J Clin Psychiatry*, 1985; **46**:222–25.

36. **Montplaisir J**, **Godbout R**. Nocturnal sleep of narcoleptic patients: revisited. *Sleep*, 1986; **9**:159–61.

37. **Scrima L**, **Hartman P**, **Johnson F H Jr**, et al. Efficacy of gamma-hydroxy-butyrate versus placebo in treating narcolepsy–cataplexy: double blind subjective measures. *Biol Psychiatry*, 1989; **26**:331–43.

38. **Scrima L**, **Hartman P**, **Johnson F**, et al. The effects of γ-hydroxy-butyrate on the sleep of narcolepsy patients: a double blind study. *Sleep*, 1990; **13**: 479–90.

39. **Lammers G**, **Arends J**, **Declerck A**, et al. Gamma-hydroxybutyrate and narcolepsy: a double-blind placebo-controlled study. *Sleep*, 1993; **6**:216–20.

40. **US Xyrem® Multicenter Study Group**. A randomized, double blind, placebo-controlled multicenter trial comparing the effects of three doses of orally administered sodium oxybate with placebo for the treatment of narcolepsy. *Sleep*, 2002; **25**:42–49.

41. **US Xyrem® Multicenter Study Group**. A 12-month, open-label, multi-center extension trial of orally administered sodium oxybate for the treatment of narcolepsy. *Sleep*, 2003; **26**:31–35.

42. **Xyrem® International Study Group**. A double-blind, placebo-controlled, study demonstrates the nightly administration of sodium oxybate significantly improves excessive daytime sleepiness in narcolepsy patients taking concurrent stimulant medications. *J Clin Sleep Med*, 2005; **1**:391–97.

43. **Black J**, **Houghton W**. Sodium oxybate improves excessive daytime sleepiness in narcolepsy. *Sleep*, 2006; **29**:939–46.

44. **Morgenthaler T**, **Kapur V**, **Brown T**, et al. Practice parameters for the treatment of narcolepsy and other hypersomnias of central origin. *Sleep*, 2007; **30**:1705–11.

45. **Thorpy M**, **Snyder M**, **Aloe F**, et al. Short-term triazolam use improves nocturnal sleep of narcoleptics. *Sleep*, 1992; **15**:212–16.

46. **Monderer R**, **Thorpy M**. Sleep disorders and daytime sleepiness in Parkinson's disease. *Curr Neurol Neurosci Rep*, 2009; **9**:173–80.

47. **Ondo W**, **Perkins T**, **Swick T**, et al. Sodium oxybate for excessive daytime sleepiness in Parkinson disease: an open-label polysomnographic study. *Arch Neurol*, 2008; **65**:1337–40.

48. **Schweitzer P**, **Hall J**, **Griffin K**, et al. Enhancing slow wave sleep with sodium oxybate reduces the behavioral and psychological impact of sleep loss. *Sleep*, 2009; **32**(Suppl):A154.

49. **Xyrem® (sodium oxybate) oral solution**. Prescribing Information. Jazz Pharmaceuticals, Inc.

50. **Wang Y**, **Swick T J**, **Carter L**, et al. Safety overview of postmarketing and clinical experience of sodium oxybate (Xyrem): abuse, misuse, dependence, and diversion. *J Clin Sleep Med*, 2009; **5**:365–71.

51. **Nicholson K**, **Balster R**. GHB: a new and novel drug of abuse. *Drug Alcohol Depend*, 2001; **63**:1–22.

52. **Carter L**, **Pardi D**, **Gorsline J**, et al. Illicit gamma-hydroxybutyrate (GHB) and pharmaceutical sodium oxybate (Xyrem): differences in characteristics and misuse. *Drug Alcohol Depend*, 2009; **104**:1–10.

53. **Seeck-Hirschner M**, **Baier P**, **von Freier A**, et al. Increase in sleep-related breathing disturbances after treatment with sodium oxybate in patients with narcolepsy and mild obstructive sleep apnea

syndrome: two case reports. *Sleep Med*, 2009; **10**:154–55.

54. **George C**, **Feldman N**, **Inhaber N**, *et al*. A safety trial of sodium oxybate in patients with obstructive sleep apnea: Acute effects on sleep-disordered breathing. *Sleep Med*, 2010; **11**:38–42.

55. **Feldman N**. Clinical perspective: monitoring sodium oxybate-treated narcolepsy patients for the development of sleep-disordered breathing. *Sleep Breath*, 2010; **14**:72–79.

56. **Zvosec D**, **Smith S**, **Hall B**. Three deaths associated with use of Xyrem. *Sleep Med*, 2009; **10**:490–93.

Section 4 Chapter 38

Therapy of Excessive Sleepiness

Caffeine and other alerting agents

William D. S. Killgore

Introduction

We live in a sleepy society. Contemporary pressures from home and work seem to demand more from us each day. For a variety of reasons, people find themselves getting up earlier, working longer hours, and staying up later. There never seems to be enough time – something's got to give. Unfortunately, it seems that sleep is often one of the first casualties when people try to make cuts in their daily schedule. One less hour of sleep is just one more hour available for work and play, we tell ourselves – and sometimes, we don't have any other choice. Besides, we console ourselves, if we start feeling a little sleepy, we can always just grab a cup of java at the corner café for a quick pick-me-up. But can caffeine really help? Does a cup or two of coffee really reduce sleepiness, sustain alertness, and improve performance – and if so, for how long and under what circumstances?

While people use a variety of strategies to combat sleepiness, including modified work/rest scheduling, sleep optimization, sleep-inducing medications, strategic use of bright light, and napping, undoubtedly the most commonly used temporary countermeasure against sleepiness is caffeine. Routinely consumed in the form of coffee, tea, soft drinks, cocoa, and chocolate, caffeine is reported to be the most commonly used psychoactive substance in the world [1]. Nearly 90% of Americans regularly use caffeine [2], and as many as 78% of automobile drivers report drinking caffeinated beverages to stave off sleepiness while driving [3]. In the United States, adults usually consume caffeine in the form of coffee, whereas children and adolescents tend to get most of their caffeine from soft drinks [2]. Individuals in the United Kingdom, Finland, and Sweden typically consume from 100 to 400 mg/day of caffeine [4], and recent survey data suggest that American caffeine users consume an average of 193 mg/day, with males between the ages of 35 and 54 being the highest users, typically consuming 336 mg/day [2]. As the amount of caffeine in an 8-ounce cup of coffee generally ranges from about 80 to 135 mg [5]; this roughly corresponds to about two to four cups of coffee per day for most American consumers. For reference, a non-exhaustive list of a few common caffeine-containing foods and beverages, as reported by the Center for Science in the Public Interest (www.cspinet.org) is provided in Table 38.1.

Pharmacology

Caffeine is effective at restoring alertness and psychomotor vigilance during periods of sleepiness [6]. While the mechanisms by which caffeine restores alertness and reduces sleepiness are not entirely understood, considerable evidence suggests that much of the alerting effect of caffeine actually comes about through stimulation of arousal-promoting neurons and inhibition of sleep-promoting neurons in the brain via blockade of adenosine receptors [4, 7]. This theory, known as the "adenosine hypothesis", is based on the finding that during wakefulness, the brain continuously breaks down adenosine triphosphate, a primary component of cellular energy reserves. With prolonged wakefulness, the consumption of adenosine triphosphate to sustain waking brain arousal slowly produces a build-up of excess extracellular adenosine as a byproduct. This accumulation is particularly notable in the cholinergic basal forebrain, a part of the brain that is heavily involved in alertness and arousal. As adenosine accumulates, it binds to A_1 receptors of cholinergic neurons, leading to a reduction in neurotransmitter release and inhibition of neuronal firing rate.

Sleepiness: Causes, Consequences and Treatment, ed. Michael J. Thorpy and Michel Billiard. Published by Cambridge University Press. © Cambridge University Press 2011.

Table 38.1 Caffeine content of select foods and beverages

Dietary source	Serving size	Caffeine (mg)	
Generic brewed coffee	8 oz	133	(range: 102–200)
Generic instant coffee	8 oz	93	(range: 27–173)
Generic decaffeinated coffee	8 oz	5	(range: 3–12)
Starbucks brewed coffee (grande)	16 oz	320	
Brewed tea	8 oz	53	(range: 40–120)
Coca-Cola classic	12 oz	35	
Diet Coke	12 oz	47	
Pepsi Cola	12 oz	38	
Mountain Dew	12 oz	54	
Sprite	12 oz	0	
Red Bull	8.3 oz	80	
Monster Energy	16 oz	160	
Spike Shooter	8.4 oz	300	
Hershey's chocolate bar	1.55 oz	9	
Hershey's special dark chocolate bar	1.45 oz	31	

Source: Center for Science in the Public Interest (www.cspinet.org).

Thus, adenosine inhibits arousal systems. Interestingly, adenosine also appears to reduce activity in GABAergic neurons, leading to a downstream disinhibition of sleep-promoting neurons in the preoptic/anterior hypothalamus. In short, prolonged wakefulness leads to a build-up of extracellular adenosine, which is sleep-promoting, whereas sleep gradually reduces adenosine concentrations [7]. Caffeine is believed to have nonselective affinity for these same adenosine receptors, particularly the A_1 and A_{2A} receptors [8]. Caffeine acts as an adenosine receptor antagonist, blocking the sleep-promoting effects caused by the accumulation of adenosine during the waking period [5] and increasing the release of cortical acetylcholine [9]. By blocking the sleep-promoting effects of adenosine, caffeine sustains alertness.

The specific neural systems most affected by caffeine are still uncertain, although it is known that A_1 and A_{2A} adenosine receptors are differentially distributed throughout the brain. The A_1 receptors tend to be found in abundance across the entire brain, with particular concentrations in several cerebral structures involved in aspects of higher cognition, including the cerebral cortex, hippocampus, thalamus, and cerebellum, whereas the A_{2A} receptors tend to predominate in dopamine-laden regions involved in reward and motor control, including the nucleus accumbens and striatum [5, 8]. Recent functional neuroimaging studies suggest that caffeine may increase task-related activation within the medial prefrontal cortex (BA 10) and right anterior cingulate gyrus (BA 32) relative to placebo during a complex working memory task [10] (see Figure 38.1). These regions are involved in attention, planning, cognitive monitoring, and problem-solving, suggesting that caffeine may exert some of its cognitive enhancing effects by increasing activation of these prefrontal regions during mentally demanding tasks.

Once ingested, orally administered caffeine is absorbed rapidly and reaches peak plasma levels within 30–120 min. The half-life of caffeine is quite variable, but has generally been suggested to range from about 3 to 6 h for a single dose in healthy individuals [11]. There appears to be considerable interindividual variability in sensitivity to the effects of caffeine. While some people are relatively insensitive to caffeine's effects, others show very low tolerance, including higher maximum plasma concentrations, slower elimination half-life, and greater sleep disturbance when given an equivalent dosage [12]. Caffeine is metabolized hepatically, with only about 1% eliminated unchanged in the urine [11]. In most

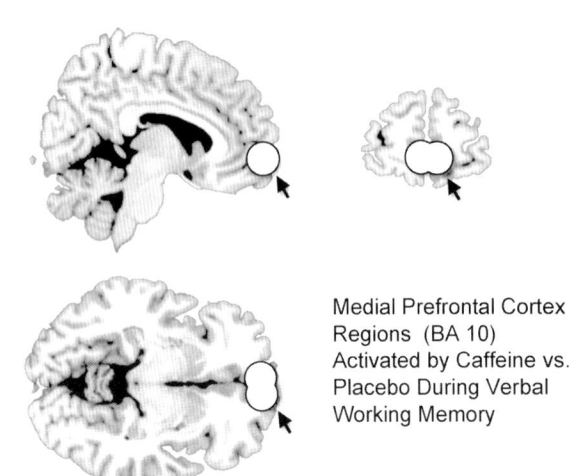

Countering daytime sleepiness

Even in normally rested individuals there are daily rhythms in alertness that fluctuate across the daytime waking period. Perhaps the most well known of these rhythms is the afternoon circadian nadir or "post-lunch dip," a mild decline in general alertness that occurs in the mid-afternoon hours, even among non-sleep-deprived individuals. This temporary fluctuation is normal and, despite mild increases in sleepiness, does not necessarily reflect insufficient nocturnal sleep [14]. Various countermeasures can be used to combat this afternoon wilt in alertness, including taking a brief nap, increasing exposure to bright light, or drinking a cup of coffee, just to name a few.

Several studies have compared the effectiveness of different countermeasures to mild daytime sleepiness. Horne and colleagues compared four conditions, including a 20-minute afternoon nap, 150 mg of caffeine in the afternoon, a normal night of sleep (mean = 7.6 h of sleep), or a full night of sleep extended for an extra 90 min, to see which was most effective at reducing objective sleepiness on the Multiple Sleep Latency Test (MSLT) and subjective sleepiness on the Karolinska Sleepiness Scale (KSS) in the afternoon. While a brief nap emerged as most effective at staving off sleepiness on the MSLT, a single 150 mg dose of caffeine was found to be a close second in effectiveness [14]. Interestingly, while objective sleep latency on the MSLT was improved by both methods, neither napping nor caffeine had any significant influence on subjective ratings of sleepiness. Another study also demonstrated the effectiveness of a nap at reducing objective and subjective sleepiness, but also found that the post-nap period was often accompanied by sleep inertia or residual sleepiness [15]. This sleep inertia was eliminated, however, by combining caffeine with a nap. Specifically, 200 mg of caffeine followed immediately by a 20-min nap during the lunch hour was highly effective at sustaining reaction time and accuracy on a working memory search task and reducing subjective sleepiness during the afternoon dip when compared to a nap alone [15]. Furthermore, caffeine plus a nap resulted in greater sustained alertness compared to other conditions, such as a nap plus bright light or a nap plus cold-water face washing. Thus, while a brief nap appears quite effective at temporarily restoring alertness during the post-lunch period, a single dose of caffeine equal to about a cup or two of coffee appears to be nearly as beneficial. The combination

Figure 38.1 Caffeine is associated with greater functional brain activation within the medial prefrontal cortex, particularly within Brodmann's Area 10 (BA 10), during a 2-back working memory task relative to placebo [10]. For graphic representation, the white circular regions represent spheres (10 mm radius) surrounding the location of maximal responsiveness to caffeine.

healthy individuals, caffeine ingestion is associated with statistically reliable increases in systolic (i.e. 3–15 mmHg) and diastolic (i.e. 4–13 mmHg) blood pressure that peak within 1–2 h after administration, although these effects are diminished in chronic caffeine users that have developed tolerance [11]. Although some aspects of autonomic arousal are increased at rest by double-blind administration of caffeine (250 mg), including skin conductance, respiration, and reduced alpha power on electroencephalogram (EEG), cardiac indices including heart rate do not appear to be significantly affected [13].

Effectiveness of caffeine as a countermeasure to sleepiness

Sleepiness can result from a number of causes, including (1) normal fluctuations in alertness that occur throughout the day, (2) more severe degradation of alertness that occurs during the overnight circadian trough, (3) increased homeostatic sleep pressure that accumulates during periods of prolonged wakefulness, or (4) some combination of these factors. We will explore the effectiveness of caffeine as a countermeasure to sleepiness in each of these situations.

of caffeine and a brief nap seems to be particularly effective.

A number of other studies have also shown that modest caffeine doses, generally equivalent to one or two cups of coffee, are effective at reducing daytime sleepiness and sustaining simple cognitive performances relative to placebo in non-sleep-deprived volunteers. Doses ranging from 75 to 150 mg of caffeine have effectively improved daytime vigilance and alertness for up to 90 min post-administration [16], while 200 mg has been shown to sustain daytime performance up to 4 h after administration in normally rested volunteers [17]. Of note, differences were not observed between habitual and non-habitual users of caffeine in these studies, despite the fact that participants were required to abstain from caffeine during the night preceding testing. This suggests that the observed effects were not likely caused by simple reversal of withdrawal symptoms among regular caffeine users.

Most people who use caffeine do so on a fairly regular basis. Thus, the question arises – does caffeine lose its effectiveness if it is consumed routinely? Tolerance to caffeine appears to be most clearly observed for subjective ratings, whereas tolerance for physiological indices is less demonstrable [18]. Cognitive studies have been contradictory regarding the effects of caffeine tolerance. Evidence suggests that some aspects of cognitive performance, such as mood and simple response time, may exhibit tolerance to repeated doses of caffeine whereas others, such as working memory and selective attention, may not [19]. In one study, normally rested subjects were pre-dosed with 200 mg of caffeine, D-ribose, or placebo every day for a week and then measured on a variety of fatigue-inducing cognitive tasks throughout a single day [20]. Even after a week of daily pre-dosing, caffeine was still more effective than placebo at improving cognitive performance, suggesting that the development of this degree of tolerance does not completely obviate the effectiveness of caffeine. D-Ribose had no effect on alertness whatsoever.

Many college students can attest to the pick-me-up given by a quick cup of coffee before class. For instance, college students administered a double-blind dose of 100 mg of caffeine an hour before a 75-min lecture reported significantly higher perceptions of being "alert," "clear minded," "energetic," and "anxious" than those receiving an identical placebo, although ratings of "efficient" and "creative" did not differ [21].

Similarly, a large double-blind study of college students found that a single cup of caffeinated coffee (100 mg) resulted in significantly lower daytime sleepiness scores on the Stanford Sleepiness Scale (SSS) and higher ratings of subjective "activation" (i.e. combined visual analogue ratings of "alert" and "vigorous" versus ratings of "tired" and "sleepy") than decaffeinated coffee, regardless of time of day. Notably, the advantage of caffeine was evident within 10 min after consumption and showed progressive improvement for up to 30 min [22], suggesting that the subjective alerting effects of caffeine are quite rapid. Interestingly, these effects occurred independently of average daily caffeine intake.

Based on the evidence reviewed so far, it appears that during daytime hours, alertness can be improved among non-sleep-deprived individuals by doses of caffeine equivalent to that found in one to two cups of coffee. But what about lower doses, such as those typical of tea or soft drinks – are they useful in sustaining daytime alertness too? For normal serving sizes, these beverages typically contain between 30 and 60 mg of caffeine [5]. For the most part, even these smaller doses of caffeine do appear to have some alerting effects. Low doses of caffeine seem to be most effective at sustaining response speed relative to response accuracy. For instance, in a sample of non-sleep-deprived subjects that had abstained from caffeine overnight, 60 mg of caffeine dissolved in tea or hot water produced significantly faster response times than placebo on tests of pattern recognition, delayed match to sample memory, and visual search, but had no effect on performance accuracy [23]. Positive effects were observed almost immediately after beverage consumption, suggesting that even low dose caffeine can improve response speed rapidly. Lieberman and colleagues compared the effectiveness of several dosages of caffeine in non-sleep-deprived volunteers, and found that morning doses as low as 32 mg were associated with improved auditory and visual vigilance (i.e. reaction time and correct detections) relative to placebo, and no dose–response function was apparent, suggesting that higher doses (up to 256 mg) did not necessarily lead to better performance [24]. Interestingly, despite the improvement in objective performance, self-reported mood variables and subjective sleepiness were unaffected by any dose of caffeine. Caffeine at even lower doses can have an effect as well. For example, Smit and Rogers found that morning caffeine doses as low as 12.5 mg can significantly

4. Therapy of Excessive Sleepiness

Table 38.2 Summary points for countering daytime sleepiness

1. Low doses of caffeine ranging from about 30 to 60 mg (e.g. amounts commonly found in tea and soft drinks) can modestly improve response speed and vigilance in normally rested persons, but such low doses may have minimal effects as sleep debt is increased.
2. Caffeine in doses of approximately 100 mg (e.g. about one cup of coffee) is generally effective for reducing afternoon sleepiness and restoring alertness for up to 90 min in non-sleep-deprived persons.
3. Doses of 200 mg (e.g. about two cups of coffee) are effective at sustaining daytime performance through the afternoon circadian nadir for up to 4 h.
4. The combination of 150–200 mg of caffeine followed by a brief nap (i.e. 20 min or less) is particularly effective at sustaining afternoon alertness and performance, and minimizes immediate post-nap grogginess.
5. The effectiveness of caffeine for countering afternoon sleepiness does not appear to differ markedly between regular consumers of caffeine and those who use it infrequently.

improve simple reaction time (most evident around 45 min after administration) relative to placebo [25].

While low to moderate doses of caffeine may be effective at improving alertness and vigilance performance during the day in normally rested individuals, there is some evidence that lower doses may be less effective, as sleep debt is increased. For example, a low dose of caffeine (i.e. 30 mg) in the context of a high sugar (i.e. 42 g) energy drink was ineffective at alleviating moderate afternoon sleepiness induced by restricting sleep to only 5 h the night preceding the experiment [26]. The energy drink was administered at 13:50 hours, following a light lunch, and vigilance testing was initiated 10 min later and continued for the next hour and a half. The energy drink failed to improve performance or subjective sleepiness ratings and actually showed worse performance than placebo after 60 min of continuous vigilance testing. The authors conclude that the high-sugar content of energy drinks may actually counter any alerting benefits of a low dose of caffeine in sleepy people.

Overall, the evidence suggests that caffeine does appear to be effective at reducing afternoon sleepiness in non-sleep-deprived individuals. Table 38.2 summarizes some of the major conclusions regarding the use of caffeine for countering normal fluctuations in daytime alertness.

Countering night shift sleepiness

In contrast to the occasional sleepiness that sometimes occurs during the afternoon dip among generally rested individuals, workers during the night shift routinely suffer from excessive sleepiness and associated impairments in performance. Night workers are particularly vulnerable to sleepiness because they are simultaneously fighting two biological mechanisms that promote sleep: (1) the homeostatic drive for sleep, and (2) the circadian rhythm of alertness. Homeostatic sleep pressure refers to the biological drive to obtain sleep, which increases monotonically the longer an individual remains awake. Like hunger, the drive to replenish the reservoir of sleep becomes stronger with each passing hour of wakefulness. For workers during a normal day shift, this increasing drive for sleep is generally offset by the upswing in the circadian rhythm of alertness that peaks in the late afternoon. Consequently, as the day progresses, day shift workers do not necessarily experience a significant increase in sleepiness. Night shift workers, in contrast, experience the combined effects of increasing homeostatic sleep pressure in conjunction with the declining phase of the circadian rhythm during the early morning hours. This convergence of two powerful biological pressures that promote sleep places night workers at particular risk for unwanted sleepiness, attention lapses, and errors on the job. Compared to day workers, night shift workers are 1.7-times more likely to report unintentionally falling asleep at work [27]. In fact, during a single night shift monitored with ambulatory EEG, 20% of workers fell asleep at some point during their shift, whereas no sleep episodes occurred for afternoon and evening shift workers in the same study [28]. Nighttime sleepiness can be particularly dangerous for workers operating heavy machinery or motor vehicles. For example, driving between the hours of 02:00 and 05:00 in the morning multiplies the probability of a motor vehicle accident by 5.6 times [29]. With up to a quarter of the population involved in some aspect of shift work [30], this represents a major public safety concern. Several studies have evaluated the effectiveness of caffeine and other countermeasures against this type of nighttime sleepiness.

Most studies on the effectiveness of caffeine as a countermeasure to night shift sleepiness have examined doses ranging between 100 and 400 mg, usually administered early in the night, near the period when many night shifts begin (e.g. between 22:00 and 02:00). For instance, Bonnet and colleagues compared caffeine, placebo, and napping, and found that a single 400 mg dose of caffeine taken at 01:30 in the morning was more effective than placebo at sustaining alertness and performance until 05:30 the same morning [31]. Lower doses of 300 and 150 mg were less effective, but still better than placebo. Overall, the authors suggested that 150–300 mg of caffeine was about as effective as a 2 to 4-h prophylactic nap, while 400 mg was as effective as an 8-h nap at sustaining performance during a single overnight session [31]. Walsh and colleagues found that caffeine doses equivalent to 4 mg/kg (i.e. approximately 280 mg for a 155 lb man) administered near 22:30 were effective at reducing objective measures of sleepiness over the next 5.5–7.5 h of a single night [32]. Interestingly, despite improvements in objective measures of sleepiness on the MSLT, subjective sleepiness scores on the SSS were unaffected by caffeine. In another study [33], low to moderate caffeine users (0.2–3.0 cups per day) were asked to abstain from caffeine use for 7 days and then engaged in a 5-day simulated night-shift study. Participants were administered either decaffeinated coffee or coffee with the equivalent of 2 mg/kg of caffeine (i.e. approximately 140 mg for a 155 lb man). The experimental beverages were given at two time points (about 22:30 and 01:30) for the first three nights, while only decaffeinated coffee was given to all participants for the last two nights. After each simulated night shift, subjects slept each day from 09:00 to 17:00. During the first three nights, subjects receiving caffeine showed less physiological sleepiness on the MSLT than the placebo group, but only showed lower subjective sleepiness on the SSS during the first night. Importantly, both groups also showed notable declines in objective alertness and performance on a simulated assembly line task over the course of each night, suggesting that the dose of caffeine used was insufficient to fully overcome the effects of sleep pressure and circadian decline in the final early morning hours of the night shift. Additionally, despite the fact that no caffeine was given for the last two nights, those subjects previously receiving caffeine for the first three days showed no differences in overnight physiological sleepiness compared to the placebo group, suggesting no adverse withdrawal effects within the caffeine group. Finally, when subjects tried to sleep during the daytime following their shifts, the caffeine group complained of subjectively poorer sleep, but PSG recordings suggested that caffeine did not adversely affect the objective quality or quantity of daytime sleep [33].

Because nighttime driving can be a particularly hazardous task when sleepy, Philip and colleagues examined the effectiveness of caffeine versus napping on actual nighttime highway driving from 02:00 to 03:30 in the morning [34]. Normally rested participants received either coffee containing 200 mg of caffeine or placebo (decaffeinated coffee) half an hour before nighttime driving, or took a 30-min nap while reclining in the driver's seat of a parked car at a rest-stop 1 h before driving. During the driving periods, subjects drove 200 km on an open highway while being continuously monitored. As might be expected, nighttime driving led to a significant increase in highway line crossings and subjective sleepiness compared to a matched period of daytime driving. However, both the caffeine and napping conditions showed significantly fewer inappropriate line crossings and less subjective sleepiness during the nighttime driving period than the placebo group, with no difference between caffeine and nap group performance. Notably, 87% of the placebo drivers showed evidence of impaired driving ability, whereas only 25% of the caffeine group and 34% of the nap drivers were similarly impaired. Measurements of sleep quality after the driving session were unaffected by caffeine or nap conditions, suggesting that these interventions can be implemented without major concern for subsequent sleep disruption. A parallel study by the same group examined the effectiveness of caffeine (200 mg) versus napping (30 min) in younger (20–25 years) compared to middle-aged (40–50 years) drivers [35]. The study parameters were identical to those described above. Just as in the previous study, nighttime driving led to significant increases in highway line crossings, with no difference between younger and middle-aged groups. Relative to placebo, a single 200-mg dose of caffeine was highly effective at reducing inappropriate line crossings for both age groups, with no significant age effect observed. Interestingly, while naps were generally as effective as caffeine, the performance enhancing effect of a nap was significantly better for the younger than the middle-aged subjects. This may have been due to the deeper and therefore more restorative sleep obtained by the younger group during the nap period. Contrary to the previous study, caffeine was associated with a slight increase in sleep latency (about 1–2 min difference) when subjects returned to their beds after the driving session. Overall sleep efficiency was unaffected by caffeine, however.

While caffeine and napping each appear to be effective at sustaining performance during the overnight shift, there is compelling evidence to suggest that they may be most effective when used in combination.

Schweitzer and colleagues subjected 67 moderate caffeine-using participants to four consecutive simulated night shifts after their caffeine intake had been restricted to one cup per day for one week [36]. Participants were given a placebo, a 2.5-h nap, a dose of caffeine (i.e. 4 mg/kg), or a nap followed by caffeine, 30 min prior to beginning the overnight shift at 23:00. All treatments were better than placebo during the first overnight shift, with the combination of a nap and caffeine yielding the best sustainment of alertness on the maintenance of wakefulness test (MWT) and performance on the PVT, although alertness and performance waned over the course of the night shift regardless of condition. Overall, the nap+caffeine condition was also most effective at sustaining some measures of executive functioning, such as verbal fluency, creative thinking, and higher-level conceptual abilities. The alerting effects of nap+caffeine were most apparent on the first night shift and appeared to degrade slightly over the next three nights. Within the same investigation, Schweitzer and colleagues also included a field study of actual night shift workers to examine whether the effects of 300 mg of caffeine taken at the start of the night shift would be enhanced by the inclusion of a 2-h nap at home in the evening about 3–4 h prior to going to work. Again, the combination of a nap+caffeine sustained PVT performance relative to placebo, suggesting that the combined intervention was effective within a real-life shift-work setting.

While naps appear to be particularly helpful in sustaining alertness and performance during periods of insufficient sleep, people often avoid them due to the feeling of grogginess, sleepiness, and impaired cognitive/psychomotor functioning that is usually present immediately upon awakening. This general feeling of post-nap sluggishness is known as "sleep inertia" and can be present from 20 min to several hours after awakening. Van Dongen and colleagues examined the potential usefulness of low doses of caffeine to minimize the effects of sleep inertia resulting from several 2-h naps taken periodically throughout an 88-h period of sustained wakefulness [37]. After 22 h of wakefulness, volunteers began taking repeated doses of either 0.3 mg/kg of caffeine or placebo every hour for the next 66 h. For the caffeine group, this was about the equivalent of a quarter cup of coffee every hour. The naps occurred at different times of day to control for circadian influences. Consistent with expectations, subjects receiving placebo showed notable sleep inertia effects on the psychomotor vigilance test. Remarkably, the subjects receiving low-dose caffeine were able to nap and showed no evidence of sleep inertia immediately upon awakening. In most cases, the performance of the caffeine group immediately post-nap was generally as good or better than during the session immediately preceding the nap.

In summary, the available evidence suggests that caffeine, in doses of 2–4 mg/kg (i.e. roughly 1–3 cups of coffee, depending on brewing method and body size) taken half an hour before or within the first couple of hours of the night shift appears to be effective at reducing sleepiness and sustaining cognitive and vigilance performance for several hours. However, the effectiveness of a single dose of caffeine is affected by several factors, including its short half-life, the duration of prior wakefulness, and the time of night. Thus, nighttime effectiveness of caffeine appears to be limited to only a few hours and declines considerably by the end of the shift. By the early morning hours, even a second moderate dose of caffeine (e.g. one cup of coffee) may be insufficient to completely counteract the combined effects of homeostatic sleep pressure and the circadian drive on alertness, making this a particularly dangerous time for operating equipment or motor vehicles. The combination of a prophylactic nap and caffeine appears to be the most effective at sustaining alertness and performance during the night shift. Table 38.3 summarizes some these points.

Countering sleepiness during prolonged sleep deprivation

Laboratory studies

A much less common scenario than occasional sleepiness caused by the afternoon dip or night shift work is the profound sleepiness that can result from prolonged periods of sleep deprivation. This situation occurs when the period of wakefulness is significantly extended for 24 h or more. While "pulling an all nighter" is usually a rare occurrence for most of the population, there are some professions, such as emergency responders, medical personnel, and military special operations forces, where a night or more of sleep deprivation can be a relatively common experience. Depending on circumstances and mission requirements, these personnel may, on rare occasions, be required to sustain effective levels of performance for extended periods lasting two or even three

Table 38.3 Summary points for countering night shift sleepiness

1. Night shift workers are particularly susceptible to sleepiness because of the combined effects of (1) the homeostatic drive for sleep, and (2) the decline of the circadian rhythm of alertness in the early morning. These two processes are normally in opposition during the day, but work in tandem to increase sleepiness during the night.
2. Doses from about 150 to 300 mg (i.e. about 1–3 cups of coffee) taken at the start of the night shift or split into multiple doses across the night are more effective than placebo for sustaining objective alertness until morning, although the effectiveness is significantly reduced near the circadian nadir.
3. Doses from 300 to 400 mg (i.e. about 3–4 cups of coffee) taken at the start of the shift generally sustain objective alertness for much of the night (between 5.5 and 7.5 h), although effectiveness may wane near the circadian nadir.
4. Nighttime driving is equally and effectively improved by a 200 mg dose of caffeine (e.g. about 2 cups of coffee) or a 30-min nap taken within a half hour before driving.
5. Combining a nap plus caffeine appears to be the most effective strategy for sustaining overnight alertness and performance.
6. Modest doses of caffeine (e.g. 200 mg) taken early in the shift appear to have little to no adverse effects on objectively measured sleep quality following the shift, although some individuals may report subjectively poorer sleep quality with caffeine.

days without the opportunity for restorative sleep. A number of studies have examined the effectiveness of caffeine and other stimulants at sustaining alertness and performance under these extreme situations. While these levels of sleep deprivation are atypical and unlikely to be encountered by most people, the information provided by such studies can provide unique insight into the limits of effectiveness of caffeine and other countermeasures to sleepiness.

The majority of laboratory studies suggest that even at durations of up to two nights of total sleep deprivation, caffeine appears to be more effective than placebo at sustaining alertness and performance. For example, a 300 mg/70 kg dose of caffeine administered after 32 h of sleep deprivation was effective at sustaining early evening alertness as measured by sleep latency, but had no effect on recovery sleep attempted about 7.5 h later [38]. Similarly, Penetar and colleagues administered double-blind doses of caffeine (150, 300, or 600 mg/70 kg) or placebo to healthy volunteers in the morning after 49 h of wakefulness and found that objective sleepiness, as defined by the latency to fall asleep with eyes closed in a darkened room, was significantly improved by the maximal dose of caffeine for 4.5 h [39]. Subjective sleepiness was also improved for all three caffeine doses relative to placebo for up to 2 h after administration. A variety of mood, vigor, and energy ratings were also elevated for between 2 and 12 h after administration, with better improvement associated with higher doses. However, caffeine at the higher doses was also associated with increased ratings of anxiety, jitteriness, and nervousness for the same time period. Another laboratory study examined the effectiveness of a single dose of 400 mg of caffeine each night at 01:30, or repeated lower doses (150 or 300 mg) every 6 h during 52 h of sleep deprivation [31]. The effectiveness of caffeine on measures of alertness and performance was most pronounced during the first night of sleep deprivation, and showed a greater effect for the higher dose of caffeine. On the first night, the 400-mg dose clearly sustained sleep latency and psychomotor performance relative to placebo for approximately 6 h but then declined to placebo levels, while the lower doses of caffeine were intermediate in effectiveness. Over the following day and next night, doses of 150–300 mg every 6 h yielded generally modest effects on performance measures, sleep latency, and mood, while a second single 400-mg dose at 01:30 improved performance briefly during the early morning hours.

A series of studies conducted by the Walter Reed Army Institute of Research examined the effectiveness of a single large dose of caffeine following various durations of prolonged sleep deprivation. Killgore and colleagues showed that a single dose of 600 mg of caffeine (the equivalent of about six cups of coffee) administered at 03:00, after 44 h of continuous wakefulness, resulted in rapid improvement of simple reaction time, speed, and minor lapses (i.e. lapses 0.5–3 s) on a psychomotor vigilance test for up to about 7.5 h compared to placebo, although its effectiveness declined rapidly as the circadian nadir approached [40] (see Figure 38.2). The magnitude of performance improvement among the caffeine group was generally indistinguishable from that of comparison groups receiving 20 mg of dextroamphetamine or 400 mg of modafinil, although the effectiveness of caffeine was much shorter lived. Importantly, this large dose of caffeine was also associated with significantly more complaints of unpleasant side-effects compared to placebo, including symptoms of nervousness (50%), excitation (75%), abdominal pain (58%), nausea (83%), and jitteriness (75%). However, when volunteers attempted

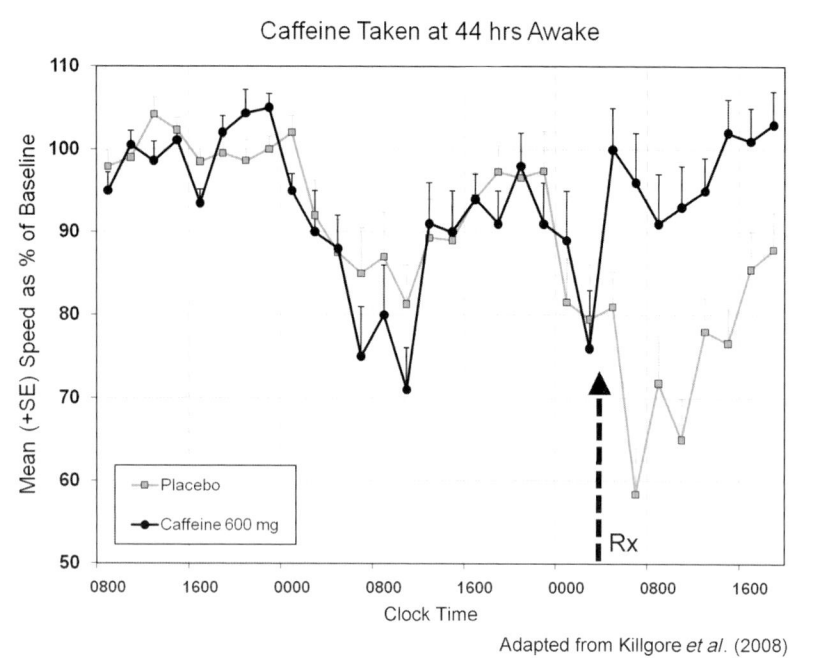

Figure 38.2 Speed of responding to a psychomotor vigilance task is shown for a period of 61 h of total sleep deprivation [40]. At 02:50 a.m., following 44 h of wakefulness (see dashed arrow), volunteers ingested either 600 mg of caffeine (black circles) or an identical placebo (gray squares). Caffeine significantly sustained psychomotor vigilance performance (as a percentage of baseline) relative to placebo for the next 7.5 h (until 10:30 a.m.).

to sleep later that evening (17 h after drug administration), caffeine had no adverse effects on recovery sleep. A companion study by Wesensten and colleagues examined the same large doses of stimulants following an even longer period of sleep deprivation. That study showed that after 54 h of wakefulness, a 600-mg dose of caffeine administered at midnight was as effective as either a 200–400 mg dose of modafinil at sustaining psychomotor vigilance speed until 11:00 the following morning [6]. Additionally, caffeine was highly effective at sustaining 10-choice reaction-time speed, speed of serial addition–subtraction, latency to stage-2 sleep on a modified MWT, and subjective ratings of sleepiness on the SSS. As shown in Figure 38.3, a third study in the series showed that a 600-mg dose of caffeine given at midnight, after 64 h awake, significantly increased sleep latency until 02:00 on a modified MWT, and was able to sustain psychomotor vigilance speed better than placebo until 06:00 that morning [41]. For psychomotor vigilance, caffeine did not differ from modafinil 400 mg or dextroamphetamine 20 mg throughout the early morning, but was significantly worse than modafinil by 06:00. For sleep latency, caffeine was generally not as effective as the other stimulants during the early morning hours. There was no significant effect of caffeine or the other stimulants on subjective sleepiness.

Field studies

As demonstrated in the preceding section, caffeine significantly improves alertness and performance in sleep-deprived people, at least when studied in highly controlled laboratory settings using fairly artificial computerized tests that may not necessarily be representative of real-world tasks. Does caffeine also improve performance of "real-life" tasks when studied in more ecologically valid situations, such as during simulated military field operations? A number of studies suggest that caffeine does indeed sustain performance of sleep-deprived personnel when tested in more realistic settings. McLellan and colleagues studied Canadian soldiers as they performed militarily relevant tasks during a 28-h period of sleep deprivation [42]. A 400-mg dose of caffeine administered in chewing gum at 21:30 reduced ratings of perceived effort during a simulated 15-min road march at 22:00 and improved the speed with which soldiers were able to build sandbag walls near midnight. This dose, when followed by 100-mg booster doses at 03:00 and 05:00 during the overnight sleep deprivation period, was more effective than placebo at sustaining the time to exhaustion during a run at 85% of maximum capacity at 07:00 in the morning [42]. Soldiers in the placebo condition showed declines in their run performance, whereas those in the caffeine condition performed comparable to their baseline levels, running an

Figure 38.3 Speed of responding to a psychomotor vigilance task is shown for a period of 85 h of total sleep deprivation [41]. At 11:50 p.m., following 64 h of wakefulness (see dashed arrow), volunteers ingested either 600 mg of caffeine (black circles) or an identical placebo (gray squares). Caffeine significantly sustained psychomotor vigilance performance (as a percentage of baseline) relative to placebo for the next 6 h (until 06:00 a.m.).

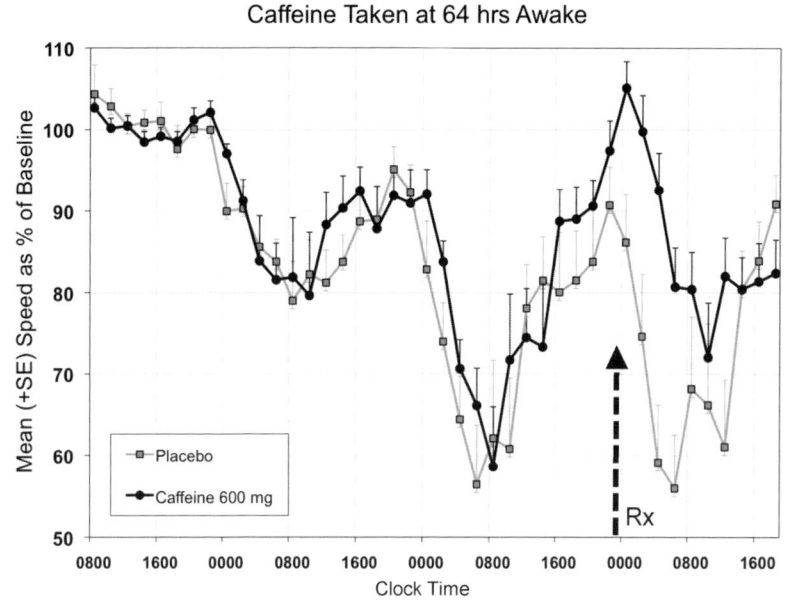

Adapted from Wesensten et al. (2005)

average of 25% longer before succumbing to exhaustion relative to their peers who received placebo. As part of the same study, soldiers completed two separate hour-long simulated marksmanship tasks, one at baseline and one at 05:00, following 22 h of wakefulness [43]. Whereas placebo was associated with significantly degraded response times to engage with targets (24% slower) and fewer shots fired at foe targets, the caffeine group engaged the targets as quickly and attempted as many shots at foes as they had on the baseline day. Other measures of marksmanship accuracy, such as the number of targets hit and shooting efficiency, were not improved by caffeine, however.

Caffeine is also effective at sustaining operational vigilance and run time performance of elite Special Forces soldiers during a night of sleep deprivation. In one study, Special Forces personnel were required to covertly observe and record periodic activities occurring in a nearby building for several hours between 02:00 and 05:45. Caffeinated gum administered in 200-mg doses at 01:45 and 03:45 effectively sustained performance on this reconnaissance vigilance task and on periodic psychomotor vigilance tests relative to placebo. A third 200-mg dose of caffeine taken at approximately 06:30 had no effect on marksmanship scores, but did lead to a 2.5% improvement, relative to baseline, in 6.3-km run times occurring near 08:00. By contrast, soldiers receiving placebo were about 2.6% slower compared to their baseline run. Similar findings have been reported by a number of field studies, suggesting that caffeine is superior to placebo at sustaining militarily relevant vigilance performance in urban operational environments, marksmanship response times, and motivated physical endurance. Further work is still needed to determine the optimal dosing schedules during overnight field operations, but available evidence suggests that multiple repeated doses of 200 mg administered bihourly appear to be effective at sustaining psychomotor vigilance during at least one night of sleep deprivation, although subjective sleepiness may not be significantly influenced [44]. Table 38.4 summarizes some of the main points of this section.

Concerns and controversies

Adverse effects on nighttime sleep

Most of the foregoing discussion focused on the use of caffeine to overcome sleepiness and sustain alertness and performance during periods when sleep is not desired or must be avoided. One obvious drawback to using caffeine is its potential to disrupt normal sleep during periods when sleep is necessary or desired. A number of factors can contribute to the unwanted effects of caffeine on sleep, including the magnitude and timing of the dose, accumulated tolerance, and

Table 38.4 Summary points for countering sleepiness during sleep deprivation

1. A single dose of caffeine between 300 and 600 mg appears to be as effective as comparable doses of other stimulants such as modafinil or dextroamphetamine in restoring psychomotor vigilance and alertness in sleep-deprived individuals, although the duration of effectiveness for caffeine is generally shorter lived due to its 3–6 h half-life.

2. Single doses of caffeine ranging from 400 to 600 mg generally sustain alertness and vigilance near baseline levels for about 4.5–7.5 h in persons deprived of sleep for up to 70 h.

3. During periods of prolonged sleep deprivation, even large doses of caffeine (e.g. 400–600 mg) have shown little if any adverse effects on subsequent recovery sleep attempted at least 8 h after ingestion.

4. High doses of caffeine (e.g. 300–600 mg) are often associated with adverse side-effects, including anxiety, jitteriness, nervousness, excitation, abdominal pain, and nausea.

5. Field studies show that 400 mg of caffeine, followed by 100–200 mg booster doses every 2–3 h, is more effective than placebo at sustaining performance on "real-life" military tasks during overnight sleep deprivation. Advantages of caffeine include a reduction in perceived effort during demanding activities, increased speed and effort at completing physical tasks, improved endurance and completion times on road runs, reduced latency to engage and fire at targets on marksmanship tasks, and improved alertness during monotonous reconnaissance missions.

individual sensitivity to the stimulant. High doses of caffeine during the day can be particularly disruptive to nocturnal sleep. In an attempt to model the physiological arousal associated with insomnia, Bonnet and Arand administered 400 mg of caffeine to subjects three times a day (i.e. roughly equivalent to 12 cups of coffee a day) for seven days [45]. Sleep efficiency, total sleep time, and percentage of slow-wave sleep were reduced, while latency to fall asleep was increased, showing clearly that excessive caffeine consumption can disrupt nocturnal sleep. Interestingly, modest tolerance to the sleep-disruptive effects developed over the course of the week-long study, suggesting that subjects showed some adaptation to the effects of high levels of caffeine on their sleep. Other studies have shown that even at lower doses (e.g. the equivalent of a single cup of coffee), caffeine may adversely affect sleep if consumed within 30 min prior to bedtime [5, 46]. Population-based studies have suggested that higher rates of caffeine use are associated with greater severity of complaints of daytime sleepiness [47], raising the possibility that greater caffeine consumption leads to impaired nocturnal sleep and greater sleepiness during the day. However, the cause and effect relationship cannot be established from such studies. It is just as possible that sleepy individuals may consume more caffeine to deal with their severe sleepiness. Regardless, it would seem prudent to avoid caffeine for at least one half-life (i.e. 3–6 h) prior to a scheduled sleep period, in order to minimize potential sleep disruption.

Caffeine withdrawal

Approximately 50% of moderate caffeine users experience symptoms of withdrawal following a period of abstinence, with symptoms typically emerging within 12–24 h after cessation [48]. This withdrawal syndrome usually peaks between 20 and 51 h and may include symptoms of headache, drowsiness–sleepiness, decreased alertness, fatigue, depressed mood, decreased contentedness, irritability, fogginess, difficulty concentrating, and reduced energy [49], as well as increased blood flow velocity in the middle and anterior cerebral arteries, and changes in EEG suggestive of increased drowsiness [18]. Perhaps one of the most vigorously debated topics in the current caffeine literature concerns whether the documented cognitive enhancing effects of caffeine truly reflect absolute improvement in alertness or, alternatively, whether such effects simply reflect a relative reversal of withdrawal symptoms, possibly as an epiphenomenon of flawed experimental design. James and Rogers have pointed out that most studies on the topic typically require participants to abstain from caffeine intake the evening prior to study participation [50]. Because the vast majority of the population regularly consumes some level of dietary caffeine [2], most subjects entering these studies are, therefore, likely to be experiencing some degree of withdrawal. Consequently, baseline alertness and performance will be reduced as a function of acute abstinence and any improvement in alertness and performance observed following caffeine administration might simply reflect a reversal of the withdrawal symptoms rather than true enhancement of performance. Indeed proponents of the withdrawal-reversal hypothesis have provided convincing evidence that when normally rested research participants have abstained from caffeine for a week or more, there may be little if any additional benefit in performance to be gained by taking caffeine [50]. Recent evidence suggests that withdrawal-reversal may indeed account for some of the effects of caffeine, particularly those involving mood and reaction time, but other aspects of working memory and selective attention do appear to be improved beyond what would be expected by the withdrawal-reversal hypothesis [19]. As touched upon in several of the preceding sections, however, many of the studies demonstrating the effectiveness of caffeine have included controls for withdrawal or statistically analyzed the relationships of caffeine effects to habitual caffeine intake. Many of these studies find that caffeine has an alertness-enhancing effect, even when withdrawal or habitual use is controlled. Because of the complexity of the issues, the nuances of the arguments, and the volume of the research involved, the scope of this chapter is insufficient to comprehensively address the topic of withdrawal reversal, and the interested reader is referred to some excellent reviews [5, 50]. Clearly, this is an area where further research is needed.

Conclusions

Sleepiness when climbing into bed for the night can be welcome, but sleepiness at work, on the road, or at times when the opportunity for sleep is not available can be disastrous or even deadly. A variety of countermeasures to sleepiness are available, including naps, physical activity, bright light, and stimulants. Caffeine is the most widely used of these countermeasures. When applied judiciously, caffeine appears to be a relatively safe, effective, and socially acceptable countermeasure to occasional unwanted sleepiness. However, like most drugs, optimal benefits from caffeine only emerge when it is used appropriately and with due consideration to both its positive and negative effects. The dose selected and timing of ingestion will depend on a number of factors, including the environment and circumstances (i.e. afternoon post-lunch dip; night shift work; overnight driving; prolonged wakefulness), the desired duration of sustained wakefulness, the availability/feasibility of other countermeasures (e.g. naps), the degree of accumulated sleep debt, individual sensitivity and accumulated tolerance to caffeine, and the schedule of future sleep episodes, just to name a few. Low doses can be effective at reducing mild sleepiness, particularly during daytime hours, while larger doses may be required during overnight shifts where the duration of wakefulness and circadian influences may act synergistically to impair alertness and performance. For sustaining overnight alertness, a dose of caffeine followed by a brief nap appears to be a particularly effective strategy. For extended periods of wakefulness, repeated doses of caffeine every 2 or 3 h during the overnight period may be necessary. Ultimately, however, caffeine is not a replacement for sleep and tolerable doses become progressively less effective at sustaining normal alertness and performance as the duration of wakefulness continues. When used sensibly and strategically, caffeine appears to provide a relatively safe and effective short-term countermeasure to occasional unwanted sleepiness.

References

1. **Gilbert R M**. Caffeine consumption. In: Spiller G A, Ed. *The Methylxanthine Beverages and Foods: Chemistry, Consumption, and Health Effects*. New York, NY: Liss, 1984: 185–213.
2. **Frary C D, Johnson R K, Wang M Q**. Food sources and intakes of caffeine in the diets of persons in the United States. *J Am Diet Assoc*, 2005; **105**:110–13.
3. **Arnold P K, Hartley L R, Corry A**, *et al*. Hours of work, and perceptions of fatigue among truck drivers. *Accid Anal Prev*, 1997; **29**:471–77.
4. **Boutrel B, Koob G F**. What keeps us awake: the neuropharmacology of stimulants and wakefulness-promoting medications. *Sleep*, 2004; **27**:1181–94.
5. **Roehrs T, Roth T**. Caffeine: sleep and daytime sleepiness. *Sleep Med Rev*, 2008; **12**:153–62.
6. **Wesensten N J, Belenky G, Kautz M A**, *et al*. Maintaining alertness and performance during sleep deprivation: modafinil versus caffeine. *Psychopharmacology (Berl)*, 2002; **159**:238–47.
7. **Porkka-Heiskanen T, Strecker R E, Thakkar M**, *et al*. Adenosine: a mediator of the sleep-inducing effects of prolonged wakefulness. *Science*, 1997; **276**:1265–68.
8. **Ferre S**. An update on the mechanisms of the psychostimulant effects of caffeine. *J Neurochem*, 2008; **105**:1067–79.
9. **Carter A J, O'Connor W T, Carter M J**, *et al*. Caffeine enhances acetylcholine release in the hippocampus in vivo by a selective interaction with adenosine A1 receptors. *J Pharmacol Exp Ther*, 1995; **273**:637–42.
10. **Koppelstaetter F, Poeppel T D, Siedentopf C M**, *et al*. Does caffeine modulate verbal working memory processes? An fMRI study. *Neuroimage*, 2008; **39**:492–99.
11. **Mort J R, Kruse H R**. Timing of blood pressure measurement related to caffeine consumption. *Ann Pharmacother*, 2008; **42**:105–10.
12. **Bchir F, Dogui M, Ben Fradj R**, *et al*. Differences in pharmacokinetic and electroencephalographic

responses to caffeine in sleep-sensitive and non-sensitive subjects. *C R Biol*, 2006; **329**:512–19.

13. **Barry R J**, **Clarke A R**, **Johnstone S J**, et al. Timing of caffeine's impact on autonomic and central nervous system measures: clarification of arousal effects. *Biol Psychol*, 2008; **77**:304–16.

14. **Horne J**, **Anderson C**, **Platten C**. Sleep extension versus nap or coffee, within the context of 'sleep debt'. *J Sleep Res*, 2008; **17**:432–36.

15. **Hayashi M**, **Masuda A**, **Hori T**. The alerting effects of caffeine, bright light and face washing after a short daytime nap. *Clin Neurophysiol*, 2003; **114**:2268–78.

16. **Haskell C F**, **Kennedy D O**, **Milne A L**, et al. The effects of L-theanine, caffeine and their combination on cognition and mood. *Biol Psychol*, 2008; **77**:113–22.

17. **Michael N**, **Johns M**, **Owen C**, et al. Effects of caffeine on alertness as measured by infrared reflectance oculography. *Psychopharmacology (Berl)*, 2008; **200**:255–60.

18. **Sigmon S C**, **Herning R I**, **Better W**, et al. Caffeine withdrawal, acute effects, tolerance, and absence of net beneficial effects of chronic administration: cerebral blood flow velocity, quantitative EEG, and subjective effects. *Psychopharmacology (Berl)*, 2009; **204**:573–85.

19. **Addicott M A**, **Laurienti P J**. A comparison of the effects of caffeine following abstinence and normal caffeine use. *Psychopharmacology (Berl)*, 2009; **207**:423–31.

20. **Ataka S**, **Tanaka M**, **Nozaki S**, et al. Effects of oral administration of caffeine and d-ribose on mental fatigue. *Nutrition*, 2008; **24**:233–38.

21. **Peeling P**, **Dawson B**. Influence of caffeine ingestion on perceived mood states, concentration, and arousal levels during a 75-min university lecture. *Adv Physiol Educ*, 2007; **31**:332–35.

22. **Adan A**, **Prat G**, **Fabbri M**, et al. Early effects of caffeinated and decaffeinated coffee on subjective state and gender differences. *Prog Neuropsychopharmacol Biol Psychiatry*, 2008; **32**:1698–703.

23. **Durlach P J**. The effects of a low dose of caffeine on cognitive performance. *Psychopharmacology (Berl)*, 1998; **140**:116–19.

24. **Lieberman H R**, **Wurtman R J**, **Emde G G**, et al. The effects of low doses of caffeine on human performance and mood. *Psychopharmacology (Berl)*, 1987; **92**:308–12.

25. **Smit H J**, **Rogers P J**. Effects of low doses of caffeine on cognitive performance, mood and thirst in low and higher caffeine consumers. *Psychopharmacology (Berl)*, 2000; **152**:167–73.

26. **Anderson C**, **Horne J A**. A high sugar content, low caffeine drink does not alleviate sleepiness but may worsen it. *Hum Psychopharmacol*, 2006; **21**:299–303.

27. **Akerstedt T**, **Knutsson A**, **Westerholm P**, et al. Work organisation and unintentional sleep: results from the WOLF study. *Occup Environ Med*, 2002; **59**:595–600.

28. **Torsvall L**, **Akerstedt T**, **Gillander K**, et al. Sleep on the night shift: 24-hour EEG monitoring of spontaneous sleep/wake behavior. *Psychophysiology*, 1989; **26**:352–58.

29. **Connor J**, **Norton R**, **Ameratunga S**, et al. Driver sleepiness and risk of serious injury to car occupants: population based case control study. *BMJ*, 2002; **324**:1125.

30. **Schwartz J R**, **Roth T**. Shift work sleep disorder: burden of illness and approaches to management. *Drugs*, 2006; **66**:2357–70.

31. **Bonnet M H**, **Gomez S**, **Wirth O**, et al. The use of caffeine versus prophylactic naps in sustained performance. *Sleep*, 1995; **18**:97–104.

32. **Walsh J K**, **Muehlbach M J**, **Humm T M**, et al. Effect of caffeine on physiological sleep tendency and ability to sustain wakefulness at night. *Psychopharmacology (Berl)*, 1990; **101**:271–73.

33. **Muehlbach M J**, **Walsh J K**. The effects of caffeine on simulated night-shift work and subsequent daytime sleep. *Sleep*, 1995; **18**:22–29.

34. **Philip P**, **Taillard J**, **Moore N**, et al. The effects of coffee and napping on nighttime highway driving: a randomized trial. *Ann Intern Med*, 2006; **144**:785–91.

35. **Sagaspe P**, **Taillard J**, **Chaumet G**, et al. Aging and nocturnal driving: better with coffee or a nap? A randomized study. *Sleep*, 2007; **30**:1808–13.

36. **Schweitzer P K**, **Randazzo A C**, **Stone K**, et al. Laboratory and field studies of naps and caffeine as practical countermeasures for sleep–wake problems associated with night work. *Sleep*, 2006; **29**:39–50.

37. **Van Dongen H P**, **Price N J**, **Mullington J M**, et al. Caffeine eliminates psychomotor vigilance deficits from sleep inertia. *Sleep*, 2001; **24**:813–19.

38. **Waters W F**, **Magill R A**, **Bray G A**, et al. A comparison of tyrosine against placebo, phentermine, caffeine, and d-amphetamine during sleep deprivation. *Nutr Neurosci*, 2003; **6**:221–35.

39. **Penetar D**, **McCann U**, **Thorne D**, et al. Caffeine reversal of sleep deprivation effects on alertness and mood. *Psychopharmacology (Berl)*, 1993; **112**:359–65.

40. **Killgore W D S**, **Rupp T L**, **Grugle N L**, et al. Effects of dextroamphetamine, caffeine and modafinil on psychomotor vigilance test performance after 44 h of continuous wakefulness. *J Sleep Res*, 2008; **17**:309–21.

41. **Wesensten N J**, **Killgore W D S**, **Balkin T J**. Performance and alertness effects of caffeine, dextroamphetamine, and modafinil during sleep deprivation. *J Sleep Res*, 2005; **14**:255–66.

42. **McLellan T M**, **Bell D G**, **Kamimori G H**. Caffeine improves physical performance during 24 h of active wakefulness. *Aviat Space Environ Med*, 2004; **75**:666–72.

43. **Tikuisis P**, **Keefe A A**, **McLellan T M**, *et al*. Caffeine restores engagement speed but not shooting precision following 22 h of active wakefulness. *Aviat Space Environ Med*, 2004; **75**:771–76.

44. **Kamimori G H**, **Johnson D**, **Thorne D**, *et al*. Multiple caffeine doses maintain vigilance during early morning operations. *Aviat Space Environ Med*, 2005; **76**:1046–50.

45. **Bonnet M H**, **Arand D** L. Caffeine use as a model of acute and chronic insomnia. *Sleep*, 1992; **15**:526–36.

46. **Karacan I**, **Thornby J I**, **Anch M**, *et al*. Dose-related sleep disturbances induced by coffee and caffeine. *Clin Pharmacol Ther*, 1976; **20**:682–89.

47. **Ohayon M M**, **Caulet M**, **Philip P**, *et al*. How sleep and mental disorders are related to complaints of daytime sleepiness. *Arch Intern Med*, 1997; **157**:2645–52.

48. **Schuh K J**, **Griffiths R R**. Caffeine reinforcement: the role of withdrawal. *Psychopharmacology (Berl)*, 1997; **130**:320–26.

49. **Juliano L M**, **Griffiths R R**. A critical review of caffeine withdrawal: empirical validation of symptoms and signs, incidence, severity, and associated features. *Psychopharmacology (Berl)*, 2004; **176**:1–29.

50. **James J E**, **Rogers P J**. Effects of caffeine on performance and mood: withdrawal reversal is the most plausible explanation. *Psychopharmacology (Berl)*, 2005; **182**:1–8.

Section 4 Chapter 39

Therapy of Excessive Sleepiness

Histamine receptor (H₃R) antagonists, hypocretin agonists, and other novel alerting agents

Meredith Broderick and Christian Guilleminault

Introduction

Histamine receptor (H₃R) antagonists, hypocretin agonists, and other novel alerting agents are the major classes of drugs being developed as potential treatments for excessive daytime sleepiness (EDS). At this stage of development, these drugs hold potential for treating EDS in the setting of narcolepsy or neurological diseases associated with EDS. A few of these drugs are being evaluated specifically for treatment of EDS in the setting of narcolepsy. However, these drugs may have a wider application for treatment of EDS as a consequence of other sleep disorders, such as idiopathic hypersomnia, obstructive sleep apnea, shift work sleep disorder, or neurological conditions associated with EDS such as Parkinson's disease or multiple sclerosis. Currently, drug development in these areas is in the preliminary stages and awaiting research that will help elucidate whether clinical use will ultimately become a reality. This chapter focuses on the development of histamine receptor (H₃R) antagonists and hypocretin agonists as emerging treatments of EDS. Other novel therapies in development for treatment of EDS including immunotherapy, thyrotrophin (TRH) analogues and promoters, and miscellaneous therapies will also be discussed.

Histamine 3 receptor (H₃R) antagonists

Histamine has long been known to have a key role in the regulation of sleep and wakefulness. Histamine has a diurnal rhythm with high levels during wakefulness and lower levels during sleep. In the brain, histaminergic neurons project from the tuberomamillary nucleus in the hypothalamus diffusely to the cortex. These neurons are the only source of histamine in the central nervous system. Histaminergic activation produces wakefulness, whereas decreased activity produces sleepiness. Recent studies have also demonstrated a relationship of hypocretin to histamine suggesting hypocretin-induced arousal requires downstream release of histamine [1]. Histaminergic neurons are also thought to integrate a number of signals from many different sources exerting a wake-promoting effect with circadian variation. In 2009, Nishino *et al.* reported a decrease in CSF histamine in patients with narcolepsy and idiopathic hypersomnia [2]. With these relationships in mind, one may hypothesize that patients with idiopathic hypersomnia may lack histamine-producing neurons in the tuberomamillary nucleus pointing to histamine as a potential treatment target for EDS.

There are four metatropic histamine receptor subtypes. They are designated H_1R–H_4R, all of which are G-protein-coupled receptors (GPCRs). The sedative effects of H_1R blockers are an example of the properties of histaminergic neurons, which explains the presence of these compounds in many over-the-counter sleeping pills. H_1R- and H_2R-based drugs are often referred to as "blockbuster drugs" because of the wide success of anti-allergy and anti-ulcer drugs that act as H_1R and H_2R antagonists, respectively. Greater than 50% of the most successful pharmaceutical treatments are drugs that act via GPCRs pathways.

The histamine H_3 receptor (H_3R) was discovered in 1983 by Arrang and colleagues and later, the H_4 receptor (H_4R) was discovered in 2000 [3, 4]. Lovenberg *et al.* cloned and described the functional expression of the H_3R in 1999 [5]. Identification of H_3R and description of its functional expression were important advances because these discoveries revealed the inhibitory effect histamine has on its own synthesis and showed that release of histamine is through a mechanism independent of H_1R or H_2R. Subsequent

---

Sleepiness: Causes, Consequences and Treatment, ed. Michael J. Thorpy and Michel Billiard. Published by Cambridge University Press. © Cambridge University Press 2011.

research in this area has shown that H_3R antagonists activate histaminergic neurons thereby increasing histamine, and producing wakefulness [6]. H_3R is not only involved in neurotransmission of histamine, but was also determined to have a critical role in the regulation of other neurotransmitters such as acetylcholine, dopamine, serotonin, and norephinephrine. H_4R is expressed in hematopoietic cells, suggesting a strong role in inflammatory and immunomodulatory processes [7].

H_3R is a presynaptic autoreceptor, which means it mediates the synthesis of histamine by reducing downstream processing of a cyclic AMP response element binding protein and limits release of histamine as well as other monamines known to have an effect on wakefulness, such as dopamine, serotonin, glutamate, GABA, and acetylcholine [1, 8]. The H_3R is densely located centrally in the hippocampus, amygdala, nucleus accumbens, globus pallidus, hypothalamus striatum, substantia nigra, and the cerebral cortex. Peripherally, H_3R are also located in the GI tract, airways and cardiovascular system. H_3R antagonists increase waking amines in the synaptic cleft, hence promoting wakefulness via post-synaptic H_1R activity. H_3R antagonists are thought to exert their effect by increasing histamine release and thereby increasing H_1 activation. This knowledge brings about enormous potential for development of H_3R antagonists and H_3 inverse agonists as potential treatments of narcolepsy, EDS, disorders of alertness, memory processing, feeding and locomotion. Accordingly, H_3R antagonists are being studied for a wide number of applications including sleep–wake disorders, ADHD, epilepsy, cognitive impairment, schizophrenia, obesity, and neuropathic pain, to name a few [8]. In fact, because of the wide applications in drug development, one of the challenges is predicting the clinical activity of different H_3R ligands. Preliminary studies suggest that differences in the targeted brain regions and the way neurotransmitter levels are affected explain these variations.

The first-generation selective H_3R ligands were agonist R-a-methylhistamine and inverse agonist thioperamide [4]. Using these two compounds, scientists were able to confirm the role of H_3R in the regulation of histamine and release of other neurotransmitters. In 1999, researchers at Johnson & Johnson cloned the cDNA encoding the human H_3R [4]. Extensive splicing of the H_3R of the H_3R gene occurs, resulting in greater than 20 isoforms. In general, many of the prototype H_3R ligands are imidazole-based compounds linked via a propyloxy group to a lipophilic terminus, although some pharmaceutical companies are developing non-imidazole-based compounds because imidazole compounds are often potent inhibitors of drug-metabolizing CYP enzymes which results in a high potential for drug interactions.

Development of a successful H_3R antagonist drug has not yet been accomplished because of the tremendous complexity of the receptor. The receptor is constitutively active, which means H_3 ligands can act as both antagonists and inverse agonists based on the presence of competing ligands and the physiological environment of the receptor. When histamine or other competing ligands are not present, the result is H_3R-mediated inhibition of norepinephrine, dopamine, serotonin, acetylcholine, and other neurotransmitters. When a competing ligand or histamine is present, presynaptic release and synthesis would theoretically be inhibited. The effect of an inverse agonist varies based on its location in the central nervous system and the concentration of histamine and competing ligands. To make things even more complicated, these variations in concentrations change with circadian regulation as well as many other physiological variations.

Most reference compounds with affinity for H_3R also possess affinity for the H_4R receptor so that a limitation of many of the first-generation H_3R ligands is a lack of receptor selectivity. Therefore, newer drugs are being developed with high selectivity for H_3R. Newer research has revealed wide variations in selectivity between species, that is, species-dependent receptor heterogeneity with an up to 1000-fold difference in rat and human binding potencies [3]. Thus, finding animal models with selectivity similar to humans so as to apply for potential clinical use is one of the challenges in current research. Another challenge in drug development is synthesizing ligands that readily pass through the blood–brain barrier. To make it even more complicated, the existence of over 20 different isoforms of H_3R have been described. Despite these challenges, preliminary research in a handful of compounds shows potential for use in treatment of excessive daytime sleepiness.

Ciproxifan is one of the prototypical H_3R ligands. H_3R antagonists thioperamide, carboperamide, and ciproxifan have been tested in rats, mice and cats and produced increases in wakefulness without rebound hypersomnolence or increasing locomotor activity [6, 9–13]. In one study, thioperamide and ciproxifan demonstrated an increase in wakefulness and cortical EEG fast activity without an increase in sleep rebound [9]. In cats and rats, thioperamide has been studied and a dose-dependent enhancement in wakefulness, decreased slow-wave sleep (SWS) and REM sleep were observed [6]. However, because of hepatotoxicity, further studies with thioperamide have not been conducted.

In addition to H_3R antagonists, H_3 inverse agonists are also being developed. H_3 inverse agonists are thought to promote wakefulness by inhibiting the H_2 autoreceptor, which then enhances histamine release [14]. Tiprolisant or BF2.649 is the first H_3 inverse agonist that passed clinical Phase II trials in the treatment of EDS in narcolepsy [6]. In rats, tiprolisant increased levels of dopamine, histamine, and acetylcholine in the prefrontal cortex and hence an awakening effect as determined by spectral analysis of electroencephalograms was observed in studies [15]. Tiprolisant has also been shown to work in synergy with modafinil in orexin -/- mice to suppress SWS and REM sleep for 3–6 h. In a pilot study single-blinded with 22 patients, receiving a placebo followed by tiprolisant for one week, the Epworth Sleepiness Score (ESS) was reduced from baseline of 17.6 by 5.9 with tiprolisant compared to 1.0 for placebo [14]. This effect is equivalent to studies done showing a therapeutic response to modafinil. The dose studied was 40 mg orally and the most frequent side-effects were headache (5), nausea (4), insomnia (2), malaise (2), and sweating (2), with 95% of side-effects occurring during the first three days of administration. The total amount of sleep was not significantly different between tiprolisant and placebo. This study did not examine the effect of tiprolisant on other symptoms of narcolepsy such as cataplexy. Other studies looking at tiprolisant for EDS in other diseases such as in Parkinson's disease are also underway. Tiprolisant has been granted orphan drug status by the European Medicine Agency for the therapeutic treatment of narcolepsy [7]. BF2.649 is another high-affinity competitive antagonist and potent inverse agonist for H_3R [8, 15].

Conessine is a naturally occurring substance shown to have potent H_3R antagonist activity. Slight modifications of conessine produce similar H_3R antagonist effects with longer half-lives, which is a limitation to clinical utility because of disruption to sleep–wake cycle with a prolonged duration of action [16]. One of the key characteristics of a successful H_3R antagonist is an ideal duration of action so that it is long enough acting to provide a clinical effect during the day, but without being so long acting so that it disrupts sleep.

JNJ-5207852 is a novel diamine-based H_3R antagonist that has been studied in rodents and which demonstrated potency and selectivity for H_3R. JNJ-5207852 was well absorbed via oral administration with good penetration of the CNS and a long half-life. It was also shown to have clear wake-promoting properties, suppression of SWS without appetite suppression, rebound hypersomnolence or increasing locomotor activity [17]. This drug is thought to have potential in the treatment of EDS in obstructive sleep apnea, multiple sclerosis, and fibromyalgia. JNJ-637940 and JNJ-10181457 have shown similar results [7]. JNJ-17216498 is an orally active agent in phase II evaluation for treatment of narcolepsy. Johnson & Johnson has also recognized the potential of combining H_3R antagonists with selective serotonin reuptake inhibitors (SSRIs) to counter the side-effects of fatigue often seen with administration of these drugs, which has led to another area of research and drug development.

GSK 189254 is another H_3R antagonist which has been tested on orexin$^{+/+}$ and orexin$^{-/-}$ mice [17]. Acute administration of GSK189254 at 10 mg/kg increased wakefulness and decreased SWS and paradoxical sleep to an equivalent dose of modafinil 64 mg/kg. It was also shown to reduce narcoleptic episodes in orexin -/- mice. It was subsequently studied in Phase II trials for narcolepsy and is also being studied in dementia and neuropathic pain [7].

These specific examples represent only a few of the many potential drugs in development targeting the H_3R. See Table 39.1 for a summary of H_3R antagonists and Table 39.2 for H_3R inverse agonists. In 2004, 8 of the 10 largest pharmaceutical companies were involved in histamine H_3R research development [4]. H_3R inverse agonists and antagonists hold great promise for treatment of narcolepsy and EDS; however, some of the current barriers are H_3R versus H_4R selectivity, protean agonism, species heterogeneity, receptor isoforms, and constitutive activity, which are all challenges in the future of H_3R drug development and research [4]. Due to the complexity of the H_3R, developing useful animal models to describe drug behavior that can be applied to clinical use in humans is another challenge. Describing the relationship to circadian factors is also a huge unknown. Another major obstacle will be developing

Table 39.1 H$_3$R antagonists

Ciproxifan
Carboperamide
Thioperamide
Conessine
JNJ-5207852
JNJ-637940
JNJ-10181457
JNJ-17216498
GSK-189254

Table 39.2 H$_3$R inverse agonists

Tiprolisant or BF2.649

drugs without dangerous side-effects after long-term usage, particularly because drugs used to treat excessive daytime sleepiness are needed in the setting of chronic conditions. The long-term effects of H$_3$R will ultimately determine if and how useful these drugs will be in the treatment of excessive daytime sleepiness in the setting of neurological disease, narcolepsy, idiopathic hypersomnia, or other chronic diseases.

Hypocretin-based treatments

One of the most important recent discoveries in narcolepsy research was the description of hypocretin deficiency to narcolepsy–cataplexy (NC). In humans, abnormally low or undetectable levels of hypocretin-1 have been reported in 95 % of patients with NC [18, 19]. If hypocretin deficiency is the main pathophysiological feature of NC, then it follows that hypocretin replacement is an important potential therapeutic strategy for excessive daytime sleepiness in NC. Direct hypocretin administration, hypocretin gene therapy, hypocretin stem cell transplantation, and hypocretin agonists are some of the strategies being investigated for drug development in treating EDS in NC.

Hypocretin neurons are widely projected to the areas of the brainstem linked to motor inhibition, which include the locus coeruleus, raphe nuclei, laterodorsal tegmental nuclei, and ventral tegmental neurons [20]. Preprohypocretin is cleaved to form hypocretin-1 and hypocretin-2 in the lateral hypothalamus. Both are medium-sized peptides thought to play a key role in the regulation of arousal, appetite, sleep architecture, neuroendocrine, and autonomic control. Hypocretin-1 is a key modulator in the arousal state and locomotor activity through its actions on the locus coeruleus [21]. Hypocretin-1 is more frequently studied than hypocretin-2 in pharmacological studies because it is more stable in the blood and CSF than hypocretin-2. Hypocretin-1 and hypocretin-2 bind to at least two known seven-transmembrane GPCRs named hypocretin receptor-1 (hcrtr1) and hypocretin receptor-2 (hcrtr2), respectively. Although they share some of the same characteristics, each has slightly different properties. Hypocretin-1 binds with two to three times the affinity to hcrtr 1 than hypocretin-2 [22]. Hypocretin-2 does not pass through the blood–brain barrier intact [23, 24].

Systemic administration of hypocretin-1 in canines with narcolepsy produces increases in activity levels, wake times, reduces sleep fragmentation, and has a dose-dependent reduction in cataplexy [25]. However, the major barrier to systemic delivery of hypocretin-1 to the hypothalamus is that it has very low permeability across the blood–brain barrier, which limits its bioavailability to the central nervous system when injected peripherally. Low permeability in turn requires high peripheral doses, increasing systemic side-effects and driving up costs, which are also obstacles in successful drug development. Intracerebroventricular hypocretin replacement, intranasal hypocretin administration, hypocretin cell transplantation, hypocretin gene therapy, and hypocretin stem cell transplantation are also being investigated to achieve the same concept, but as a mean of bypassing the obstacles with peripheral administration.

In narcoleptic mice, intracerebroventricular (ICV) replacement of hypocretin-1 has been studied and observed as being effective; however, it was not effective when injected into hcrtr2-mutated Dobermans [23]. Intranasal delivery of hypocretin bypasses the blood–brain barrier with the added benefits of onset of action within minutes and fewer peripheral side-effects [22]. Intranasal delivery works because of the connections between the central nervous system to the outside environment through the olfactory and trigeminal nerves. The mechanism of action is extracellular, so there is no dependence on receptors or axonal transport for drug delivery. Studies looking at cerebrospinal fluid levels after intranasal administration have shown detectable levels after intranasal delivery of hypocretin [22, 26]. One study looking at intranasal delivery of hypocretin in the awake state found that after administration concentrations were highest in the hypothalamus and the trigeminal nerve [22].

An alternative solution to the poor permeability of hypocretin-1 through the blood-brain barrier is to develop hypocretin peptide analogues. These peptide analogues could be designed to possess greater stability in the blood, greater CNS penetration, and selectively targeted for hcrtr1 or hcrtr2 [18]. Only the C-terminal of the hypocretin proteins is necessary for biological activity and selectivity for the receptors [27, 28]. Researchers have determined the minimal sequences required for receptor activation by synthesizing different combinations of C-terminally and N-terminally truncated peptides in addition to fragments of central sequences of hypocretin-1 and hypocretin-2 [29]. They found that full sequences of hypocretin-1 were necessary to activate receptors, while hypocretin-2 fragments containing the C-terminus remained active so long as more than 19 amino acids were present. Several analogues that selectively activate hcrtr1 have also been reported. With this knowledge, future studies can be directed at finding a peptide analogue with the right combination of selective activation that also minimizes peripheral side-effects. Then, additional studies will need to be done in order to determine the right application of these drugs, because it is unclear whether hypocretin agonists would only be effective when used in patients with absent or low hypocretin-1 levels, such as in NC, or if they would be widely applicable for treatment of EDS in other diseases, such as idiopathic hypersomnolence, obstructive sleep apnea, Parkinson's disease, and multiple sclerosis. Investigation will also need to be conducted to determine whether sensitivity to peptide analogues persists for a long time, or if there is a limited time window to begin treatment due to disappearance and remodeling of a receptor if it is not stimulated.

Gene therapy is another possible mechanism for hypocretin replacement therapy. Gene therapy aimed at stimulating the production of hypocretin could theoretically address the deficiency of hypocretin in NC or as a therapeutic modality in treatment of EDS. Studies examining the possibility of genetic rescue in mice with ablated hypocretin neurons found that ectopic transgenic expression of hypocretin prevents cataplexy even in the setting of hypocretin neuron ablation [30]. This study suggests that deficiency or absence of hypocretin-1 does not confer a permanent loss of function. The study highlights hypocretin gene therapy with viral vectors as a potential future treatment for narcolepsy–cataplexy. Additional evidence examining the molecular genetics of narcolepsy has suggested a potential relationship between monoaminergic genes and immune-related genes, which could also serve as a target for gene therapy [31].

Hypocretin cell transplantation is another possibility in the development of treatment in excessive daytime sleepiness. Normal subjects have approximately 70 000 hypocretin neurons and in narcolepsy–cataplexy, 85–95% of hypocretin neurons are lost. This corresponds to a CSF hypocretin-1 level of less than 30% of normal. Therefore, a minimum of 10% of hypocretin-producing cells that need to be replaced for a therapeutic effect [18, 32]. Transplantation is limited by graft survival and immune reactions [20]. Studies in rats show survival of hypocretin-containing rat neurons implanted in the pontine reticular formation were unsuccessful unless enriched transplant medium was used in which case survival was extended to 36 days [33]. Transplant of hypocretin grafts are also limited by supplies of hypocretin neurons and cost-effectiveness because assuming limited survivability, repeat treatments will be needed. The barrier of graft survivability, graft reactions, and cost could be reduced if genetically engineered cells or employing stem cell techniques were used instead.

Other novel therapies for excessive sleepiness

Immunotherapy and thyrotrophin releasing hormone (TRH) agonists are two other novel therapies being investigated for utility in the treatment of EDS. The leading theory explaining the destruction of hypocretin producing neurons in the setting of narcolepsy is that they are destroyed by an autoimmune process which has led some investigators to explore immunotherapy as a treatment for narcolepsy such as corticosteroids, plasmapheresis, and intravenous immunoglobulin (IVIg) because of their use in the treatment of other autoimmune disorders [34, 35]. The case studies reported have mixed results, suggesting a therapeutic benefit may be limited by whether it is administered close to the onset of disease. If destruction of hypocretin-producing neurons is due to an autoimmune process, it is irreversible and, therefore, immunotherapy would theoretically only be effective if used before destruction occurred, although some theories suggest hypocretin-producing cells are inactivated with disease onset and immunotherapy directly reduces symptoms. None of the current literature reports long-term follow-up, and even when immunotherapy is effective it is often discontinued because of unwanted side-effects.

Thyrotrophin releasing hormone is a tripeptidic hormone (L-pyroglutamyl-L-histidyl-L-prolineamide) distributed throughout the central nervous system. TRH stimulates release of thyroid-stimulating hormone and prolactin. TRH receptor-1 is found predominantly in the hypothalamus while TRH receptor-2 is more widespread and located in the reticular nucleus of the thalamus [36]. TRH may also have stimulant, antidepressant, and neurotrophic effects, making it a potential treatment modality for excessive sleepiness [37].

Three TRH analogues were tested by Nishino et al. for effectiveness in treating excessive sleepiness in canine narcolepsy [38]. All three compounds had a significant impact on the frequency of cataplexy, whereas only two had benefit in excessive sleepiness. Free T3 and T4 levels were not altered and no significant side-effects were noted. Oral CG-3703 was an active compound and at two weeks was shown to reduce cataplexy and excessive sleepiness in a dose-dependent manner. The effective dose in producing wakefulness was similar to a reasonable dose of D-amphetamine. They found a trend of needing increasing doses of CG-3703 with prolonged exposure to elicit the same therapeutic benefit. The mechanism of action CG-3703 in producing an alerting effect is due to enhancement of dopaminergic effects. Another application of TRH agonists to obtain an alerting effect is to inhibit the breakdown of TRH by blocking the TRH-degrading enzyme [39].

Antidepressants are classically used in the narcolepsy with cataplexy (NC) for the treatment of cataplexy. However, not all antidepressants are effective in reducing cataplexy, but may be useful in the treatment of EDS. DOV 216,303 is one antidepressant being developed that blocks norepinephrine, serotonin, and dopamine. DOV 216,303 was tested in 7 subjects and in doses up to 100 mg per day for 10 days was safe and tolerated [40]. Duloxetine, a novel serotonin-norepinephrine reuptake inhibitor (SNRI), was examined in a pilot study in three patients, one of whom was treated with a combination of duloxetine and modafinil and two others were treated with monotherapy [41]. All three showed REM sleep suppression, increase in REM latencies, and improvement in EDS on post-treatment polysomnography and multiple sleep latency testing. Another SNRI, reboxetine 10 mg by mouth, was studied in a pilot study of 12 patients who showed measurable improvement in excessive daytime sleepiness (EDS) as determined by the Epworth Sleepiness Scale (ESS) and MSLT after 2 weeks of treatment. Atomoxetine, another SNRI, 40 mg by mouth 3 times daily was given for 4 weeks in another study and demonstrated improvement in EDS and cataplexy starting on day 6 of treatment [42]. The idea of developing dual or triple monoamine uptake inhibitors may facilitate treatment of EDS and cataplexy simultaneously with one agent. This would be effective in improving adherence to therapy, and decreasing cost of treatment in the setting of NC. GABAergic hypnotics known to increase slow-wave sleep are currently being studied and include gaboxadol and tiagabine [43, 44]. Ritanserin 5 mg, ritanserin 10 mg, or placebo were compared for 28 days and both doses of ritanserin increased the quantity of slow-wave sleep and reduced NREM stage 1 sleep. SR 46349B, another 5-HT2 antagonist, was administered 3 h prior to bedtime at a dose of 1 mg by mouth. SR 46349B increased the amount of slow-wave sleep and reduced the amount of stage 2 sleep [45]. These two 5-HT2 antagonists presumably increase the quality of sleep as a means of improving excessive sleepiness and may be applicable in the treatment of EDS. Two hypocretin antagonists in development are postulated to improve consolidation of sleep in patients with narcolepsy, SB649868 by GlaxoSmithKline and ACT-078573 by Actelion. In the future, other potential targets for reducing EDS will likely involve developing novel neuropeptides and targeting proteins like circadian clock proteins, specific ion channels such as prokineticin or neuropeptide S [46, 47].

Conclusions

There are many exciting developments in the treatment of excessive sleepiness specific to narcolepsy with cataplexy and for other chronic conditions with EDS. Some of the major areas of drug development are histamine (H$_3$) antagonists, hypocretin agonists, immunotherapy, and thyrotrophin (TRH) analogues and promoters.

References

1. **Barbier A J**, **Bradbury M J**. Histaminergic control of sleep–wake cycles: recent therapeutic advances for

sleep and wake disorders. *CNS Neurol Disord Drug Targets*, 2007; **6**:31–43.

2. **Nishino S**, **Sakurai E**, **Nevsimalova S**, et al. Decreased CSF histamine in narcolepsy with and without low CSF hypocretin-1 in comparison to healthy controls. *Sleep*, 2009; **32**:175–80.

3. **Hancock A A**. The challenge of drug discovery of a GPCR target: analysis of preclinical pharmacology of histamine H3 antagonists/inverse agonists. *Biochem Pharmacol*, 2006; **71**:1103–13.

4. **Wijtmans M**, **Leurs R**, **de Esch I**. Histamine H3 receptor ligands break ground in a remarkable plethora of therapeutic areas. *Expert Opin Investig Drugs*, 2007; **16**:967–85.

5. **Lovenberg T W**, **Roland B L**, **Wilson S J**, et al. Cloning and functional expression of the human histamine H3 receptor. *Mol Pharmacol*, 1999; **55**:1101–07.

6. **Lin J S**, **Sakai K**, **Vanni-Mercier G**, et al. Involvement of histaminergic neurons in arousal mechanisms demonstrated with H3-receptor ligands in the cat. *Brain Res*, 1990; **523**:325–30.

7. **Tiligada E**, **Zampeli E**, **Sander K**, et al. Histamine H3 and H4 receptors as novel drug targets. *Expert Opin Investig Drugs*, 2009; **18**:1519–31.

8. **Sander K**, **Kottke T**, **Stark H**. Histamine H3 receptor antagonists go to clinics. *Biol Pharm Bull*, 2008; **31**:2163–81.

9. **Le S**, **Gruner J A**, **Mathiasen J R**, et al. Correlation between ex vivo receptor occupancy and wake-promoting activity of selective H3 receptor antagonists. *J Pharmacol Exp Ther*, 2008; **325**:902–09.

10. **Monti J M**, **Jantos H**, **Ponzoni A**, et al. Sleep and waking during acute histamine H3 agonist (BP2.99) or H3 antagonist carboperamide (MR 16155) administration in rats. *Neuropsychopharmacology*, 1996; **15**:31–35.

11. **Parmentier R**, **Anaclet C**, **Guhennec C**, et al. The brain H3-receptor as a novel therapeutic target for vigilance and sleep–wake disorders. *Biochem Pharmacol*, 2007; **73**:1157–71.

12. **Soya A**, **Song Y H**, **Kodama T**, et al. CSF histamine levels in rats reflect the central histamine neurotransmission. *Neurosci Lett*, 2008; **430**:224–29.

13. **Toyota H**, **Dugovic C**, **Koehl M**, et al. Behavioral characterization of mice lacking histamine H(3) receptors. *Mol Pharmacol*, 2002; **62**:389–97.

14. **Lin J S**, **Dauvilliers Y**, **Arnulf I**, et al. An inverse agonist of the histamine H(3) receptor improves wakefulness in narcolepsy: studies in orexin–/– mice and patients. *Neurobiol Dis*, 2008; **30**:74–83.

15. **Ligneau X**, **Perrin D**, **Landais L**, et al. BF2.649 [1-{3-[3-(4-Chlorophenyl)propoxy]propyl}piperidine, hydrochloride], a nonimidazole inverse agonist/antagonist at the human histamine H3 receptor: preclinical pharmacology. *J Pharmacol Exp Ther*, 2007; **320**:365–75.

16. **Covel J A**, **Santora V J**, **Smith J M**, et al. Design and evaluation of novel biphenyl sulfonamide derivatives with potent histamine H(3) receptor inverse agonist activity. *J Med Chem*, 2009; **52**:5603–11.

17. **Barbier A J**, **Berridge C**, **Dugovic C**, et al. Acute wake-promoting actions of JNJ-5207852, a novel, diamine-based H3 antagonist. *Br J Pharmacol*, 2004; **143**:649–61.

18. **Mignot E**, **Lammers G J**, **Ripley B**, et al. The role of cerebrospinal fluid hypocretin measurement in the diagnosis of narcolepsy and other hypersomnias. *Arch Neurol*, 2002; **59**:1553–62.

19. **Nishino S**, **Ripley B**, **Overeem S**, et al. Hypocretin (orexin) deficiency in human narcolepsy. *Lancet*, 2000; **355**:39–40.

20. **Thorpy M**. Therapeutic advances in narcolepsy. *Sleep Med*, 2007; **8**:427–40.

21. **Hagan J J**, **Leslie R A**, **Patel S**, et al. Orexin A activates locus coeruleus cell firing and increases arousal in the rat. *Proc Natl Acad Sci USA*, 1999; **96**:10 911–16.

22. **Hanson L R**, **Taheri M**, **Kamsheh L**, et al. Intranasal administration of hypocretin 1 (orexin A) bypasses the blood–brain barrier and target the brain: a new strategy for the treatment of narcolepsy. *Drug Deliv Tech*, 2004; **4**:1–10.

23. **Fujiki N**, **Yoshida Y**, **Ripley B**, et al. Effects of IV and ICV hypocretin-1 (orexin A) in hypocretin receptor-2 gene mutated narcoleptic dogs and IV hypocretin-1 replacement therapy in a hypocretin-ligand-deficient narcoleptic dog. *Sleep*, 2003; **26**:953–59.

24. **Kastin A J**, **Akerstrom V**. Orexin A but not orexin B rapidly enters brain from blood by simple diffusion. *J Pharmacol Exp Ther*, 1999; **289**:219–23.

25. **John J**, **Wu M F**, **Siegel J M**. Systemic administration of hypocretin-1 reduces cataplexy and normalizes sleep and waking durations in narcoleptic dogs. *Sleep Res Online*, 2000; **3**:23–28.

26. **Born J**, **Lange T**, **Kern W**, et al. Sniffing neuropeptides: a transnasal approach to the human brain. *Nat Neurosci*, 2002; **5**:514–16.

27. **Asahi S**, **Egashira S**, **Matsuda M**, et al. Development of an orexin-2 receptor selective agonist, [Ala(11, , D-Leu(15)]orexin-B. *Bioorg Med Chem Lett*, 2003; **13**:111–13.

28. **Zeitzer J M**, **Buckmaster C L**, **Parker K J**, et al. Circadian and homeostatic regulation of hypocretin in a primate model: implications for the consolidation of wakefulness. *J Neurosci*, 2003; **23**:3555–60.

29. **Lang M, Soll R M, Durrenberger F,** et al. Structure–activity studies of orexin A and orexin B at the human orexin 1 and orexin 2 receptors led to orexin 2 receptor selective and orexin 1 receptor preferring ligands. *J Med Chem*, 2004; **47**:1153–60.

30. **Mieda M, Willie J T, Hara J,** et al. Orexin peptides prevent cataplexy and improve wakefulness in an orexin neuron-ablated model of narcolepsy in mice. *Proc Natl Acad Sci USA*, 2004; **101**:4649–54.

31. **Dauvilliers Y, Tafti M.** Molecular genetics and treatment of narcolepsy. *Ann Med*, 2006; **38**:252–62.

32. **Thannickal T C, Moore R Y, Nienhuis R,** et al. Reduced number of hypocretin neurons in human narcolepsy. *Neuron*, 2000; **27**:469–74.

33. **Arias-Carrion O, Murillo-Rodriguez E, Xu M,** et al. Transplantation of hypocretin neurons into the pontine reticular formation: preliminary results. *Sleep*, 2004; **27**:1465–70.

34. **Peyron C, Faraco J, Rogers W,** et al. A mutation in a case of early onset narcolepsy and a generalized absence of hypocretin peptides in human narcoleptic brains. *Nat Med*, 2000; **6**:991–97.

35. **Zeitzer J M, Nishino S, Mignot E.** The neurobiology of hypocretins (orexins), narcolepsy and related therapeutic interventions. *Trends Pharmacol Sci*, 2006; **27**:368–74.

36. **Heuer H, Schafer M K, O'Donnell D,** et al. Expression of thyrotropin-releasing hormone receptor 2 (TRH-R2) in the central nervous system of rats. *J Comp Neurol*, 2000; **428**:319–36.

37. **Riehl J, Honda K, Kwan M,** et al. Chronic oral administration of CG-3703, a thyrotropin releasing hormone analog, increases wake and decreases cataplexy in canine narcolepsy. *Neuropsychopharmacology*, 2000; **23**:34–45.

38. **Nishino S, Arrigoni J, Shelton J,** et al. Effects of thyrotropin-releasing hormone and its analogs on daytime sleepiness and cataplexy in canine narcolepsy. *J Neurosci*, 1997; **17**:6401–08.

39. **Schomburg L, Turwitt S, Prescher G,** et al. Human TRH-degrading ectoenzyme cDNA cloning, functional expression, genomic structure and chromosomal assignment. *Eur J Biochem*, 1999; **265**:415–22.

40. **Beer B, Stark J, Krieter P,** et al. DOV 216,303, a "triple" reuptake inhibitor: safety, tolerability, and pharmacokinetic profile. *J Clin Pharmacol*, 2004; **44**:1360–67.

41. **Izzi F, Placidi F, Marciani M G,** et al. Effective treatment of narcolepsy–cataplexy with duloxetine: a report of three cases. *Sleep Med*, 2009; **10**:153–54.

42. **Niederhofer H.** Atomoxetine also effective in patients suffering from narcolepsy? *Sleep*, 2005; **28**:1189.

43. **Krogsgaard-Larsen P, Frolund B, Liljefors T,** et al. GABA(A) agonists and partial agonists: THIP (Gaboxadol) as a non-opioid analgesic and a novel type of hypnotic. *Biochem Pharmacol*, 2004; **68**:1573–80.

44. **Mathias S, Wetter T C, Steiger A,** et al. The GABA uptake inhibitor tiagabine promotes slow wave sleep in normal elderly subjects. *Neurobiol Aging*, 2001; **22**:247–53.

45. **Landolt H P, Meier V, Burgess H J,** et al. Serotonin-2 receptors and human sleep: effect of a selective antagonist on EEG power spectra. *Neuropsychopharmacology*, 1999; **21**:455–66.

46. **Cheng M Y, Bullock C M, Li C,** et al. Prokineticin 2 transmits the behavioural circadian rhythm of the suprachiasmatic nucleus. *Nature*, 2002; **417**:405–10.

47. **Xu Y L, Reinscheid R K, Huitron-Resendiz S,** et al. Neuropeptide S: a neuropeptide promoting arousal and anxiolytic-like effects. *Neuron*, 2004; **43**:487–97.

Section 4 Chapter 40

Therapy of Excessive Sleepiness

Behavioral and psychiatric treatments for sleepiness

Shelby F. Harris and Michael J. Thorpy

Introduction

Effective treatment of excessive daytime sleepiness (EDS) is often influenced by the underlying cause. This chapter presents an overview of many behavioral strategies implemented to combat EDS. These techniques are varied in their approach and can include the use of appropriate timing of light therapy for circadian rhythm disorders, scheduled naps, CPAP compliance for sleep-related breathing disorders, extension of bed and/or wake times, and psychotherapeutic techniques for EDS secondary to psychiatric disorders. A brief discussion of general strategies to help combat and cope with EDS in all patients, regardless of the underlying cause, is also included.

Sleepiness due to narcolepsy

EDS can significantly interfere with a patient's quality of life, and impact one's ability to work, socialize and drive. People with narcolepsy often lack the energy to participate in daily activities. Although patients may fall asleep during times of inactivity or boredom, they may also do so during inappropriate or dangerous times such as at work, mid-conversation, driving. After brief sleep episodes, patients often feel refreshed until the next episode.

Proper treatment strategies are highly important given the significant negative impact narcolepsy can have in the daily life of patients. Pharmacological methods are considered the primary treatment for managing symptoms of narcolepsy, and behavioral methods play a large role in adjunctive treatment.

Scheduled naps

Naps can be beneficial although difficult to incorporate into a patient's daily routine. Studies have examined the role of naps as they relate to improvement of alertness for patients, with some suggesting that one extended nap provides maximum benefit for longer, sustained wakefulness [1–4].

Short, intermittent naps have also been reported as beneficial and may be a feasible option for certain patients. Rogers and colleagues investigated three different sleep schedules and their effects on EDS in narcolepsy patients taking stimulants [5]. The best response was found in patients where nighttime sleep was regularized with two 15-min naps added as compared to patients on a study-imposed regular schedule with no naps or those with the patients' habitual sleep patterns with two naps added.

Patients with narcolepsy should plan a sleep–wake schedule by tracking the times of maximal wakefulness and sleepiness. This allows patients to customize their nap schedules to yield optimal response.

Dietary changes

Few studies have investigated the relationship between EDS and diet. Some patients alter their food intake to decrease EDS. Patients with narcolepsy have reported activities ranging from avoiding lunch, binge eating before bedtime, avoiding carbohydrates, increasing protein, or increasing caffeine [6, 7].

Conflicting data exist as to whether dietary alterations increase daytime alertness. Bruck and colleagues found that ingestion of glucose increases sleepiness in those with narcolepsy [8], whereas others have suggested that the contents of a lunchtime meal had no direct effects upon EDS in this population [9].

A number of studies have reported an increased body mass index and/or increased frequency of type II diabetes in patients with narcolepsy [10–12]. One study suggests that lower metabolic rates, most likely due to hypocretin deficiency, and differences in eating

Sleepiness: Causes, Consequences and Treatment, ed. Michael J. Thorpy and Michel Billiard. Published by Cambridge University Press. © Cambridge University Press 2011.

Table 40.1 Basic sleep hygiene strategies

Maintain a regular bedtime and waketime seven days per week
Exercise regularly, but not within 3 h of bedtime
Do not clock-watch
Maintain a comfortable bedroom temperature at all times
Avoid alcohol and large meals within 3 h of bedtime
Avoid nicotine, especially within 3 h of bedtime and during any nocturnal awakenings
Keep the bedroom very dark and quiet
Limit caffeine intake after noon
Allow for at least 45 min to 1 h of wind-down time before bedtime
Do not engage in stressful activities before bedtime

habits could account for higher BMIs found in patients with narcolepsy [13]. As a result, patients should be counseled on nutrition and daily caloric intake.

Caffeine can have an alerting effect, but it has not been studied as a means of treating sleepiness in patients with narcolepsy. Most narcoleptics report that caffeine has minimal effect on EDS and caffeine should be avoided in the evening, as it may aggravate nocturnal sleep disturbance [14].

Exercise

Even though patients report feeling more alert when they are active, it is often difficult for narcoleptics with EDS to motivate themselves to exercise. The alerting effects of physical activity in this population have not been studied; however, studies in sleep-deprived individuals have shown that exercise can be effective at improving alertness. While further research should be done to study the effects of exercise on EDS in narcolepsy, patients should be encouraged to do light aerobic exercise.

Disrupted nocturnal sleep

Sleep maintenance insomnia is commonly seen in patients with narcolepsy. Lack of consolidated nocturnal sleep can influence daytime alertness. Symptoms of insomnia often appear within five years after the occurrence of excessive daytime sleepiness [15].

Behavioral strategies for consolidating nighttime sleep in patients with narcolepsy are similar to those recommended for patients suffering from insomnia. Refer to Table 40.1 for a listing of basic sleep hygiene strategies.

Stimulus control instructions should also be discussed with the patient given the increased time spent awake in bed [16]. These instructions are identical to those provided to patients with insomnia and include: (a) go to bed only when sleepy but not before your standard bedtime, (b) get out of bed once you realize you are awake at any point during the night (it is advised to refrain from clock-watching as this can be mentally stimulating), (c) sit somewhere outside of the bedroom in dim light until sleepy again, (d) while sitting outside of the bedroom, engage in pleasurable but non-stimulating activities so one doesn't focus upon the time passing, (e) return to bed only when sleepy, and (f) keep a fixed wake time every day regardless of how much sleep was obtained the night before.

The step of leaving the bedroom and returning to bed may be repeated several times over the course of the night for the first week or two if the patient has significantly broken nocturnal sleep. Helping the patient generate a list of relaxing activities (e.g. practice relaxation exercises, listen to relaxing music, read a magazine, folding laundry) can be useful in helping the patient to get out of bed even when the patient does not want to.

Relaxation techniques (such as muscle relaxation strategies, diaphragmatic breathing, imagery, and mindfulness) may prove useful. Limited research exists to show that these exercises increase and consolidate nocturnal sleep time.

General behavioral strategies for work, home, school

Patients with narcolepsy report difficulties with completing everyday chores. Nearly one-third of patients with narcolepsy describe difficulties with caring for children and cooking, and 11% of patients had difficulties with ironing [17]. Daytime sleepiness can often cause serious injuries from burns due to falling asleep while smoking, ironing, or cooking.

Patients are advised to avoid situations where sleepiness is likely to occur. Common triggers for sleepiness often include excessive warmth, sedentary activities, and boredom. Many patients report that standing (rather than sitting), being outdoors, and seeking cool environments can be effective ways of promoting wakefulness. Creativity is often necessary to help combat EDS. For example, many patients have found it alerting to increase background noise levels or chewing on ice.

As many as 66% of patients with narcolepsy report a history of falling asleep while driving, and 37% had major accidents while 67% had near motor vehicle accidents [18]. Although these rates are alarmingly high, there are no widely accepted guidelines on driving for patients with narcolepsy. Patients have adopted a number of strategies to help remain alert when they are driving. Strategies such as taking extra stimulant medication before driving, using a manual shift car, not driving long distances during the night, and stopping for coffee and taking a short nap have all been adopted to help increase alertness. Patients are advised against avoiding social situations, driving with the car windows open or while using an alarm, smoking cigarettes, and inducing pain while behind the wheel.

Patients should be advised to solicit family support with household chores and only engage in these activities when most alert. In addition, the patient should be advised against driving, bathing, swimming and using heavy machinery or household appliances during times of sleepiness.

Insufficient Sleep Syndrome (ISS)

ISS is considered to be the most common cause of daytime sleepiness and fatigue, with patients exhibiting difficulties in memory, attention, and psychomotor performance. The clinician should work with the patient to determine the cause of insufficient sleep, as it can often be poor sleep hygiene (e.g. not allowing for wind-down time, texting late at night) or self-imposed sleep deprivation (e.g. long work hours, wanting to stay up to say hello to a loved one who works late). Extension of bed and wake times is the primary treatment of choice. Psychoeducation regarding proper sleep hygiene and working with the patient to see the pros and cons of the current situation are all necessary to help allow for more time in bed to sleep. Stress and time management skills can also be taught to help alleviate any excessive pressure to work late into the night.

Sleepiness related to positive airway pressure (PAP) non-compliance

A number of studies have evaluated the efficacy of PAP in the overall treatment of EDS [19–21]. Patel and colleagues conducted a meta-analysis that found PAP to be effective in improving EDS [22]. Several studies compared 1 month of PAP use to control placebo pill, noting that PAP reduced overall EDS [23–24]. Jenkinson et al. compared 1 month of optimal pressure PAP therapy to a PAP machine set at the lowest pressure with holes cut in the mask (also known as "sham PAP"). Results from this study indicate that PAP was associated with EDS improvements across all measures [25]. Randomized, age- and gender-matched trials between no treatment and PAP have shown reduced sleepiness as far out as 3 months with use [26, 27].

Not all studies have found PAP to reduce EDS to levels that are within normal limits. While PAP may not be a foolproof method for significantly reducing EDS in all patients, it is currently the best method to treat sleep-disordered breathing (SDB). PAP non-compliance may be one confounding factor yielding mixed results in reducing overall EDS. Some have suggested that the baseline severity of both the SDB and EDS may moderate the overall efficacy of PAP in reducing EDS. Redline and colleagues noted that EDS in mild obstructive sleep apnea (OSA) patients was not objectively different post-treatment from those with placebo pill, weight loss advice, or a nasal dilator strip, but indicated that improvements with EDS related to PAP treatment was found on subjective measures [28].

Poor adherence to PAP is common among those who are prescribed the treatment. Twenty-five percent of patients discontinue PAP within the first year, and many more tend not to use the treatment as indicated [29–31]. Kribbs and colleagues investigated PAP compliance by monitoring actual pressure and use throughout the day. Patients were not aware of the monitoring and were found to overestimate actual use of PAP. During the first 3 months of treatment, less than 50% of patients used PAP for at least 4 h per night on 70% of the nights monitored. Only 6% used treatment optimally on at least 70% of the nights. The frequency and duration of PAP use in the first month of treatment reliably predicted use in the third month [29].

Reasons for PAP non-compliance are varied and often include poor mask fit, nasal congestion, partner complaints, feeling suffocated, cost, and inconvenience. Non-complaince predictors include history of uvulopalatopharyngoplasty, oxygen desaturation, AHI severity, weight, sex, age and education. Research eliciting specific predictors is inconsistent, with several studies finding no differences in PAP pressure level, AHI, and EDS [32–34]. Patients educated on OSA and the benefits of PAP, especially those who believed PAP was likely to help with their OSA, were more likely to follow through with treatment [35]. Subjective improvements in daytime and nocturnal symptoms with treatment may help continue ongoing use of PAP. The most consistent indicator of PAP compliance is perceived benefits from use [36].

Research aimed at increasing PAP compliance is varied and relies on psychological and behavioral techniques as their base. General strategies for increasing PAP compliance are discussed below.

Educational

Psychoeducation and self-efficacy regarding OSA and PAP have been linked to increased compliance [37]. Education-based treatments have been investigated, including those designed to provide psychoeducation, videos, telephone support, support groups, and educational literature [37–44]. These treatments focus upon providing information to new PAP users about how to best utilize the treatment and provide solutions to common side-effects. Results have been inconsistent in improving PAP adherence, but need to be interpreted with caution because many of these studies are limited by small sample sizes and lack of a control group.

Cognitive behavioral (CBT) interventions

An emerging line of research utilizing specific CBT strategies for PAP compliance exists. Richards *et al.* compared CBT interventions plus treatment as usual (mask fitting and basic education) to treatment as usual in 100 patients. The CBT group included sessions with both the patient and their partner, and incorporated elements of cognitive therapy to modify erroneous beliefs regarding PAP treatment. Videos of PAP using role models were shown to the group and relaxation strategies were taught to reduce anxiety regarding wearing the mask. Patients in the CBT group used PAP 2.9 more hours over 28 days in comparison to controls. Richards suggests that the treatment group may have increased patient confidence in PAP use and the inclusion of the partner in treatment further enhanced results. Results should be interpreted cautiously, as there was no time-matched therapist group and partner involvement was not controlled [45].

A new line of research in PAP compliance incorporates elements of the Transtheoretical Model (TTM) and social cognitive theory (SCT) to enhance treatment outcomes. SCT [46] posits that perceived self-efficacy (confidence in utilizing the treatment) is a major determinant of whether and to what extent one will initiate and continue treatment and to what extent one will continue to do so when complications are encountered. SCT emphasizes the importance of the influence both personal and environmental factors can have upon behavior change. TTM [47] suggests that ambivalence is key in behavior change and that patients fall along a continuum of various stages of readiness to change. These stages include precontemplation (not thinking about behavior change), contemplation (actively thinking about behavior change but not making any changes), preparation (beginning to make changes), action (actively engaged in behavior change) and maintenance (maintaining any changes that were made). The pros and cons of engaging in the new behavior are investigated to encourage change.

Motivational Interviewing (MI) [48] is an efficacious treatment for behavior change in various disorders, especially drug and alcohol dependence. MI is a client-centered therapy designed to increase readiness for behavior change and is based on both SCT and TTM. MI has been applied to PAP compliance (Motivational Enhancement Therapy, MET) [49], addressing patient ambivalence about PAP use. MET consists of two 45-min in-person sessions with a 15-min follow-up phone call. The first session discusses the advantages and disadvantages of treatment (decisional balance), reviews the pre- and post-treatment PSG report in detail, as well as any other health complaints. The decisional balance exercise helps patients to discuss benefits of not using PAP and helps move them from the precontemplation stage to contemplation, action, etc. In session 2, the patient's thoughts regarding PAP use since session 1, any difficulties are assessed and realistic goals for PAP use are developed. Important life goals that the patient has set for himself are reviewed and a discussion of how PAP use can facilitate some of these goals is initiated. A follow-up phone call promotes benefits.

Aloia *et al.* compared MET, a brief in-person educational treatment, and standard care (material informing patients of consequences of OSA and treatment benefits), in a total of 160 patients (aged 25–86) with OSA, with a number of patients placed on flexible

Table 40.2 Sample PAP exposure hierarchy

1. Connect the PAP unit to the mask and hose. Hold the mask over your face and breathe in and out (without PAP on) while awake.
2. Connect the PAP unit to the mask and hose. Hold the mask over your face and breathe in and out (with PAP on) while awake.
3. Strap mask onto your head, and, with PAP on, breathe with PAP on for 5 min.
4. Strap mask onto your head, and, with PAP on, breathe with PAP on for 10 min.
5. Use PAP during a scheduled nap at home.
6. Use PAP during initial 3–4 h of nighttime sleep.
7. Use PAP throughout an entire night of sleep.

pressure delivery. Although MET and the educational treatment were found to be superior (though not statistically significant) in comparison to standard clinical care, MET was most efficacious when flexible pressure PAP treatment was utilized [50].

This newly proposed treatment for PAP compliance is still being refined and limited data exist evaluating its effectiveness. Nevertheless, self-efficacy and coping skills (both suggested to be important in adherence to PAP) are found to predict PAP use [51–53].

Desensitization

Although MET has shown promise in increasing PAP compliance, it does not address patients who complain of intense anxiety, panic or suffocation related to PAP use. Edinger and Means investigated PAP non-compliant patients with claustrophobia. Treatment consisted of graded exposure therapy to disconnect the association between anxiety and PAP use [54]. Patients acclimated to the PAP at various steps along individually tailored exposure hierarchies. As a patient practices each step on the hierarchy, he should continue the exercise until his anxiety comes to a peak and then reduces by at least half. Discontinuing the exercise at the peak of anxiety (as many patients will be tempted to do) will only serve to negatively reinforce the phobia. Patients are then encouraged to move on to the next step on the exposure hierarchy once their peak anxiety for a particular step is significantly lowered (refer to Table 40.2 for a sample hierarchy). Edinger and Means report that 92% of their patients treated with exposure therapy used PAP significantly longer than at baseline (either more hours per night or more days per week) [54].

Excessive sleepiness and psychiatric disorders

Psychologically driven treatment

Research investigating behavioral treatments for excessive sleepiness comorbid with psychiatric disorders is in its infancy. A psychologically based treatment for insomnia has been suggested as excessive sleepiness in psychiatric disorders may be maintained by factors such as avoidance, anhedonia and sleep-state misperception [55, 56]. Billiard *et al.* investigated the sleep of two groups on polysomnography (PSG), idiopathic hypersomnia and psychiatric hypersomnia, over a two-day study period. Results from this study suggest that a majority of patients in the psychiatric group spent significant time lying in bed, but no objective sleep was measured on PSG. These findings contrast with those from the idiopathic hypersomnia group who had shortened sleep latencies on MSLT and extended total nocturnal sleep time on PSG (7.68 h in psychiatric group, 9.92 h in idiopathic group) [57]. Others also obtained similar results comparing the sleep of patients with narcolepsy to bipolar patients with excessive sleepiness. Bipolar patients were found to have PSG and MSLT scores comparable to healthy young adults even though patients complained of significant sleepiness. Patients with narcolepsy had significantly reduced sleep latencies and marked daytime sleepiness on MSLT [58]. These studies lend support for a psychologically driven treatment for excessive sleepiness related to psychiatric disorders. Patients do not objectively appear to be pathologically sleepy during the day and do not have markedly longer nocturnal sleep. Targeting the extreme fatigue, excessive time in bed, anhedonia and avolition is warranted.

Excessive sleepiness is commonly reported in diagnoses such as major depressive disorder, bipolar disorder, atypical depression, dysthymia and seasonal affective disorder. Despite the particular psychiatric condition, several basic behavioral sleep–wake principles should be reviewed. Nocturnal sleep periods should be structured with established bedtimes and waketimes that allow for at least 8 h in bed. The practitioner should ensure that the patient follows basic stimulus control procedures and proper sleep hygiene.

Kaplan and Harvey outline a cognitive–behavioral therapy program for the treatment of EDS in psychiatric disorders. Their brief treatment (consisting of

4–8 sessions) includes various components. They suggest a functional analysis of the excessive sleepiness including "antecedents, behaviors and consequences of hypersomnia" ([56], p. 283). Motivational interviewing to elucidate the pros and cons of treating the excessive sleepiness is included, as well as overall goal setting, focusing on both short- and long-term goals. The authors also propose using psychoeducation as a tool, giving information on circadian rhythms, sleep inertia, sleepiness and fatigue. Finally, wind-down and wake-up periods, behavioral experiments (actually testing out beliefs related to excessive sleepiness and fatigue) and relapse prevention are all incorporated into the treatment package. As this treatment was recently developed, outcome research investigating the effects of psychological interventions upon psychiatric-related excessive sleepiness is still unavailable.

Light therapy

Bright light therapy has been shown to reduce excessive sleepiness in patients with Seasonal Affective Disorder (SAD) and Major Depression (MD) [59]. Significant limitations exist within the light therapy literature, most notably the lack of standardization of methods across many of the studies. The use of bright light in bipolar disorder (BD) is still debated as researchers gain a better understanding of the circadian disruption. Some suggest that early morning bright light may induce mania or mixed episodes and midday bright light alleviates depressive symptoms [60, 61]. While bright light treatment may be efficacious in the overall relief of MD, SAD and BD, its positive effects on excessive sleepiness are only observed in SAD [62].

Behavioral treatment of circadian rhythm disorders

Delayed Sleep Phase Syndrome (DSPS)

Bright light therapy (>2000 lux) for 1–2 h in the morning (after core body temperature reaches its minimum) has been shown to phase advance sleep onset time and reduce morning sleepiness [63]. There are ample data evaluating the relationship between light intensity and gradient of phase shift, but there are few data that evaluate how much phase shift is accomplished by light exposure of varying durations. In order to properly utilize this treatment, a full understanding of the patient's phase response curve is necessary. Administration of light too early in the morning (before core body temperature reaches its minimum) can result in a further delay of sleep onset. Bright light should be avoided in the early evening through bedtime to further initiate a phase advance.

Chronotherapy has also been shown to help DSPS. Introduced by Czeisler and colleagues in 1981, this treatment was proposed to take advantage of the DSPS patient's natural ability to phase delay [64]. Patients are encouraged to delay both bedtime and waketime by 3 h each day until they come around to a suitable sleep–wake schedule. Although there is research in support of the treatment [65], various modifications to the treatment exist, which make generalizing its effectiveness difficult [66]. A number of practical problems arise from this treatment, as the patient often needs to block out one week to make sure he can sleep during the daytime without interruption.

Regardless of what treatment option is utilized, basic principles of stimulus control and sleep hygiene must be enforced. Further, the patient must utilize proper zeitgeibers to help with sleep onset and awakening. For example, many patients with DSPS tend to be most active in the evening (saving the nighttime for working and other activities), so the clinician should help the patient switch these activities to the morning and daytime. Emphasis on wind-down time before bed as well as usage of dim light can help reinforce the sleep–wake schedule.

Advanced Sleep Phase Syndrome (ASPS)

The treatment of ASPS is essentially the reverse of that for DSPS. Regardless of the treatment option being utilized, the patient with ASPS is encouraged to follow basic sleep hygiene and stimulus control procedures. They are also counseled against winding down too early in the afternoon/early evening and activities are planned to help the patient further delay the bedtime. Evening bright light treatment (generally between 7pm and 9pm), combined with limiting early morning bright light, is the most utilized and researched. This has been shown to delay circadian rhythms and early afternoon sleepiness enough to allow for a more appropriate bedtime and waketime [67–69].

Moldofsky and colleagues utilized chronotherapy to capitalize on the ASPS patient's propensity towards sleepiness earlier in the evening/late afternoon. The patient is encouraged to progressively advance sleep time by 2 h every 2 days until the desired bedtime and waketime are both reached [70]. As with chronotherapy for DSPS, this treatment is limited due to issues of practicality.

Shift Work Disorder (SWD)

A successful treatment for SWD is one that has the patient's circadian rhythms properly match his work–sleep schedule. Behavioral treatments implemented depend upon the type of shift that the patient works. Regardless of the shift that is worked, various environmental and social elements must be controlled as well. If possible, a steady sleep–wake schedule should be protected 7 days per week.

During the times for sleep, the patient must limit interruptions (e.g. phone calls, housework and errands). Having others help out with these responsibilities is important to keeping the sleep time and environment protected. The bedroom should be kept dark and quiet, with blackout shades and a white noise machine or earplugs used if necessary. In addition, the patient must follow proper sleep hygiene and stimulus control procedures.

Rotating shifts generally require a clockwise rotation, where the patient is instructed to delay his work schedule later every shift or few shifts, from day to evening to night and back to day. In night shift workers, bright light exposure has been successfully utilized to align the circadian rhythm with the sleep–wake schedule necessary for work [68, 71]. Light exposure should begin early in the shift and end 2 h before the end of the shift (sunglasses can aid in blocking light). The patient is encouraged to avoid bright light during the commute home and light intensities ranging from 1200 to 10 000 lux have been investigated, as well as various durations for the light exposure (ranging from 20-min per hour pulses up to 6 h continuously). Some patients exhibit comorbid insomnia, and the initiation of CBT strategies can prove helpful (e.g. cognitive therapy, stimulus control, sleep hygiene and restriction of time in bed and relaxation techniques). Daytime sleep should be initiated soon after returning home from work.

Jet Lag Type (JLT)

The type of treatment required for JLT is dependent upon the direction of travel. During westward travel, difficulty maintaining sleep is commonly reported. During eastward travel, sleep onset is problematic for many. Patients adapt to westward travel better than eastward travel. General strategies to always follow include wearing comfortable clothing, avoiding alcohol, excessive food, and caffeine during the flight. Once the patient reaches his travel destination, he should remain on the local time, including eating, sleeping, and exercising according to the local clock. Ear plugs and eye masks should be used during travel if necessary.

Use of bright light exposure depends upon the direction of travel. If traveling eastward, bright light in the early morning should be avoided, with bright light encouraged in the evening. Westward travelers should do the opposite [72]. Depending on the direction of travel, the patient can gradually delay or advance his bedtime and waketimes for one week before travel to facilitate the patient's adjustment to the destination time.

Irregular Sleep–Wake Type (ISWT)

The goal of treatment for ISWT is to consolidate nocturnal sleep. Although ISWT is a difficult disorder to treat successfully, several strategies have been found useful. Strategies include increasing bright light exposure during the morning and afternoon and limiting light and noise during the evening. The clinician should work with the patient to increase structured activities (e.g. exercise and socializing) during the daytime to further separate day from night [73].

Non-entrained Type (NT)

Most of the studies on treatment for NT have been conducted in blind people utilizing sleep hygiene, maintenance of a fixed sleep–wake schedule, increasing scheduled daytime activities and low doses of melatonin [74]. Little research exists on behavioral treatments in the sighted with NT. The clinician should focus upon behavioral strategies indicated above, creating regular sleep–wake and work schedules and increasing bright light exposure at fixed times daily.

Basic strategies for every patient presenting with EDS

Techniques considered to be beneficial, regardless of the underlying cause, include having a frank discussion regarding the threats of driving while sleepy. Clinicians should brainstorm with their patients any options to prevent against drowsy driving. Such techniques can include taking a short nap before driving, pulling over while driving to nap, letting another person drive, and strategic use of caffeine. Proper sleep hygiene, stimulus control, and allowing for at least 8 h in bed for sleep should all be reviewed in detail.

Conclusion

EDS is a common symptom found in numerous sleep, medical and psychiatric disorders which can greatly impact one's daily functioning. Although pharmacological methods are often considered for the management of EDS, behavioral methods play a large role in both adjunctive and primary treatment. Patients often have residual sleepiness that is not effectively managed by pharmacological methods alone and the addition of behavioral interventions can prove useful. EDS can often interfere with work and home lives, and these difficulties can lead to depression and anxiety as well as significant problems with family, peers, and employers.

Behavioral treatment strategies utilized by the clinician to address EDS are greatly influenced by the underlying cause. Techniques chosen can vary from appropriate timing of light therapy for circadian rhythm disorders, scheduled naps, PAP compliance for sleep-related breathing disorders, extension of bed and/or wake times for insufficient sleep, and psychotherapeutic techniques for excessive sleepiness secondary to psychiatric disorders. Behavioral techniques to be utilized in all patients should include sleep hygiene, stimulus control, and avoidance of drowsy driving and dangerous activities.

References

1. **Guilleminault C**, **Stoohs R**, **Clerk A**. Daytime somnolence: therapeutic approaches. *Neurophysiol Clin*, 1993; **23**:23–33.
2. **Rogers A E**, **Aldrich M S**. The effect of regularly scheduled naps on sleep attacks and excessive daytime sleepiness associated with narcolepsy. *Nurs Res*, 1993; **42**:111–17.
3. **Mullington J**, **Broughton R**. Scheduled naps in the management of daytime sleepiness in narcolepsy–cataplexy. *Sleep*, 1993; **16**:444–56.
4. **Helmus J**, **Rosenthal L**, **Bishop C**, *et al*. The alerting effects of short and long naps in narcoleptic, sleep-deprived and alert individuals. *Sleep*, 1997; **20**:251–57.
5. **Rogers A E**, **Aldrich M S**, **Lin X**. A comparison of three sleep schedules for reducing daytime sleepiness in narcolepsy. *Sleep*, 2001; **24**:385–91.
6. **Chabas D**, **Fouton C**, **Gonzalez J**. Eating disorder and metabolism in narcoleptic patients. *Sleep*, 2007; **30**:1267–73.
7. **Bruck D**. Food consumption patterns in narcolepsy. *Sleep*, 2003; **26**(Abstract suppl):A272–73.
8. **Bruck D**, **Armstrong S**, **Coleman G**. Sleepiness after glucose in narcolepsy. *J Sleep Res*, 1994; **3**:171–79.
9. **Pollack C P**, **Green J**. Eating and its relationship with subjective alertness and sleep in narcoleptic subjects living without temporal cues. *Sleep*, 1990; **13**:467–78.
10. **Honda Y**, **Doi Y**, **Ninomiya R**, *et al*. Increased frequency of non-insulin dependent diabetes mellitus among narcoleptic patients. *Sleep*, 1986; **1**:254–59.
11. **Schuld A**, **Beitinger P A**, **Dalal M**, *et al*. Increased body mass index in male narcoleptic patients, but not in HLA-DR2-positive healthy male volunteers. *Sleep Med*, 2002; **3**:335–39.
12. **Dahmen N**, **Bierbrauer J**, **Kasten M**. Increased prevalence of obesity in narcoleptic patients and relatives. *Eur Arch Psychiatry Clin Neurosci*, 2001; **251**:85–89.
13. **Chabas D**, **Foulon C**, **Gonzalez J**, *et al*. Eating disorder and metabolism in narcoleptic patients. *Sleep*, 2007; **30**:1267–73.
14. **Wright K P Jr**, **Badia P**, **Myers B**, *et al*. Combination of bright light and caffeine as a countermeasure for impaired alertness and performance during extended sleep deprivation. *J Sleep Res*, 1997; **6**; 26–35.
15. **Billiard M**, **Besset A**, **Cadihac J**. The clinical and polygraphic development of narcolepsy. In: Guilleminault C, Lugaresi E, Eds., *Sleep/Wake Disorders: Natural History, Epidemiology and Long-Term Evolution*. New York, NY: Raven Press, 1983: 171–85.
16. **Bootzin R R**. Stimulus control for the treatment of insomnia. Proceedings from the 80th Annual Convention of the American Psychological Association, 1972; **7**:395–96.
17. **Tiexera V G**, **Faccenda J F**, **Douglas N J**. Functional status in patients with narcolepsy. *Sleep Med*, 2004; **5**:477–83.
18. **Broughton R**, **Ghanem Q**, **Hishikawa Y**, *et al*. Life effects of narcolepsy in 180 patients from North America, Asia, and Europe compared to matched controls. *Can J Neurol Sci*, 1981; **8**:299–304.
19. **Chokoverty S**. Editor's corner. *Sleep Med*, 2000; **1**:173.
20. **Davies R J**, **Stradling J R**. The efficacy of nasal continuous positive airway pressure in the treatment

of obstructive sleep apnea syndrome is proven. *Am J Respir Crit Care Med*, 2000; **161**:1775–76.

21. **Engelman H M**, **Kingshott R N**, **Wraith P K**, et al. Randomized placebo-controlled crossover trial of continuous positive airway pressure for mild sleep apnea/hypopnea syndrome. *Am J Respir Crit Care Med*, 1999; **159**:461–67.

22. **Patel S R**, **White D P**, **Malhotra A**, et al. Continuous positive airway pressure therapy for treating sleepiness in a diverse population with obstructive sleep apnea: results of a meta-analysis. *Arch Intern Med*, 2003; **163**:565–71.

23. **Engelman H M**, **Martin S E**, **Deary I J**, et al. Effect of continuous positive airway pressure treatment on daytime function in sleep apnoea/hypopnoea syndrome. *Lancet*, 1994; **343**:572–75.

24. **Engelman H M**, **Martin S E**, **Kingshott R N**, et al. Randomised placebo controlled trial of daytime function after continuous positive airway pressure (CPAP) therapy for the sleep apnoea/hypopnoea syndrome. *Thorax*, 1998; **53**:341–45.

25. **Jenkinson C**, **Davies R J**, **Mullins R**, et al. Comparison of therapeutic and subtherapeutic nasal continuous positive airway pressure for obstructive sleep apnoea: a randomized prospective parallel trial. *Lancet*, 1999; **353**:2100–05.

26. **Lamphere J**, **Roehrs T**, **Wittig R**, et al. Recovery of alertness after CPAP in apnea. *Chest*, 1989; **96**:1364–67.

27. **Engelman H M**, **Cheshire K E**, **Deary I J**, et al. Daytime sleepiness, cognitive performance and mood after continuous positive airway pressure for the sleep apnoea/hypopnoea syndrome. *Thorax*, 1993; **48**:911–14.

28. **Redline S**, **Adams N**, **Strauss M E**, et al. Improvement in mild sleep-disordered breathing with CPAP compared with conservative therapy. *Am J Resp Crit Care Med*, 1998; **157**:858–65.

29. **Kribbs N B**, **Pack A I**, **Kline L R**, et al. Objective measurement of patterns of nasal CPAP use by patients with obstructive sleep apnea. *Am Rev Resp Dis*, 1993; **147**:887–95.

30. **Reeves-Hoche M K**, **Hudgel D W**, **Meck R**, et al. Continuous versus bilevel positive airway pressure for obstructive sleep apnea. *Am J Respir Crit Care Med*, 1995; **151**:443–49.

31. **Sin D D**, **Mayers I**, **Man G C**, et al. Long-term compliance rates to continuous positive airway pressure in obstructive sleep apnea: a population-based study. *Chest*, 2002; **121**:430–35.

32. **Alacron A**, **Leon C**, **Maimo A**, et al. Compliance with nasal continuous positive airway pressure (CPAP) treatment in sleep apnea–hypopnea syndrome. *Arch Bronchoneumol*, 1995; **31**:56–61.

33. **Edinger J D**, **Carwile S**, **Miller P**, et al. Psychological status, syndromatic measures, and compliance with nasal CPAP therapy for sleep apnea. *Percept Mot Skills*, 1994; **78**:1116–18.

34. **Engleman H M**, **Martin S E**, **Douglas N J**. Compliance with CPAP therapy in patients with the sleep apnoea/hypopnoea syndrome. *Thorax*, 1994; **49**:263–66.

35. **Smith S S**, **Lang C P**, **Sullivan K A**, et al. The development of two new tools for assessing knowledge and beliefs about OSA and CPAP. *Sleep Med*, 2004; **5**:359–67.

36. **Engleman H M**, **Wild M R**. Improving CPAP use by patients with the sleep apnoea–hypopnoea syndrome (SAHS). *Sleep Med Rev*, 2003; **7**:81–99.

37. **Chervin R**, **Theut S**, **Bassetti C**. Compliance with nasal CPAP can be improved by simple interventions. *Sleep*, 1997; **20**:284–89.

38. **Fletcher E**, **Luckett R**. The effect of positive reinforcement on hourly compliance in nasal continuous positive airway pressure users with obstructive sleep apnea. *Am Rev Resp Disord*, 1991; **143**:936–41.

39. **Golay A**, **Girard A**, **Grandin S**, et al. A new educational program for patients suffering from sleep apnoea syndrome. *Patient Educ Counsel*, 2006; **60**:220–27.

40. **Hoy C**, **Vennelle R**, **Kingshott R**, et al. Can intensive support improve continuous positive airway pressure use in patients with sleep apnea/hypopnea syndrome? *Am J Resp Crit Care Med*, 1999; **159**:1096–100.

41. **Hui D**, **Chan J**, **Choy K**, et al. Effects of augmented continuous positive airway pressure and support on compliance and outcome in a Chinese population. *Chest*, 2000; **117**:1410–16.

42. **Likar L**, **Panciera T**, **Erickson A**, et al. Group education sessions and compliance with nasal CPAP therapy. *Chest*, 1997; **111**:1273–77.

43. **Murphy P W**, **Chesson A L**, **Walker L**, et al. Comparing the effectiveness of video and written material for improving knowledge among sleep disorders clinic patients with limited literacy skills. *South Med J*, 2000; **93**:297–304.

44. **Smith S S**, **Lang C P**, **Sullivan K A** et al. A preliminary investigation of the effectiveness of a sleep apnea education program. *J Psychosom Res*, 2004; **56**:245–49.

45. **Richards D**, **Bartlett D**, **Wong K**, et al. Increased adherence to CPAP with a group cognitive behavioral treatment intervention: a randomized trial. *Sleep*, 2007; **30**:635–40.

46. **Bandura A**. *Social Foundations of Thought and Action. A Social Cognitive Theory*. Englewood Cliffs, NJ: Prentice Hall, 1986.

47. **Prochaska J O, Redding C A, Evers K E**. The transtheoretical model and stages of change. In: Glanz K, Lewis F M, Rimer B K, Eds. *Health Behavior and Health Education*. San Francisco, CA: Jossey-Bass, 1997: 60–84.

48. **Miller W R, Rollnick S**. *Motivational Interviewing: Preparing People for Change* (2nd Ed). New York, NY: Guilford, 2002.

49. **Aloia M S, Arnedt J T, Riggs R L**, *et al*. Clinical management of poor adherence to CPAP: Motivational Enhancement. *Behav Sleep Med*, 2004; **2**:205–22.

50. **Aloia M S, Smith K, Ernedt J T** *et al*. Brief behavioral therapies reduce early positive airway pressure in discontinuation rates in sleep apnea syndrome: preliminary findings. *Behav Sleep Med*, 2007; **5**:89–104.

51. **Stepnowsky C J, Marler M R, Palau J**, *et al*. Social cognitive correlates of CPAP adherence in experienced users. *Sleep Med*, 2006; **7**:350–56.

52. **Weaver T E, Maislin G, Dinges D F**, *et al*. Self efficacy in sleep apnea: instrument development and patient perceptions of obstructive sleep apnea risk, treatment benefit, and volition to use continuous positive airway pressure. *Sleep*, 2003; **26**:727–32.

53. **Stepnowsky C J, Bardwell W A, Moore P J**, *et al*. Psychologic correlates of compliance with continuous positive airway pressure. *Sleep*, 2002; **25**:758–62.

54. **Edinger J D, Means M K**. Graded exposure therapy for addressing claustrophobic reactions to continuous positive airway pressure: a case series report. *Behav Sleep Med*, 2007; **5**:105–16.

55. **Jacobsen N, Martell C, Dimidjian S**. Behavioral activation treatment for depression: returning to contextual roots. *Clin Psychol Sci Pract*, 2001; **8**:255–70.

56. **Kaplan K, Harvey A**. Hypersomnia across mood disorders: a review and synthesis. *Sleep Med Rev*, 2009; **13**:275–85.

57. **Billiard M, Dolenc L, Aldaz C**, *et al*. Hypersomnia associated with mood disorders: a new perspective. *J Psychosom Res*, 1994; **38**(Suppl 1):41–47.

58. **Nofzinger E A, Thase M E, Reynolds C F**, *et al*. Hypersomnia in bipolar depression: a comparison with narcolepsy using the multiple sleep latency test. *Am J Psychiatry*, 1991; **148**:1177–81.

59. **Golden R, Gaynes B, Ekstrom R**, *et al*. The efficacy of light therapy in the treatment of mood disorders: a review and meta-analysis of the evidence. *Am J Psychiatry*, 2005; **162**:656–62.

60. **Sit D, Wisner K, Hanusa B H**, *et al*. Light therapy for bipolar disorder: a case series in women. *Bipolar Disord*, 2007; **9**:918–27.

61. **Terman M**. Evolving applications of light therapy. *Sleep Med Rev*, 2007; **11**:497–507.

62. **Lam R W**. *Seasonal Affective Disorder and Beyond: Light Treatment for SAD and Non-SAD Conditions*. Washington, DC: American Psychiatric Press, 1998.

63. **Rosenthal N E, Joseph-Vanderpool J R, Levendosky A A**, *et al*. Phase-shifting effects of bright morning light as a treatment for delayed sleep phase syndrome. *Sleep*, 1990; **13**:354–61.

64. **Czeisler C A, Richardson G S, Coleman R M**, *et al*. Chronotherapy: resetting the circadian clocks of patients with delayed sleep phase insomnia. *Sleep*, 1981; **4**:1–21.

65. **Duffy J F, Rimmer D W, Czeisler C A**. Association of intrinsic circadian period morningness–eveningness, usual wake time and circadian phase. *Behav Neurosci*, 2001; **115**:895–99.

66. **Lack L C, Wright H R**. Clinical management of delayed sleep phase disorder. *Behav Sleep Med*, 2007; **5**:57–76.

67. **Lack L, Shumacher K**. Evening light treatment of early morning insomnia. *Sleep Res*, 1993; **22**:224–27.

68. **Crowley S J, Lee C, Tseng C Y**, *et al*. Combinations of bright light, scheduled dark, sunglasses and melatonin to facilitate circadian entrainment to night shift work. *J. Biol Rhythms*, 2003; **18**:513–23.

69. **Lack L, Wright H, Kemp K**, *et al*. The treatment of early-morning awakening insomnia with 2 evenings of bright light. *Sleep*, 2005; **28**:616–23.

70. **Moldofsky H, Musisi S, Phillipson E A**. Treatment of a case of advanced sleep phase syndrome by phase advance chronotherapy. *Sleep*,1986; **9**:61–65.

71. **Burgess H J, Sharkey K M, Eastman C I**. Bright light, dark and melatonin can promote circadian adaptation in night shift workers. *Sleep Med Rev*, 2002; **6**:407–20.

72. **Herxheimer A, Waterhouse J**. The prevention and treatment of jet lag. *BMJ*, 2003; **326**:296–97.

73. **Ancoli-Israel S, Martin J L, Kripke D F**, *et al*. Effect of light treatment on sleep in circadian rhythms in demented nursing home patients. *J Am Geriatr Soc*, 2002; **50**:282–89.

74. **Sack R L, Brandes R W, Kendall A R**, *et al*. Entrainment of free-running circadian rhythms by melatonin in blind people. *N Engl J Med*, 2003; **323**:1070–77.

Index

Accreditation Council for Graduate Medical Education (ACGME) 209
acromegaly 368–69
actigraphy
  children 266
  delayed sleep phase disorder (DSPD) 179
  military personnel 218
  sleep time measurement 249
activity
  sleep latency and 57
  sleepiness during 39
acute disseminated encephalomyelitis (ADEM) 357
adenosine 221–22, 430–31
  related genes 107
adenosine receptors, caffeine actions 430–31
adolescents
  motor vehicle crash risk 86
  sleep delay 177
  see also young adults
adrenergic agonists 244
advanced sleep phase disorder (ASPD) 176–83
  causes of sleepiness 179–80
  daytime sleepiness 179–80
  depression 283
  description 178–79
  treatment of sleepiness 180–83, 457–58
African trypanosomiasis 354
age differences
  adjustment to shift work 195
  countermeasures taken by drowsy drivers 88
  daytime napping 295
  excessive daytime sleepiness 292
  motor vehicle crash risk 86
  sleep duration 252
  see also adolescents; older adults; young adults

aggressive behavior, Kleine–Levin syndrome 139, 141
agomelatine, depression 287
aircrew 187, 188, 189, 235
alcohol 46, 242, 393
alerting agents 430–41
  novel 444–49
  see also armodafinil; modafinil; sodium oxybate; stimulants
alertness
  caffeine-mediated 432–39
  defined 262
  hypothalamo-pituitary–thyroid axis and 368
  post-lunch dip 432–33
  three-process model 194, 252
Alexander the Great 216–17
alprazolam 244
Alzheimer's disease (AD) 294–95
amantadine 144, 244
American Academy of Sleep Medicine (AASM)
  categories of sleepiness severity 39
  MSLT protocol 51
  MWT protocol 53, 54
amphetamines 401–05
  abuse 401–02, 405
  children 270
  idiopathic hypersomnia 132
  mechanism of action 402
  Parkinson's disease 308, 309
  pharmacokinetics 402–03
  toxicity/adverse effects 403–04, 405
  treatment of daytime sleepiness 403
  see also dextroamphetamine; methamphetamine
analgesics 392–93
androgens 369–70
Angelman syndrome 337, 338
angiitis, hypothalamic CNS 355
anti-anxiety drugs 387–88
anti-Ma2 encephalitis 353

antidepressants
  depression 287
  narcolepsy 121, 271, 449
  novel 449
  restless legs syndrome/periodic limb movements 242
  sedating 388–89, 390, 392
antiepileptic drugs (AEDs) 244, 358, 390–91, 392
antihistamines 386, 391–92, 444
antihypertensive drugs 392
antipsychotic drugs (neuroleptics) 242, 390
anxiety disorders 41, 169, 171
apomorphine 392
arachnoid cyst 353
armodafinil 408–15, 418
  mode of action 416
  narcolepsy 122, 411, 414
  obstructive sleep apnea 410–11
  safety and tolerability 416–17
  shift work disorder 197, 411, 412–13
Arnold–Chiari malformation 359
arousal
  cognitive performance and 72
  disruption in Parkinson's disease 301–02
  dopaminergic regulation 302–05
  insomnia 172
  sleep latency effects 57
ascending arousal system (AAS) 116, 117
asthma, bronchial (BA) 380
astrocytoma, pilocytic 352
atomoxetine 121, 449
attention deficit hyperactivity disorder (ADHD) 346
attentional deficits
  health care workers 207
  obstructive sleep apnea 155–56, 157
  sleepiness 73–75

462

Index

attentional tests, obstructive sleep apnea 156, 161–62
autistic spectrum disorders 345–46
automatic behavior 113
autonomic symptoms 127, 140, 157

baclofen 422, 425
Baddeley's logical reasoning task 31–32
Battle of Gaugamela (331 BC) 216–17
behavioral correlates, sleep duration 252
behavioral problems
  Kleine–Levin syndrome 138–39, 141
  sleepiness in children 269
behavioral treatment 452–59
  circadian rhythm disorders 457–58
  CPAP non-compliance 454–56
  idiopathic hypersomnia 132
  insomnia 169, 170, 171
  insufficient sleep syndrome 454
  narcolepsy 119, 452–54
  psychiatric disorders 456–57
benzodiazepines 386–87, 388
  Parkinson's disease 307
  restless legs syndrome/periodic limb movements 243–44
beta-adrenergic antagonists 392
BF 2.649 (tiprolisant) 309, 446
bilevel positive airway pressure (BiPAP) 324
biological clock *see* body clock
bipolar disorder 41, 131, 456
  PER3 gene polymorphisms 283
  treatment 279, 286–87, 288, 457
blind people 458
blink behavior, motor vehicle drivers 83, 84, 187, 192
blood tests 45–46
body clock 176, 227–29, 281
  adjustment to jet lag 230–33
  age-related changes 178–79
  roles 228–29
brain malformations, structural 359
brain maturation, sleep loss and 269
brain tumors 352–54
brainstem tumors 353
brofaromine 121, 122

bromocriptine 243, 306, 392
bupropion 244, 308, 309
burnout 188, 192
bus drivers 94
buspirone 388

cabergoline 243, 307
caffeine 430–41
  containing foods/beverages 430, 431
  effectiveness in countering sleepiness 432–34, 439
  jet lag 231
  narcolepsy 121, 453
  nocturnal sleep disruption 439–40
  pharmacology 430–32
  shift workers 212, 434–36, 437
  tolerance 433
  withdrawal 440–41
Calwell v. Hassan 95
Campbell v. James Gordon Hitchcock 94
canine narcolepsy, familial 16, 21–22, 23
cannabis use 46
car manufacturing workers 190
carbamazepine 244
carbidopa/levodopa (Sinemet) 243
carboperamide 445–46
cardiovascular disease 162, 296, 297
cataplexy 16
  clinical features 112–13
  differential diagnosis 115
  drugs aggravating 122
  like drop attacks, Coffin–Lowry syndrome 339–40
  Niemann–Pick C disease 342
  pathophysiology 20, 118
  pharmacotherapy 121
  see also narcolepsy
catechol-O-methyltransferase (COMT) gene polymorphism 104–05
catecholamines, narcolepsy 22
central nervous system (CNS) causes of sleepiness 351–59
central sleep apnea (CSA) 154
  congenital hypothyroidism 367, 368
centrofacial dysgenesia 340
cephalometric X-rays 46

cerebral blood flow
  narcolepsy 32, 33, 34
  sleep deprivation 30
cerebral metabolism
  depression 282–83
  narcolepsy 32
  sleep deprivation 29, 30
cerebral perfusion, narcolepsy 32
cerebrovascular disease 355–56
Charcot–Marie–Tooth disease (CMT) 348–49
Childhood Sleep Habits Questionnaire 265–66
children 262–72
  assessment of sleepiness 263–65, 268
  causes of sleepiness 262–63, 264
  clinical presentation of sleepiness 262
  consequences of sleep loss 78, 269
  measures of sleepiness 68–69, 264–65, 268
  prevalence of sleepiness 262
  treatment of sleepiness 269–70, 271, 272
cholinergic receptors, narcolepsy 22
chromosomal abnormalities 335–40
chronic fatigue syndrome 131, 415
chronic obstructive pulmonary disease (COPD) 380
chronobiotics 231, 232
chronotherapy 180–81, 287–88, 457–58
chronotypes (larks and owls) 177, 234
ciproxifan 445–46
circadian misalignment 179, 204, 230
circadian pacemaker, endogenous *see* body clock
circadian rhythm sleep disorders 176–79
  behavioral treatment 457–58
  extrinsic 177
  history-taking 39
  intrinsic *see* advanced sleep phase disorder; delayed sleep phase disorder
  post-traumatic 330
  Sanfilippo syndrome 341
  Smith–Magenis syndrome 339
  see also jet lag; shift work disorder

463

Index

circadian rhythms 226–27
  depression and 279, 280, 281, 282
  dopamine systems 303
  endogenous and exogenous
    components 226–27
  hemodialysis patients 378
  interactions with time awake
    229–30
  long sleepers 252–53
  regulation 228–29
cirrhosis of liver 379
clock genes/proteins 227
clomipramine 121
clonazepam 122, 243
clonidine 244, 392
cocaine abuse 46
Coffin–Lowry syndrome 339–40
cognitive assessment tests 45
cognitive–behavioral therapy (CBT)
  CPAP noncompliance 455–56
  insomnia 169, 170, 171
cognitive deficits
  excessive sleepiness and 10
  Kleine–Levin syndrome 138
  myotonic dystrophy 319, 319
cognitive effects of sleepiness 72, 79
  children 269
  differential vulnerability 102–04
  genetic markers of vulnerability 104
  healthcare workers 204–05
  neuroimaging markers of
    vulnerability 107–08
cognitive evoked potential responses
  (P300) 129
cognitive performance
  after extended sleep 253
  circadian rhythm 229
  effects of caffeine 432–34, 438, 439,
    440–41
Cold War (1945–1991) 217
coma 351
commercial vehicle drivers
  employer liability 94
  medical examination 95, 96
  physician liability 95, 96
  work scheduling 86–87, 94
  see also train drivers; truck drivers
conessine 446
continuous positive airway pressure
  (CPAP)
  diabetes 372
  narcolepsy 122

obstructive sleep apnea 163–64,
  408–11
  effect on co-morbidities 163
  fitness to drive after 162
  management of non-compliance
    454–56
  residual excessive sleepiness
    163–64
conversion disorders 41, 131
coronary heart disease (CHD) 296
corticosteroids 371
cortisol, circadian rhythm 280–81
CPAP see continuous positive airway
  pressure
cranial irradiation 354
craniopharyngioma 352, 353
Cushing's syndrome 371
cystic fibrosis (CF) 380
cysticercosis 354, 354
cytokines
  hemodialysis patients 378
  infection and inflammation
    354–55, 375
  liver failure 379–80
  myotonic dystrophy 323
  obesity and 376
  obstructive sleep apnea 158, 159

daytime sleepiness
  caffeine as countermeasure 432–34
  defined 3, 262
  excessive see excessive daytime
    sleepiness
  long sleepers 252
  model, advanced and delayed phase
    disorders 180
  see also hypersomnia
Daytime Sleepiness Scale (DSS) 317
death see mortality
decision-making tasks 73, 76
delayed sleep phase disorder (DSPD)
  176–83
  adolescent form 177
  causes of sleepiness 179–80
  daytime sleepiness 179–80
  depression 177, 283
  description 177–78
  post-traumatic 330
  treatment of sleepiness 180–83, 457
dementia 10, 294–95
dementia with Lewy bodies (DLB)
  306

demyelinating diseases 356–57
depression
  advanced and delayed sleep phase
    disorders 177, 283
  epilepsy and 359
  excessive sleepiness 279–89
    circadian rhythm disturbances
      279, 280, 281, 282
    clinical findings 41, 280–81
    diagnosis 284–85, 286
    epidemiological studies 10
    genetics 283
    management 286–89, 415,
      456–57
    pathophysiology 281–82, 283
  healthcare workers 208
  insomnia pharmacotherapy 169,
    171
  myotonic dystrophy 319, 319
  obstructive sleep apnea 159
  older adults 293
  restless legs syndrome 239
  vs. Kleine–Levin syndrome 142
  with narcolepsy 114
derealization, Kleine–Levin syndrome
  138, 140
desensitization, CPAP users 456
dextroamphetamine 401, 403
  narcolepsy 120, 121
  Parkinson's disease 309
  see also amphetamines
diabetes mellitus 162, 371–72
diaries, sleep 42
dietary changes, narcolepsy 452–53
diphenhydramine 391
diurnal changes
  histamine CSF levels 24, 25
  hypocretin/orexin system 20, 24
DMPK gene 323
doctors see physicians
dopamine agonists
  Parkinson's disease 306, 307
  restless legs syndrome 241, 242–43
  sedating effects 392
dopamine D2 receptors, narcolepsy
  22, 32
dopamine receptors 302, 304
dopamine transporter (DAT) 304
  modafinil binding 415–16
  narcolepsy 32
  Parkinson's disease 305
dopaminergic (DA) system
  γ-hydroxybutyrate interactions 422

Index

idiopathic hypersomnia 22–23, 131–32
narcolepsy 21–22, 23, 32
Parkinson's disease 301–02, 305
restless legs syndrome 241
sleep–wake state modulation 302–05

DOV 216, 303 449

Down syndrome 335–36

doxepin 388

driver support systems, technological 88

driving 82–83, 89
awareness of sleepiness while 93, 191
caffeine use 435
dangerous or reckless 92–94
employer liability 94
history-taking 39
indicators of sleepiness 83–84
narcolepsy 85, 454
night shift workers 85–86, 187, 188–89
obstructive sleep apnea 159–62
Parkinson's disease 307
physician liability 95–96
real road, vs. simulators 84–85
sleep-related crashes see motor vehicle crashes, sleep-related

driving simulators
indicators of sleepiness 83–84
obstructive sleep apnea 161–62
shift work studies 187
vs. real road driving 84–85

drop attacks, Coffin–Lowry syndrome 339–40

drowsiness see sleepiness

drug abuse, serum or urine screening 45–46

drugs, sedating 46–47, 294, 386–94

Duchenne muscular dystrophy (DMD) 347, 348

duloxetine 392, 449

dynorphin 16

dysthymic disorder 41, 131

ecstasy (MDMA) 45–46

EDS see excessive daytime sleepiness

educational interventions, CPAP compliance 455

elderly see older adults

electrocardiogram (EKG) 46

electroencephalography (EEG) 46
children 268
cognitive effects of sleepiness 73, 75
depression 284–86
Kleine–Levin syndrome 142–43
menstrual-related hypersomnia 148
motor vehicle drivers 84
nap tests 50
polysomnography 43
shift workers 186–87
see also polysomnography

electromyography (EMG) 43, 46

electrooculography (EOG) 43, 84, 186–87

emotional state
cataplexy triggers 112
effects of sleepiness 76

employers, liability for sleep-related injuries 94–95

encephalitis, anti-Ma2 353

end stage kidney disease 376–78

endocrine disorders 364–72

entacapone 244

epilepsy 96, 358–59

Epstein–Barr virus (EBV) infection 354

Epworth Sleepiness Scale (ESS) 42, 63, 65–66
children 68, 264–65
clinical use 41
development 61
epidemiological studies 11
fitness to drive assessment 161
myotonic dystrophy 316–17
normative data 65, 65
obstructive sleep apnea 154–55, 156
older adults 292
Parkinson's disease 307, 310
post-traumatic sleepiness 330–31
shift workers 186
vs. clinical judgment 66

escitalopram 169, 171

eszopiclone 169, 170–71

etanercept 158, 159

ethnocultural differences 11

European Working Time Directive 209, 211

evoked potentials 268

EVT201 169

examination, physical 42–43

excessive daytime sleepiness (EDS)
associated factors 10
causes 36–38
clinical evaluation 38–46
definitions 3, 4, 36, 251
differential diagnosis 114–15
epidemiology 3–11, 37–38
historical aspects 14, 15
laboratory investigations 43–46
management 46–47
prevalence 4–5, 7

executive functioning
effects of sleepiness 73, 75–76
sleep-deprived children 269
see also working memory

exercise, narcolepsy 453

Exxon Valdez disaster (1989) 94–95, 190

falls 296

family history 41

fatigue
circadian rhythm 229
myotonic dystrophy 317, 318–19
narcolepsy 113, 122
post-traumatic 330, 331
primary insomnia 168
travel 225, 226
vs. sleepiness 36, 39–40, 67–68, 186, 351

Federal Aviation Administration (FAA) 44–45

fluoxetine 169, 171

folate 244

four-process model of sleep/wakefulness 252

fragile X chromosome 336, 337

frontal assessment battery 45

functional impairment
myotonic dystrophy 318
older adults 294, 295

functional magnetic resonance imaging (fMRI)
cognitive effects of sleepiness 74, 75, 78
sleep deprivation 31–32
vulnerability to sleep loss and 107–08

functional neuroimaging 29–34
depression 282–83
healthy human sleep 29

465

functional neuroimaging (*cont.*)
  markers of vulnerability to sleep loss 107–08
  narcolepsy 32–33, 34
  sleep deprivation 29–30, 31, 32

gabapentin 244, 391, 392

gaboxadol 449

γ-aminobutyric acid (GABA) 421, 422

γ-hydroxybutyrate (GHB) 421–23
  clinical use in narcolepsy 422–23
  neurobiology 421–22
  pharmacokinetics 422
  see also sodium oxybate

gamma-hydroxybutyric (GHB) aciduria 341

gangliocytoma, third ventricle 353

gender differences
  countermeasures taken by drowsy drivers 88
  sleep duration 252

gene therapy, narcolepsy 123, 448

generalized anxiety disorder 169, 171

genetic disorders 335–49

germinoma, suprasellar 353

GHB *see* γ-hydroxybutyrate

glandular fever (infectious mononucleosis) 354

Goldenhar syndrome 340

growth hormone (GH) 323, 368

GSK 189254 446

Guillain–Barré syndrome 131

healthcare workers 204–12
  circadian misalignment 204
  mood disturbances 208
  sleep deprivation 204–05
  work hours 204, 209–12
    authors' recommendations 211
    challenges to reform 212
    concerns about reducing 210–11
    current US regulations 209
    recommended US changes 210
    safety and 190, 205–08
    see also nurses; physicians-in-training

heart failure (HF) 381–82

heart rate 57, 297

heavy goods vehicle (HGV) drivers *see* truck drivers

hemodialysis (HD) 376–78

hepatic encephalopathy 379

hereditary motor and sensory neuropathy (HMSN) 348–49

hippocampus 77

histamine 23–25, 444
  cerebrospinal fluid (CSF) 25
  hypocretin interactions 23–24, 25
  idiopathic hypersomnia 25, 26, 132
  narcolepsy 14–15, 22, 23, 25, 26

histamine-1 receptor (H_1R) antagonists 386, 391–92, 444

histamine-2 receptor (H_2R) antagonists 392, 444

histamine-3 receptors (H_3R) 444–45
  antagonists 122, 444–47
  inverse agonists 309, 446, 447
  ligand development 445

history, clinical
  chief complaint 38, 40
  family/social history 41
  medical history 40–41
  psychiatric disorders 41
  sleep history 39

HLA associations
  Kleine–Levin syndrome 143
  menstrual-related hypersomnia 149
  myotonic dystrophy 324
  narcolepsy 119, 268

HLA DQB1*0602 allele
  narcolepsy 119, 268
  vulnerability to sleep loss 105–06

hours of service (HOS) regulations 86–87, 94
  nurses 210
  physicians-in-training 209, 210

human immunodeficiency virus (HIV) infection 354

Hunter syndrome 341

Hurler syndrome 341

hydrocephalus, obstructive 353

hypercapnia, myotonic dystrophy 322

hyperparathyroidism, secondary 378

hyperphagia, Kleine–Levin syndrome 138–39

hyperprolactinemia 371

hypersexuality, Kleine–Levin syndrome 138–39

hypersomnia
  children 269–71, 272
  definition 3–4, 262
  historical allusions 14, 15
  idiopathic *see* idiopathic hypersomnia
  Kleine–Levin syndrome 138
  long sleep 250
  menstrual-related *see* menstrual-related hypersomnia
  not due to a substance or known medical condition 130–31
  pathophysiology 14–15, 19
  post-infectious 131
  post-traumatic 131, 330
  prevalence 7
  psychiatric 131, 456
  recurrent 40, 138, 147
  symptomatic (secondary) 14, 351–59
  use of term 36

hypertension 162, 163, 297

hypnagogic hallucinations (HH) 113
  Kleine–Levin syndrome 138
  myotonic dystrophy 320
  pathophysiology 118
  pharmacotherapy 121

hypnotic medications 386–87
  insomnia 169, 170–71
  jet lag 231–32

hypocretin (orexin)
  based treatments 447–48
  discovery 16, 19
  replacement therapy 16, 119, 447–48

hypocretin-1 (orexin A) 19, 447
  cerebrospinal fluid (CSF)
    children 268
    diurnal pattern 20, 24
    idiopathic hypersomnia 19, 132
    myotonic dystrophy 324
    narcolepsy with cataplexy 16, 18, 114
    narcolepsy without cataplexy 16, 115
    restless legs syndrome 241
    symptomatic narcolepsy 21
    traumatic brain injury 332
  replacement therapy 447–48
  structure 17

hypocretin-2 (orexin B) 19, 447
  cerebrospinal fluid 115–16
  structure 17

hypocretin agonists 123, 448

hypocretin deficiency
  histamine and 25, 26

knockout mouse model 16
  narcolepsy-cataplexy 14, 16–18, 19–21, 115–16
  symptomatic narcolepsy 14, 21
hypocretin gene therapy 123, 448
hypocretin neurons 16, 17, 19–20, 116
  cell transplantation 123, 448
  postnatal cell death 16–18, 19, 21, 448–49
  potential autoantigens 119
  sleep regulation 20
  traumatic loss 332, 333
hypocretin receptor 1 (Hcrtr1) 17, 19, 23, 447
hypocretin receptor 2 (Hcrtr2) 17, 19, 447
  defects 16, 21
  distribution 17, 23
  histaminergic interactions 23
hypocretin (orexin) receptors 17, 19
  agonists 123, 448
  antagonists 287, 449
hypocretin (orexin) system 14–15, 17
  CNS disease 352
  histamine interactions 23–24, 25
  narcolepsy 115–16
  Parkinson's disease 305
  sleep regulation 19–20, 118
hypogonadism, male 369–70
hypothalamo-pituitary–adrenal (HPA) axis 280–81
hypothalamo-pituitary–thyroid (HPT) axis 364–65, 368
hypothalamus
  CNS disease involving 352
  dysfunction in Prader–Willi syndrome 337–38
  histamine neurons 23
  hypocretin and histamine interactions 23–25
  hypocretin neurons 16, 19–20
  neoplasms involving 352–53
  suprachiasmatic nucleus 227, 281
  traumatic injury 332
  ventrolateral preoptic nucleus (VLPO) 116–17
hypothyroidism 365–66, 368
  congenital 367–68
  latent (subclinical) 130, 268, 365–67
hypoxemia, nocturnal, obstructive sleep apnea 157–59
hypoxic encephalopathy 355

idiopathic hypersomnia (IH) 126–33
  clinical features 127
  clinical variant 130
  demographics 127
  diagnosis 40, 127–29
  differential diagnosis 115, 128, 130, 131
  historical background 126–27
  Multiple Sleep Latency Test (MSLT) 51, 53, 127–29
  natural history 129
  pathophysiology 19, 22–23, 25, 26, 131–32
  predisposing factors 131
  spectrum 129–30
  treatment 132
  with long sleep time 127–28, 129–30
  without long sleep time 127, 129, 130
idiopathic pulmonary fibrosis (IPF) 380
imipramine 121
immunotherapy, narcolepsy 448–49
individual differences
  jet lag 234–35
  sleep-related motor vehicle crashes 85–86
  tolerance of shift work 195–96
  vulnerability to sleep loss 102–03, 104
industry, shift workers 190
infants, sleep times 262
infections 131, 354–55, 375
infectious mononucleosis (IM) 354
inflammation
  infection-related 354–55, 375
  obstructive sleep apnea 158, 159
inflammatory disorders 357–58
insomnia
  24-hour hyperarousal 172
  daytime sleepiness 168–73
    effects of therapy 168–69, 171, 172–73
    objective data 53, 57, 168, 171–72
    self-report data 68, 168, 171
    subgroup differences 172
  epilepsy 358
  long sleepers 250, 252
  narcolepsy 453
  polysomnography 43
  post-traumatic 330
  road traffic crash risk 85
  sleep onset 177

insufficient sleep syndrome (ISS) 7–8, 131, 454
insulin-like growth factor binding protein 3 (IGFBP3) 16, 18
insulin resistance 162, 163, 372, 375–76
Intern Sleep and Patient Safety Study 207–08, 211
interns *see* physicians-in-training
intravenous immunoglobulins (IVIg) 122–23
iron
  deficiency, restless legs syndrome 241
  therapy, restless legs syndrome 242
irregular sleep–wake type 458

Japan, Heian period (794–1184 AC) 14, 15
jet lag 225–26
  individual differences 234–35
  management 230–32, 233, 234, 458
  problems associated with 230
  vs. travel fatigue 226
JNJ-5207852 446

Karolinska Drowsiness Score (KDS), motor vehicle drivers 84
Karolinska Sleepiness Scale (KSS) 42, 63, 64
  clinical use 41
  shift workers 188–89, 192
  vs. objective measures 64
ketamine, oral 244
Kleine–Levin syndrome (KLS) 136–45, 147
  benign vs. severe forms 140
  brain imaging 142
  case report 136–37
  clinical features 137–39, 140
  clinical forms 140–41
  complications 141
  course 141
  diagnosis 138, 141–42
  differential diagnosis 141–42
  epidemiology 137
  investigations and pathology 142–43, 144
  management 144, 145
  secondary 140
Kluver–Bucy syndrome 142

Index

lapse hypothesis (Williams *et al*) 73–74

learning 76–78, 208–09

legal consequences *see* medico-legal consequences

levodopa
  Parkinson's disease 306, 308
  restless legs syndrome 241, 243

lifestyle modification
  childhood narcolepsy/hypersomnias 270
  restless legs syndrome 242

light, body clock adjustment 228

light therapy
  advanced and delayed phase sleep disorders 181–82, 457
  dementia 295
  jet lag 232, 233, 458
  psychiatric disorders 288, 457
  shift work disorder 197, 458

linea nigricans 263–64

lithium 144, 279, 286–87

liver failure 378–80

locus coeruleus (LC) 303

long sleep
  biological basis 252–53
  defined 249
  negative effects 253–54, 257

long sleepers 131, 249–58
  behavioral and socio-psychological correlates 252, 255
  genetic factors 253
  morbidity/mortality 251–52
  sleepiness 254–58
  terminology and concepts 249–50

Lyme disease 354

lymphoma, primary CNS 353

lysosomal storage disorders 341–44

Maastricht Cohort Study 92

Maggie's Law, New Jersey 93–94

magnetic resonance imaging (MRI) 46

Maintenance of Wakefulness Test (MWT) 53–54
  American Academy of Sleep Medicine (AASM) protocol 53, 54
  agreement with other measures 56–57
  children 267
  clinical use 44–45, 54, 55
  motor vehicle drivers 161
  normative data 53, 55
  obstructive sleep apnea 155, 156, 161
  Parkinson's disease 306–07
  premenstrual syndrome 150

marijuana use 46

Mayes v. Goodyear Tire and Rubber Co. 94

mazindol 120, 122

McDonnell, Maggie 93–94

measures of sleepiness
  children 68–69, 264–68
  depression 284
  motor vehicle drivers 83–84
  Parkinson's disease 306–07
  sleep duration context 250–51
  see also objective measures of sleepiness; subjective measures of sleepiness

medical conditions
  causing excessive sleepiness 37
  physician's duty to report certain 95–96

medical errors, sleep-related 190, 206
  extended work hours and 190, 206
  reduced work hours and 207–08, 210–11

medical history 40–41

medications, sedating 46–47, 294, 386–94

medico-legal consequences 92–96
  employer liability 94–95
  personal liability 92–94
  physician liability 95–96

melatonin
  advanced and delayed sleep phase disorders 182
  body clock adjustment 228
  circulating, night shift workers 196
  genetic syndromes 339, 341, 343
  idiopathic hypersomnia 132
  jet lag 232, 233
  narcolepsy 122
  shift work disorder 197
  sleep onset and 229

melatonin agonists 182, 287

memory 76–77, 78, 208–09
see also working memory

meningitis 354

menopause 169, 171, 370–71

menstrual cycle
  hormonal changes 147
  sleepiness associated with 149–51

menstrual-related hypersomnia 140–41, 147–49, 151
  clinical features 147–48
  history 147
  laboratory investigations 148
  management 144–45, 149
  pathophysiology 148–49

metabolic disorders 375–82
  inherited nervous system 340–44
  myotonic dystrophy 323

metabolic syndrome 375–76

metal metabolism, inherited disorders of 344

methadone 244

methamphetamine 401, 403
  narcolepsy 53, 120, 121
  neurotoxicity 404, 405
  see also amphetamines

methyl-4-phenyl-1, 2, 3, 6-tetrahydropyridine (MPTP) 305, 308

methylenedioxymethamphetamine (MDMA; ecstasy) 45–46

methylphenidate 401–05
  children 270
  idiopathic hypersomnia 132
  mechanism of action 402
  misuse 402, 405
  myotonic dystrophy 325
  narcolepsy 120, 121, 122
  pharmacokinetics 403
  toxicity/adverse effects 403–04
  treatment of daytime sleepiness 403

migraine medications 393

military 76, 215–23
  nighttime operations 216
  sleep research 217–23
  tactics using sleep deprivation 215–16

military personnel (soldiers)
  caffeine studies 438–39
  chronic sleep restriction 218–19
  mild traumatic brain injury 222–23
  post-traumatic stress disorder 223
  sleep restriction studies 219–20, 221, 222

mini mental status examination (MMSE) 45

mirtazapine 390

Möbius syndrome 340

modafinil 408–15, 418
 children 270
 depression 287, 415
 idiopathic hypersomnia 132
 mode of action 415–16
 myotonic dystrophy 325
 narcolepsy 33, 34, 53, 54, 120–21, 122, 410, 413–14
 obstructive sleep apnea 408–10
 off-label uses 414–15
 Parkinson's disease 308–09, 414
 post-traumatic sleepiness 332
 safety and tolerability 416–17
 shift work disorder 197, 410, 411–12

monoamines
 human and canine narcolepsy 21–22, 23
 idiopathic hypersomnia 22–23, 131–32

mood, circadian rhythm 229, 280

mood disorders
 healthcare workers 208
 history-taking 41
 see also bipolar disorder; depression; seasonal affective disorder

mortality
 daytime napping and 296–97
 excessive daytime sleepiness and 10, 293–94
 obstructive sleep apnea 162–63
 prolonged sleep deprivation 60
 road traffic crashes 82
 sleep duration and 251–52

motivational interviewing 455–56

motor vehicle crashes, sleep-related 82–83
 countermeasures 86–87, 89
 driver liability 92–94
 employer liability 94
 healthcare workers 85–86, 206
 history-taking 39
 obstructive sleep apnea 85, 159–61, 162
 physician liability 95, 96
 risk groups and individual differences 85–86
 shift workers 85–86, 190–91

motor vehicle driving see driving

MPTP (methyl-4-phenyl-1, 2, 3, 6-tetrahydropyridine) 305, 308

MSLT see Multiple Sleep Latency Test

mucopolysaccharidoses 341

multiple sclerosis (MS) 356–57, 414–15

Multiple Sleep Latency Measurement 50

Multiple Sleep Latency Test (MSLT) 44, 50–53
 AASM protocol 51
 children 266–67
 clinical use 43, 52–53
 delayed sleep phase disorder 179
 depression 284
 development 50
 epidemiological studies 10–11
 idiopathic hypersomnia 51, 53, 127–29
 insomnia 53, 168
 motor vehicle drivers 161
 myotonic dystrophy 321, 324
 normative data 52
 obstructive sleep apnea 53, 155, 161
 Parkinson's disease 301, 306–07
 post-traumatic sleepiness 330–31
 shift workers 188, 196
 vs. other objective measures 56–57
 vs. subjective measures 64–65, 66, 67

muscarinic cholinergic receptors, narcolepsy 22, 32, 33–34

muscle relaxants, skeletal 393

MWT see Maintenance of Wakefulness Test

myocardial infarction (MI) 296, 297

myotonic dystrophy (DM1) 268, 316–25
 clinical findings 316–17, 318, 319, 320
 genetics 323
 laboratory investigations 320–22
 management of sleepiness 324–25
 metabolic abnormalities 323
 pathogenesis of sleepiness 323–24
 sleep-related breathing disorders 322–23, 324–25

myxedema 365, 367
 see also hypothyroidism

N-methyl-D-aspartate (NMDA) antagonists 244

naps
 caffeine plus 432–33, 435–36
 children 262
 delayed sleep phase disorder 179–80
 dementia 294
 drowsy drivers 88
 idiopathic hypersomnia 127

 involuntary 36, 39
 night shift workers 197
 older adults 295–97
 scheduled, narcolepsy 119, 452

narcolepsy 111–23
 animal models 16
 associated symptoms 113, 122
 behavioral modification 119, 452–54
 caffeine use 121, 453
 children 267, 268, 269–71, 272
 differential diagnosis 40, 114–15, 128, 130
 Maintenance of Wakefulness Test 54
 motor vehicle driving 85, 454
 MPTP-induced parkinsonism 305
 Multiple Sleep Latency Test (MSLT) 44, 51, 52–53
 Parkinson's disease 301, 305, 307–08
 pathophysiology 14–15, 16–18, 19, 20–22, 23, 25, 26, 115–18
 pharmacotherapy 120–22
  associated symptoms 122
  disturbed nocturnal sleep 122, 422–25
  excessive sleepiness 120–21, 410, 411, 413–14, 423–24, 425
  functional neuroimaging studies 33–34
  future prospects 122–23
  initiation 122
  novel alerting agents 446
  REM sleep dissociation phenomena 121–22
 polysomnography 44
 prevalence 8–9, 10
 secondary (symptomatic) 14
  CNS disorders 351–59
  hypocretin involvement 21
 treatment 119–23
 with cataplexy 111
  autoimmune etiology 119
  clinical features 15–16, 111–14
  comorbidity 113–14
  diagnosis 16, 114
  epidemiology 111
  genetic aspects 118–19
  hypocretin measurement 114
  pathophysiology 16–21
 without cataplexy 16, 111
  diagnosis 115
  pathophysiology 21

nefazodone 388

nerve conduction velocity (NCV) studies 46

Index

nervous system
  genetic programming malformations 335–40
  inherited metabolic and degenerative diseases 340–45
neuroanatomy of sleepiness 351–52
neurochemistry 14–26
neurocysticercosis 354
neurodegenerative diseases, inherited 340–41, 344–45
neurodevelopmental disorders, with genetic component 345–46
neuroimaging
  clinical evaluation 46
  functional see functional neuroimaging
  Kleine–Levin syndrome 142, 143
  markers of vulnerability to sleep loss 107–08
  sleep deprivation studies 73
neuroleptics (antipsychotics) 242, 390
neurological disorders
  causing sleepiness 351–59
  Kleine–Levin syndrome 140
neurological examination 42–43
neuromuscular diseases, inherited 346–49
neuronal activity-regulated pentraxin (NARP) 16
neuronal ceroid lipofuscinosis (NCL) 342–43, 344
Niemann–Pick C disease 268, 341–42
night shift workers 186
  adjustment under special conditions 189
  caffeine use 212, 434–36, 437
  countermeasures 196–97
  driving 85–86, 187, 188–89
  physiological sleepiness 187, 188
  rotating shifts 194–95
  survey studies of sleepiness 186
  see also shift work disorder; shift workers
nighttime military operations 216
non-24-hour sleep/wake disorder 181
non-alcoholic fatty liver disease (NAFLD) 379, 380
non-rapid eye movement sleep see NREM sleep
non-entrained sleep–wake rhythm 458

non-invasive assisted ventilation (NIAV) 324–25
norepinephrine (NE) system
  depression 284
  idiopathic hypersomnia 22–23, 131–32
  narcolepsy 22, 23
Norrie disease 340
North Sea oil platform workers 189
NREM sleep 15
  depression 285
  functional imaging 29
  idiopathic hypersomnia 132
  narcolepsy 15–16
nuclear power plant accidents 190
nurses
  melatonin rhythm 196
  work hours 190, 206, 210

obesity 375–76
  diabetes 372
  hypothalamic tumors 352–53
  impaired driving ability 161
  Kleine–Levin syndrome 141
  management 122
  narcolepsy 113, 452–53
  obstructive sleep apnea 159
objective measures of sleepiness 50–58
  agreement between 56–57
  children 265, 266–68
  depression 284
  early development 50
  insomnia 53, 57, 168
  motor vehicle drivers 83–84, 161
  myotonic dystrophy 321
  obstructive sleep apnea 155, 156
  shift workers 186–87, 188
  vs. subjective measures 64–65, 66, 67
obstructive airways disease (OAD) 380
obstructive sleep apnea (OSA)
  children 263–64
  cognitive deficits 75
  comorbid conditions 159
  CPAP see under continuous positive airways pressure
  diabetes 372
  Down syndrome 336
  epilepsy 358
  fitness to drive assessment 161–62
  hypothyroidism 365, 366–67
  idiopathic hypersomnia with 128, 129

mucopolysaccharidoses 341
narcolepsy with 114, 122
older adults 294, 297
Parkinson's disease 306, 307–08
polysomnography 43–44
post-menopausal women 370–71
Prader–Willi syndrome 337
sleepiness due to 154–64
  clinical features 40, 42, 154–57
  differential vulnerability 103
  impaired driving ability 85, 159–62
  pathophysiology 157–58, 159, 160
  physician liability 95, 96
  predicting comorbidities 162–63
  treatment options 163–64, 408–10, 411
sodium oxybate safety 426
Stanford Sleepiness Scale 63
obtundation 351
occupational accidents/injuries see work-related accidents/injuries
older adults
  advanced sleep phase disorder 178–79
  daytime sleepiness 292–98
    causes 293
    consequences 293–94
    insomnia 168, 171, 172
    prevalence 4, 292, 293
    treatment 294
  long sleepers 254, 255, 257
  motor vehicle crash risk 86
  napping 295–97
  periodic limb movements of sleep 240
opiate abuse 45
opioids 244, 392–93
oral contraceptive pill 149
orexin see hypocretin
overtime work, shift workers 195
Oxford Sleepiness Resistance (OSLER) test 50, 54–55
  agreement with other measures 56
  clinical use 45, 55
  obstructive sleep apnea 155, 156, 161
oxycodone 244

pain medications 392–93
paraneoplastic disorders 353
Parkinson's disease (PD) 301–10, 392
  awareness of sleepiness 38

470

determinants of sleepiness 305–06
follow-up management 310
general approach and management 307–08
measurement of sleepiness 306–07
prevalence of sleepiness 301
treatment of sleepiness 308–09, 310, 414, 425

Pediatric Daytime Sleepiness Scale (PDSS) 63, 68–69, 264–65

Pediatric Sleep Questionnaire (PSQ) 63, 68, 265–66

pedunculopontine tegmental nucleus (PPN) 305, 310

percutaneous injuries, healthcare workers 206

performance testing 45, 50

pergolide 243, 392

PERIOD3 (PER3) gene polymorphisms 104, 105, 106, 107, 108, 234, 283

periodic limb movement disorder (PLMD) 238–45
clinical features 40, 239–40
diagnostic criteria 240
management 241–44

periodic limb movements of sleep (PLMS) 238, 240
idiopathic hypersomnia and 128, 129
myotonic dystrophy 322
narcolepsy with 114, 122
Parkinson's disease 301, 306, 307–08

personality, myotonic dystrophy 319

personality disorders, delayed sleep phase disorder 177

phase–response curves (PRCs) 228

phenotype, defined 102–03

physical examination 42–43

physicians
liability for sleep-related injuries 95, 96
work hours and safety 206–07

physicians-in-training (interns and residents)
acute and chronic sleep deprivation 204–05
learning and sleep restriction 208–09
mood disturbances 208
motor vehicle crashes 85–86, 206
objective sleepiness 187

sleep and circadian determinants of performance 204
sleep inertia 205
terminology 204
work hours 190, 204
authors' recommendations 211
challenges to reform 212
concerns about reducing 210–11
current US regulations 209
recommended US changes 210
safety issues 190, 205–06, 207–08

Pierre–Robin syndrome 340

pilots 44–45

pineal gland tumors 353

Pittsburgh Sleep Quality Index (PSQI) 41

pituitary adenomas 353, 368

police operations 76

polycystic ovary syndrome (PCOS) 376

polysomnography (PSG) 43–44
children 267–68
delayed sleep phase disorder 177–78, 179
depression 284–85, 286
idiopathic hypersomnia 127–29
Kleine–Levin syndrome 143, 144
menstrual-related hypersomnia 148
myotonic dystrophy 320–22, 324
shift workers 186–87, 188
sleep time measurement 249
see also sleep architecture

Pompe disease 341

positive airway pressure (PAP) *see* continuous positive airway pressure

positron emission tomography (PET) 29, 30

post-concussion syndrome (PCS) 222–23

post-lunch dip, alertness 432–33

post-traumatic hypersomnia 131, 330

post-traumatic sleepiness 329–33
clinical findings 330–31
diagnostic investigations 331, 332
management 332–33
natural history 331
pathogenesis 331–32, 333

post-traumatic stress disorder (PTSD) 223

power station operators 187

Prader–Willi syndrome 268, 337, 338

pramipexole 242, 301, 306, 392

prazosin 122

prefrontal cortex (PFC)
effects of sleepiness 73, 75–76
hypoxic damage 164

pregabalin 391, 392

premenstrual syndrome (PMS) 149–51

prepro-orexin gene knockout mice 16

presenting complaint, history of 38, 40

primary biliary cirrhosis (PBC) 378–79, 380

Profile of Mood States (POMS) Vigor and Fatigue scales 62, 67

progesterone 148–49

prolactin 149, 371

psychiatric disorders 37
behavioral interventions 456–57
history-taking 41
hypersomnia 131, 456
vs. Kleine–Levin syndrome 142

psychological problems, Kleine–Levin syndrome 139–40, 141

psychometric performance tests 45, 50

psychomotor vigilance test (PVT) 45, 73–74, 75
differential vulnerability to sleep loss 102–03
premenstrual syndrome 151
sleep restriction studies 219, 220–21, 222

psychostimulants *see* stimulants

psychotherapeutic drugs, sedating 387–90

psychotic disorders 41

pulmonary disease, chronic 380–81

pulmonary fibrosis, idiopathic (IPF) 380

pulmonary function tests 46, 323

pupillography 55–56, 268

PVT *see* psychomotor vigilance test

quality of life
myotonic dystrophy 318
obstructive sleep apnea 164
restless legs syndrome 239

R v. Gill 93

radiotherapy, cranial 354

ramelteon 182

rapid eye movement sleep *see* REM sleep

reaction times 73–74, 75
  effects of caffeine 433–34
  obstructive sleep apnea 161–62
  see also psychomotor vigilance test

reboxetine 449

Regina v. Hundal 92–93

relaxation techniques 453

REM sleep 15
  depression 280, 285
  dopaminergic regulation 305
  functional imaging 29
  hypocretin ligand deficiency and 20–21
  short sleep latency in narcolepsy 15–16

REM sleep behavior disorder (RBD)
  narcolepsy with 114, 122
  Parkinson's disease 301, 306

renal insufficiency 376–78

residents, hospital *see* physicians-in-training

restless legs syndrome (RLS) 238–45
  clinical features 40, 238–39
  diagnostic criteria 238
  genetics 241
  laboratory investigations 45, 46, 241
  management 241–42, 244
  natural history 240–41
  pathology 241
  physical examination 42–43
  primary 238
  secondary 238

reticular ascending system (RAS), tumors involving 353

retirement (from work) 293

Rett syndrome 345

Rip Van Winkle effect 253

ritanserin 449

road traffic crashes *see* motor vehicle crashes

ropinirole 242–43, 301, 306, 392

rotigotine 243, 392

rumble strips 88–89, 191, 192

Sanfilippo syndrome 341

sarcoidosis 357–58

schizophrenia 41

School Sleep Habits Survey (sleepiness scale) 68

seasonal affective disorder (SAD) 280, 286, 457

sedating medications 46–47, 294, 386–94

sedentary situations 39, 68

seizures 46

Selby (UK) train disaster (2001) 94

selective norepinephrine reuptake inhibitors (SNRIs) 121, 390, 449

selective serotonin reuptake inhibitors (SSRIs) 121, 271, 287, 390

selegiline 121, 122, 244

self-report measures of sleepiness *see* subjective measures of sleepiness

serotonergic (5-HT) changes
  depression 283–84
  menstrual-related hypersomnia 149
  narcolepsy 21–22, 23
  obstructive sleep apnea 372

serotonin-2 (5-HT2) antagonists 449

sex chromosomal abnormalities 336–37

shift work 186
  duration of shifts 195
  individual differences in tolerance 195–96
  monotonous 195
  permanent and rotating shifts 194–95, 196–97
  special cases 194–95

shift work disorder (SWD) 103, 196
  countermeasures 196–97
  treatment 197, 410, 411–13, 458

shift workers 186–97
  caffeine use 212, 434–36, 437
  causes of sleepiness 193, 194
  dangerous levels of sleepiness 192–93
  modeling sleepiness 194
  momentary subjective sleepiness 188, 189
  motor vehicle crash risk 85–86, 190–91
  performance and accidents at work 189–91, 192
  physiological sleepiness 186–87, 188
  strength of sleepiness 191–92, 193

survey studies of sleepiness 186
see also healthcare workers; night shift workers; truck drivers

single photon emission computed tomography (SPECT)
  Kleine–Levin syndrome 142, 143
  narcolepsy 22, 32–33, 34

sleep
  circadian rhythm 229
  functional neuroimaging 29
  physiology 15–16
  regulation *see* sleep–wake regulation

Sleep, Activity, Fatigue and Task Effectiveness (SAFTE) model 218

sleep apnea
  acromegaly 368–69
  Down syndrome 336
  Maintenance of Wakefulness Test (MWT) 54, 55
  Multiple Sleep Latency Test (MSLT) 53
  myotonic dystrophy 322–23, 325
  Oxford Sleepiness Resistance (OSLER) test 55
  stroke 355
  testosterone and 369–70
  see also central sleep apnea; obstructive sleep apnea

sleep architecture
  depression 284–85, 286
  hypothyroidism 365
  male hypogonadism 369–70
  myotonic dystrophy 320–21
  obstructive sleep apnea 157, 158
  Parkinson's disease 301
  see also polysomnography

sleep banking 221

sleep behavior, nocturnal 39

sleep debt 220

sleep deprivation (SD) 101–08
  biomarkers of vulnerability 104–08
  brain maturation and 269
  caffeine use 436–38, 439, 440
  causing death 60
  chronic partial *see* sleep restriction, chronic
  cognitive effects 72, 73–74, 75–76, 77, 78
  functional imaging studies 29–30, 31, 32
  genetic markers of vulnerability 105, 106, 107
  historical studies 61

individual differences in response 102–03, 104
as military tactic 215–16
neuroimaging markers of vulnerability 107–08
prefrontal cortex activation and 73
prevalence 101–02
risks 101–02
sodium oxybate therapy 425–26
therapy, for depression 287–88
total, vs. chronic sleep restriction 221–22

sleep-disordered breathing (SDB)
  acromegaly 368
  CPAP non-compliance 454–56
  depression and 280
  diagnosis 40
  differential diagnosis 130
  genetic disorders 336, 346–48
  heart failure 381–82
  hypothyroidism 365, 366–67
  myotonic dystrophy 322–23, 324–25
  post-menopausal women 370–71
  sleepiness due to 154–64
  sodium oxybate and 426
  stroke and 355
  see also obstructive sleep apnea; sleep apnea

sleep disorders characterized by excessive sleepiness 36, 37
  differential diagnosis 40
  older adults 293, 294
  Parkinson's disease 307–08
  prevalence 7–10

sleep drunkenness 126, 127

sleep duration (quantity)
  behavioral and socio-psychological correlates 252
  biological basis 252–53
  excessive 3
    idiopathic hypersomnia 127–28
    Kleine–Levin syndrome 143
    long sleepers 131
    menstrual-related hypersomnia 148
    prevalence 4
    see also hypersomnia
  history-taking 39
  idiopathic hypersomnia with normal 129
  inadequate 101–02
    advanced and delayed sleep phase disorders 179
    see also sleep deprivation; sleep restriction, chronic
  infants and children 262

measurement issues 249–50
mortality/morbidity and 251–52
motor vehicle crash risk and 86
myotonic dystrophy 319–21
narcolepsy 113
shift workers 193
variability 258
see also long sleep; long sleepers

sleep efficiency see sleep quality

sleep episodes, short see naps

sleep fragmentation
  myotonic dystrophy 320–21
  narcolepsy 113
  obstructive sleep apnea 157, 158
  shift workers 193

sleep history 39

sleep hygiene 46, 242, 453

sleep hypoventilation syndrome 154

sleep inertia
  benefits of caffeine 432–33, 436
  healthcare workers 205

sleep latency
  delayed sleep phase disorder 178
  factors affecting 57
  fitness to drive criteria 161
  idiopathic hypersomnia 128, 129
  measures see Maintenance of Wakefulness Test; Multiple Sleep Latency Test
  MSLT vs. MWT 56–57
  narcolepsy 113
  premenstrual syndrome 150

sleep logs 42, 264

sleep monitoring see polysomnography

sleep-onset REM periods (SOREMPs) 15–16
  idiopathic hypersomnia 128, 129
  myotonic dystrophy 321–22
  narcolepsy 267
  Parkinson's disease 301, 305

sleep paralysis 113
  myotonic dystrophy 320
  pathophysiology 118
  pharmacotherapy 121

sleep position 39

sleep propensity
  circadian rhythm 229
  effects of jet lag 230
  increased daytime 3, 180

sleep quality
  advanced and delayed sleep phase disorders 177–78, 179

assessing 39
jet lag 230
long sleepers 252
myotonic dystrophy 320
older adults 293

sleep questionnaires 41, 265–66

sleep-related breathing disorders see sleep-disordered breathing

sleep restriction, chronic (CSR)
  failure of adaptation to 219–20
  healthcare workers 204–05
  long sleepers 251
  military research 219–20, 221, 222
  public health concerns 102
  soldiers on operations 218–19
  vs. total sleep deprivation 221–22
  see also sleep deprivation

sleep-switch 116–18

sleep–wake cycle 176, 229
  disturbances in dementia 294–95
  effects of alterations 230
  history-taking 39
  irregular pattern 458
  non-entrained 458

sleep–wake predictor (three-process model of alertness; TPM) 194, 252

sleep–wake regulation 116–18
  disturbances, idiopathic hypersomnia 132
  dopaminergic modulation 302–05
  flip-flop model 281
  hypocretin/orexin system 19–20, 118
  neuroanatomy 351–52
  sleep switch concept 116–18
  see also two-process model of sleep regulation

sleepiness
  after extended sleep 253–54, 257
  biological function 60
  circadian rhythm 229
  clinical evaluation 66–68
  daytime see daytime sleepiness
  defined 36, 262
  excessive daytime see excessive daytime sleepiness
  harmful effects 60
  jet lag 230
  long sleepers 254–58
  measures see measures of sleepiness
  menstrual cycle-associated 149–51
  severity assessment 39, 154
  terms used by patients 36
  vs. fatigue 36, 39–40, 67–68, 186

sleeping sickness 354

473

Smith–Magenis syndrome 339

snoring, history-taking 40

social cognitive theory (SCT), CPAP compliance 455

social history 41

socio-psychological correlates, sleep duration 252

sodium oxybate (SXB; SO) 421–27
  cataplexy 122
  clinical development 421, 423–24, 425, 426
  idiopathic hypersomnia 132
  narcolepsy 120, 121, 122, 271–72, 423–24, 425
  Parkinson's disease 425
  safety 426
  sleep-deprived subjects 425–26
  see also γ-hydroxybutyrate

soldiers see military personnel

solvent exposure 382

somatoform disorder, undifferentiated 131

somnolence see sleepiness

SOREMPs see sleep-onset REM periods

Spillane v. Wasserman 96

spinal muscular atrophy (SMA) 348

spinocerebellar ataxias (SCA) 345

SR 46339B 449

Stanford Sleepiness Scale (SSS) 62–63, 64
  children 264–65
  clinical use 41, 63
  development 61
  vs. objective measures 64

state boundary control, loss of, narcolepsy 118

state instability hypothesis 74

Sternberg working memory task (SWMT) 31, 76, 107–08

stimulants 401–05
  children 270
  idiopathic hypersomnia 132
  Kleine–Levin syndrome 144
  myotonic dystrophy 325
  narcolepsy 120
  obstructive sleep apnea 164

stimulus control instructions, narcolepsy 453

stroke 355–56

stupor
  idiopathic 142
  vs. sleepiness 351

subjective measures of sleepiness 60–69
  assessing fitness to drive 161
  children 68–69, 264–65, 266
  depression 284
  history 61
  insomnia 168
  obstructive sleep apnea 154–55, 156
  shift workers 186, 188, 189
  vs. objective measures 64–65, 66, 67

subthalamic stimulation 309–10

suprachiasmatic nucleus (SCN) 227, 281

surgical treatment, Parkinson's disease 309–10

sympathetic activation
  arousal from daytime napping 297
  obstructive sleep apnea 158, 159
  sleep latency effects 57

syringomyelia 359

systemic lupus erythematosus (SLE) 358

T-cell receptor alpha locus polymorphism 119

tasimelteon 182

task impurity problem 76, 79

temazepam 243

temperature, body
  circadian rhythm 226, 227
  long sleepers 252–53
  sleep onset and 229

testosterone 369–70

thalamus, dopamine neurons 302–03

thioperamide 445–46

three-process model of alertness (TPM) 194, 252

thyroid function tests 45, 268

thyroid hormone 364–65
  replacement therapy 367–68

thyroid-stimulating hormone (TSH) 364–65

thyrotropin releasing hormone (TRH) 368, 449
  agonists 449

tiagabine 449

time awake
  interactions with circadian rhythms 229–30
  performance effects 229

time-on-task effects
  cognitive performance 74–75
  motor vehicle driving 86
  shift work 193–94

time-zone transitions 225–35
  see also jet lag

tiprolisant 309, 446

topiramate 391

Tourette syndrome 346

toxin exposure 375, 382

train drivers 85, 187

tramadol 244–45

transcranial magnetic stimulation (TMS), depression 288–89

transtheoretical model (TTM), CPAP compliance 455

traumatic brain injury (TBI)
  mild (mTBI), soldiers 222–23
  sleepiness after see post-traumatic sleepiness

travel fatigue 225, 226

trazodone 388

Treacher–Collins syndrome 340

triazolam 244, 425

tribbles homolog 2 (trb2) 119

tricyclic antidepressants (TCAs)
  narcolepsy 121, 271
  sedating effects 388

triiodothyronine (T3) 364–65

triptans 393

truck drivers
  differential vulnerability to sleepiness 103
  employers' liability for crashes 94
  night driving 85, 86, 187, 188–89
  sleep-related crashes 94, 190

trypanosomiasis, African 354

tuberomammillary nucleus (TMN) 23

two-process model of sleep regulation 252
  advanced and delayed sleep phase disorders 180
  depression 281, 282
  shift work 194

Index

Ullanalina Narcolepsy Scale 41
upper airway, evaluation 42, 46
upper airway resistance syndrome (UARS) 130, 154
uremia 376–78
urine tests 45–46

vagus nerve stimulation (VNS) 359
valproic acid 244
vascular disease, CNS 355–56
venlafaxine 121
ventrolateral preoptic nucleus (VLPO) 116–17
vigilance
  effects of caffeine 433–34, 438, 439
  effects of sleepiness 73–74, 75
  histaminergic control 23, 24
viral infections 131, 354

visual Analogue Scale (VAS) of sleepiness 41, 43, 61–62, 64
vitamin B_{12} 182–83

Walter Reed Sleep/Performance Management System (SPMS) 218
weight, body 40
Williams syndrome 338–39
Wilson disease (WD) 344
work hours
  healthcare workers *see under* health-care workers
  motor vehicle crash risk and 85–86
  regulations *see* hours of service (HOS) regulations
  shift work 186
work performance, shift workers 189–91

work-related accidents/injuries 92
  employers' liability 94–95
  healthcare workers 206
  shift workers 189–91
working memory
  effects of sleepiness 76
  functional neuroimaging studies 31, 32, 107–08

Yamino Soushi 14, 15
Yerkes–Dodson law 72
young adults
  daytime sleepiness in insomnia 168, 171, 172
  long sleepers 254, 255, 257, 258
  motor vehicle crash risk 86
  see also adolescents

zeitgebers 228, 231
zolpidem 169, 171, 387
zopiclone 387

475